Health and safety
Occupational therapy
Occupational health

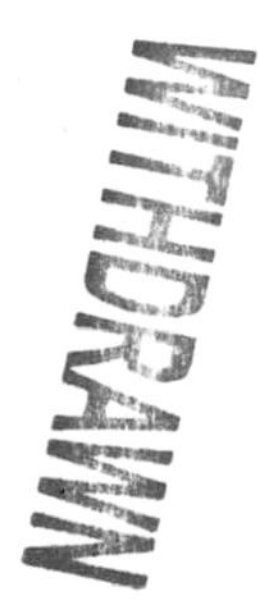

The Latest Evolution in Learning.

Evolve provides online access to free learning resources and activities designed specifically for the textbook you are using in your class. The resources will provide you with information that enhances the material covered in the book and much more.

Visit the Web address listed below to start your learning evolution today!

LOGIN: http://evolve.elsevier.com/Sanders/ergonomics/

Evolve Student Learning Resources for *Sanders: Ergonomics and the Management of Musculoskeletal Disorders, ed 2*, offers the following features

- **WebLinks**
  Links to helpful websites.
- **Study Questions**
  Study questions are provided for each chapter.
- **References**
  Gives links to Medline Abstracts for key references in the main text.

Think outside the book...evolve.

Ergonomics and the Management of Musculoskeletal Disorders

Ergonomics and the Management of Musculoskeletal Disorders

Edited by

MARTHA J. SANDERS, MA, MSOSH, OTR/L

Assistant Professor of Occupational Therapy
Department of Occupational Therapy
Quinnipiac University
Hamden, Connecticut

SECOND EDITION

With 20 Contributing Authors

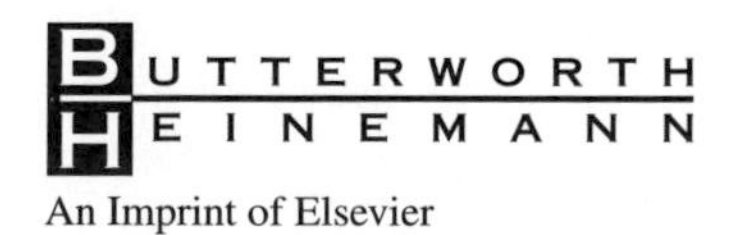

An Imprint of Elsevier

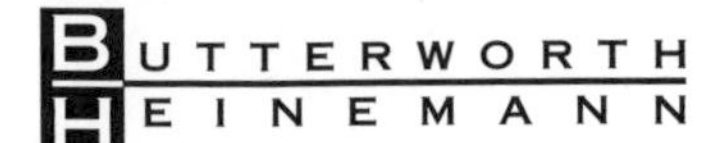

An Imprint of Elsevier

11830 Westline Industrial Drive
St. Louis, Missouri 63146

ERGONOMICS AND THE MANAGEMENT OF MUSCULOSKELETAL DISORDERS, SECOND EDITION 0-7506-7409-1

NOTICE

Occupational therapy and ergonomics are ever-changing fields. Standard safety precautions must be followed, but as new research and clinical experience broaden our knowledge, changes in treatment may become necessary or appropriate.

Previous edition copyrighted 1997

International Standard Book Number 0-7506-7409-1

Publishing Director: Linda Duncan
Managing Editor: Kathy Falk
Associate Developmental Editor: Melissa Kuster Deutsch
Publishing Services Manager: Patricia Tannian
Project Manager: Sarah Wunderly
Designer: Gail Morey Hudson
Cover Design: Jyotika Schroff

Printed in United States of America

Last digit is the print number: 9 8 7 6 5 4 3 2 1

Contributors

CHERYL ATWOOD, BS
Yarns for Ewe
Bethlehem, Connecticut

NANCY BAKER, ScD, OTR/L
Assistant Professor
Department of Occupational Therapy
School of Health and Rehabilitation Science
University of Pittsburgh
Pittsburgh, Pennsylvania

DONALD CLARK, MS, PT
Private Practice
Westerly, Rhode Island

CHARLES F. DILLON, MD, PhD
Research Medical Officer
Department of Health and Human Services
Centers for Disease Control
Division of Health Examination Statistics/NHANES
Hyattsville, Maryland

SUSAN V. DUFF, EdD, PT, OTR/L, CHT, BCP
Clinical Research Director
Clinical Research Department
Shriners Hospitals for Children
Philadelphia, Pennsylvania
Clinical Faculty Associate
Physical Therapy Program
New York Medical College
Valhalla, New York

DOROTHY FARRAR EDWARDS, PhD
Program in Occupational Therapy
Washington University School of Medicine
St. Louis, Missouri

MELANIE T. ELLEXSON, MBA, OTR/L, FAOTA
Assistant Professor
Chicago State University
Chicago, Illinois

ROBERT O. HANSSON, PhD
Professor of Psychology
University of Tulsa
Tulsa, Oklahoma

BARBARA J. HEADLEY, MS, PT
Innovative Systems for Rehabilitation Inc.
Boulder, Colorado

CARYL D. JOHNSON, OTR/L, CHT
Johnson Hand Therapy Services
New York, New York

JAMES H. KILLIAN
Graduate Student
Industrial-Organizational Psychology
University of Tulsa
Tulsa, Oklahoma

JAMES W. KING, MA, CHT, OTR/L
Regional Manager
Alliance Imaging
Waco, Texas

BRENDAN C. LYNCH, MA
Graduate Student
Clinical Psychology
University of Tulsa
Tulsa, Oklahoma

MICHAEL MELNIK, MS, OTR
Prevention Plus
Minneapolis, Minnesota

TIM MORSE, PhD
Training Coordinator
Ergotechnology Center of Connecticut
Division of Occupational and Environmental Medicine
University of Connecticut Health Center
Farmington, Connecticut

RICHARD K. SCHWARTZ, MS, OTR
Richard K. Schwartz Consulting Services, Inc.
Industrial Medicine and Risk Management
San Antonio, Texas

JUDY SEHNAL, MS, OTR/L, CPE
Executive Technical Consultant
The Hartford
Hartford, Connecticut

ROBYN STRICOFF, OTR/L, CHT
Occupational Solutions
Monroe, Connecticut

CLAUDIA MICHALAK-TURCOTTE, CDA, RDH, MSDH, MSOSH
Associate Professor
Department of Allied Dental
Tunxis Community-Technical College
Farmington, Connecticut
Department of Allied Dental—Dental Hygiene
University of Connecticut School of Dental Medicine
Farmington, Connecticut

NICK WARREN, ScD, MAT
Coordinator, Ergotechnology Center of Connecticut
Division of Occupational and Environmental Medicine
University of Connecticut Health Center
Farmington, Connecticut

Preface

The second edition of *Ergonomics and the Management of Musculoskeletal Disorders* (previously, *Management of Cumulative Trauma Disorders*) has added much depth and breadth to the first edition to reflect the major changes in the political, medical, ergonomic, and research arenas relative to managing musculoskeletal disorders. The name of this book has been changed to reflect the adoption of the term *musculoskeletal disorder* (MSD) by the National Institute of Occupational Safety and Health.

Seven new chapters have been added and seven new expert contributors have added incredible new information and experience to the book. The context of work is now framed in the history of work, all the while maintaining a client-centered perspective. An update on the regulatory status and incidence of MSDs supports our need to continue our work toward preventing such disorders. The medical chapters offer cutting-edge information on arthritis-related MSDs, heretofore rarely acknowledged in MSD literature. The entire context of ergonomics is expanded and discussed from a contemporary perspective that incorporates not only job design, but also the organization of work and characteristics of the individual. Ergonomics is taken out of the exclusive arena of work and applied to home and leisure environments, acknowledging that MSD management is not limited to medical and industrial environments. Finally, special populations that provide challenges for MSD management, older workers and daycare workers, are presented in this edition.

As before, *Ergonomics and Management of Musculoskeletal Disorders* is organized to present information in earlier chapters that is sequentially developed and applied in later chapters.

Although we should take pride that the overall number of musculoskeletal disorders has begun to decline, much work still needs to be done to prevent, minimize, and treat workers who have developed MSDs in the workplace. A collaborative approach of all disciplines is crucial to our further understanding and management of MSDs.

Martha J. Sanders

This book is dedicated to
the families and colleagues of all contributors
whose support made this book possible.

More specifically
my family has been a great source of clarity and drive.
Thanks to
Dad
who instilled in us the self-fulfilling nature of work
Mom
whose compassion compels my quest for clients' health and happiness
Peter
whose focus allows us to plan and finish a project
Jeffrey
whose balance makes us remember to have fun
Wendy
whose creativity allows us to express ideas with new flair
Jimmy
whose broad scope allows us to expand into new horizons
Paul
whose breadth of knowledge invites new applications for traditional content.
But a special thanks to
Addie and **Tai**
who taught us about perseverance.

Acknowledgements

Many individuals gave their time to the creation of this second edition. Again, thanks to the contributors for fitting in this professional writing with daily life. A second thanks to Norma Keegan, Interlibrary Loan Director at Quinnipiac University, who gracefully supplied me with reams of research studies for both the first and second editions. A special thanks to Ruthanna Terreri and Cheryl Atwood, who provided the patience and expertise for many of the photos in this book.

Contents

PART I
Systems Involved in MSD Management: Worker, Medical, and Regulatory Perspectives

1 Musculoskeletal Disorders: A Worldwide Dilemma, 3
2 The Individual Worker Perspective, 15
3 The Medical Context, 29
4 MSD: The Regulatory Perspective, 44

PART II
Conditions Related to MSDs: Diagnosis and Intervention

5 Pathomechanics of MSDs, 63
6 Treatment of MSD and Related Conditions, 89
7 Joint Injury and Arthritis in the Spectrum of Workplace MSDs, 132

PART III
Ergonomic Risk Factors Related to MSDs in Business and Industry

8 The Expanded Definition of Ergonomics, 151
9 Physiologic Risk Factors, 160
10 Biomechanical Risk Factors, 191
11 Job Design, 230
12 Psychosocial Factors, 265

PART IV
Developing and Implementing Worksite Programs

13 Job Analysis and Worksite Assessment, 283
14 Reducing Injuries, Claims, and Costs, 299
15 Employment Examinations, 324
16 Implementing an Effective Injury Prevention Process, 342
17 Outcome Assessment of Prevention Programs, 363

PART V
Managing MSDs in Home and Leisure Environments

18 Ergonomics in the Home, 389
19 Ergonomics of Child Care, 405
20 Ergonomics of Leisure Activities, 419

PART VI
Specific Programs for High-Risk Populations

21 The Older Worker, 437
22 Preventing Work-Related MSDs in Dental Hygienists, 448
23 Managing MSDs in Performing Artists, 474
24 Addressing Musculoskeletal Disorders at Computer Workstations, 494

PART ONE

Systems Involved in MSD Management: Worker, Medical, and Regulatory Perspectives

CHAPTER 1

Musculoskeletal Disorders: A Worldwide Dilemma

Martha J. Sanders

Our society prides itself on the belief that technical advancements in information processing, manufacturing technology, and medical science will enhance the quality of life for all individuals. Logic dictates that if we work more efficiently, we will be more productive and, therefore, more satisfied with our personal work, our wages, and the use of our leisure time. Unfortunately, the basic assumptions that underlie this logic are gradually being undermined by the hidden costs of doing business in today's highly technical society. The hidden costs that we address are the escalating incidents of stress-related and musculoskeletal disorders (MSDs) for the thousands of workers responsible for our soaring productivity.

Today, we are witnessing what has been termed an *industrial epidemic* (Schenck, 1989)—that is, an overwhelming increase in reports of work-related disorders that affect not only industry productivity and labor costs but also the quality of workers' lives both inside and outside the workplace. The problem has dramatic repercussions. As employment positions become less secure, workers are less willing to perform jobs that jeopardize their health and limit future earning potential. As businesses become increasingly competitive, employers complain that the cost of MSDs reduces profits by increasing workers' compensation costs and decreasing productivity. The cost of managing these disorders reverberates from the factory or office floor to the medical and often legal arenas, all of which remove the employee farther from work and drive our health care costs even higher.

The differences in focus among industrial, medical, insurance, and legal systems exacerbates the problem. Each system possesses a unique set of goals, languages, and procedures that can alienate other provider systems. Although each provider contributes a valuable perspective, one provider cannot effectively remediate MSDs to the exclusion of other systems. Clearly, in the management of MSDs, the whole is truly greater than the sum of the parts.

The perspective of this book is that effective prevention and management programs for MSDs must thoroughly integrate all professional perspectives. The values of individual workers and worker cultures must be integrated with the medical, corporate, and insurance systems so that long-term solutions can be reached. Although health care practitioners and ergonomic consultants will enter the arena of MSD management from medical, insurance, industrial, or even educational systems, all practitioners will need to appreciate the contribution of other systems and be prepared to work with representatives from those systems toward a thorough, comprehensive MSD management plan.

This book systematically examines the means by which health care practitioners and consultants can effect change to facilitate safer, more productive, and stimulating workplaces. Contextual background from the individual worker, medical, and industrial/regulatory perspectives are presented to sensitize health care practitioners to the concerns of each participant.

From all perspectives, worker health is a priority in our efforts. If companies are to survive, managers need to maximize productivity and minimize medical costs. If workers are to maintain quality of work and home life, workers need to take responsibility for protecting their health. If medicine is to alleviate disability, health professionals must step beyond the clinics into the "real world" of industry and business. Cooperatively, we must balance productivity with health, consider long-term gains versus short-term profit, and reexamine the value of work for today's worker.

From the high-speed assembly lines to the propagating computer terminals, modern tools of the trade certainly have improved our standard of living. But what about our quality of work life? Are we any better off than we were at the turn of the century? As Eli Ginzberg (1982) eloquently stated, "It remains to be seen whether or not the potential of modern technology will turn out to be a blessing."

HISTORY OF MUSCULOSKELETAL DISORDERS

The occurrence of MSDs in industry is not new. In 1717, Bernardo Ramazzini, the father of occupational medicine, first introduced to physicians the common musculoskeletal disorders that arose from eighteenth-century occupations in his treatise *De Morbis Artificum Diatriba* ("The Diseases of Workers") (translated by Wright, 1940). Ramazzini observed that many diseases or conditions appeared to be related to his patients' exposures to hazardous work environments. At that time, however, physicians rarely asked patients about their jobs. Ramazzini, therefore, initiated one of the first systematic attempts to attribute specific diseases or conditions to factors in workers' environments. Ramazzini documented the musculoskeletal, respiratory, dermatologic, and emotional problems exhibited by his patients. He then observed workers at their jobs and related specific aspects of the environment (such as hazardous materials, airborne toxins, and excessive physical demands) to these medical conditions. In essence, Ramazzini laid the foundation for occupational health practices today. Ramazzini (1717) opens his treatise with the following overview.

Various and manifold is the harvest of diseases reaped by certain workers from the crafts and trades that they pursue; all the profit that they get is fatal injury to their health. That crop germinates mostly, I think, from two causes. The first and most potent is the harmful character of the materials that they handle for these emit noxious vapors and very fine particles inimical to human beings and induce particular diseases; the second cause I ascribe to certain violent and irregular motions and unnatural postures of the body, by reason of which the natural structure of the vital machine is so impaired that serious diseases gradually develop therefrom (p. 15).

Ramazzini poignantly describes the morbidity of many acquired conditions and the futile reward of illnesses that many workers suffered as a result of enduring hazardous work environments. He describes the conditions that resulted from specific occupations. He wrote the following about sedentary workers.

[M]en and women who sit while they work at their jobs, become bent, hump-backed and hold their heads like people looking for something on the ground; this is the effect of their sedentary life and the bent posture as they sit ... and sew ... (p. 282).

He described scribes and notaries this way.

[T]he maladies that afflict the clerks afore said arise from three causes: First, constant sitting, secondly the incessant movement of the hand and always in the same direction, thirdly the strain on the mind from the effort not to disfigure the books by errors or cause loss to their employers when they add, subtract, or do sums of arithmetic ... Furthermore, incessant driving of the pen over paper causes intense fatigue of the hand and the whole arm because of the continuous and almost tonic strain on the muscles and tendons, which in course of time results in failure of power of the right hand (pp. 421, 423).

Of painters he reported that "their sedentary life and melancholic temperament may be partly to blame, for they are almost entirely cut off from intercourse with other men and constantly absorbed in the creations of their imagination" (p. 67). He noted of bakers, "[N]ow and again, I have noticed bakers with swelled hands, and painful, too; in fact, the hands of all such workers become thickened by the constant pressure of kneading the dough" (p. 229).

Ramazzini identified hazards in workers' environments that we have come to associate with the risk factors for MSDs today. He recognized not only the physical demands such as "violent and irregular motions," "bent posture," "incessant use of the hands," and "tonic strain on the muscles," but also the emotional or mental demands that contribute to work-related fatigue, such as "melancholic temperament," "sedentary life," and "strain on the mind." Still, disorders of workers were treated on an individual basis, and workers had relatively few choices about whether to work in the face of such disorders.

MUSCULOSKELETAL DISORDERS IN THE TWENTIETH CENTURY

As the Industrial Revolution gained momentum and assembly-line pacing, predetermined motion and time standards, long hours at work, and the performance of repetitive tasks became the norm, the serious and problematic nature of work-related diseases became increasingly apparent. When workers' compensation laws were introduced in 1911 and then amended in 1914 and expanded to cover conditions such as tenosynovitis, insurance companies began to record and further examine these injuries as related to their clients' occupations (Conn, 1931; Hagan, Montgomery, & O'Reilly, 2001).

Physicians became instrumental in determining whether these disorders were actually related to work. Physicians therefore began to compile data that equated musculoskeletal symptoms with workplace factors. Conn (1931) examined rubber company workers who had tenosynovitis and determined that new "high-speed hand operations," "increased intensity of effort," and being new to the job clearly predisposed individuals to disorders such as tenosynovitis. Hammer (1934), who attempted to delineate the tolerances, or number of repetitions that human tendons could withstand before tenosynovitis developed, concluded that tenosynovitis would occur in human tendons if repetitions exceeded 30 to 40 per minute, or 1500 to 2000 manipulations per hour. Hammer noted certain hand symptoms consistent with carpal tunnel syndrome, but this condition was not explored further until Phalen reported on it in 1947.

Flowerdew and Bode (1942) raised the issue of improper training and physical conditioning as contributors to tenosynovitis in some workers. Among a group of 52 military personnel assigned to farm work in Great Britain, 16 developed tenosynovitis of the wrist and finger extensors shortly after starting intensive manual work. Fourteen of these 16 individuals had no previous manual labor experience. Blood (1942), a medical officer at a company in Great Britain, agreed that "newcomers to a repetitive stereotyped job are particularly vulnerable, but ... cases crop up among employees who have had years of experience at these jobs, particularly after returning to work following a holiday or sick leave" (p. 468). Blood attributed a 50% increase in cases of tenosynovitis from 1940 to 1941 to an influx of new workers in his industry.

As automation progressed and manual work became lighter and more efficient, musculoskeletal problems related specifically to office work became apparent. In the 1950s, new office equipment such as high-speed typewriters and keypunch operations streamlined tasks by eliminating movements not directly related to the job (such as retrieving the typewriter carriage after each line). Automation eliminated both the brief rest periods inherent in operating the old machinery and the need for workers to use several different muscle groups to accomplish a task. Physically, jobs became sedentary, static, and, unvarying; people relied on localized muscles to perform the work. Mentally, the work routines became highly monotonous, although detailed work demanded high levels of concentration. Workers lost a sense of the overall task to which they were contributing (Giuliano, 1982).

By the mid-1950s, the musculoskeletal and mental fatigue problems associated with operating new and repetitive machines were clear. The Fifth Session of the International Labor Organization Advisory Committee on Salaried Employees and Professional Workers reported the serious physical consequences created by mechanized work (ILO Advisory Committee, 1960). Clerical workers complained of low-back and neck pain; keypunch operators complained of "painful nerves" in the hands; accounting-machine operators complained of fatigue, eye strain, pain and stiffness in cervical and lumbar regions, and numbness in the right hand (Maeda, Hunting, & Grandjean, 1980). Although these disorders crossed national boundaries, peaks in reporting occurred at different times for each country.

Occupational Cervicobrachial Disorder in Japan

In Japan, a dramatic increase in musculoskeletal disorders was reported between 1960 and 1980. Comparatively high prevalence of hand and arm pain was first reported in keypunch operators (17% of the occupational sample). Later, typists (13%), telephone operators (16%), office keyboard operators (14%), and assembly-line workers (16%) reported pain in the hands and arms that interfered with their abilities to perform their jobs (Maeda, 1977; Ohara, Itani, & Aoyama, 1982). The claims rose to such a proportion that, in 1964, the Japanese Ministry of Labour issued guidelines for keyboard operators, demanding that workers spend no more than 5 hours per day on the keyboard, take a 10-minute rest break every hour, and perform fewer than 40,000 keystrokes per day. In companies that implemented these preventive measures, the prevalence of arm and hand disorders decreased from an overall prevalence of 10% to 20% down to 2% to 5% (Ohara et al., 1982). However, the overall number of individuals who received compensation for hand and arm disorders in the private sector in Japan increased from 90 in 1970 to 546 in 1975 (Maeda, 1977).

In 1971, Japan formed the Japanese Committee on Cervicobrachial Syndrome to define the syndrome and fully identify contributing factors. The committee proposed the name *occupational cervicobrachial disorder* (OCD) and defined the problem as a functional or organic disorder (or both) resulting from mental strain or neuromuscular fatigue due to performing jobs in a fixed position or with repetitive movements of the upper extremity (Keikenenwan Shokogun Iinkai [Japanese Association of Industrial Health], 1973).

The Japanese committee then conducted a mass screening of individuals in private industry to further delineate the causative factors for OCD. Researchers concluded that "how the workers use their muscular and nervous systems at work" and "how the task is organized into the work system as a whole" underlie the condition (Maeda, 1977, p. 200). Researchers specifically identified static loading of the postural muscles, dynamic loading of localized arm and hand muscles, and lack of active rest breaks during the day as factors contributing to OCD. The condition was found to advance with excessive workload and insufficient recovery from fatigue.

The Japanese committee astutely regarded visual eye strain and mental fatigue as being related to OCD. It urged physicians to further investigate the relationship between sleep disturbance, chronic fatigue, and symptoms of OCD (Maeda, 1977). A 20-year review of the disorder by Maeda analyzed the progression of the disease in Japan and posed questions about exposure or dose-effect relationships. Maeda, Horiguchi, and Hosokawa (1982) found that OCD first peaked in individuals within 6 to 12 months of starting a new job (possibly due to overwork of untrained individuals) and then peaked again between 2 and 3 years (possibly due to chronic fatigue of muscles). Maeda identified the fundamental controversy that exists today: whether OCD is caused by factors solely within the workplace or by psychological factors such as personal anxiety or workplace stress that becomes magnified by the physical aspects of the workplace.

Other countries subsequently began to examine the incidence of musculoskeletal disorders related to office work. In each country, a gross rise in workers' compensation claims for musculoskeletal disorders served as the catalyst for research of the problem. Specific task forces were established in each country to study MSDs within the socioeconomic context of that country. Most countries followed a similar chronologic pattern of first recognizing acute hand and arm pain in workers, then identifying problems related to static posturing of the shoulder and cervical regions, and finally relating specific medical problems to workplace factors.

REPETITIVE STRAIN INJURY IN AUSTRALIA

In the 1970s and 1980s, Australia observed a dramatic increase in the number of telecommunications workers who reported symptoms of arm pain or muscular fatigue (Chatterjee, 1978; Ferguson, 1971a; McDermott, 1986). Ferguson (1971a) first investigated the prevalence of telegraphists' cramp in 517 male workers in the Australian telegraph service and found that 20% of the workers complained of an occupational cramp or occupational myalgias. Ferguson reported that 75% of these workers had a history of neurosis and complained of work overload or job dissatisfaction. Ferguson therefore attributed the cramp more to psychological and social factors within the workplace than to the physical performance of the job.

In a later study of 77 female workers in an electronics assembly plant who were diagnosed with tendinitis, Ferguson (1971b) acknowledged the awkward and repetitive nature of electronics jobs as contributing to workers' symptoms. However, Ferguson questioned the validity of the initial diagnosis of tendinitis and the necessity for the excessive medical leave (more than 4 months) for workers with this condition. Ferguson (1971b) advocated early return to work and medical surveillance in addition to ergonomic changes.

The term *repetitive strain injury* (RSI) was adopted among Australian medical investigators in the early 1980s, although most did not believe that the term adequately described the condition (Ireland, 1992; McDermott, 1986; Stone, 1983). Within years, RSI had affected Australian telegraphists and typists, tradesmen, and assembly-line, clerical, data-processing, and postal workers. McDermott (1986) explained that the number of occupational claims for RSI in Australia increased generally from 300% to 400% in data-processing, accounting, and postal services from the mid-1970s to the early 1980s. The Commonwealth Government of Australia, in response to the spiraling cost of RSI in that country, set up a task force on RSI, seeking input from the National Occupational Health and Safety Commission. This task force concluded that a combination of ergonomic and psychological factors contributed to the problem (McDermott, 1986).

Clearly, investigators in Australia resisted relating RSI to biomechanical factors within the workplace and struggled with the definition of RSI as a separate disease entity as opposed to a grouping of conditions with similar occupational etiologies. Ireland (1992), a researcher from Australia, still contends that musculoskeletal pain relates only to workers' psychological stress, because no objective medical tests (e.g., nerve conduction or electromyography) can diagnose the condition definitively. Despite the strong association of RSI with psychological factors, few studies attempted to evaluate the psychological aspects of RSI.

Occupational Disorders in Europe

The Nordic countries have long been involved in industrial health care. Whereas most of the research in musculoskeletal problems initially focused on factors related to low-back pain,

Swedish researchers began to examine upper-extremity musculoskeletal disorders related to work in the 1980s in response to increasing complaints of neck and shoulder pain among blue-collar workers (Bjelle, Hagberg, & Michaelson, 1981; Dimberg et al., 1989; Kvarnstrom, 1983).

Kvarnstrom (1983) and Bjelle et al. (1981) examined the records of workers on long-term sick leave in large industrial plants in Sweden and noted the increasing magnitude of neck and shoulder problems. Kvarnstrom found that 48% of all workers on long-term sick leave had musculoskeletal conditions; neck and shoulder problems were the most common disorders among light-manufacturing workers. When Kvarnstrom (1983) studied the demographic, work task, and social factors related to shoulder problems in 112 workers, the variables related to the presence of shoulder pain were as follows: older workers were affected more often; female workers were 10 times more likely than male workers to suffer shoulder pain; light-manufacturing jobs were most often associated with shoulder pain; piece-rate incentives were positively correlated with shoulder pain; and immigrants were at higher risk than other workers for developing shoulder pain. Some factors could be explained by the relationship among variables. For example, women tended to be clustered in the higher-risk jobs, and immigrant workers, because of their limited language skills, did not have the opportunity for proper training or job rotation.

When cases were matched with controls, Kvarnstrom (1983) found that a group piece-rate system, shift work, and regard for the work as repetitive, monotonous, and stressful were significant among case subjects. More case subjects than controls cited a poor relationship with their supervisors, although no difference in relationships with their peers was seen between groups. Finally, Kvarnstrom noted a significant association of shoulder pain with social factors, including being married, having a sick spouse, having children at home, working alternate shifts from one's spouse, and having few leisure activities. Researchers discussed the heavy burden placed on workers with both job and home responsibilities (see Chapter 2). This study heralded the beginning of many future studies to systematically examine the relationship between physical and psychosocial factors in the development of MSDs.

Nordic researchers recognized the difficulty in comparing studies from country to country because of a lack of uniform terminology and criteria for diagnosis (Kuorinka et al., 1987; Kvarnstrom, 1983). The Nordic Council of Ministers therefore supported a project to develop a standardized Nordic questionnaire for the purposes of collectively recording and compiling information. The Standardized Nordic Questionnaire, now widely used and translated into four Nordic languages, is meant as a screening for musculoskeletal disorders of the low back, neck, and shoulder complaints related to ergonomic exposures (Kuorinka et al., 1987). Using this questionnaire, the estimated prevalence of hand and wrist disorders in Sweden ranged from 18% among Swedish scissor makers to 56% among Swedish packers (Luoparjärvi, Kuorinka, Virolainen, & Holmberg, 1979).

Throughout Europe, the European Union has exerted strength in the formation of Occupational Safety and Health laws that emphasize social policy, improvements to quality of life, protection of the environment, and a minimum common standard for working conditions in member countries (Batra & Hatzopoulou, 2001).

Musculoskeletal Disorders in North America

The United States witnessed a gradual rise in MSDs from 1980 to 1986. The incidence then rose tremendously from less than 50,000 in 1985 to 330,000 in 1994 (BLS, 1992, 2002). The incidence has fallen steadily over the past 6 years to 241,800 in 2000, most likely because of ergonomic changes and early intervention. (See

Chapter 4 for a compete discussion.) In the United States, carpal tunnel syndrome (CTS) was the initial focus of investigation. The occupational causes of CTS were first investigated by Armstrong and Chaffin (1979) in two groups of female seamstresses, one with a known history of CTS and one with no previous history. Researchers found that women with a history of CTS used more force and wrist deviation when performing the work tasks than those with no history of CTS. Researchers questioned whether the differences in work methods between the groups was the cause or the effect of CTS in the affected women.

In an effort to delineate risk factors in an industrial population, Silverstein, Fine, & Armstrong (1987) investigated the relationship between force and repetition in a job task and the prevalence of CTS in 652 industrial workers. Results of a physical examination and interview indicated that workers in high-force, high-repetition jobs were 15 times more likely to have CTS than workers in low-force, low-repetition jobs (Silverstein et al., 1987). (See Chapter 10 for a complete discussion.) This study became the hallmark for identifying biomechanical risk factors and drawing an association between exposures and musculoskeletal conditions.

As the reported incidence of MSDs skyrocketed, researchers began to document and examine the prevalence of MSD in specific high-risk occupations. Self-reported studies indicated upper-extremity symptoms among the following occupational samples: 62.5% of female supermarket checkers (Margolis & Kraus, 1987), 63% to 95% of dental hygienists (Atwood & Michalak, 1992; Shenkar, Mann, Shevach, Ever-Hadani, & Weiss, 1998), and 82% of electricians (Hunting, Welch, Cuccerini, & Seiger, 1994), to name a few. A compilation of well-documented research attributed the high prevalence of MSDs to job tasks involving postural loads at the neck and shoulders, awkward postures, and long hours of repetitive and static work along with organizational factors (Bernard, 1997). (See Chapter 10 for a complete discussion).

However, a group of physicians in the mid-1990s argued that solely psychosocial issues and the sociopolitical climate were causal in the etiology of MSDs, particularly with regard to the incidence of CTS in keyboard users. This group attributed the rise in CTS to workers' frustrations with their jobs, difficulty coping with nondescript, short-lived pain, and the contagion of inflammatory self-reports (Hadler, 1996). Hadler contended that typical exposures experienced during keyboard tasks were not excessive or hazardous to the worker and were unrelated to health outcomes.

Silverstein, Silverstein, and Franklin (1996) countered this argument citing a well-researched body of evidence indicating dose-response relationships between biomechanical risk factors in the workplace and the development of MSDs. Although Silverstein et al. shared Hadler's concern for the management of MSDs and some physicians' preponderance toward surgery, their distinct beliefs about the causes of MSDs also represent divergent beliefs on prevention.

Finally, in 1997 in the United States, the National Institute for Occupational Health and Safety (NIOSH) adopted the term *work-related musculoskeletal disorder* (WMSD), or MSD, to replace the term *cumulative trauma disorder* (Bernard, 1997; NIOSH, 1997). This change represented an effort to accommodate the wide range of disorders associated with work exposures. Ongoing efforts continue to establish an ergonomics standard as part of the federal OSHA legislation. (See Chapter 4 for a complete discussion.)

GLOBAL APPRECIATION FOR THE IMPACT OF WORK-RELATED STRESS

As industrialized nations have identified that stress is contributory to the overall MSD etiology, more global legislative efforts are addressing the impact of stress on workers, identifying the sources of work-related stress, and advocating that institutions take responsibility for minimizing stress by examining their organizational frameworks (Levi, Sauter, & Shimomitsu, 1999; Sanders, 2001).

In the United States, NIOSH (1999) published its monograph on stress prevention strategies for the workplace, stating that "because work is changing at whirlwind speed ... perhaps now more than ever, job stress poses a threat to the health of workers and in turn, to the health of organizations" (p. 10). NIOSH upholds that workplaces should address not only the biomechanical aspects of a job but also the psychosocial aspects focusing on providing worker control, skill-enhancing, and decision-making opportunities. Levi et al. (1999) contend that the widely used routine of providing stress management skills to help individual workers cope with stressful situations is merely a short-term approach to solving greater, more complex problems for the entire organization (Levi et al., 1999). (See Chapters 8 and 12 for further discussions of work-related stress.)

Initiatives have been taken throughout the world to encourage employers to look internally to minimize stresses in work environments. In the United Kingdom, the reduction of work-related stress is part of a greater proposal by the Health and Safety Commission to promote health across all industrial and governmental sectors from line workers to administrative levels (Health and Safety Commission, 1999). The European Parliament Resolution in 1999 urged employers to adapt work to the workers' abilities, thus minimizing the disparity between work demands and workers' capacities. The influence of limited job autonomy, job variety, and worker participation on worker health has rung loud and clear in current programming (Levi et al., 1999).

The culmination of these legislative efforts is the Tokyo Declaration, a treatise developed by worldwide experts on stress research in response to mounting evidence as to the profound influence of stress in industrialized nations. Researchers expressed concern about the effects of technological changes in worklife (i.e., increasing cognitive workloads) on individuals and their abilities to function to their maximum potential given these demands. The philosophy of the Declaration, "Investment for Health," implies that a commitment to individual workers will also bring about social benefits. The Declaration endorses developing measurement tools to measure psychosocial stress, examining health outcomes based on stress exposures, monitoring psychosocial health stress, providing education and training, and creating a system for gathering and disseminating information (Tokyo Declaration, 1999).

THE ROLE OF ERGONOMICS IN INDUSTRIAL DEVELOPING COUNTRIES

Whereas ergonomics has traditionally consulted with businesses in industrially advanced countries (IACs), the role of ergonomics in industrially developing countries (IDC) is being expanded with regard to productivity and health and safety (Ahasan, Mohiuddin, Vayrynen, Ironkannas, & Quddus, 1999; Brunette, 2002; O'Neill, 2000). An IDC is a country whose existence is based on either commercializing natural resources or on simply surviving. In both cases, the infrastructure is rarely adequate to sustain the characteristically high population growth. Although nutrition and basic safety are clearly lacking, it is suggested that musculoskeletal injuries in IDCs are also growing at a higher rate than in IACs. This is not surprising, since legislation in IDCs is either nonexistent or ineffective at controlling health and safety risks (O'Neill, 2000; Stubbs, 2000). Arguments for developing prevention programs for MSDs in IDCs will need incentives such as economic growth, social responsibility, or perhaps research opportunities to advance quality of work and quality of life in these countries.

O'Neill (2000) more specifically discusses ergonomic issues currently at the forefront in IDC manufacturing, the agriculture industry, and in transporting materials. In agriculture, the greatest constraints to crop production are land preparation and weeding. Both require high-energy activities and laborious work, usually within a limited amount of time. Interventions to reduce work intensity in IDCs have included better hoe designs for weeding, and improved designs of animal-drawn equipment.

In factories, heat stresses, poor air quality (from fumes, dusts, and particulates), and awkward postures and noise are commonly found. Ahasan et al. (1999) illustrate these issues in examining jobs at a metal working plant in Bangladesh. Although many ergonomic interventions have been employed, attitudinal barriers and access to adequate training resources and support from the international community are still lacking. Finally, transporting materials using people as transporters takes its toll in human injury and energy costs. For example, head loading, a prevalent mode of transporting goods over hilly terrain, involves carrying loads up to 15 lb over distances of 10 miles several times per week. The practices of transporting goods and people are in dire need of innovations to increase efficiency.

To date, researchers have found that high-end ergonomic interventions employed in industrially advanced countries (IAC) are rarely feasible in IDCs. In fact, simple interventions may have even greater potential to affect the health, productivity, and quality of life for workers in such countries. The challenge to devising acceptable solutions and transferring technology to IDCs is to understand and integrate the cultural dimensions into the recommendations. Cultural dimensions refer not only to the physical attributes of the workers (such as anthropometrics, typical postures) but also the cognitive, social, and conceptual aspects. For example, human factor information usually conveyed by color must be reassessed relative to the stereotypes of a country (e.g., in the United States red means "stop"); attitudes toward wearing protective equipment must be addressed, explained, and supported by workers.

Brunette (2002) suggests that corporate social responsibility should be a vehicle for promoting improved working conditions in developing countries. Partnerships between universities and multinational corporations (MNC) may increase awareness of ergonomic factors and begin to create an infrastructure that will allow implementation of ergonomic recommendations in IDCs. Above all, the recommendations must emanate from multidisciplinary teams with close collaboration between ergonomic and occupational health practitioners in the cultural context (O'Neill, 2000; Stubbs, 2000).

GLOBAL TRENDS IN THE TWENTY-FIRST CENTURY AND IMPLICATIONS FOR ERGONOMICS

Globalization has created large multinational companies (MNC) whose strong occupational health and safety programs have positively impacted the working lives of their employees in IDCs (Rantanen, 1999). It is hoped that these corporate standards along with the support from the international community may influence the future legislative development of national ergonomic and safety standards in developing countries (Ahasan et al, 1999).

Flexibility in Work Structure

Decentralization of the large companies into smaller networks creates a reliance on outsourcing or contracting work to smaller companies. This practice has created work organizations with increasing numbers of temporary, "e-lance," and "tele-" workers. Such variability in work structure affects the ability to reach, train, and track the injury status of self-employed workers and workers in small to midsize companies over a long period of time (Rantanen, 1999).

The Aging Population

As a whole, the world is aging because of increasing life expectancy and decreasing population growth in IACs. Since people will be working longer to support themselves, researchers in both the United States and Europe must contend with new situations: How can we keep an older population actively engaged and productive in the workforce in light of the new job demands? What are the effects of aging on physical and mental work capacity? Can we develop age-related criteria for using information technology (Rantanen, 1999; Westgaard, 2000)? Illmarinen (1997) has offered a model to promote and maintain work capacities of older employees. The model is based on factors from the work environment, organization, and individual functioning.

New Technology

Information and communication technologies (ICT) have become integral to the existence of industrialized countries in an astonishingly short time. Research has just begun to address the burgeoning questions of how the new technology will interact with and sustain the work ability, aspirations, and long-term productivity of workers (Rantanen, 1999; Westgaard, 2000). Critical areas for ergonomic growth and research will include understanding the ICT demands on the visual and auditory systems, cognitive ergonomics for intensive computer work, and physical demands and organization of ICT work.

CHALLENGES FOR RESEARCHING MSDs IN THE TWENTY-FIRST CENTURY

Rapid and significant changes in work life over the last decade have created new challenges for MSD research that will demand more innovative means to studying these conditions. In 1983, Kvarnstrom noted the existing epidemiologic struggles in compiling and comparing data between countries and occupational groups.

- Studies from different time periods are difficult to compare because of differences in the social roles of health and illness.
- Socioeconomic differences between study groups may invalidate comparisons.
- The gender bias in different populations and occupations affects results (e.g., women tend to be clustered in high-risk jobs).
- Reporting systems for epidemiologic studies differ among countries.
- Inclusion criteria for diagnostic categories and the quantification of risk factors differ among studies.

The preceding challenges have been surpassed by even broader concerns created by our accelerated use of technology, globalization, and changes in the structure of work and worker demographics (also see Chapter 2 for further discussion). Research challenges exist not only in comparing data from country to country, but also in gathering data, identifying exposures, and measuring health outcomes.

Research Baselines and Follow-Up

The process of establishing a baseline of occupational exposures as a means of measuring the impact of exposures over time and the efficacy of interventions is more difficult than in previous times (Rantanen, 1999; Stubbs, 2000). As indicated, the once stable core of homogenous full-time workers who formed the basis for epidemiological studies has been replaced by a population of workers who enjoy flexibility in employment structures, patterns, and locations. Even the regular monitoring of employees will demand new models. Research designs may need to include shorter periods of follow-up and accommodations for diverse populations and international migration. Rantanen (1999) suggests a "smart" card to follow the worker throughout the career irregardless of type and location of employment.

Exposure Measures

Ergonomic exposures typically include several types of hazards based on physical demands and changes in work organization (i.e., work schedules, work teams, work locations). New exposure concepts are surfacing related to our primarily service-oriented society and the continued prevalence of human-to-human interaction between service workers and clients

(Rantanen, 1999). The emotional load in caring occupations, threat of violence, and dealing with anger are issues yet to be identified and addressed in most classic MSD research designs.

Health Outcomes

The traditional means of measuring occupational outcomes have been the presence or absence of musculoskeletal injury. However, Rantanen (1999) suggests that our new work life has spurred interest in the functional and behavioral aspects of the workplace such as functional capacities, innovation, work motivation, the capacity to handle clients, and psychological overload (to name a few). These outcomes cannot easily be measured by traditional means; therefore, new methods will have to be identified.

SUMMARY

In summary, researchers throughout the world have come to recognize the contribution of biomechanical factors and psychosocial factors (including workplace stressors) to the overall development of MSDs in the individual worker. Research and legislation in industrialized countries has demonstrated continued commitment to minimizing ergonomic hazards for workers and has acknowledged the strength of multidisciplinary, participative approaches to interventions. As interested health care practitioners we all must encourage both research and social responsibility to improve worker health throughout the world.

REFERENCES

Ahasan, M. R., Mohiuddin, G., Vayrynen, S., Ironkannas, H., & Quddus, R. (1999). Work-related problems in metal handling tasks in Bangladesh: Obstacles to the development of safety and health measures. *Ergonomics, 42*(2), 385-396.

Armstrong, T. J., & Chaffin, D. B. (1979). Carpal tunnel syndrome and selected attributes. *Journal of Occupational Medicine, 21*(7), 481-486.

Atwood, M. J., & Michalak, C. (1992). The occurrence of cumulative trauma disorders in dental hygienists. *Work, 2*(4), 17-31.

Batra, P., & Hatzopoulou, A. (2001). The European Union's policy in the occupational and health sector. In W. Karwowski (Ed.), *International encyclopedia of ergonomics and human factors.* London: Taylor & Francis. p 48-51

Bernard, B. (Ed.) (1997). *Musculoskeletal disorders and workplace factors.* Cincinnati, OH: U.S. Department of Health and Human Services, Public Health Service, Centers for Disease Control, National Institute for Occupational Safety and Health. DHHS (NIOSH) Publication #97-141.

Bjelle, A., Hagberg, M., & Michaelson, G. (1981). Occupational and individual factors in acute shoulder-neck disorders among industrial workers. *British Journal of Industrial Medicine, 38*(4), 356-363.

Blood, W. (1942). Tenosynovitis in industrial workers. *British Medical Journal, 2*, 468.

Brunette, M. (2002). Improving working conditions in developing countries. *Human Factor and Ergonomic Society Bulletin, 45*(12), 2.

Bureau of Labor Statistics, Department of Labor (1992). *Surv occup injuries illness.* Washington, DC: Department of Labor.

Bureau of Labor Statistics, Department of Labor (2002). *Industry injury and illness data, 2000.* Washington, DC: U.S. Bureau of Labor Statistics. Available: http://stats.bls.gov/iif/oshsum.htm [Retrieved March 15, 2003].

Chatterjee, D. E. (1978). Repetition strain injury—a recent review. *Journal of the Society of Occupational Medicine, 37*(4), 100-105.

Conn, H. R. (1931). Tenosynovitis. *Ohio State Medical Journal, 27*, 713-716.

Dimberg, L., Olafsson, A., Stefansson, E., Aagaard, H., Oden, A., Andersson, G. et al. (1989). The correlation between work environment and the occurrence of cervicobrachial symptoms. *Journal of Occupational Medicine, 31*(5), 447-453.

Ferguson, D. (1971a). An Australian study of telegraphists' cramp. *British Journal of Industrial Medicine, 28*(3), 280-285.

Ferguson, D. (1971b). Repetition injuries in process workers. *Medical Journal of Australia, 2*(8), 408-412.

Flowerdew, R. E., & Bode, O. B. (1942). Tenosynovitis in untrained farm-workers. *British Medical Journal, 2*, 367.

Ginzberg, E. (1982). The mechanization of work. *Scientific American, 247*(3), 67-75.

Giuliano, V. E. (1982). The mechanization of office work. *Scientific American, 247*(3), 149-164.

Hadler, N. (1996). A keyboard for Daubert. *Journal of Occupational and Environmental Medicine, 38*(5), 469-476.

Hagan, P. E., Montgomery, J. F., & O'Reilly, J. T. (2001). *Accident prevention manual for business and industry-Administration & Programs* (12th Ed.). Itasca, IL: National Safety Council.

Hammer, A. (1934). Tenosynovitis. *Medical Record, 140*, 353-355.

Health and Safety Commission (1999). *Managing stress at work*. London.

Hunting, K. L., Welch, L. S., Cuccerini, B. A., & Seiger, L. A. (1994). Musculoskeletal symptoms among electricians. *American Journal of Industrial Medicine, 25*(2), 149-163.

Illmarinen, J. (1997). Aging and work: Coping with strengths and weaknesses. *Scandinavian Journal of Work, Environment and Health, 23* (suppl), 3-5.

The International Labour Organization Advisory Committee (1960). Effects of mechanisation and automation in officers, III. *International Labour Review, 81,* 350.

Ireland, D. C. R. (1992). The Australian experience with cumulative trauma disorders. In L. H. Millender, D. Louis, & B. P. Simmons (Eds.), *Occupational disorders of the upper extremities*. New York: Churchill Livingstone.

Keikenenwan Shokogun Iinkai (1973). Nihon sangyo-eisei gakkai keikenwan shokogun iinkai hokokusho (Report of the committee on occupational cervicobrachial syndrome of the Japanese Association of Industrial Health). *Jpn J Ind Health, 15,* 304-311.

Kuorinka, B., Jonsson, B., Kilbom, A., Vinterberg, H., Biering-Sorensen, F., Andersson, G. et al. (1987). Standardised Nordic questionnaires for the analysis of musculoskeletal symptoms. *Applied Ergonomics, 18*, 233-237.

Kvarnstrom, S. (1983). Occurrence of musculoskeletal disorders in a manufacturing industry with special attention to occupational shoulder disorders. *Scandinavian Journal of Rehabilitation Medicine, 8,* 1-61.

Levi, L., Sauter, S. L., & Shimomitsu, T. (1999). Work-related stress—it's time to act. *Journal of Occupational Health Psychology, 4*(4), 394-396.

Luoparjärvi, T., Kuorinka, I., Virolainen, M., & Holmberg, M. (1979). Prevalence of tenosynovitis and other injuries of the upper extremities in repetitive work. *Scandinavian Journal of Work, Environment and Health, 5* (Suppl 3), 48-55.

Maeda, K. (1977). Occupational cervicobrachial disorder and its causative factors. *Journal of Human Ergology, 6,* 193-202.

Maeda, K., Horiguchi, S., & Hosokawa, M. (1982). History of the studies on occupational cervicobrachial disorder in Japan and remaining problems. *Journal of Human Ergology, 11,* 17-29.

Maeda, K., Hunting, W., & Grandjean, E. (1980). Localized fatigue in accounting machine operators. *Journal of Occupational Medicine, 22*(12), 810-816.

Margolis, W., & Kraus, J. F. (1987). The prevalence of carpal tunnel symptoms in female supermarket checkers. *Journal of Occupational Medicine, 29*(12), 953-956.

McDermott, F. T. (1986). Repetition strain injury: A review of current understanding. *Medical Journal of Australia, 144*(4), 196-200.

National Institute for Occupational Health and Safety (1997). *Elements of ergonomics programs: A primer based on workplace evaluations of musculoskeletal disorders*. DHHS (NIOSH) Publication No. 97-117. U.S. Cincinnati, OH: Department of Health and Human Services.

National Institute for Occupational Health and Safety (1999). *Stress at work*. DHHS (NIOSH) Publication No. 99-101. Cincinnati, OH: U.S. Department of Health and Human Services.

Ohara, H., Itani, T., & Aoyama, H. (1982). Prevalence of occupational cervicobrachial disorder among different occupational groups in Japan. *Journal of Human Ergology, 11,* 5-63.

O'Neill, D. H. (2000). Ergonomics in industrially developing countries: Does its application differ from that in industrially advanced countries? *Applied Ergonomics, 31,* 631-640.

Phalen, G. S. (1947). The carpal-tunnel syndrome. *Journal of Bone and Joint Surgery (Am), 48*(2), 211-228.

Ramazzini, B. (1717). *De Morbis Artificum Diatriba*. In W. Wright (Trans, 1940). *The diseases of workers*. Chicago: University of Chicago Press.

Rantanen, J. (1999). Research challenges arising from changes in worklife. *Scandinavian Journal of Work, Environment and Health, 6*(special issue), 473-483.

Sanders, M. J. (2001). Minimizing stress in the workplace: whose responsibility is it? *Work, 17*(3), 263-265.

Schenck, R. R. (1989). Carpal tunnel syndrome: the new "industrial epidemic." *AAOHN Journal, 37*(6), 226-231.

Shenkar, O., Mann, J., Shevach, A., Ever-Hadani, P., & Weiss, P. L. (1998). Prevalence and risk factors of upper extremity cumulative trauma disorders in dental hygienists. *Work, 11,* 263-275.

Silverstein, B. A., Fine, L. J., & Armstrong, T. J. (1987). Occupational factors and carpal tunnel syndrome. *American Journal of Industrial Medicine, 11*(3), 343-358.

Silverstein, M., Silverstein, B. A., & Franklin, G. M. (1996). Evidence for work-related musculoskeletal disorders: A scientific counterargument. *Journal of Occupational and Environmental Medicine, 38*(5), 477-484.

Stone, W. E. (1983). Repetitive strain injuries. *Medical Journal of Australia, 2,* 616-618.

Stubbs, D. A. (2000). Ergonomics and occupational medicine: Future challenges. *Occupational Medicine, 50*(4), 277-282.

The Tokyo Declaration on work-related stress and health (1999). *Journal of Occupational Health Psychology, 4*(4), 397-402. (Also can be retrieved at http:/new.workhealth.org//newstokyo.html)

Westgaard, R. H. (2000). Work-related musculoskeletal complaints: some ergonomics challenges upon the start of a new century, *Applied Ergonomics, 31,* 569-580.

CHAPTER 2

The Individual Worker Perspective

Nancy A. Baker
Martha J. Sanders

Nick is a 47-year-old meat cutter who developed a chronic lateral epicondylitis after cutting meat for 25 years. After 3 years of intermittent therapy that brought little relief, Nick finally underwent surgery and embarked on a gradual return-to-work program. Within 3 months, the pain had returned. When the therapist revisited Nick at his job, the therapist advised Nick to stretch periodically and to "slow down." Nick stated, "I can't. That's what I'm known for. I'm the best because I'm fast, with or without a bum elbow. We'll have to think of something different."

The causes of musculoskeletal disorders (MSD) are complex and include personal, biomechanical, and psychosocial factors. Although an initial evaluation of a job may involve identifying factors in the workplace design or administrative procedures that can contribute to the development of MSDs, these are not the only areas that need assessment. We must consider that the worker is an individual in the work environment, an individual with unique beliefs and values about work. Workers' beliefs and values about work and what work requires of them have been associated with musculoskeletal discomfort at work (Baker, Jacobs, & Tickle-Degnen, 2003) and may well influence a worker's choice to accept and implement recommendations to improve the workplace. Understanding workers' beliefs and values about work may be one way to identify appropriate interventions and facilitate the acceptance by workers of appropriate workplace interventions.

This chapter presents an overview of the theoretical and practical constructs that underlie the beliefs and values associated with work in the United States. In this chapter we define "work," identify how historical context has shaped present work beliefs, and discuss some work beliefs and values. The chapter also addresses the concept of work groups as minicultures that shape workers' values, skills, and behaviors relative to work. Finally, trends in the social context of work, such as worker demographics, worker aging, downsizing, and job security issues, are addressed.

DEFINITION OF WORK

What is *work*? Many definitions of work exist, but there is no comprehensive definition that suits all purposes. At its most basic level, the term *work* refers to any activity in which an individual expends energy (Oxford English Dictionary, 1989). However, this definition is too broad to clarify the nature of work. Work is frequently defined as an activity that is done for financial recompense (Ruiz-Quintanilla & England, 1996). Unfortunately, this definition ignores the importance of nonfinancial work roles as well as people who work for little or no pay (Friedson, 1990). Another definition of work describes it as an activity that is obligatory, directed by others, and done in a specific place and at a specific time (Hearnshaw, 1954). Work, therefore, is the opposite of leisure; it is an activity that must be done and, by implication, is onerous. Yet work can be creative, self-fulfilling, and even enjoyable. Work has been described as a means to contribute to society (Ruiz-Quintanilla & England, 1996; Jahoda, 1981). It is also a strong role identity that provides rewards beyond income (Burke, 1991; Jahoda, 1981; Roberson, 1990). What becomes obvious from all these specifications of work is that work is difficult to define because it has many aspects. Each person will, therefore, define work differently based on the beliefs and values that he or she most identifies with it.

A Historical Perspective of Work

Our present beliefs and values about work have their antecedents in the history of work. Americans have a love-hate relationship with work (Tausky, 1992). This attitude can be traced back through the varied historical beliefs about working. (See Applebaum, 1992 for a complete history of working.) The nature of work has shifted radically throughout the centuries, from that of performing daily tasks engaged in for survival to the modern exchange economy in which work is perceived as a means to an end (Applebaum, 1992; Primeau, 1996; Ruiz-Quintanilla & England, 1996; Wilcock, 1998). The dichotomous nature of work, however, has been present in all but the earliest agrarian societies. Work began as a means of survival and became at various times throughout the ages a means of categorizing social class, of monetary exchange, of fulfilling spiritual obligations, and of developing personal growth and self-esteem.

The concept of the type of work as distinct to social classes was evident with the Greek and Roman aristocrats. Aristocrats did no manual labor, instead participating in government, war, and leisure pursuits. They viewed all manual labor, except farming, as degrading (Applebaum, 1992; Wilcock, 1998). With the advent of Christianity, manual work was viewed as spiritual, a way to serve God (Applebaum, 1992; Ruiz-Quintanilla & England, 1996), and also as a punishment for original sin (Thomas, 1999). All were expected to perform manual tasks regardless of class structure. The social class structure was gradually reintroduced in the Middle Ages as commerce and the formation of guilds gained momentum. In general, however, work was still a subsistence undertaking.

The idea of working hard to achieve material wealth and "salvation" was introduced in the mid-1500s with the advent of Protestantism, particularly Calvinism. Protestants believed that each person had a "calling," or a specific work role within God's scheme. If that work was performed well, one was worshiping God. If the person did well financially, it demonstrated that the individual was one of "the chosen." Hence, individuals worked long hours and accumulated wealth for wealth's sake in order to demonstrate that they had achieved salvation (Hill, 1996). Calvinist Protestants' beliefs about work eventually became known as the Protestant work ethic (Weber, 1958). These beliefs included concepts that work was itself good, that hard work would overcome all obstacles, that success was measured by both effort and material wealth, and that frugality was a virtue (Buchholz, 1978). The belief that work, in and of itself, was good and linked to success was an idea that would shape many modern work beliefs.

During the Industrial Revolution (early 1700s) the nature of work changed dramatically. Prior to the Industrial Revolution, craftsmen worked alone or in small conclaves dedicated to the production of a product. They primarily worked at home, used hand tools to craft the goods, and paced their work based on their own abilities. After the Industrial Revolution, workers were essentially machine tenders and paced their work to match the pace of the machine (Applebaum, 1992; Primeau, 1996; Ruiz-Quintanilla & England, 1996). Men, women, and children worked outside the home and were paid a wage for their labor. Each worker did only one small aspect of the job, since, according to

Frederick Taylor's *Principles of Scientific Management*, production was more efficient when jobs were divided into small, repetitive subdivisions (Liebler & McConnell, 1999; Parker, Wall, & Cordery, 2001). Workers' lives were structured around the time clock with limited leisure time.

In the 1940s, behavioral and organizational theorists initiated a shift in industrial focus from emphasis on work tasks to emphasis on the worker. The Human Relations Approach to management identified work as a means to fulfill workers' social and motivational needs (Liebler & McConnell, 1999). Thus, jobs became increasingly enriched, and work became associated with self-actualization and personal growth (Parker et al., 2001).

Over the last 50 years, the perception and structure of work has been shifting again (Ryan, 1995). The information age has caused many workers to move from manufacturing to the service arena. Because the products of service work are often intangible, intellectual property and consumer satisfaction become the end product rather than manufactured goods. As such, work is often not proscribed by time or place. Work can now occur virtually anywhere that one is able to think. The strict demarcation between working time and home time has also blurred, with telecommuting becoming an alternative to onsite work. Rapid communication allows workers to work not only outside the office but also across the globe from corporate headquarters. Finally, workers rarely stay at one job for their entire careers but shift from position to position (Ryan, 1995). These new working parameters are likely to change many of the beliefs about working, particularly those associated with work as a constrained activity.

BELIEFS AND VALUES ABOUT WORK

Beliefs are statements that individuals hold as true. Beliefs shape the values of an individual and culture; these values, in turn, form the basis for individual behavior and opinions (O'Toole, 1992). Our present-day beliefs and values about work are grounded both in the historical perspective of work and in socialization experiences (Hasselkus & Rosa, 1997; Trombly, 1995). The historical perspective provides the ontological background from which we develop our beliefs and expectations about work and what the worker role will bring to us. Examples of specific beliefs about working based on historical experiences include work as a burden, a constraint, a reciprocal arrangement, a means of self-actualization, and a means to contribute to society (Ruiz-Quintanilla & England, 1996). Early socialization experiences draw upon what workers have learned about working from their parents, friends, and society and what they have experienced in the working role.

Workers also develop values that relate to the proper way to perform work and execute the worker role. These values are also influenced by early socialization and become firmly embedded in a worker's role performance and self-perception as a worker. The introductory case of Nick illustrates the powerful influence of these behavioral values on work performance. Nick believed that he was a model worker. He felt that he was respected among his fellow workers because he valued efficient work and was the speediest, most efficient meat cutter. Although pacing himself at work might have decreased his elbow pain, admiration from his fellow workers and the ability to execute his values was integral to his self-esteem and identity as a meat cutter and therefore not an acceptable mode of intervention.

VALUES OF A WORK CULTURE

The concept of work values relates not only to individual workers but also to groups of workers in the same job or profession (referred to as *work groups*). Work groups share similar values or ideas about the "right way to do the job." These ideas may relate to the quality of the job, how the job is performed, the priorities for performing tasks, or even to the unspoken rules of conduct that govern how and when workers ask each other for help or complain about pain. Social networks between workers are believed to have a significant impact on individuals' attitudes toward work and on their tendency to report symptoms or painful conditions arising from work-related tasks (Finholt, 1994).

In addition to sharing similar values, work groups share similar tools, daily routines, language, and symbols that reflect their jobs. In other words, work groups are "minicultures" that develop from shared work experiences among their members. In the context of work, institutions that shape culture include the workplace environment, supervisor and peer relationships, roles, and work-related responsibilities. The culture of the work group influences and gradually shapes workers' perspectives on performing or modifying their jobs (Hosteded, 1996).

The ability of group culture to shape workers' attitudes toward work is clearly shown in Ashforth and Keiner's (1999) analysis of workers who do "dirty" work (i.e., work that is physically, socially, or morally repugnant to most of society). They reported that although most literature would suggest that "dirty" work should cause its members to have low self-esteem and a poor social identity, the opposite tends to be true. They hypothesized that "dirty" workers develop a strong work culture, which has a strong element of "us versus them." This strong culture allows them to reframe their work to emphasize its importance to society, recalibrate the job to change the values that are viewed as important, and reframe the job to focus on its positive aspects. By the end of an indoctrination period, most "dirty" workers who remain on the job have attained the common language and attitude that allows them to perform the work. The worker is assimilated into the culture of the job.

WORK CULTURE ASSIMILATION

Individuals become assimilated into a work culture through various channels, including technical training, formal orientations, and informal experiences. New workers learn technical skills through educational programs, vocational training, on-the-job training, and trial and error. They learn the *formal* workplace rules such as punctuality, work quality, and productivity standards through company orientations, policy and procedure manuals, and yearly performance reviews. New workers learn the important, yet unspoken, *informal* "do's and don'ts" of the job through conversation with seasoned workers, by modeling others, and by observing usual and unusual events (Van Maanen, 1976). These informal channels may exert the greatest impact on work attitudes as demonstrated by the "dirty jobs" study (Ashforth & Kreiner, 1999).

Initially, new workers are concerned with performing and complying with work role expectations. However, over time, individuals contribute their own talents and perspectives to both the task and to interactive aspects of the job, so that the work culture subtly changes with the input of new workers (Jablin, 1987; Van Maanen, 1976). (For further reading about organizational socialization, see Van Maanen, 1976 and Jablin, 1987.)

Cultural assimilation is so insidious that individuals are generally unaware of the elements of their own culture (Hall, 1973). However, workers' attitudes toward injury prevention can be affected at every step of the assimilation process through establishing a "safety culture" that provides positive feedback, injury awareness, and support from management and peers (Krause, 1997). (See Chapter 15 for a complete discussion.) The better we understand the work culture, work role assimilation, workers' routines, daily priorities, and relationships with other work groups, the better will we understand workers' attitudes and behaviors toward accepting or rejecting intervention strategies.

An ethnographic interview is one means to learn about workers' cultures, including their environments, daily routines, and tools. An ethnographic interview enables health care and ergonomic practitioners to answer such questions as the following.

- Can one worker realistically ask another worker for help, or is this considered to be a "cop-out"?
- Can workers be expected to slow down or pace themselves if pay depends on piece-rate incentives?
- What determines *quality* for certain work groups both personally and professionally?
- What aspects of a particular job should *not* be changed?

These seemingly simple questions offer much information about workers' values and how they perceive their work role.

Appendix 2-1 offers a semistructured interview that seeks to understand workers' cultures on the basis of the interview techniques described by Spradley (1979). The interview begins with a "grand tour" of the worker's physical environment, then narrows the scope to the worker's specific work area and work tasks. Next, the interview addresses such job assimilation issues as training and "learning the ropes" and ends with a discussion of his employer's response to a work-related injury, the worker's social relationships, and work values. The goal of the interview is to provide a context for understanding the workplace demands. Ultimately, health care practitioners seek to understand aspects of the job that are important to the worker.

Spradley (1979) advocates that interviewers use the technical words or jargon particular to a work group to encourage workers to explain their jobs more vividly. Although the interview was designed for an individual worker, it can be adapted for a group interview format. Readers will find that "stories" relative to unexpected events at work add particular insight into understanding a worker's perspectives.

THE CHANGING SOCIAL CONTEXT OF WORK: TRENDS IN WORK

As discussed earlier, beliefs and values about working are not static; they shift and change depending on social and historic events that frame a worker's career. The social context reflects not only the attitudes or values of society toward work during a certain period but also the worker demographics, the industry or technology trends that shape employees' jobs, and the public policy mandates that affect managing work-related conditions. The following section discusses changes in the social context of work that will influence our understanding of workers' values, roles, and services needed.

Worker Demographics

Worker demographics have been changing since the 1950s. In the 1950s the workforce was predominately male (70.4%), white (essentially 100%), and older (87% of men between 55 and 64 worked). Job categories were as follows: 41% worked in manufacturing, mining, construction, or transportation; 13% worked in government; and 37% worked in areas such as trade, finance, or service (Kutscher, 1993). By 1992, 46% of the workforce was female and 22% of the workforce was a minority; 27% worked in manufacturing, mining, construction, or transportation; 17% worked in the government; and 62% worked in areas such as trade, finance, or service (see Figure 2-1). Only 67% of men between 55 and 64 worked (Kutscher, 1993), although this trend seems to be slowing. With the baby boom population aging, there will be greater numbers of older workers in the workforce over the next few years. Another demographic characteristic of the present workforce is that a higher percentage has a college education. In 1960, 9.7% of males and 5.8% of females had a college education; in 2000, 27.8% of all males and 23.6% of all females had a college education (U.S. Census Bureau, 2001). This level of education is becoming more nec-

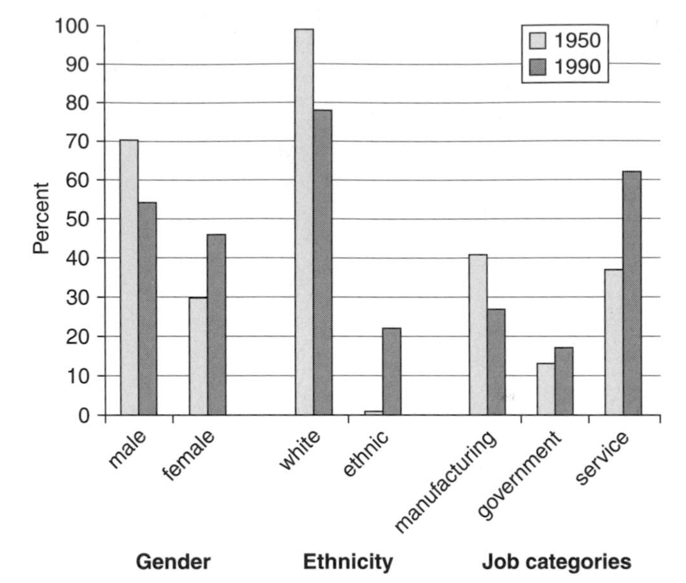

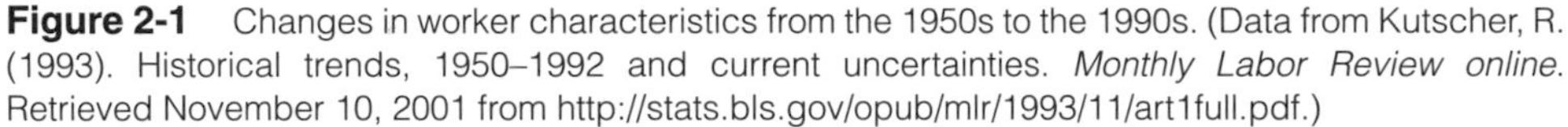

Figure 2-1 Changes in worker characteristics from the 1950s to the 1990s. (Data from Kutscher, R. (1993). Historical trends, 1950–1992 and current uncertainties. *Monthly Labor Review online.* Retrieved November 10, 2001 from http://stats.bls.gov/opub/mlr/1993/11/art1full.pdf.)

essary for a service-based working force (Hill, 1996; Ryan, 1995).

The Aging Workforce

The trend in aging baby boomers suggests that older workers are a growing percentage of the workforce. Older workers can contribute a strong work ethic, good judgment, and valuable insights about job safety and training. However, employers must acknowledge that older workers may need environmental modifications to maintain productivity (e.g., brighter lighting, less background noise, a temperature-controlled atmosphere, and flexible working parameters) (Connolly 1991; Coy & Davenport 1991). Employers must also realize that although older workers as a group have fewer injuries, they present a higher *risk* for injuries because of repeated exposure over time and changes in the body's resilience, reaction time, and depth perception. They generally take a longer time to recover from injuries. Isernhagen (1991) suggests ergonomic job task modifications for older workers that demand less lifting and impact on joints and slower reaction times as well as environmental modifications (see Chapter 21 for a complete discussion).

The Culturally Diverse Workforce

As we approach a global economy, there will be increasing numbers of companies owned by foreign subsidiaries with a greater percentage of workers coming from diverse ethnic backgrounds (Naisbitt & Aburdene, 1990). This diversity brings creativity and manpower to a company. However, it also brings a need to understand other ethnic cultures' perceptions of the worker role, work environment, and the beliefs and values of individuals.

Differences in language and cultural mores present a challenge to professionals who strive to provide health care, work incentives, and opportunities for career growth. For example, traditional Japanese workers work in cohesive groups that collectively solve problems. Hence, they are rarely singled out for individual praise or punishment. Japanese workers develop strong social bonds with supervisors and are accustomed to more personal, paternal, and supervisory styles of management than the strictly business relationship common with supervisors in the United States. Evidence exists that Japanese workers have a higher sense of organizational commitment that may be partly due to their system that rewards workers based on seniority rather than job content (Lincoln, 1996). Japanese workers tend to view working as more of an economic exchange through life commitment, whereas a greater percent of those in the United States are more inclined to view working as a means to contribute to society and develop a sense of identity (England & Whitely, 1990). U.S. managers may encounter workers from a variety of ethnic backgrounds and must realize that classically American rewards based on individual achievement and ambition may be ignoring the greater human needs and work potential of their employees.

Salimbene (2000) presents guidelines for successful interactions with individuals from different ethnic backgrounds when discussing work-related health care issues. These tips are broad and not specific to any one ethnic background (see Box 2-1).

BOX 2-1
Guidelines for Successful Interactions with Individuals from Varied Ethnic Backgrounds Regarding Health Care Issues

- *Begin the interaction more formally with workers who were born in another country.* Use the last name when initially addressing workers. It is a uniquely American tradition to address individuals by their first names.
- *Don't automatically treat someone as you would like to be treated.* Culture determines the norms for polite, caring behaviors.
- *Don't be "put off" if the worker fails to give eye contact.* In some countries it is disrespectful to look directly at another person.
- *Don't make any assumptions regarding the worker's beliefs regarding illness and health.* Encourage individuals to share their beliefs.
- *Present information in a succinct manner.* Provide only essential information at first so as not to confuse the worker.
- *Recheck workers' understandings of your words.* A worker may interpret instructions in a radically different manner than you intended.

Compiled from Salimbene, S. (2000). What language does your patient hurt in? A practical guide to culturally competent patient care. St. Paul, MN: EMC Paradigm.

Use of Self-Managed and Self-Leading Work Teams

Self-managed work teams are those that have the direct responsibility for product set-up, process, and outcome (Manz, 1996). Workers in self-managed teams perform a variety of work tasks and are given discretion over their work methods, task scheduling, and task assignment. General goals for self-managed teams are to increase production for the company while increasing quality of life for the employees. In fact, self-managed teams bear a resemblance to the job design in pre-assembly-line days in which each individual clearly influenced the final product. *Self-leading* teams further increase worker control by making workers responsible for strategically defining goals and establishing process and productivity standards that govern the system (Manz, 1996). The skills and capacities of each worker in self-managed and self-leading work teams ultimately affect the entire team and work process. Therefore, an injured worker in such an environment may perceive different work values and perspectives on returning to work than those of a worker in a more typical work environment. This concept needs to be understood for workers returning to work after an injury.

Americans with Disabilities Act and the Culture of Ableness

The Americans with Disabilities Act (ADA) was designed to present opportunities for qualified workers with disabilities to enter or return to workplaces provided with the necessary job accommodations. The ADA focuses on providing "reasonable accommodations" and making public buildings accessible for workers with physical or emotional disabilities (U.S. Department of Justice,

1991) (See Chapters 13 and 15 for further discussion.) Although critics were initially concerned about the ADA's cost to companies, research has suggested that about two thirds of all job accommodations cost less than $500 and that these costs were often more than recouped through lower job training costs, insurance claims, increased worker productivity, and reduced rehabilitation costs after injury on the job. The estimated savings was $50 for every $1 spent (Blanck, 2000).

Despite the success of many interventions, there are still issues with developing reasonable accommodations within companies. Harlan and Robert (1998) have suggested that some employers and managers still have a standard of ableness that is not related to actual ability. This standard is related to beliefs about the "right" way to work, which has its underpinnings in the historical concepts of working discussed previously. They report that some employers have prevented workers with disabilities from receiving reasonable accommodations through a variety of strategies: denying the need for accommodation; renouncing responsibility for accommodation; withholding legal information about the ADA; and using intimidation to force the worker to work within the able-bodied work culture. Health care practitioners should familiarize themselves with the ADA and advocate implementation of the law for qualified workers.

Job Security

Today's workers are rightfully skeptical about their job futures. Few organizations are insulated from economic pressures, and the potential for layoffs is real in many companies. For this reason, some workers may be hesitant to report injuries for fear of losing their jobs, or they may not report work-related injuries because they do not get reimbursed their total salary (or the total costs of an injury) (Morse, Dillon, Warren, Levenstein, & Warren, 1998). In fact, when Morse et al. (1998) examined the incidence of chronic upper extremity pain in a random Connecticut sample, they found that only 10.6% of those who reported a work-related injury had filed a workers' compensation claim. Thus, underreporting may be a common practice.

Downsizing

Business has become more competitive. One result of this competition is the increase of organizational restructuring and downsizing (Ryan, 1995). The process of downsizing companies has affected workers from high-performing, high-salaried executives to loyal, skilled machinists. For those remaining on the job, downsizing can create a grossly overworked and stressed workforce. Production workers are forced to increase the speed of their tasks without sacrificing quality, and managers are responsible for a multitude of departmental responsibilities and tasks. Open communication, however, may be the buffer for the negative effects of downsizing. A recent large-scale study on the effect of downsizing (Pepper & Messinger, 2001) found that workers who felt that the process was equitable and that communication was open had fewer symptoms and health problems. Workers who remained and who had low-decision/high-demand jobs reported increased symptoms. These results suggest that during downsizing, employers should emphasize fair proceedings and communicate openly about what is going on. It also suggests that managers need to monitor work demands carefully after downsizing. Health care practitioners can assist with this process and encourage employers to acknowledge that both white-collar and blue-collar workers are at risk of developing a stress-related disorder or MSD.

SUMMARY

This chapter has provided an overview of the beliefs and values associated with work and has also discussed how these beliefs and values may be integral to managing workers with injuries. Although individuals' beliefs and values about work may vary, there are underlying themes that are common to many workers. These beliefs will shape workers' perceptions and interactions within the working environment. Clinicians must be sensitive to a worker's beliefs and values in order to shape an intervention that can best reduce disability and return that worker to productive work.

The following case exemplifies the strong bonds and self-identity some workers associate with work. Health care professionals need to understand this relationship in order to provide client-centered treatment and vocational planning (Sanders, 1994).

Barbara Ann was a 59-year-old woman who worked at a steel mill for 17 years prior to developing carpal tunnel syndrome and degenerative changes in her right thumb carpometacarpal joint. Her job as a Z-mill operator demanded that she perform repetitive pinching and grasping of tight machine controls, lifting of 50-pound metal cylinders, and operating 40-pound shears. After undergoing surgery and developing reflex sympathetic dystrophy, it was clear that Barbara Ann would not be able to return to this physically demanding job. Although she had described the work environment as noisy, hot, and "awful smelling," when she was given the option of being retrained as a travel agent (her avocational passion), she declined. "We'll have to find something at the mill. I was the first female Z-mill operator in the United States, and a steel worker is who I am." Mill life was central to her identity.

REFERENCES

Applebaum, H. (1992). *The concept of work: Ancient, medieval, and modern*. Albany, NY: State University of New York Press.

Ashforth, B. E., & Keiner, G. E. (1999). "How can you do it?": Dirty work and the challenge of constructing a positive identity. *Academy of Management Review, 24*, 413-434.

Baker, N. A., Jacobs, K., & Tickle-Degnen, L. (2003). The association between the meaning of working and musculoskeletal discomfort. *International Journal of Industrial Ergonomics, 31*, 235-247.

Blanck, P. D. (2000). Economics of the employment provisions of the ADA. In P. D. Blanck (Ed.), *Employment, disability, and the Americans with Disabilities Act* (pp. 201-227). Evanston, IL: Northwestern University Press.

Buchholz, R. A. (1978). An empirical study of contemporary beliefs about work in American society. *Journal of Applied Psychology, 63*, 219-227.

Burke, J. J. (1991). Identity processes and social stress. *American Sociological Review, 56*, 836-849.

Connolly, J. K. (1991). Consideration for the visually impaired older worker. *Work, 2*(1), 19-28.

Coy, J. A., & Davenport, M. (1991). Age changes in the older adult worker: Implications for injury prevention. *Work, 2*(1), 38-46.

England, G. W., & Whitely, W. T. (1990). Cross national meanings of working. In A. P. Brief & W. R. Nord (Eds.), *Meanings of occupational work* (pp. 65-105). Lexington, MA: Lexington Books.

Finholt, T. (1994, December). *Psychosocial factors of upper extremity limb disorders.* Proceedings from the International Conference on Occupational Disorders of the Upper Extremity, San Francisco, CA.

Freidson, E. (1990). Labors of love in theory and practice: A prospectus. In K. Eriksen & S. P. Vallas (Eds.), *The nature of work: Sociological perspectives* (pp. 149-161). New Haven, CT: Yale University, Columbia University Press.

Hall, E. (1973). *The silent language*. Garden City, NJ: Anchor Books.

Harlan, S. L., & Robert, P. M. (1998). The social construction of disability in organizations. *Work and Occupations, 25*, 397-432.

Hasselkus, B. R., & Rosa, S. A. (1997). Meaning and occupation. In C. Christiansen & C. L. Baum (Eds.), *Enabling function and well-being* (2nd ed.). Thorofare, NF: SLACK.

Hearnshaw, L. S. (1954). Attitudes to work. *Occupational Psychology, 28*(3), 129-139.

Hill, R. B. (1996). Historical context of the work ethic. Retrieved November 28, 1999 from www.coe.uga.edu/~rhill/workethic/hist.htm.

Hosteded, G. (1996). Cultural constraints in management theories. In R. M. Steers, L. W. Porter, & G. A. Bigley (Eds.), *Motivation and leadership at work.* New York, NY: McGraw-Hill.

Isernhagen, S. J. (1991). An aging challenge for the nineties: Balancing the aging process against experience. *Work, 2*(1), 10-18.

Jablin, F. M. (1987). Organizational entry, assimilation and exit. In F. M. Jablin (Ed.), *Handbook of organizational communication.* Newbury Park, CA: Sage Publications.

Jahoda, M. (1981). Work, employment, and unemployment. *American Psychologist, 36*, 184-191.

Krause, T. R. (1997). *The behavior-based safety process* (2nd ed.). New York, NY: John Wiley & Sons.

Kutscher, R. (1993). Historical trends, 1950-1992 and current uncertainties. *Monthly Labor Review Online*. Retrieved November 10, 2001 from http://stats.bls.gov/opub/mlr/1993/11/art1full.pdf.

Liebler, J. G., & McConnell, C. R. (1999). *Management principles for health professionals* (3rd ed.). Gaithersburg, MD: Aspen Publishers, Inc.

Lincoln, J. R. (1996). Employee work attitudes and management practice in the U.S. and Japan: Evidence from a large comparative survey. In R. M. Steers, L.W. Porter, & G.A. Bigley (Eds.), *Motivation and leadership at work*. New York, NY: McGraw Hill.

Manz, C. C. (1996). Self-leading work teams: Moving beyond self-management myths. In R. M. Steers, L.W. Porter, & G.A. Bigley (Eds.), *Motivation and leadership at work*. New York, NY: McGraw Hill.

Morse, T. M., Dillon, C., Warren, N., Levenstein, C., & Warren, A. (1998). The economics and social consequences of work-related musculoskeletal disorders: The Connecticut upper extremity surveillance project. *International Journal of Occupational and Environmental Health, 4*(4), 209-216.

Naisbitt, J., & Aburdene, P. (1990). *Megatrends 2000: Ten new directions for the 1990s*. New York: Avon Books.

O'Toole, M. (Ed.) (1992). *Encyclopedia & dictionary of medicine, nursing, and allied health* (5th ed.). Philadelphia: W.B. Saunders Co.

Oxford English Dictionary (OED) (1989) (2nd ed.). Oxford, UK: Clarendon Press.

Parker, S. K., Wall, T. D., & Cordery, J. L. (2001). Future work design research and practice: Towards an elaborated model of work design, *Journal of Occupational and Organizational Psychology, 74*, 413-440.

Pepper, L., & Messinger, M. (2001). The impact of downsizing and reorganization on employee health and well-being at the DOE Nevada Test Site. Retrieved from the National Institute for Occupational Safety and Health web site (www.cdc./gov/niosh/pdfs/2001-133g16-3pdf) October 8, 2001.

Primeau, L.A. (1996). Work and leisure: Transcending the dichotomy. *The American Journal of Occupational Therapy, 50*, 569-577.

Roberson, L. (1990). Prediction of job satisfaction from characteristic of personal work goals. *Journal of Organizational Behavior, 11*, 29-41.

Ruiz-Quintanilla, S.A., & England, G.W. (1996). How working is defined: structure and stability. *Journal of Organizational Behavior, 17*, 515-540.

Ryan, C. P. (1995). Work isn't what it used to be: Implications, recommendations, and strategies for vocational rehabilitation. *Journal of Rehabilitation*, October/November/December, 8-15.

Salimbene, S. (2000). *What language does your patient hurt in? A practical guide to culturally competent patient care*. St. Paul, MN: EMC Paradigm.

Sanders, M.A. (1994). Women's socialization into non-traditional heavy work. *Work, 4*(2), 93-102.

Spradley J. (1979). *The ethnographic interview*. New York: Harcourt Brace Jovanovich.

Tausky, C. (1992). Work is desirable/loathsome. *Work and Occupation, 19*, 3-17.

Thomas, K. (1999). *The Oxford book of work*. New York: Oxford University Press.

Trombly, C.A. (1995). Occupation: purposefulness and meaningfulness as therapeutic mechanisms. *The American Journal of Occupational Therapy, 49*(10), 960-972.

U.S. Census Bureau (2001). Table No. 216. Educational attainment by race, Hispanic origin and sex: 1960 to 2000. *Statistical Abstract of the United States: 2001*. Retrieved June 14, 2002, from http://www.census.gov/prod/2002pubs/01statab/educ.pdf.

U.S. Department of Justice, Civil Rights Division, Office of the Americans with Disabilities Act (1991). *ADA highlights: Title II state and local government services*. Washington, DC: Government Printing Office.

Van Maanen, J. (1976). Breaking in: Socialization to work. In E. Dublin (Ed.), *Handbook of work, socialization and society*. Chicago: Rand McNally.

Weber, M. (1958). The Protestant work sect and capitalism. In H. H. Gerth & C. Wright Mills (Eds. and Trans.), *From Max Weber* (pp. 302-322). New York: Oxford University Press. (Original work published 1904)

Wilcock, A. A. (1998). *An occupational perspective on health*. Oxford: Clarendon Press.

APPENDIX 2-1

Ethnographic Worker Role Interview

Name: ______________________ **Date:** ______________

Job Title: ______________________

Employer: ______________________

I am interested in learning about your job.

Where do you work? ______________________

How long have you worked there? ______________________

What are your hours? ______________ Your shift? ______________

Can you tell me what you do on your job?

____

____

I am (am not) familiar with your company. Can you give me a minitour of the inside of your plant (building)?

____

Draw the facility if possible.

How is your work area organized (set up)? Are there other people who share your desk (machine, workstation, platform)?

____

Do you work with other employees or independently? ______________________________

Although your job probably varies from day to day, can you describe a *typical* day, beginning with the time at which you arrive at work and ending with the time at which you leave?

____

____

Now, I would like to ask you a few questions about the specific tasks (jobs, duties) that you do.

After you have punched in (checked in), checked your schedule (requisition sheet, assignment list, e-mails), and have gone to your work area, what are the steps for each task that you do?

____

____

Can you estimate what percentage of your time you spend in each part of your job?

____

Is that everything you do, or are there other tasks that people *expect* you to do to help others or to fill in?

____

Now I want you to think back to when you first began the job.

What attracted you to this job? ______________________________

____

How did you get the job? ______________________________

____

What was the first day like? ______________________________

____

____

Did you feel ready for the job? What skills did you already have for the job? What skills did you need to learn? ______________________________

____

____

How did you learn the job as a whole (e.g., your responsibilities, the schedules, the work flow)?

____

____

____

What do you think is the most important part of your job? ______

______

______

(Note technical words or terms here that are specific to this job.)

______

______

How do you know if you are doing a good job? ______

______

______

You said that initially you were attracted to the job because ______

Is that still the reason you are working here? Are there other reasons for staying?

______

______

Can you tell me about a time (incident) at work when you felt especially proud of something that you did? Was there a time when someone tested you and you were right?

______

______

Can you tell me about an incident that made you so frustrated that you wanted to quit?

______

______

It seems there are positive aspects to your job. What else do you like about your job?

______

______

Other than (refer to previous question), what are the aspects of your job that you do not like?

______

Do you find that workers support each other, or are they really out for themselves? Please explain.

______

______

I am interested in how you get along with your supervisor(s). Do they seem concerned with how much work you do, how well you like your job, how comfortable you are, or your chances for a raise or promotion?

______

Did you ever have a work-related injury? If so, please describe what happened.

Did you lose work time because of the injury?

If so, can you tell me how your supervisor and your peers responded to you when you returned?

I would like to understand how you manage your job and home responsibilities. How does work fit with your personal life?

What types of responsibilities or obligations do you have at home?

How do you organize your schedule to manage all your responsibilities? Are there other people on whom you can rely for help?

How do other people in your occupation (job) manage their responsibilities?

Finally, I'm curious about how your parents or other people influenced your job.

What type of work do (did) your parents (caregivers) do?

Did you watch or observe them at their jobs?

Was there anything that you learned from your parents (caregivers) that you always will remember about work?

CHAPTER 3

The Medical Context

Charles F. Dillon[1]

Musculoskeletal disorders (MSDs) present a challenge to the medical professions; accurate diagnosis and treatment are often difficult. MSDs represent a variety of possible underlying pathologies. These are superimposed on a patient's complex upper-extremity functional anatomy in the setting of occupational ergonomic exposures. Some consider MSDs an enigma, not only because of diagnostic difficulties but also because they may develop insidiously and with seemingly nonlocalized symptoms. Clinical medicine traditionally focuses on identifying disease and its risk factors as inherent in the individual patient. However, even where MSDs are well localized, the critically important ergonomic risk factors are in the external environment, not directly observable in traditional clinical encounters. Diagnosis and treatment can be challenging, especially since ergonomic risk factor and soft-tissue evaluation requires specialized skills not usually provided in medical training.

This chapter presents a medical perspective on MSD classification and diagnosis. Its purpose is to provide a practically oriented general introduction to the medical evaluation of upper-extremity MSD. This presentation derives from the experience of contemporary multidisciplinary specialty MSD clinics (Barthel, Miller, Deardorff, & Portenier, 1998; Keller, Corbett, & Nichols, 1998; Piligian et al., 2000; Tong, Haig, Theisen, Smith, & Miller, 2001). The emphasis is on non-surgical or "conservative" management of MSD cases. In individual, carefully selected cases, surgery can make an important contribution, but because of the multifactorial nature of MSDs, it is increasingly apparent that surgery is not preferable to rehabilitative care for the great majority of patients (Dobyns, 1991; Millender, 1992).

GENERAL PERSPECTIVES ON MSDs

MSD Terminology

Terms such as MSDs, cumulative trauma disorders, and repetitive strain disorders are umbrella terms signifying a set of gradual-onset, upper-extremity disorders related to repetitive activities (e.g., work, sports, music, or other physical tasks). The definition doesn't include acute injuries from direct trauma. The terms have the disadvantage of prejudging the origins of MSDs and in specific instances are misleading or inaccurate. While it is likely that a set of MSDs result from repetitive use with cumulatively accrued injury, this isn't invariably the case. Also, underlying the debate on MSDs is an unstated assumption on the part of some that work is inherently risky, leading inevitably to chronic musculoskeletal

[1]Dr. Charles Dillon authored this work in his private capacity. No official support or endorsement by the CDC or the federal government is intended or should be inferred.

dysfunction. This is unfortunate, since there is good evidence that, in general, work activity promotes good physical and psychological health. The issue facing MSD practitioners is to define with clarity potentially injurious situations and to help employers and patients identify useful, injury-preventing alternatives.

There has been a proliferation of acronyms for MSDs (see Box 3-1), motivated by a perceived need to increase clarity. Presently, there isn't general agreement on terminology. The term *MSD* was recently introduced as a generic cover term (NIOSH, 1997). The term *repetitive strain injury* was adopted in Australia in reference to soft-tissue conditions, specifically with stress as a contributory factor (Chatterjee, 1987). The term *overuse syndrome* is used most widely in relation to sports injuries or hobby-related rather than work activities (Herring & Nilson, 1987). *Occupational cervicobrachial disorder* is used widely throughout Japan, Germany, and Scandinavia. It refers specifically to constrained postures as the causal factor (Maeda, Horiguchi, & Hosokawa, 1982).

MSD Pathogenesis

An MSD conceptual model has been developed (Armstrong et al., 1993; Putz-Anderson, 1988; Tanaka & McGlothlin, 1993) wherein each cycle of a work activity has the potential to cause microinjury in the involved soft-tissue structures. One repetition may not produce inflammation or pain, but if adequate time is not allowed for tissue recovery, over a period of time microinjuries can accumulate, producing trauma to a specific area of the body. (See Chapter 8 for a complete discussion on MSD models.) More recently, it has become evident that prolonged static postures pose substantial risk of injury and may result in MSDs (Colombini et al., 2001; Novak & MacKinnon, 1997, 2002). The physiological basis of chronic muscle injury has recently been reviewed (Sjogaard & Sjogaard, 1998). Thus, a worker on a specific high-risk job may be asymptomatic for years while accruing job-related injury. Recent authors have provided extensive reviews of biomechanical risk factors for MSDs (Armstrong, 1990; Kilbom et al., 1996; Muggleton, Allen, & Chappell, 1999). Although an MSD may develop anywhere in the body, disorders of the upper extremity are the most frequently reported (Armstrong, 1990; Forde, Punnett & Wegmen, 2002).

BOX 3-1
Current Terms and Acronyms for Upper-Extremity Disorders in the Medical Literature

Cumulative Trauma Disorders (CTD)
Repetitive Strain Injury (RSI)
Occupational Cervicobrachial Disorder (OCD)
Overuse Syndrome
Work-Related Disorders
Musculoskeletal Disorders (MSD)
Repetitive Trauma Disorders
Regional Musculoskeletal Disorders
Work-Related Musculoskeletal Disorders (WRMSD)
Upper-Extremity Musculoskeletal Disorders (UEMSD)

Common Characteristics of MSDs

Despite the variety of nomenclature, common characteristics for occupational MSDs have been described worldwide in epidemiologic studies. These provide a common focus on the design of the work environment. Characteristics include the following (Armstrong, 1991; Kvarnstrom, 1983; Putz-Anderson, 1988).

- The causes of MSDs are multifactorial, involving personal, work-related, and non-work-related factors.
- MSDs involve both mechanical and physiologic mechanisms.
- MSDs are related to the intensity and duration of work.
- MSDs may also be related to a short, repetitive work cycle, to static work performed in uncomfortable positions, or to a stressful work environment.
- Symptoms can be poorly localized, nonspecific, and episodic.
- MSDs develop insidiously; they may occur after weeks, months, or years on the job.
- MSDs recuperate slowly; they may require weeks, months, or years for recovery.

The Workplace Setting of MSDs

The traditional "office-patient-based" medical model is linear and problem-oriented: diagnose the problem and its causes, and then treat the patient. It is assumed that patients will comply with treatment recommendations. Traditional office medical evaluations, however, have a significant bias: Disease risk factors inherent in the patient (e.g., anthropomorphic or heritable characteristics, co-morbid illness, physiological variations) are most often the primary focus of attention. They are more readily identified and seemingly more objective than external disease risk factors not directly observed in the office medical encounter.

MSDs, by definition, however, involve causal ergonomic risk factors external to the medical clinic that are deeply embedded in the patient's work situation. Integration of external risk factor data into medical treatment models, implying a public health approach, has historically been difficult to achieve. Examples are the hygiene control of infectious disease in the nineteenth century, tuberculosis control in the early twentieth century, and dietary and lifestyle interventions for heart disease and stroke in the late twentieth century. Even in the twenty-first century, however, the principal concern of medical providers is the pathophysiologic processes inherent in the patient. External factors such as workplace ergonomics or socioeconomic problems are treated as separate and distinct from the medical process. This impacts diagnosis, therapy, and outcomes, and it creates problems, especially psychological stress, for MSD patients. In fact, treatment outcomes for MSDs often hinge on a myriad of external issues (e.g., union agreements, unpaid bills, insurer treatment authorizations, arranging for light-duty work, and unraveling the maze of workers' compensation laws).

The traditional medical model, therefore, falls short because it treats work-related MSDs out of context. Clearly, the problem of MSD tissue pathology and treatment cannot be separated from workplace, social, and legal issues. The effective MSD diagnosis and treatment involves both medical intervention and skill for arranging follow-through in industry, insurance, and rehabilitation (Dobyns, 1987; Millender, 1992). Dobyns (1991) explains that practitioners must make a cognitive shift in examining workers with MSDs by addressing physical and socioeconomic issues with equal regard. This requires time and patience, and by definition it is poorly compensated. It is, however, the only approach that will serve patients realistically and lead to adequate treatment outcomes.

MSD DIAGNOSIS

The Traditional MSD Diagnostic System

MSDs encompass a variety of conditions relating to ergonomic risk factors. The specific diagnosable condition depends on the part of the body involved and the type of work performed. A wide range of conditions may be considered as MSDs, including peripheral entrapment neuropathies (carpal or cubital tunnel syndrome), tenosynovitis, epicondylitis, ganglion cysts, myalgias, myofascial pain syndrome, and others (see Chapter 5). In a review of MSD literature, Moore (1994) found that the great majority of MSDs involve the muscle-tendon unit (e.g., tenosynovitis and myofascial pain syndromes). MSDs of nerves, joints, and the vasculature are less common, but as a group they have more serious implications in terms of patient morbidity.

The list of recognized MSD diagnoses currently in general clinical use (codified in the International Classification of Diseases, 9th Revision, Clinical Modification ICD9-CM) is relatively short and in many cases lacks specificity (see Table 3-1). As employed by medical providers, this is essentially a standardized commercial listing used to classify patients for the purpose of insurance billing. Within this short list only a select few diagnoses have gained any real currency among medical providers and insurers, chief among these being carpal tunnel syndrome, lateral epicondylitis, tenosynovitis, and

Table 3-1

Specific Upper-Extremity MSD Recognized in the International Classification of Diseases, 9th Revision, Clinical Modification, 6th Edition (ICD9-CM)

MSD	ICD9-CM Code
Shoulder	
Rotator cuff syndrome	726.10
Bicipital tenosynovitis	726.12
Elbow and forearm	
Medial epicondylitis	726.31
Lateral epicondylitis	726.32
Olecranon bursitis	726.33
Cubital tunnel syndrome	354.2
Hand and Wrist	
Trigger finger	727.03
de Quervain's disease	727.04
Other tenosynovitis of the hand and wrist	727.05
Ganglion of joint	727.41
Ganglion of tendon sheath	727.42
Carpal tunnel syndrome	354.0

Note: Even within designated codes, ICD9-CM is often nonspecific—that is, the many tenosynovitis syndromes of the hand and wrist are classified in a single nonspecific category (727.05). Cubital Tunnel Syndome is coded as a peripheral mononeuropathy, together with metabolic, traumatic, and toxic peripheral ulnar mononeuropathies. ICD9-CM generally permits surrogate coding of any disorder. For example, Hand-Arm Vibration Syndrome can be classified under Raynaud's Disease (443.0). ICD9-CM also permits coding of nonspecific symptoms—for example, Pain in Limb (729.5) or Paresthesias (782). Department of Health & Human Services, Centers for Disease Control & Prevention, Health Care Financing Administration. (2001, October). *International Classification of Diseases, 9th Revision, Clinical Modification*, 6th Edition, Official Version (DHHS Publication No. 01-1260). [CD]. Hyattsville, MD: National Center for Health Statistics.

ganglion cyst, the set of disorders traditionally treated by surgery.

The merits of the traditional MSD classification system are as follows.

- Medical research and practice are focused on a small number of diagnoses (most especially carpal tunnel syndrome) that have been studied intensively.
- Its practical utility is in efficiently triaging a subset of MSD patients through the medical-insurance system.

The limitations of the traditional system are as follows.

- In the minds of the general public and ordinary medical practitioners, disorders such as carpal tunnel syndrome and lateral epicondylitis have become synonymous with MSDs. This is unfortunate, since prevalence studies indicate that these are among the less common MSDs, even in high-risk occupations.
- A strong economic incentive is created for medical providers to focus on only a select few MSD diagnoses. When an uncommon ICD9-CM code or a diagnosis not specifically codable to ICD9-CM is submitted to an insurer, adjustors may deny the claim or delay it for administrative review. This can significantly impact treatment.
- A corollary is that the traditional system has little capability to specify detailed diagnoses for the majority of specific anatomic units. The possibility of specific diagnosis is virtually eliminated for entire subunits of the upper extremity functional anatomy (e.g., the muscle units, joints, and the vascular system).
- As a matter of expediency, providers are encouraged to identify and treat just one "well-localized" disorder per patient encounter, selected from a short list of "acceptable" MSD diagnoses. This encourages providers to ignore other physical findings and leave any additional problems unaddressed—a situation leading to "treatment failures." Alternately, practitioners may act altruistically, identifying and treating multiple problems but only receiving reimbursement for treating a single disorder.
- The traditional insurance claims model for musculoskeletal conditions is the acute injury, which has well-developed time limits on claims. Conflict often develops because MSDs may have insidious onset and episodic relapses, a situation more characteristic of chronic illness than acute injury.

Regulatory Definitions for MSDs

Federal regulatory agencies responsible for addressing the workplace MSD problem employ working definitions for MSDs that include medical, ergonomic, and administrative criteria.

These are practical MSD definitions designed to permit standardized monitoring of workplace safety conditions and are more comprehensive than traditional medical definitions. For example, in the Occupational Safety and Health Administration (OSHA) MSD reporting procedures (OSHA, 1990), to qualify as an OSHA-recordable MSD, a condition must have either persisting symptoms (pain, paresthesias, numbness) or there must be one or more physical findings (redness, loss of motion, deformity, swelling, or positive physical examination tests). The MSD must be judged to be work-related, and action must be taken as a result of the condition (medical treatment beyond first aid, lost workdays, less than full-duty status, or transfer to another job; see Chapter 4).

Research Definitions of MSDs

In individual studies, researchers have developed specific criteria for MSD diagnoses (Silverstein, Fine, & Armstrong, 1986; Silverstein, Fine, & Stetson, 1987). Research definitions for MSDs typically use both inclusion and exclusion criteria and define a characteristic period and frequency within which symptoms must manifest. Exclusion criteria exclude cases due to acute injury or nonoccupational conditions. Typical inclusion criteria include the presence of persistent symptoms (1 week or longer, or occurring 20 or more times in 1 year); characteristic physical examination signs of muscle, tendon, or nerve disorders; and onset of symptoms occurring during work on the job in question. Examples of case exclusion criteria are evidence of acute traumatic onset of symptoms or of systemic disease that could explain the worker's symptoms.

Consensus Diagnostic Classifications for MSD

Various medical specialties (orthopedics, neurology, physical and rehabilitation medicine, radiology, occupational medicine, sports medicine) have developed detailed knowledge of certain MSD diagnoses, such as carpal tunnel syndrome. This expert knowledge, however, is generally held compartmentalized within the subspecialties. Also, subspecialists often disagree as to the criteria for diagnoses of MSDs. Further, effective communication and cooperation among medical subspecialists are rare, which leads to a somewhat fractionated overall clinical approach to this important group of disorders.

Thus far there have been relatively few attempts to establish consensus classifications and standardized diagnostic protocols for the entire range of MSDs, although some work has been done (Harrington, Carter, Birrell, & Gompertz, 1998; Harris, 1997; Waris et al., 1979). Considerable attention has been devoted to individual, high-profile disorders, and useful standards have been developed for carpal tunnel syndrome (Katz et al., 1991; Rempel et al., 1998). Historically in medicine the development of consensus standards has been a notoriously difficult and lengthy process, even for apparently well-delineated syndromes such as rheumatoid arthritis. For example, shoulder impingement syndrome case definitions have been extensively studied but without any useful results (Stiens, Haselkorn, Peters, & Goldstein, 1996). It is perhaps most significant that there is no serious ongoing interdisciplinary initiative in the medical profession to develop comprehensive consensus criteria for MSD case definitions as there is in other areas of musculoskeletal medicine.

MSD Symptom Questionnaire Surveys

Musculoskeletal symptoms, particularly pain, are a valid area of study in their own right. Although the experience of pain is inherently subjective, there are valid, standardized protocols available for obtaining symptom data from patients and workplace survey respondents. Symptom survey data can be analyzed as an outcome in and of itself, although it is demonstrated that persistent and severe symptoms are associated with increased probability of positive physical examination findings and diagnosable disease (Baron, Hales & Hurrell, 1996; Silverstein et al., 1997). When performing symptom surveys it is essential to employ instruments with high validity and reliability (Von Korf, 1992), and the instrument should be validated for the route of administration (personal versus telephone interview, self-administration). Pain diagrams and numerical or visual analog (VAS) pain rating scales are preferred (Jensen & Karoly, 1992). The Nordic Musculoskeletal Questionnaire (NMQ) and other validated questionnaires in general use have recently been reviewed (Baron, Bales, & Hurrell, 1996; Palmer, Smith, Kellingray, & Cooper, 1999; Salerno, Copley-Merriman, Taylor, & Shinogle, 2002).

MSD Diagnostic Protocols

A comprehensive, thorough medical examination protocol needs to be employed for MSD patients. Such evaluation protocols have been developed at MSD multidisciplinary specialty clinics (Barthel et al., 1998; Keller et al., 1998; Pascarelli & Hsu, 2001, Piligian et al., 2000; Tong et al., 2001, University of Michigan Department of Environmental & Industrial Health, 1984). The aim is to obtain anatomically precise clinical findings as a guide to therapy (Ranney, Wells, & Moore, 1995). These protocols typically include the following.

- *Questionnaire data:* Structured data collection on patient demographics, general medical and occupational history, MSD risk factors, the historical development of symptoms, questions (and pain diagram) geared toward localizing pain and other symptoms, questions relating to features of traditional MSD diagnoses, and psychometric scales such as the McGill Pain Questionnaire (Melzack & Katz, 1992) or the SF-36 (Brazier et al., 1992).
- *Physical examination protocol:* An upper-quarter evaluation from the neck to the fingertips. This includes detailed exam of muscles, joints, nerves, and the vascular system. Muscle assessment includes swelling, atrophy, lengthening or contracture, range of motion assessment, strength testing (noting pain on resistance testing), and pain on palpation. Detailed diagnosis-specific provocative tests are performed (Tinel's, Phalen's, Hawkins and Neer tests, etc.).
- *Examination tests:* Measured hand grip and pinch strength; monofilament testing.
- *Laboratory tests:* These are used selectively as indicated for specific cases. They include electrodiagnostic ("EMG") studies, radiologic imaging studies (x-ray, MRI), vascular studies, and so forth.

A systematic medical evaluation protocol produces a patient-specific list of symptoms and coordinated physical findings. Typically, one or more "traditional" MSD diagnoses are identified, along with several "nontraditional" ones. Not all findings carry equal weight in terms of morbidity, and some findings may prove to be transient based on follow-up evaluation. Nevertheless, such protocols provide a sounder basis for developing a biomechanical and ergonomic explanation for the MSD patient's injuries and for planning and monitoring therapy. Most important for the MSD patient, it also provides a detailed explanation of symptoms that are experienced and a logical plan for alleviating them. MSD patients should not be dismissed as having vague or nonphysiologic complaints without this type of evaluation. Systematic, protocol-based MSD evaluations are lengthy and in practice are performed as intake exams and for final follow-up assessment. Specific findings are followed for interval exams. A clinical example is helpful to define the approach.

Case Presentation and Exam Findings

A 34-year-old, right-handed woman is employed for 10 years as a bookkeeper for an accounting firm. Her work consists of computer accounting applications. For two months she has experienced annoying sharp pains, tingling, and periodic numbness in the right index and middle fingertips. She also has pain in the right forearm, elbow, and shoulder. Symptoms are prominent at the start of her workday but even more so in the afternoons as the workday progresses. She feels better after work and on the weekends. There isn't any history of endocrine disorders, smoking, obesity, hand or arm injuries, arthritis, or off-work risks for MSDs. The findings on her physical exam include a positive right Phalen's and Median Nerve Compression Test, but negative Tinel's test. Palpation shows nodules at the A-1 pulley area of the right index finger and thumb. These show clicking on exam but are not tender, and there is no triggering. Crepitation is noted in the flexor tendon sheaths of the right palm. Resistance testing of the right index and middle finger flexor profundus tendons elicits pain. There is palpable pain at the right thumb carpometacarpal joint and a positive "grind" test there, but no bony abnormality or subluxation of the joint is present. In the right forearm, muscle tenderness in the flexor compartment is noted. At the right elbow, there is marked tenderness at the medial epicondyle of the humerus, but negative resistance testing of the flexor carpi ulnaris and radialis and pronator teres muscles. The pronator teres is, however, foreshortened and contracted, preventing forearm supination beyond 50 degrees. There is some pain with resistance testing of the palmaris longus. The exam of the upper arms, shoulder, and neck is normal except for the following: a tendency to internal rotation of the shoulders; the pectoralis minor muscles are contracted right greater than left, with corresponding limitation of forward shoulder elevation; and the right pectoralis minor is painful to palpation. Monofilament testing shows no abnormalities, and an x-ray of the right hand is negative. Electrodiagnostic studies, however, are consistent with right carpal tunnel syndrome.

Diagnostic Summary

Carpal tunnel syndrome, right
Flexor tenosynovitis, right index and middle fingers
Right thumb carpometacarpal (CMC) joint strain
Trigger digit (incipient), right thumb and index finger
Medial epicondylitis, right
Forearm myofascial pain, right flexor compartment
Forearm muscle contracture, right pronator teres
Shoulder muscle contracture, bilateral pectoralis minor

This patient presents with widespread regional symptoms in the hands, forearm, elbow, and shoulder. If these symptoms were not comprehensively investigated, this could certainly raise the question of whether the patient was a credible historian or invite speculation on possible psychological disorders as explanations for her symptoms. A detailed evaluation, however, develops an explanation for each symptom. Note that the first two diagnoses would be considered definite under the traditional MSD evaluation paradigm. The cooccurrence of these is not random, since both share common ergonomic risk factors (for example, repetitive finger flexion and hand gripping) and frequently cooccur. Unilateral disease would be uncommon in carpal tunnel syndrome resulting from nonoccupational causes such as thyroid disease or diabetes. The remaining diagnoses listed are nontraditional. Disorders of joints or muscle units or range-of-motion abnormalities caused by pathologic muscle contracture are not traditionally recognized. Incipient trigger digit exam abnormalities would be dismissed because locking of the digits has not occurred yet.

The complete list of diagnoses, even though it does include clinical problems of varying severity, provides detailed data that can be checked against the onsite ergonomic data for this patient. In this particular instance, multiple diagnoses (carpal tunnel syndrome, flexor tenosynovitis, trigger digit) point to tasks requiring repetitive finger flexion or hand-grip. In an office computer worker, these most commonly relate to computer keying and hand gripping with computer mouse use. Most often, however, multiple work tasks with similar ergonomic risks are additive in contributing to injury. In the typical office setting other typical manual office tasks involving repetitive finger flexion and hand grip include the use of handheld staplers and staple removers, handwriting, and, for bookkeepers, the use of calculators. These are activities typically performed with the dominant hand.

The nontraditional MSD diagnoses have ergonomic correlates. The CMC joint strain classically is related to forceful gripping, but in this case it appeared related to a repetitive control-function keyboard maneuver wherein the thumb is used in a rocking motion to activate the control key, with the index finger reaching to activate the function keys at the top of the keyboard. This maneuver not only strained the thumb CMC joint but likely also caused a median nerve traction injury, exacerbating the patient's carpal tunnel syndrome symptoms.

The medial epicondylitis, which appeared driven principally by activation of the palmaris longus, appeared related to computer mouse use, since that muscle is typically first recruited to provide the initial 10 to 15 degrees of wrist flexion. Onsite ergonomic evaluation revealed that the patient was resting her forearms and elbows on her desk, a position that serves to functionally disconnect the forearms and hands from the upper arms and shoulders. Such a "disconnect" syndrome is a mechanically disadvantageous situation, inasmuch as it forces an increased level of forearm and hand muscle recruitment over what would ordinarily be the case. Prolonged static posturing likely led to the observed proximal muscle contractures. Computer work is generally performed in a pronated forearm posture. Pronator teres contracture and accompanying supination lag typically result from this (there was not any evidence on exam for pronator syndrome complicating her carpal tunnel syndrome). Internal rotation of the shoulders and accompanying muscle contracture is frequently observed in computer workers and appears to result principally from the fact that keyboard width is less than shoulder breadth (biacromial diameter). In order to operate the keyboard, the hands and forearms, and secondarily the shoulders, must be kept internally rotated.

Multiple MSD Symptoms and Diagnoses

Given the preceding example, one can legitimately ask whether all MSD patients can be expected to have multiple symptoms and multiple diagnoses. The answer is that most MSD patients in fact have multiple symptoms and that multiple MSD diagnoses are also common, depending on MSD duration and severity.

In the medical literature, some skepticism has been engendered about the validity of MSD patients' self-reported symptoms and the validity of self-reported data generally. Such authors consider multiple presenting MSD symptoms illegitimate or a sign of malingering or a psychological disorder. This appears to be an aberration and is contradictory to generally accepted medical practice, where it has been clearly demonstrated that the clinical interview, based on the patient's self-reported history and symptom profile, typically has more value diagnostically than physical examination or laboratory data. Further, self-reported data are a well-accepted basis for diagnosing and managing many important disorders such as arthritis, cardiac angina, migraine headache, and so on.

The fact is that MSD patients with multiple symptoms are the rule rather than the exception. This is easily demonstrated by taking a careful clinical history in an initial patient encounter. Also, if standardized intake questionnaires are administered to new patients, many will indicate symptoms at multiple levels in the upper extremities. This is also a well-demonstrated phenomenon in numerous questionnaire prevalence field studies. There has, however, been little serious research as to why this is the case.

One clear reason why many MSD patients typically report multiple symptoms is that they may in fact have multiple medical problems, as the previous clinical example illustrates. Such multiple problems may vary in severity and importance, but are often a sufficient explanation for the variety of a patient's presenting symptoms. Another explanation for MSD patients reporting widespread or multiple symptoms at different anatomical levels is that the anatomical structures themselves are "widespread" or may serve multiple functions that cross traditional anatomical zones. Here are some examples.

- A patient with flexor tendinitis of the fingers typically experiences pain radiating up and down the entire course of the muscle tendon unit, which extends from the proximal volar forearm to the fingertips. Symptoms are routinely reported in the fingers, hand, wrist, and forearm.

- A patient with proximal biceps tendinitis may experience pain both intrinsically at the shoulder (the proximal course of the tendon is intraarticular) and along the course of the muscle-tendon unit, which extends almost half a meter to the proximal forearm. A combination of shoulder, upper arm, and, occasionally, elbow pain is reported.
- Muscles such as the trapezius and levator scapulae have dual roles in controlling both shoulder and neck motion. Pain from these muscles may result from ergonomic stressors on the neck, the shoulder, or both, and may rationally be perceived as a somewhat ill-defined combination of neck and shoulder pain.

MSD patients may legitimately experience symptoms at multiple sites in cases of neurological or vascular pain. Here, pain originating from one location is well known to be transmitted to multiple sites based on the distribution of these structures (Butler & Jones, 1991). Severe pain may also be referred to other anatomic areas on a nonneurological basis (Simons, Travell, & Simons, 1998).

In clinical practice, multiple MSD diagnoses are present in substantial numbers of patients. Multiple MSDs in a patient are most likely in cases with long-standing symptoms or severe disease. In these settings, multiple diagnoses may result from related or multiple ergonomic risk factors, or occur as secondary complications to the original injury. A case example will help clarify this.

Case Presentation and Findings

A 37-year-old, right-handed factory assembler has sharp pain at the anterior aspect of his right shoulder. He works on an assembly line with pneumatic tools, bolting parts on steel frame assemblies. This is a machine-paced task. His pain has been present for a year and a half, and it has steadily worsened, now involving the right upper arm and neck. He experiences pain principally at work but also at night if he sleeps on his right side. He doesn't report any swelling. There is no prior history of injury to the neck or shoulder, and he is otherwise healthy. He is a nonsmoker and has no personal or family history of arthritis. He has seen his primary care physician and a specialist previously and was treated with a local steroid injection that transiently benefited his shoulder symptoms but ultimately did not abate them. He is on light duty at work. Physical examination of the right shoulder shows normal range of motion except for mild limitation in external rotation but some palpable rotator cuff tenderness and a positive Hawkins impingement sign. There is no exam evidence for bicipital tendinitis or AC joint pain, but there is mild relative laxity of the joint as compared to the left but without any subluxation. Apprehension sign is negative. Scapular stability appears abnormal on the right as compared to the left; some scapular elevation and protraction are evident. There is some weakness in the supraspinatus and deltoid muscles. Muscle atrophy is not evident, but muscle bulk is comparable right to left. The cervical spine exam shows some loss of cervical lordosis, increased paracervical muscle tension, a positive Spurling's test, and right-sided C5 neuroforaminal tenderness. The exam of the arm and hand is normal except for minimal right-sided biceps weakness and an equivocally decreased biceps deep-tendon reflex. The sensory exam is intact. X-ray of the shoulder is unremarkable. A cervical MRI shows a moderate right-sided C5 disc herniation and no evidence of arthritis or degenerative disease.

Diagnostic Summary

Cervical disc herniation (right C5)
Scapular stabilization abnormality, right
Shoulder impingement syndrome, right

This patient shows a constellation of findings most consistent with related primary and secondary MSDs. Although one cannot be entirely certain from a retrospective evaluation, it is most probable that the cervical disc lesion is the initial injury, which in turn caused secondary weakness in the right C5 innervated shoulder and arm muscles, with scapular instability and shoulder tendon impingement syndrome later resulting. From the exam findings of mild diffuse muscle weakness, it can be supposed that the collective problems were relatively longstanding. This patient may also have previously been treated successfully for proximal bicipital tendinitis, given the medical history.

A work-site ergonomic evaluation shows risk factors consistent with the MSD. In his work, he stands facing the assembly line and, because of his height, has his neck in chronic flexion while doing manual tasks. He turns his head from side to side constantly to coordinate receiving and sending parts along the assembly line. There is little heavy lifting with this job, but he uses an extended reach maneuver to place parts weighing up to 2 pounds on the metal assembly and stabilize them while he uses unsupported pneumatic tools to fix them in place.

Stages of MSDs

It is obligatory to classify MSD patients as to their initial stage at presentation. A categorization based on three major groups is a useful guide: primary MSD cases with recent onset of symptoms, secondary cases presenting over a year after onset of first symptoms or with particularly severe symptoms, and tertiary cases with long-standing symptoms (years) and extensive prior medical evaluation and treatment. Multiple diagnoses should be routinely expected in secondary and tertiary stage patients—both multiple primary disorders and secondary MSD complications. A detailed clinical evaluation of MSD patients in these groups is particularly important because it provides the best chance to therapeutically address the entirety of the patient's problems. Experience shows that tertiary stage patients are particularly difficult to treat (Himmelstein et al., 1995).

It is important to recognize that the MSD medical literature is distorted in perspective by the different types of patient populations in the various medical practices. Primary care doctors and general occupational medicine clinics will typically see predominantly Stage 1 MSD patients, with a mixture of Stage 2 and 3. Medical specialists and multidisciplinary clinics may have a filtered group of referral patients, primarily Stage 2 and 3. Literature publications from these different clinical settings gives quite different perspectives on MSDs. Finally, patient selection bias also affects the insurance perspective on MSDs. Some element of dishonesty is nearly universal, and while practicing physicians may periodically see patients who are malingering or deliberately falsifying claims, insurers and medical specialists typically see a much higher prevalence of this type of conduct, which colors their general perspective on MSDs.

Nonoccupational MSD Risks and MSD Differential Diagnosis

To avoid misdiagnosis and treatment failure, medical professionals treating MSD patients must understand the differential diagnoses for specific conditions. Soft-tissue musculoskeletal disorders similar to MSDs can occur as extra-articular manifestations of arthritis syndromes, viral infections, or nutritional disorders. Endocrine disorders such as hypothyroidism, diabetes, and hyperparathyroidism can also produce similar conditions. Practitioners should be knowledgeable about the MSDs that characteristically result from common sports and hobbies (tennis, racket sports, bicycling, swimming, golf, etc.) (Metz, 1999; Richmond, 1994). Patients should be routinely screened about such off-work activities. Nonoccupational factors may in fact be the primary cause of a patient's symptoms. It is often the case, however, that comorbid conditions and ergonomic risks common to both at- and off-work activities act synergistically to cause a patient's MSD.

PSYCHOSOCIAL AND ORGANIZATIONAL ISSUES IN MSD DIAGNOSIS:

The Twentieth-Century MSD Debate

Although it is generally agreed that environmental, ergonomic, and personal factors combine to produce the MSDs, some physicians historically contested the notion that MSDs exist or could be at all work-related. One group of physicians asserted that MSDs are an iatrogenic disorder heavily influenced by personal issues (Hadler, 1989). Others contended that MSDs are related to the psychological stress of the work task rather than to the physical components of the work activity (Ireland, 1992). In these writings, the various nonoccupational risk factors known to be associated with MSDs are also typically emphasized, including endocrine disorders, pregnancy, obesity, and medical history. This was despite data indicating that MSD prevalence is low in populations not exposed to repetitive tasks (Battevi, Menoni, & Vimercati, 1998). Somewhat paradoxically, few of these authors seemed to contest the existence of MSDs originating from ergonomic or biomechanical risk factors in off-work activities, such as sports or hobbies. However, the opinion of expert scientific consensus bodies (National Research Council, 1998) supports the concept of work-related MSDs, as does the general body of the scientific literature relating to employed persons (Bernard, 1997; Malchaire, Cook, & Vergracht, 2001).

In this twentieth-century debate on MSD work-relatedness, the major focus of both supporters and critics was on the analysis of MSD cases reported through the workers' compensation insurance system and on into regulatory surveillance systems. For purposes of debate, this group of reported cases was generally considered to represent the entire universe of MSD cases. In the debate, advocates of an MSD-workplace association focused principally on proving the validity of the set of cases as MSDs, whereas detractors generally asserted the contrary, seeking either to negate or minimize the scope of the overall MSD problem. Among detractors, employee abuse of the workers' compensation system (a "moral hazard" risk) and employee psychological disorders were prominent explanations for widespread MSD prevalence.

During this time, however, industry-based field studies and other reports routinely demonstrated the existence of large numbers of workers with MSDs and other work injuries (even including occupational fatalities) who had never reported their condition to their employers, to regulators, or to workers' compensation insurers (Biddle, Roberts, Roseman, & Welch, 1998; Chaffin, 1979; Hensler et al., 1991; Rossignol, 1994; Silverstein, Stetson, Keyserling, & Fine, 1997; Yassi, Sprout, & Tate, 1996). More recent population-based studies both confirm this phenomenon and provide a more comprehensive assessment. It is evident from this body of work that the prevalence of workplace injuries, including MSDs, is far larger than that ever reported to existing workers' compensation systems by at least an order of magnitude in some studies (Morse, Dillon, Warren, Hall, & Hovey, 2001; Pransky, Snyder, Dembe, & Himmelstein, 1999; Rosenmann et al., 2000). It is a particularly telling point that the great majority of workers with MSDs (but also other work-related injuries) seek their medical treatment privately, never inform their employers, and do not file workers' compensation claims. Substantial numbers of these workers lose time from work or change jobs because of their injuries. From this, it seems clear that the bulk of MSD patients have no particular wish to enter, much less take advantage of, the workers' compensation insurance system. It would be difficult to label this group of employees as psychiatric cases or malingerers. The overall scope of the MSD problem, therefore, is far larger than originally defined. This phenomenon has implications for the MSD patients who may bear the costs of medical treatment on their own. It also has important economic implications for employers—for example, the major medical cost shifting from workers' compensation to private sector insurers, loss of productivity, production quality problems, and significant rates of "unexplained" turnover of experienced, trained workers (Dillon, 2001).

Psychological, Socioeconomic, and Work Organizational Factors and MSD Diagnosis

Psychiatric disorders present themselves in all medical patient populations, and an MSD confers no special immunity to these types of problems. There are no population-based studies that suggest that psychiatric disorders are more prevalent in patients with MSD symptomatology than in other medical patient groups (e.g., general practice medicine). In all types of medical practices it is known that somatization disorder and related but much less common disorders (somatoform pain disorder and conversion disorder) are more commonly found than in the general population (Barsky & Borus, 1995; Forman, Palmeri, & Menza, 1993; McCahill, 1995). Practitioners should learn the criteria for these disorders and screen for them in their patient population, obtaining psychiatric consultation when a problem is suspected.

Multidisciplinary MSD evaluation centers routinely employ psychologists or psychological social workers as part of their evaluation team. This is for the purpose of screening for primary psychiatric disorders but also for evaluation and counseling regarding the patient's coping skills and support network. The possibility of development of a psychiatric disorder secondary to the MSD is also evaluated. Anxiety and depression disorders, for example, can occur as secondary complications of a protracted Stage 2 or 3 MSD case and significantly interfere with attempts at therapy if left untreated. Secondary psychiatric disability is particularly common in the situation where medical treatment is interrupted, delayed, or denied by insurers, and it often has long-lasting implications.

Socioeconomic factors such as higher educational attainment, income, and the degree of family and work supervisor support can powerfully affect MSD outcomes and the likelihood of disability. This is not substantially different from experience with the general range of medical disorders, such as chronic arthritis, heart disease, or cancer, where socioeconomic disparities in the general population explain much of the variance in morbidity and in treatment success rates. In the MSD literature, there has been a feeling that a high rate of treatment failures brings into question the accuracy or legitimacy of MSD diagnosis. The reevaluation of diagnosis is in fact a mandatory first step in the setting of treatment failure. For MSDs, however, treatment failures most often reflect the lack of control of factors external to the medical encounter. Examples are failure to identify or control pertinent workplace ergonomic risks; interruption of treatment; insurance factors; problems with communication of treatment plans to patient's employers, insurers, and rehabilitation facilities; or problems with patient compliance with the treatment regimen.

SUMMARY

MSDs represent a unique group of syndromes. It is important, however, to understand that despite the role of external workplace and ergonomic influences, the problems inherent in MSD diagnosis and management are not intrinsically different from those encountered in other musculoskeletal conditions or, in fact, for the general range of medical disorders. The development of diagnostic criteria, valid case definitions, and effective treatment protocols has generally proved to be a formidable task in all areas of modern medicine. For work-related MSDs these issues clearly need to be more formally addressed by continuing scientific research on consensus standards.

REFERENCES

Armstrong, T. J. (1990). Ergonomics and cumulative trauma disorders of the hand and wrist. In J. M. Hunter, L. H. Schneider, E. J. Mackin, & A. D. Callahan (Eds.), *Rehabilitation and surgery of the hand* (3rd ed.). St. Louis: Mosby.

Armstrong, T. J. (1991, December). *Cumulative trauma work place factors.* Presented at the Occupational

Orthopedics Meeting. New York: American Academy of Orthopedic Surgeons.

Armstrong, T. J., Buckle, P., Fine, L. J., Hagberg, M., Jonsson, B., Kilbom, A. et al. (1993). A conceptual model for work-related neck and upper-limb musculoskeletal disorders. *Scandinavian Journal of Work, Environment and Health, 19,* 73-84.

Baron S., Hales T., & Hurrell J. (1996). Evaluation of symptom surveys for occupational musculoskeletal disorders. *American Journal of Industrial Medicine, 2*(6), 609-617.

Barsky, A. J., & Borus, J. F. (1995). Somatization and medicalization in the era of managed care. *JAMA, 274,* 1931-1934.

Barthel, H. R., Miller, L. S., Deardorff, W. W., & Portenier, R. (1998). Presentation and response of patients with upper extremity repetitive use syndrome to a multidisciplinary rehabilitation program: A retrospective review of 24 cases. *Journal of Hand Therapy, 11,* 191-199.

Battevi, N., Menoni, O., & Vimercati, C. (1998). The occurrence of musculoskeletal alterations in worker populations not exposed to repetitive tasks of the upper limbs. *Ergonomics, 41,* 1340-1346.

Bernard, B.P. (1997) Musculoskeletal disorders and workplace factors: a critical review of epidemiologic evidence for work-related musculoskeletal disorders of the neck, upper extremity and low back. U.S. Department of Health and Human Services (DHHS) Publication No. 97-141. Center for Disease Control and Prevention, National Institute for Occupational Safety and Health, Cincinnati, OH.

Biddle, J., Roberts, K., Roseman, D., & Welch, E. (1998). What percentage of workers with work-related illnesses receive workers' compensation benefits. *Journal of Occupational Medicine, 40,* 325-331.

Brazier, J. E., Harper, R., Jones, N. M. O'Cathain, A., Thomas, K. J., Usherwood, T. et al. (1992). Validating the SF-36 health survey questionnaire: New outcome measure for primary care. *British Medical Journal, 305*(6846), 160-164.

Butler, D. S., & Jones, M. A. (1991). *Mobilization of the nervous system*. London: Churchill-Livingstone.

Chaffin, D. B. (1979). Manual materials handling, the cause of overexertion illness and injury in industry. *Journal of Environmental Pathology and Toxicology, 2,* 67-73.

Chatterjee, D. S. (1987). Repetition strain injury—a recent review. *Journal of the Society of Occupational Medicine, 37,* 100-105.

Colombini, D., Occhipinti, E., Delleman, N., Fallentin, N., Kilbom, A., & Grieco, A. (2001). Exposure assessment of upper limb repetitive movements: A consensus document developed by the Technical Committee on Musculoskeletal Disorders of International Ergonomics Association (IEA) endorsed by International Commission on Occupational Health (ICOH). *Giornale Italiano di Medicina de Lavoro ed Ergonomia, 23,* 129-142.

Dillon, C. F. (2001). Management perspectives for workplace ergonomics. In W. Karwowski (Ed.), *International encyclopaedia of ergonomics and human factors* (pp. 1694-1698). New York: Taylor and Francis.

Dobyns, J. H. (1987). Role of the physician in worker's compensation injuries. *Journal of Hand Surgery 12,* 826-829.

Dobyns, J. H. (1991). Cumulative trauma disorder of the upper limb. *Hand Clinics, 7,* 587-595.

Forde, M. S., Punnett, L., & Wegman, D. H. (2002). Pathomechanisms of work-related musculoskeletal disorders: conceptual issues. *Ergonomics, 45*(9), 619-630.

Forman, N., Palmeri, B.A., & Menza, M.A. (1993). Somatoform disorders: Diagnosis and treatment. *New Jersey Medicine, 90,* 119-122.

Hadler, N. M. (1989). Work-related disorders of the upper extremity: I. Cumulative trauma disorders—a critical review. *Occupational Problems in Medical Practice, 4,* 1-8.

Harrington, J. M., Carter, J.T., Birrell, L., & Gompertz, D. (1998). Surveillance case definitions for work related upper limb syndromes. *Occupational and Environmental Medicine, 55,* 264-271.

Harris, J. S. (Ed.). (1997). *Occupational medicine practice guidelines. Evaluation and management of common health problems and functional recovery in workers.* Beverly, MA: OEM Press.

Hensler, D. R., Marquis, M. S., Abrahamse, A. F., Berry, S. H., Ebener, P.A., Lewis, E. G. et al. (1991). *Compensation for accidental injuries in the United States*. Santa Monica, CA: RAND Corporation.

Herring, S.A., & Nilson, K. L. (1987). Introduction to overuse injuries. *Clinics in Sports Medicine, 6,* 225-239.

Himmelstein, J. S., Feuerstein, M., Stanek, E. J. III, Koyamatsu, K., Pransky, G. S., Morgan, W. et al. (1995). Work-related upper-extremity disorders and work disability: Clinical and psychosocial presentation. *Journal of Occupational and Environmental Medicine, 37,* 1278-1286.

Ireland, D. C. R. (1992). The Australian experience with cumulative trauma disorders. In L. H. Millender, D. H. Louis, & B. P. Simmons (Eds.), *Occupational disorders of the upper extremity*. London: Churchill Livingstone.

Jensen, M., & Karoly, P. (1992). Self-Report scales and procedures for assessing pain in adults. In D. C. Turk & R. Melzack (Eds.), *Handbook of pain assessment* (pp. 135-151). New York: The Guilford Press.

Katz, J.N., Larson, M. G., Fossel, A. H., & Liang, M. H. (1991). Validation of a surveillance case definition of carpal tunnel syndrome. *American Journal of Public Health, 81,* 189-193.

Keller, K., Corbett, J., & Nichols, D. (1998). Repetitive strain injury in computer keyboard users: Pathomechanics and treatment principles in individual and group intervention. *Journal of Hand Therapy, 11,* 9-26.

Kilbom, S., Armstrong, T., Buckle, P., Fine, L., Hagberg, M., Haring-Sweeney, M. et al. (1996). Musculoskeletal disorders: Work-related risk factors and prevention. *International Journal of Occupational and Environmental Health, 2,* 239-246.

Kvarnstrom, S. (1983). Occurrence of musculoskeletal disorders in a manufacturing industry with special attention to occupational shoulder disorders. *Scandinavian Journal of Rehabilitation Medicine, 8,* 1-61.

Maeda, K., Horiguchi, S., & Hosokawa, M. (1982). History of the studies on occupational cervicobrachial disorder in Japan and remaining problems. *Journal of Human Ergology, 11,* 17-29.

Malchaire, J., Cock, N. & Vergracht, S. (2001). Review of the factors associated with musculoskeletal problems in epidemiological studies. *International Archives of Occupational and Environmental Health, 74* (2), 79-90.

McCahill, M. E. (1995). Somatoform and related disorders: Delivery of diagnosis as first step. *American Family Physician, 52,* 193-204.

Melzack, R., & Katz, J. (1992). The McGill pain questionnaire: Appraisal and current status. In D. Turk & R. Melzack (Eds.), *Handbook of pain assessment* (pp. 152-168). New York: The Guilford Press.

Metz, J. P. (1999). Managing golf injuries. *Physician and Sportsmedicine, 27,* 41-56.

Millender, L. H. (1992). Occupational disorders of the upper extremity: Orthopedic, psychosocial and legal implications. In L. H. Millender, D. H. Louis, & B. P. Simmons (Eds.), *Occupational disorders of the upper extremity*. London: Churchill Livingstone.

Moore, J. S. (1994, December). *The epidemiological context of upper extremity disorders associated with work.* Presented at the International Conference on Occupational Disorders of the Upper Extremities, University of California Center for Occupational and Environmental Health and University of Michigan Center for Occupational Health and Safety Engineering, San Francisco, CA.

Morse, T., Dillon, C., Warren, N., Hall, C., & Hovey, D. (2001). Capture-recapture estimation of unreported work-related musculoskeletal disorders in Connecticut. *American Journal of Industrial Medicine, 39,* 636-642.

Muggleton, J. M., Allen, R., & Chappell, P. H. (1999). Hand and arm injuries associated with repetitive manual work in industry: a review of disorders, risk factors and preventive measures. *Ergonomics, 42,* 714-739.

National Research Council. (1998). *Work-related musculoskeletal disorders: A review of the evidence*. Washington DC: National Academy Press.

Novak, C. B., & MacKinnon, S.E. (1997). Repetitive use and static postures: A source of nerve compression and pain. *Journal of Hand Therapy, 10,* 151-159.

Novak C. B., MacKinnon S. E. (2002). Multilevel nerve compression and muscle imbalance in work-related neuromuscular disorders. *American Journal of Industrial Medicine, 41*(5), 343-352.

OSHA—Occupational Safety and Health Administration, U.S. Department of Labor (1990). *Ergonomic program management guidelines for meatpacking plants*. Washington, DC: U.S. Department of Labor/OSHA 3123.

Palmer K., Smith G., Kellingray S. & Cooper C. (1999). Repeatability and validity of an upper limb and neck discomfort questionnaire: the utility of the standardized Nordic questionnaire. *Occupational Medicine (Oxford, England), 49*(3), 171-175.

Pascarelli, E. F., & Hsu, Y. P. (2001). Understanding work-related upper extremity disorders: Clinical findings in 485 computer users, musicians, and others. *Journal of Occupational Rehabilitation, 11,* 1-21.

NIOSH (National Institute for Occupational Safety & Health). (1997). *Elements of ergonomic programs a primer based on evaluations of musculoskeletal disorders*. DHHS (NIOSH) Publication No. 97-117.

Piligian, G., Herbert, R., Hearns, M., Dropkin, J., Landsbergis, P., & Cherniack, M. (2000). Evaluation and management of chronic work-related musculoskeletal disorders of the distal upper extremity. *American Journal of Industrial Medicine, 37,* 75-93.

Pransky, G., Snyder, T., Dembe, A., & Himmelstein, J. (1999). Under-reporting of work-related disorders in the workplace: A case study and review of the literature. *Ergonomics, 42,* 171-182.

Putz-Anderson, V. (1988). *Cumulative trauma disorders: A manual for musculoskeletal diseases of the upper limbs*. Philadelphia: Taylor & Francis.

Ranney, D., Wells, R., & Moore, A. (1995). Upper limb musculoskeletal disorders in highly repetitive industries: precise anatomical findings. *Ergonomics, 38,* 1408-1423.

Rempel, D., Evanoff, B., Amadio, P. C., deKrom, M., et al. (1998). Consensus criteria for the classification of carpal tunnel syndrome in epidemiologic studies. *American Journal of Public Health, 88*(10), 1447-1450.

Richmond, D. R. (1994). Handlebar problems in bicycling. *Clinics in Sports Medicine, 13,* 165-173.

Rosenmann, K. D., Gardiner, J. C., Wang, J., Biddle, J., Hogan, A., & Reilly, M. J. (2000). Why most workers with occupational repetitive trauma do not file for workers' compensation. *Journal of Occupational and Environmental Medicine, 42,* 25-34.

Rossignol, M. (1994). Completeness of provincial workers' compensation files to identify fatal occupational injuries. *Canadian Journal of Public Health, 85,* 244-247.

Salerno, D. F., Copley-Merriman, C., Taylor, T. N., Shinogle, J., & Schulz, R. M. (2002). A review of functional status measures for workers with upper extremity disorders. *Occupational and Environmental Medicine, 59*(10), 664-670.

Silverstein, B.A., Fine, L., & Armstrong, T. J. (1986). Hand-wrist cumulative trauma disorders in industry. *British Journal of Industrial Medicine, 43*(11), 779-784.

Silverstein, B.A., Fine, L., & Stetson, D. (1987). Hand-wrist disorders among investment casting plant workers. *Journal of Hand Surgery, 12,* 838-844.

Silverstein, B.A., Stetson, D. S., Keyserling, W. M., & Fine, L. J. (1997). Work-related musculoskeletal disorders: comparison of data sources for surveillance. *American Journal of Industrial Medicine, 31,* 600-608.

Sjogaard, G., & Sjogaard, K. (1998). Muscle injury in repetitive motion disorders. *Clinical Orthopaedics and Related Research, 351,* 21-31.

Simons, D. G., Travell, J. G., & Simons, L. S. (1998). *Travell & Simons' myofascial pain and dysfunction: The trigger point manual* (2nd ed.). Baltimore: Williams & Wilkins.

Stiens, S.A., Haselkorn, J. K., Peters, D. J., & Goldstein, B. (1996). Rehabilitation intervention for patients with upper extremity dysfunction: Challenges of outcome evaluation. *American Journal of Industrial Medicine, 29,* 590-601.

Tanaka, S., & McGlothlin, J. D. (1993). A conceptual model for prevention of work-related carpal tunnel syndrome (CTS). *International Journal of Industrial Ergonomics, 11,* 181-193.

Tong, H. C., Haig, A. J., Theisen, M. E., Smith, C., & Miller, Q. (2001). Multidisciplinary team evaluation of upper extremity injuries in a single visit: The UPPER Program. *Occupational Medicine (Oxford, England), 51,* 278-286.

University of Michigan Department of Environmental & Industrial Health. (1984). *Evaluation of upper extremity & low back cumulative trauma disorders: A screening manual.* Ann Arbor: School of Public Health.

Von Korf, M. (1992). Epidemiological and survey methods: Chronic pain assessment. In D. C. Turk & R. Melzack (Eds.), *Handbook of pain assessment* (pp. 391-408). New York: The Guilford Press.

Waris, P., Kuorinka, I., Kurppa, K., Luopajarvi, T., Pesonen, K., Nummi, J., et al. (1979). Epidemiologic screening of occupational neck and upper limb disorders. Methods and criteria. *Scandinavian Journal of Work, Environmental and Health, 5*(suppl 3), 25-38.

Yassi, A., Sprout, J., & Tate, R. (1996). Upper limb repetitive strain injuries in Manitoba. *American Journal of Industrial Medicine, 30,* 461-472.

CHAPTER 4

MSD: The Regulatory Perspective

Tim Morse

In a profit-driven economy managers are under continuous pressure to deliver goods in a predetermined time, of sufficient quality, at the lowest cost. Health and safety regulations are sometimes viewed by employers as a hindrance to these goals for the following reasons: They appear to create obstacles to getting the job done in the shortest amount of time (i.e., guards on machines, rest breaks, fall protection), they are sometimes inflexible or not seen to be applicable to particular industries or jobs, they create paperwork and recording burdens, and they create anxiety that regulators may walk into the workplace and fine them for regulations that they do not understand (Dorman, 1996; McCaffrey, 1982; Noble, 1986). Processes to prevent musculoskeletal disorders (MSDs) can be viewed as part of the health and safety regulatory process. MSDs are complex because they occur over time and can be caused by multiple factors and not just work. Employers sometimes feel that they have to pay workers' compensation for conditions that are not caused by work.

How should employers respond to the problem of MSDs? The answer requires understanding the magnitude of the problem (both in terms of human costs and economic costs), the indirect impacts on employers, union or worker pressures, other benefits (e.g., productivity) from ergonomic programs, and regulatory imperatives (including Occupational Safety and Health Administration [OSHA], Americans with Disabilities Act [ADA], and workers' compensation). Once they understand these issues, many employers embrace ergonomic programs as profitable programs that improve worker productivity as well as worker health, and that not only meet but exceed regulatory requirements.

This chapter covers the magnitude of the problem of MSD, the social and economic impact of MSD, how employers can use data to estimate their incidence in relation to other companies, how to estimate costs of MSD in a company, and an overview of the regulatory environment, including OSHA, workers' compensation, ADA, and voluntary standards.

MAGNITUDE OF THE PROBLEM

Injury and Illness Statistics

OSHA tracks both acute traumatic injuries and more chronic illnesses, although MSD tends to fall somewhere in the middle with some acute conditions, such as strains and sprains, and some more chronic conditions, such as carpal tunnel syndrome and tendinitis. This chapter will focus on cumulative, chronic conditions, except where noted.

OSHA requires a record of new injury and illness cases that are work-related (work caused or contributed to the condition or significantly aggravated a preexisting condition). OSHA surveys those conditions each year to produce an estimate of the magnitude of the problem.

The primary MSD category is for conditions associated with "repeated trauma," which include "noise-induced hearing loss, tenosynovitis, bursitis, Raynaud's phenomena, and other conditions due to repeated motion, vibration, or pressure" (Bureau of Labor Statistics, 1986). This category includes most of the upper-extremity conditions (and some lower-extremity) that are not due to acute events such as strains and sprains. OSHA also breaks out tendinitis and carpal tunnel syndrome specifically in their data.

In 2000, OSHA reported 241,800 illnesses associated with "repeated trauma" for the United States, with 69% in the manufacturing sector

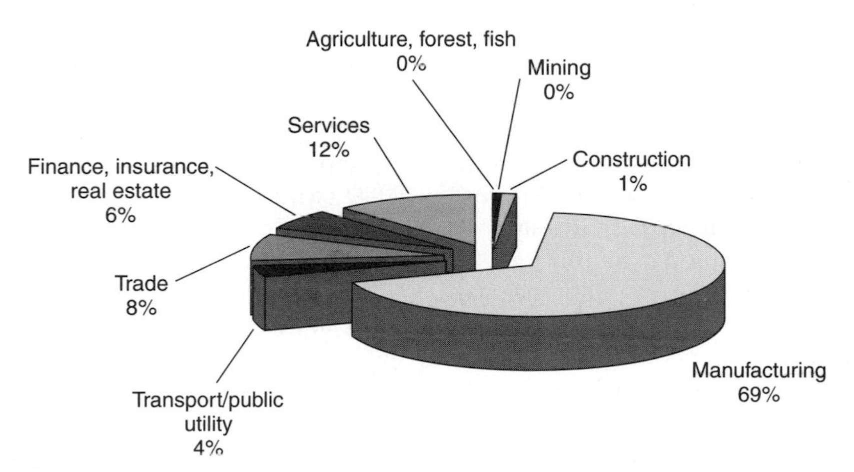

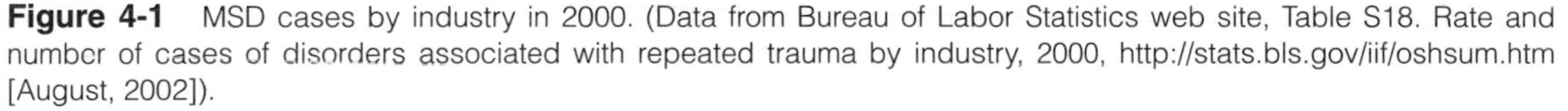
Figure 4-1 MSD cases by industry in 2000. (Data from Bureau of Labor Statistics web site, Table S18. Rate and number of cases of disorders associated with repeated trauma by industry, 2000, http://stats.bls.gov/iif/oshsum.htm [August, 2002]).

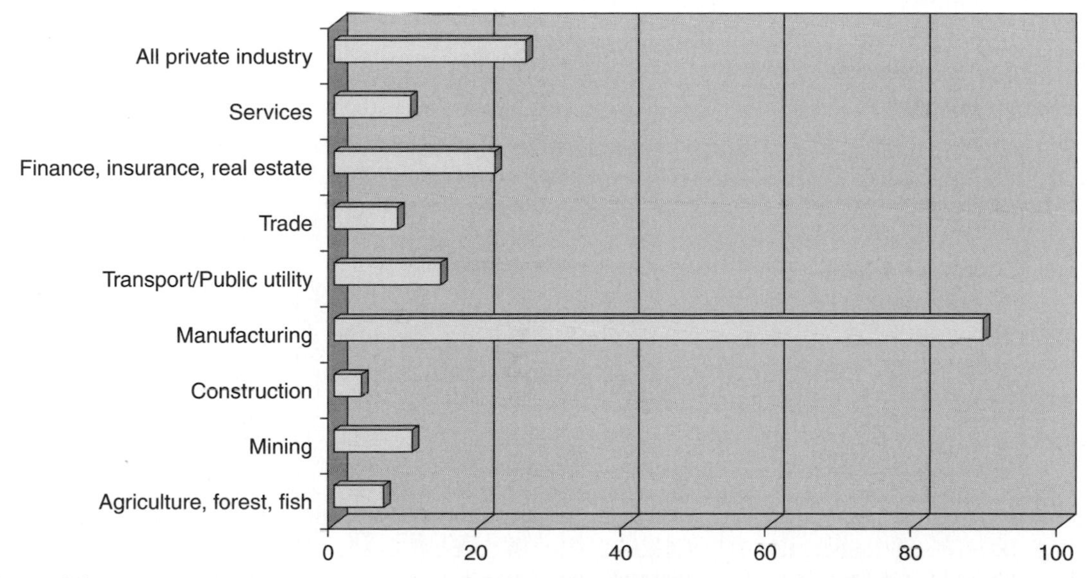

Figure 4-2 Rate of repetitive trauma by industry in 2000. (Data from Bureau of Labor Statistics web site, Table S14. Rate and number of cases of disorders associated with repeated trauma by industry, 2000, http://stats.bls.gov/iif/oshsum.htm [August, 2002]).

(Figure 4-1), which also has by far the highest rate (Figure 4-2) (Bureau of Labor Statistics, 2002). The rate had been declining slightly over the previous 5 years, dropping from 33.5 per 10,000 workers in 1996 to 26.3 in 2000 (and continuing to drop to 23.8 in 2001), after steep increases in the late 1980s to the 1990s (Figure 4-3).

Food products and manufacturing generally had the highest rates, led by meatpacking plants (with a stunning 812 cases per 10,000 workers), motor vehicle manufacturing (727), poultry processing (374), automotive trim (329), and textiles (286) (Table 4-1). The industries with the highest *number* of cases are a little different, since that depends both on the rates and the number of people employed in the industry (Table 4-2). These are led by auto manufacturing, meat products, hospitals, aircraft manufacturing, grocery stores, plastic manufacturing, metal forgings, telephone communications, textile products, and doctors' offices.

OSHA reported just under 30,000 carpal tunnel syndrome cases that involved lost time from work (1.7% of all lost-time cases). They also received reports on approximately 15,000 cases of tendinitis, 1000 cases of tenosynovitis, and 30,000 cases of other musculoskeletal disorders that involved lost time.

MSD cases tend to be very costly, largely because of extensive lost time. While the overall average (median) for lost time cases was 6 days, tendinitis and other musculoskeletal disorders averaged a median of 10 to 11 days away from work, and carpal tunnel syndrome averaged 27 days. Cases caused by repetitive motion averaged 19 days of lost time.

Women comprise approximately 33% of all lost-time cases (and work about 41% of the hours), but comprise 63.9% of repetitive trauma cases.

The preceding figures are for MSD caused by repetitive trauma. The broader category of MSD (which can also benefit from ergonomics programs) also includes acute cases. OSHA reported 577,814 MSD cases overall, of which 77% are strains, sprains, and tears; 5.5% are back pain; and 4.7% are hernias (Figure 4-4).

Underreporting of MSDs

Studies indicate that these *reported* MSDs are only a subset of work-related MSDs. Several studies have shown that there is extensive underreporting, with estimates of only 10% to 25% of cases being reported to the Bureau of Labor Statistics (BLS) or workers' compensation (Morse, Dillon, Warren, Hall, & Hovey, 2001; Morse, Dillon, Warren, Levenstein, & Warren,

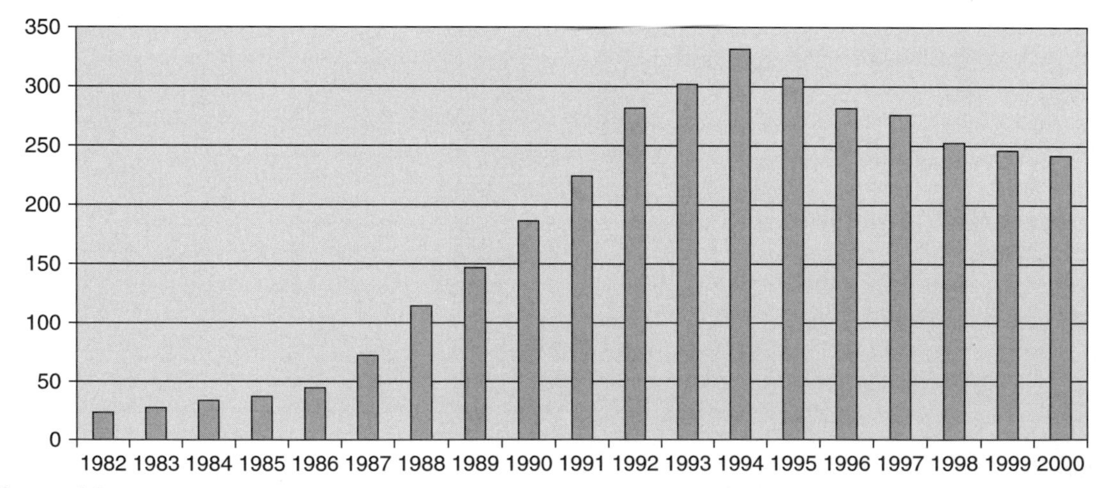

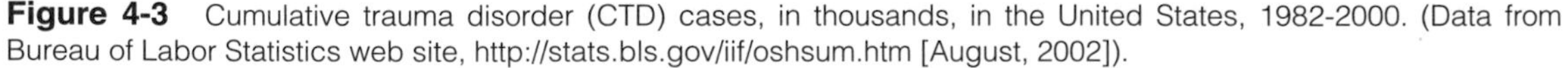
Figure 4-3 Cumulative trauma disorder (CTD) cases, in thousands, in the United States, 1982-2000. (Data from Bureau of Labor Statistics web site, http://stats.bls.gov/iif/oshsum.htm [August, 2002]).

Table 4-1
Industries with Highest Cumulative Trauma Rates, U.S., OSHA, 2000

Industry	SIC	Employment	Rate	Number
Meat packing plants	2011	148.1	812.0	12.6
Motor vehicles and car bodies	3711	353.5	726.9	25.7
Poultry slaughtering and processing	2015	253.2	374.0	9.5
Automotive and apparel trimmings	2396	62.8	328.7	2.0
Fabricated textile products, n.e.c.	2399	30.0	286.0	0.8
Sausages and other prepared meats	2013	103.8	274.2	3.0
Public building and related furniture	253	53.7	273.7	1.5
Engine electrical equipment	3694	67.4	258.2	1.8
Men's footwear, except athletic	3143	16.0	256.7	0.4
Automotive stampings	3465	122.6	240.9	3.1
Dental equipment and supplies	3843	15.7	232.1	0.4
Men's and boys' trousers and slacks	2325	39.7	224.8	0.8
Motor vehicle parts and accessories	3714	549.7	221.1	12.5
Leather tanning and finishing	311	10.9	199.2	0.2
Aircraft	3721	233.8	187.8	4.4
Pens and mechanical pencils	3951	8.3	179.4	0.1
Motor homes	3716	21.9	179.0	0.4
Dolls and stuffed toys	3942	4.7	178.8	0.1
Household appliances, n.e.c.	3639	12.9	170.8	0.2
Commercial lighting fixtures	3646	28.6	169.8	0.5
Household vacuum cleaners	3635	11.9	169.4	0.2
Men's and boys' work clothing	2326	25.5	169.3	0.4
Household refrigerators and freezers	3632	28.6	160.8	0.5
Ship building and repairing	3731	97.1	154.7	1.5
Hosiery, n.e.c.	2252	34.3	149.0	0.5
All private industry		**110,064.9**	**26.3**	**241.8**

Rates per 10,000 workers; employment and number of cases in thousands.
Data from OSHA http://stats.bls.gov/iif/oshwc/osh/os/ostb0997.txt, accessed 6/24/02

1998). Cases are more likely to be reported if they are more serious (such as requiring surgery), diagnosed by a physician, or if they involve a unionized workplace (Morse, Punnett, Warren, Dillon, & Warren, 2003). Liss, Armstrong, Kusiak, and Gailitis (1992) and Katz et al. (1998) estimate unreported carpal tunnel cases at 1.5 to 10 times those reported through workers' compensation systems. Maizlish, Rudolph, Dervin, and Sankaranarayan (1995) performed a county-level study of work-related carpal tunnel cases in California and found carpal tunnel cases to be underreported by a factor of 5.8. Silverstein, Stetson, Keyserling, and Fine (1997) found substantial underreporting of MSD based on comparisons of health surveillance interview and physical examination compared to reporting on OSHA 200 logs.

Yassi, Sprout, and Tate (1996) found that workers' compensation cases in Manitoba for upper-extremity MSD lost more time from work than a control group of other (acute) upper-limb musculoskeletal injuries (71.4 days for MSD versus 33.6 days for controls), cost more ($5569 versus $2480), and were less likely to be able to return to the same job (67.3% versus 81%). Additionally, they found that although 13% of MSD cases returned to modified work with the same employer, a larger percentage of cases than controls were unable to return to any type of

Table 4-2
Industries with the highest number of MSD cases, U.S., OSHA, 1999–2000

Industry	SIC code	2000 annual average employment (000)	Number (000)	
			1999	2000
Motor vehicles and equipment	371	1,016.5	39.3	39.3
Meat products	201	505.1	25.5	25.2
Hospitals	806	3,958.2	6.7	8.2
Aircraft and parts	372	463.1	7.3	6.0
Grocery stores	541	3,069.2	4.1	5.4
Miscellaneous plastics products, n.e.c.	308	744.9	3.9	4.7
Metal forgings and stampings	346	254.9	4.1	3.9
Telephone communications	481	1,155.3	4.1	3.6
Miscellaneous fabricated textile products	239	214.3	2.6	3.5
Offices and clinics of medical doctors	801	1,936.9	3.6	3.3

Data from OSHA: http://stats.bls.gov/news.release/osh.t04.htm

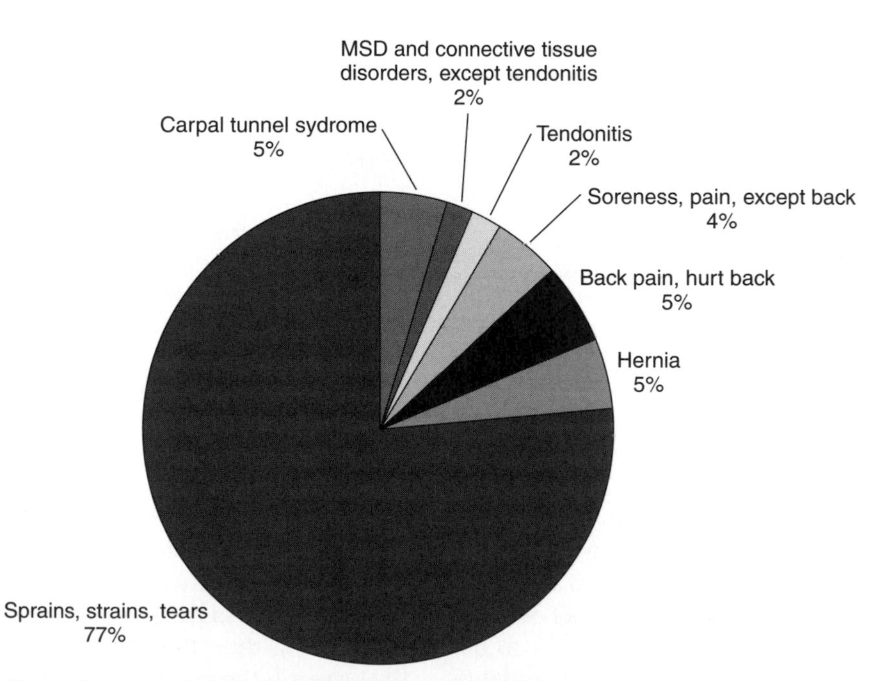

Figure 4-4 Types of musculoskeletal disorders with days away from work, acute and cumulative in the United States in 2000. (Data from Bureau of Labor Statistics web site, Charts, Musculoskeletal disorders by selected worker and case characteristics, 2000, http://stats.bls.gov/iif/oshcdnew.htm [August, 2002]).

work at all (2.9% versus 0.5%). MSD cases were also more likely to recur on return to work (18.9% versus 9.6%).

HOW TO USE INJURY DATA

How would an employer or worker understand whether his or her workplace is higher or lower than average, or be able to track whether rates are getting better or worse? Although the answer has some complications based on the underreporting issue, there are some fairly easy ways to approach these questions.

The first step is to understand the data that are available. This is typically in two forms: the OSHA injury and illness log and workers' compensation data. Definitions for the two differ somewhat, but there is extensive overlap.

The OSHA record-keeping system is now built around the OSHA 300 form, which went into effect in 2002 (updating the OSHA 200 Form) (OSHA, 2001). Most employers need to maintain this form and post a summary for the month of February. Employers with fewer than 10 employees and most companies in retail, service, finance, insurance, and real estate industries are exempt from the record keeping (although *not* from other OSHA regulations), unless they are asked to participate in the OSHA annual survey.

All new work-related cases (where work caused or contributed to the illness or significantly aggravated a preexisting condition) must be recorded. New cases include those in which the condition existed previously but the person had fully recovered. There are specific instructions in the OSHA standard (1904.12) for MSD, which are similar to the general reporting requirements, although they are under review as of this writing. Cases must be recorded if they result in days away from work, or restricted work or transfer to another job, or medical treatment beyond first aid. Restricted work, which often occurs with MSD, includes keeping the worker "from performing one or more of the routine functions of his or her job, or from working the full workday that he or she would otherwise have been scheduled to work" (Section 1904.7(b)(4)). Routine functions are those that the employee regularly performs at least once per week. This definition includes a physician recommendation for those restrictions even if the person actually works his or her usual job. These definitions apply the same for diagnosed conditions such as carpal tunnel syndrome and for symptoms such as pain, tingling, or burning.

Injury and illness records can be useful both in reviewing actual *numbers* of cases as well as *rates* per 100 (or 10,000) workers. The actual numbers are used as an indicator of the overall magnitude of the problem. These will indicate the areas or jobs that are causing the most problems overall, but they are often driven by the number of people that are employed in those areas or jobs. So, for example, a manufacturing company that also includes a very large office workforce may find that people working on computers account for the greatest number of MSDs—say, accounting for 10 cases out of 200 office workers. However, it may turn out that certain manufacturing jobs (such as a small assembly operation) have a much higher *rate* of MSDs—say, 5 cases out of 20 assembly workers (25%, or 2500 per 10,000 workers) compared to 5% or 500 per 10,000 workers in the office area. Areas with the highest rates tend to offer opportunities for interventions with the biggest "bang for the buck," since investigations and interventions can be much more concentrated.

The OSHA 300 log can be compared to overall averages and to specific Standard Industrial Classification (SIC) subcategories (such as nursing homes or engine manufacturing) through the OSHA web site at www.osha.gov (the OSHA standards may also be found there, such as the record-keeping standard mentioned previously, as well as related interpretations of the standards). The averages may be found in the statistics section of the web site under "BLS Industry Injury and Illness Data" for the current year, and then "Illnesses by Type/Incidence

Rates by Detailed Industry." The industry type is located by SIC code (there is also an SIC look-up table on the web site if help is needed).

For an employer to accurately compare the rates from his or her company, the employer needs to use the same definitions as OSHA. OSHA standardizes its rates based on 200,000 hours worked per one worker per year. To standardize rates, an employer would add up the hours worked for all the employees at the company in the entire year and divide by 200,000 to get the full-time equivalent (FTE) number of workers. The employer would then divide the number of MSDs by the number of FTEs, then multiply by 100 to get a percent or by 10,000 to get a rate per 10,000. This number can then be compared to the OSHA averages for all employers or for a specific industry.

Workers' compensation records can also be used for comparisons, although typically this must be done through the insurer because national data (or even state data in most cases) are not available for comparison. One advantage of workers' compensation data is that cost data can typically be obtained from the insurer, which can give at least the direct compensated costs combined with reserves for future anticipated costs (see following). Definitions of compensable MSD vary from state to state, and it may be difficult to obtain compensation when a short time is allowed for filing a claim after an exposure or other legal obstacles. States also have different waiting periods for lost-time compensation, and insurers have somewhat different approaches to accepting or contesting MSD cases. These all make comparisons more difficult, but they can still be useful to get general comparisons and to help understand overall costs. Workers' compensation reports can also include medical-only claims as well as lost-time cases.

Early reporting systems have been used very effectively by many large employers, such as an award-winning program developed by Travelers Insurance Company (for their own employees) and the ErgoCenter at UConn Health Center that decreased surgery rates by over 90% and greatly decreased compensation costs (*CTDNews*, 1997). The programs are designed to encourage workers to report the earliest signs and symptoms of MSD. Once a report is made, the worker is given conservative medical treatment (usually inexpensive and effective, since symptoms are much more easily treated in early stages) combined with an ergonomic evaluation and intervention of the workstation. These typically result in no or very little lost or restricted time because both the symptoms and causes are simultaneously remedied. However, such systems will cause a very noticeable spike in reported cases in the first year or so, although the severity and costs for the cases will tend to be very low, and reports will tend to drop dramatically the next year. The U.S. Veterans Health Administration has used a metric of at least a 5:1 ratio of reported to lost time claims as an indicator that its early reporting and ergonomic intervention system is successful.

Many of the "safety bingo" approaches popular among employers, which use incentives such as prizes or free donuts as a reward for low or no reported injuries or illnesses, are at odds with such an early reporting system, since they create powerful incentives among both supervisors and coworkers to avoid reporting until after the month (or longer) is over. This can result in cases not being reported to the employer until they are far advanced, frequently resulting in extensive lost time and medical costs (including surgery or extensive physical and occupational therapy).

ECONOMIC AND SOCIAL ASPECTS OF MSDs

The most important reason for prevention of MSD is the humanitarian one—MSDs are preventable conditions that can have dramatic consequences on workers. The loss of use of the hands and arms can have a profound effect on almost every aspect of life: work, child care, home maintenance, hobbies such as playing a musical instrument, sewing, crafts, or sports.

The Connecticut Upper-Extremity Surveillance Project (CUSP) study found an 8 to 35 times higher likelihood of problems in activities of daily living for those with MSD than for controls (Figure 4-5). Social impacts were also widespread (Table 4-3). MSD cases were half as likely to have been promoted in the previous 12 months (OR = 0.45), but were twice as likely to have been divorced (OR = 1.9) or to have moved for financial reasons (OR = 2.4) (Morse et al., 1998).

However, costs of MSD to employers are also an important issue in prevention, particularly because there is still a paucity of regulation on ergonomics. An appreciation of costs provides motivation to invest in ergonomics programs and can also assist in targeting specific interventions. Typically, there is a lot of overlap between the humanitarian incentive and the economic, since MSDs tend to be expensive. A Liberty Mutual study found a large difference between the *mean* cost of $8,070 and a *median* cost of $824 (that is, the cost of the individual in the middle if all the cases were arranged from lowest to highest cost) for upper-extremity MSD workers' compensation payouts (Webster & Snook, 1994). This difference underlines the concept that it is the few very expensive cases that drive the overall costs. The majority of cases are quite inexpensive to treat and to fix from an ergonomic standpoint, and it is therefore important to detect and treat cases early.

Table 4-3

Odds Ratios of Social Effects of MSD, with 95% Confidence Intervals, Cases vs. Controls, CUSP Study, CT, 1993

	Odds Ratio	Lower CI	Upper CI
Promoted	0.45	0.28	0.74
Stress at home	1.31	0.95	1.82
Divorce	1.91	1.01	3.58
Move for financial reasons	2.41	1.2	4.86
Lose home	3.44	1.14	10.35
Lose car	2.45	1.04	5.74
Lose health insurance	1.91	0.99	3.71

Data from Morse, T. F., Dillon, C., Warren, N., Levenstein, C., & Warren, A. (1998). The economic and social consequences of work-related musculoskeletal disorders: The Connecticut Upper-Extremity Surveillance Project (CUSP). *International Journal of Occupational and Environmental Health, 4*(4), 209–216.

In the CUSP study a high proportion of medical bills for MSD were paid from general health insurance: 71% of respondents said medical visits and procedures were paid for by general health insurance, 8% out-of-pocket, and

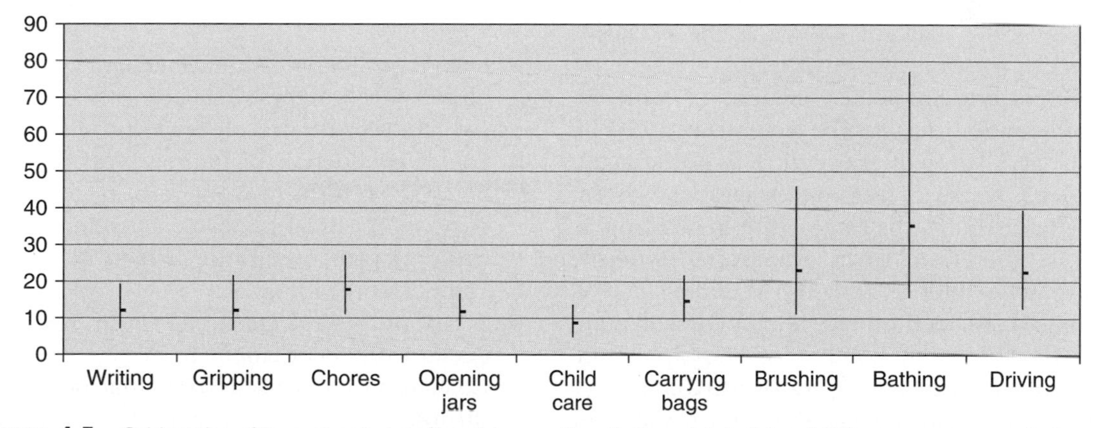

Figure 4-5 Odds ratios of "some" or "a lot of" problems with activities of daily living, MSD cases versus controls, with 95% confidence intervals, CUSP study, CT, 1993. (Data from Morse, T. F., Dillon, C., Warren, N., Levenstein, C., & Warren, A. [1998]. The economic and social consequences of work-related musculoskeletal disorders: The Connecticut Upper-Extremity Surveillance Project [CUSP]. *International Journal of Occupational and Environmental Health*, *4*[4], 209–216.)

only 21% from workers' compensation. In addition, 5.8% of MSD cases received benefits under sick time or disability, and 2.4% from unemployment, attributed to the condition. Out-of-pocket expenses were estimated at $489 per case per year, costing workers $15 million to $71 million in out-of-pocket expenses per year for Connecticut alone (Morse et al., 1998).

Compiled anecdotal evidence has found that employers who institute ergonomic programs dramatically save workers' compensation costs. A U.S. Government Accounting Office (GAO) study of five employers found reductions of 35% to 91% in workers' compensation costs for MSD, resulting from both reductions in numbers of new conditions (ranging from 2.4 to 6.1 percentage point reductions in rates), as well as better medical management and return to work programs (Government Accounting Office, 1997).

The most basic cost driver is workers' compensation. Workers' compensation provides for medical treatment, reimbursement of a proportion of lost-time costs (typically two-thirds of gross pay or 75% of net pay) while workers are out of work due to the injury or illness, and some benefits (different state-to-state) for permanent partial disability. In exchange for this benefit, workers are not allowed to sue their employers (in most situations in most states) for anything else, such as pain and suffering due to negligence, a concept known as the exclusive remedy provision (Boden, 2000).

Calculating the dollar amount of workers' compensation that can be potentially saved by employers through prevention is not straightforward because it is an insurance system designed to buffer the employer from catastrophic losses. Therefore, small employers (typically those with under $200,000 in annual payroll costs) are charged insurance premiums that are just based on the number of employees and the type of business, with no savings if they have an excellent safety record and no penalty for a terrible record (although they may have a harder time finding an insurer). Larger employers do have premium modifications ("mod factors"), based on their history of injuries and illnesses, that can range up to about 50% of the base premium costs and that are averaged over the previous 3 years. Therefore, if a large company with a 50% mod factor is able to reduce claims by $100,000 each year, they may see premiums go down by only $16,667 in the first year, $33,333 the second, and $50,000 in the third. In most states large companies are able to self-insure. These companies realize fairly immediately any cost saving from prevention programs, although they typically still will reinsure against very large claims and so will not have 100% recovery.

The direct cost for workers' compensation costs is not the only cost associated with occupational injuries and illnesses. There are a wide variety of indirect costs, typically estimated at 3 to 7 times the direct cost of claims (Andreoni, 1986; Oxenburgh, 1997; Punnett, 1999). These indirect costs include the following.

- Paperwork and human resources time associated with processing workers' compensation claims, physician notes, sick time, insurance, scheduling changes, OSHA forms, and so on
- New hires to replace injured workers
- Training of replacement worker for injured worker's job
- Less work by other workers because of injury event, discussion of event, supervision of new workers
- Lower production for replacement workers or for other workers having to work overtime (which has considerably lower productivity)
- Lower production of injured worker when he or she returns to work (light or restricted duty, more breaks, slower movements because of pain, medication effects from pain killers, or orthotics)
- Scrap or rework resulting from inexperienced workers or fatigue from overtime
- Costs of unrecognized MSDs that do not go through workers' compensation (general health insurance, sick time, early retirement)
- Lost wages not reimbursed (cost to workers, since they only receive 75% of net wages)

- Household production for disabled worker (mowing lawn, maintenance, child care)

There are several ways to estimate costs resulting from MSDs and therefore the potential savings from ergonomic interventions. These range from very basic, seat-of-the-pants estimates to get a rough idea of the costs to highly detailed economic analyses that factor in most of the employer-based costs noted previously that can be used to evaluate the impact of major investments.

The simplest approach would be to take the average cost of an MSD (for example, the $8,070 per case estimated by Liberty Mutual; the article includes a state breakdown; see Webster & Snook, 1994), multiply it by 5 to account for indirect costs (or roughly $40,000 per MSD case including direct and indirect costs), and multiply that by the number of MSDs in the company based on workers' compensation or OSHA log data. For small companies, it makes sense to get an average based on the past 5 years' experience to get a more stable number. Alternately, the insurer for the company may be able to provide the actual costs for MSD claims, which could be used for the base amount. The cost provided by the insurer will probably include both actual historic costs (what they actually paid out to the worker and for medical costs) as well as an estimate of future costs (reserves). When reviewing the numbers the employer should note that the costs for more recent claims will not typically be complete (for example, they may not include any payments for permanent partial disability if there are permanent effects from the MSD) and may therefore look considerably lower if they don't include reserves, or they may look higher if reserves are overestimated.

Another approach for more stable numbers for small employers would be to take the industry average of MSDs from the BLS statistics for the specific industry and multiply that by the average cost of an MSD. It should be recalled that the BLS numbers for repetitive trauma also include non-MSDs such as noise-induced hearing loss (although MSD dominates the category) and typically does not include the very numerous lower-extremity (i.e., back) conditions nor more acute musculoskeletal injuries, both of which may be significantly affected by ergonomic programs.

If costs were derived from the company's actual costs from workers' compensation or actual number of MSDs, then these can be compared to industry benchmarks derived from the BLS figures. Figures can also be broken down by job or area to provide a guide for setting priority areas for ergonomic analysis and intervention.

COST-BENEFIT ANALYSIS

Estimates of costs can be used to justify ergonomic interventions and programs. One basic principle of safety interventions is that the savings improve the bottom line directly; a $10,000 savings in payout for injuries is the same as an increase of $100,000 in sales if there is a 10% profit margin on sales.

Oxenburgh (1997) provides the most comprehensive approach to costing out MSD in relation to the costs of ergonomic interventions (cost-benefit) for individual companies. The model compares costs before an ergonomic intervention to costs after the intervention. The intervention can be either actual and done historically to document the savings of an intervention that was already made, or hypothetical to estimate potential saving from an intervention being considered. The latter is quite similar to the approach used by companies to estimate the potential impact of productivity improvements in order to get approval to implement changes.

The example Oxenburgh used was that of a factory that makes parts that need to be sanded very smooth. This operation was done by four people by hand, all day long, resulting in extensive hand problems both from the sanding done with the right hand as well as the gripping of the part done with the left hand. As workers became disabled, others had to pick up the work and started working extensive overtime, which led to even more hand problems. Because of worker fatigue, parts were not getting sanded sufficiently, which led to a lot of defective and rejected parts. The ergonomic intervention was to mount the part on an inexpensive potter's wheel that both held and spun the part so that there was much less strain on the hands. As a result, injury costs, overtime, and defective parts were greatly reduced, with a payback period for the intervention of only 0.9 years (about a month; see Table 4-4).

His model is based on productive hours worked per employee, which adjusts for vacations, illnesses, and so forth. This figure is then multiplied by wage costs, which include wages, fringe, and overhead costs, to derive an average wage cost per employee per productive hour. Overhead costs include insurance costs that could be adjusted for workers' compensation insurance savings (though Oxenburgh's example does not include this, since it would not get picked up until the next year). Turnover and training costs get entered in if there was extensive training needed for the job (such costs were minimal in the specific example). Next, overtime and lowered production is accounted for (productivity loss per employee per productive hour). Lowered production also accounts for losses caused by defects in parts that are rejected. Once all the factors are included, the differences in costs before and after the ergonomic intervention are compared to the cost of the intervention to get a payback period.

Table 4-4

Example of a Cost-benefit Summary Table for an Ergonomic Intervention. Example of a Small Workshop, Net Change in Costs

	Base Situation Year 1	After Changes (Potter's Wheel) Year 2
Group 1: Productive hours/employee/year	1670 hours	1840 hours
Group 2: Wage and salary costs	$21.83	$19.81
Group 3: Turnover and training costs	$0.00	$0.00
Group 4: Productivity losses	$7.40	$1.04
Cost/employee/productive hour	**$29.23**	**$20.85**

Although there was a high labor turnover, management considered that the training costs were small as the employees were unskilled. Administration costs were absorbed into other costs. For this reason and in this particular example the training and turnover costs have been ignored. Including them would give a faster payback period but, since the payback period was so rapid in any case, the error in omitting the turnover and training costs is, in practice, negligible. (Data from Oxenburgh, M. [1997]. Cost-benefit analysis of ergonomics programs. *American Industrial Hygiene Association Journal, 58,* 150–156.)

Ergonomics is in general an area where one can often advance a humanitarian goal at the same time as improving productivity and profits. In the example above, MSDs had a dramatic effect on workers' hand function as well as on the economics of the firm for which they worked. However, there will be situations where the cost of investment will be more than the return; these situations can be dealt with as pure humanitarian decisions in a workplace with a philosophy of "safety first" or absorbed by the cost savings achieved by other ergonomic interventions. The response to such challenges must also take into account the regulatory environment.

THE REGULATORY ENVIRONMENT

There currently are not extensive regulations regarding ergonomics, although there was one put in place by OSHA under the Clinton administration but subsequently revoked by Congress under the Bush administration. There are currently four primary aspects to regulation: other OSHA standards, state regulations, nonbinding private standards, and the ADA.

OSHA

OSHA proposed a standard in 1999 (which never went into effect) and then enacted a new comprehensive standard on ergonomics in late 2001. Although the standard had been in process for over 10 years and had gone through an extraordinarily extensive public hearing and comment process, it was revoked in the only instance of the use of the Congressional Review Act. This act allows Congress to revoke a standard shortly after enactment, without hearings or committee review, with a simple majority vote. This was done in the days immediately following the inauguration of George W. Bush, in the short period that both houses of Congress were Republican-controlled (before James Jeffords of Vermont left the Republican Party and put the Senate under Democratic control). The revocation means that OSHA cannot put in place another ergonomic standard without approval of Congress. There are as of this writing some Congressional initiatives to require a new standard, but it appears that the Bush administration is planning on continuing a primarily nonregulatory approach to ergonomics. Some employers have found the overturned standard to provide a very good template for developing voluntary programs in ergonomics (see following).

Currently, OSHA's primary regulatory tool for ergonomics falls under what is called the "General Duty Clause" of the original OSHA act, which states that the employer must "furnish to each of its employees employment and a place of employment which are free from recognized hazards that are causing or likely to cause death or serious physical harm" (Section 5(a)(1) of the OSHA Act). OSHA has been interpreting that to mean that if there is evidence (primarily from reports of MSD) that there are ergonomic problems, that those problems must be addressed. OSHA has issued significant fines in some industries (notably in food processing, especially in poultry factories) around ergonomic issues based on the General Duty Clause. That has been reemphasized in the Bush administration, which has announced an approach that also includes education of employers and issuing guidelines for specific high-hazard industries (OSHA has guidelines and extensive information available on its web site).

There are a few other OSHA standards that have some application for ergonomics. The record-keeping standard (Section 1904 of the OSHA General Industry Standards) requires that work-related MSDs be recorded on an OSHA 300 log, which must be posted every February (see preceding). The Access to Medical and Exposure Records Standard (Section 1020) states that any medical or exposure records (or analyses) that are done by the employer must, upon request, be shared with the union (with employee permission for medical records) and affected workers.

State Standards

State standards are a complex and rapidly changing landscape. As of this writing, there are two states (California and Washington) with ergonomics standards that have been passed, both of which have been the subject of litigation. California has a standard requiring an ergonomics program where work-related MSDs have occurred. Washington has a more comprehensive and prevention-based law that is being phased in. In the absence of a national standard, it is likely that there will be increased efforts to enact other state-based standards.

Voluntary Standards

There are several national organizations that issue consensus standards that are frequently used by employers as voluntary guidelines. OSHA sometimes has used such standards to support citations under the General Duty Clause as well as where there is no specific OSHA standard. The two most prominent voluntary standard-setting organizations in occupational health and safety are the American Conference of Governmental Industrial Hygienists (ACGIH) and the American National Standards Institute (ANSI).

The ACGIH Hand Activity Level Standard

The ACGIH is well known for issuing threshold limit values (TLVs), which are recommended maximums for exposure to chemical hazards and are frequently used by industry as internal standards. (Since the OSHA chemical standards are rarely if ever updated due to an extremely cumbersome regulatory process, the TLVs tend to reflect more recent studies.)

ACGIH has used a similar approach for ergonomics in trying to set a maximum for hand activities. The standard, which has been approved by ACGIH, is called the HAL (Hand Activity Level) standard. The HAL is computed by graphing the *average* number of hand repetitions on one axis, combined with the *maximum* hand force on the other axis. There is a line drawn on the graph that is the border between safe and risky hand activity (Figure 4-6). It is designed only for monotask jobs—that is, jobs that use the same hand motions over and over.

Average hand motions are rated on a 10-point scale from "hands idle most of the time; no regular exertions" (0) to "steady motion/exertion; infrequent pauses" (6) to "rapid steady motion/difficulty keeping up or continuous exertion" (10). The normalized peak force is then estimated, also on a 10-point scale, either by force measurement (as a percent of "maximum voluntary contraction," which is the measured maximum force the worker can exert), a Borg scale (from "nothing at all" [0], through moderate [3], strong [5], up to "extremely strong/almost max" [10]), or by an observation method ("barely noticeable or relaxed effort" [0.5] to "obvious effort but unchanged facial expression" [4] to "uses shoulder or trunk for force" [10]). These ratings are then graphed with force on one axis and activity on the other axis. The graph has a line (the TLV line) drawn from the point where activity = 1 and force = 7 to the point where both are 10. Everything above the line is considered out of standard and potentially hazardous. A second line goes from the point where activity = 1 and force = 5 to the point where both are 10; this is the "action limit." Tasks that lie between the action limit and the TLV are considered to be questionable; below the action limit is considered to be acceptable (Figure 4-6).

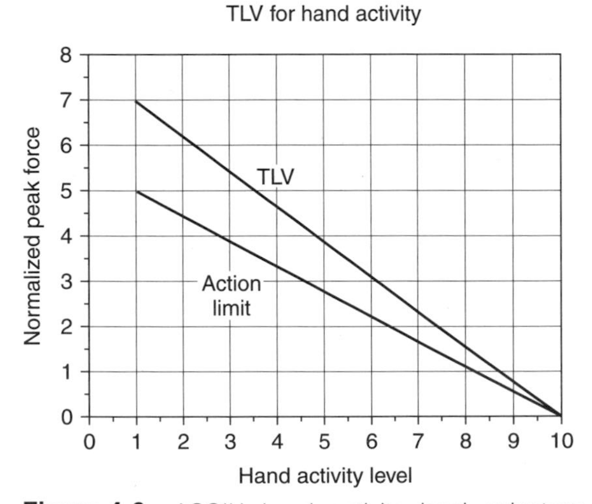

Figure 4-6 ACGIH hand activity level voluntary standard for mono-task jobs, American Conference of Governmental Industrial Hygienists.

The National Safety Council/American National Standards Institute Ergonomic Program Standard

The National Safety Council has undertaken an effort, which is still in progress, to create an ergonomics program standard (NSC Z-365) under ANSI. A draft of the voluntary standard said that an ergonomic control program *shall* have components for management responsibility, training, employee involvement, surveillance, evaluation and management of MSD cases, job analysis, and job design and intervention. The components also *shall* have training as appropriate; the opportunity for employees to participate; prompt evaluation by a health care provider when MSDs are reported; job analysis when an MSD is found to be work-related; evaluations of trends across jobs; consideration of force, posture, vibration, repetition, and other risk factors; and reduction of risk factors as much as technically and practically feasible. In addition, program components *should* have a written program, encourage notification of problems, use job surveys when cases are reported or with turnover or job change, and have the health care provider include an occupational history and consideration of activities, give a diagnosis and opinion on job-relatedness, include work organization factors, and evaluate the program.

The National Institute for Occupational Safety and Health Lifting Equation

The National Institute for Occupational Safety and Health (NIOSH) has a guideline for lifting that is useful in ergonomic analysis and is widely accepted by ergonomists and industry. Their lifting equation, which is fairly complex, uses data from actual lifting tasks to provide the maximum weight that is safe to lift. It begins with a premise that most workers can safely lift a maximum of 51 pounds on a regular basis under ideal lifting conditions. If the conditions are less than ideal, then the maximum weight is reduced. The conditions include that the grip for the load is less than 10 inches in front of the worker, the lifts are no lower than about knuckle height (30 inches above the floor) and no higher than about the shoulders, the vertical travel distance is 10 inches or less, lifting is not too frequent (no more than 0.2 lifts per minute) and has sufficient breaks, there is no twisting, and there is an excellent grip. Each of these factors is weighted. The actual equation can be obtained at the NIOSH web site (http://www.cdc.gov/niosh/homepage.html), and electronic versions are available at http://www.industrialhygiene.com/calc/lift.html and http://www.ccohs.ca/oshanswers/ergonomics/niosh/calculating_rwl.html. An easy way to use the equation is with a free computer program called ErgoEaser, which is available from the U.S. Department of Energy web site at http://nattie.eh.doe.gov/others/ergoeaser/download.html. The program also includes a useful computer workstation ergonomic evaluation tool.

Americans with Disabilities Act

The ADA provides for both easier access to buildings for people with disabilities (such as ramps and elevators) and also for protection of employment (and encouragement of employment) for people with disabilities.

The law requires that anyone with a covered disability (which includes some work-related disabilities) who would be able to perform the essential functions of a job must be given "reasonable accommodations" that allow them to perform those functions. The ADA is administered by the Equal Employment Opportunity Commission (EEOC) under the Justice Department. The definitions of covered disabilities have been narrowed by Supreme Court decisions, so disabilities that affect only certain work tasks may not be covered (Toyota Motor Manufacturing, Kentucky, Inc. v. Williams, decided January 8, 2002). Reasonable accommodations may include rest breaks, ergonomic interventions (such as improving reaches, reducing force requirements, or allowing better posture), and job rotations. Employers only have to do what is economically feasible, which is interpreted that large employers (such as the government) have to do more than what would be required for small employers (also refer to Chapters 13 and 15).

WORKERS' COMPENSATION

Workers' compensation is a system for paying medical costs and lost wages to workers who are injured or made ill from their job, with total benefit payouts for the United States estimated at $45.9 billion in 2000 (just over 1% of payroll) and covering 126.6 million workers (Mont, Burton, Reno, & Thompson, 2002). It is a state-based system, so the benefits differ somewhat from state to state (AFL-CIO, 2001). It is a no-fault system, so it does not matter if it was the worker's fault or the employer's fault. If the injury or illness was caused by or significantly aggravated by the job (defined as more than 50% sure, or more likely than not), then benefits must be paid. The "significantly aggravated" aspect is particularly important for occupational illnesses such as MSD, since they can be caused by multiple events. There is an exclusive remedy provision to the law, so that if workers are covered by the workers' compensation law, then they are typically prohibited from suing the employer for tort liability such as for negligence.

Workers' compensation pays for all medical costs associated with the injury or illness. It also pays usually either two-thirds of gross pay or 75% of net pay (varies state by state) while the worker is unable to work because of the condition. There are also typically additional monetary benefits if the worker has any permanent disability.

States vary in their coverage of chronic conditions such as MSD. There is often a statute of limitations (such as one year) for filing a claim, which is sometimes defined as beginning at the time of first exposure. If it is several years after the exposure began that a work-related condition is diagnosed by a physician, then the claim may not be able to meet that timeline, and the claim may be denied. Other states have the timeline start at the time of the diagnosis or the last date of exposure, whichever is later, which makes a successful claim more likely. Since MSDs are by definition cumulative and there is no specific date or time of injury, claims are typically more difficult to win than acute injury claims even if there is not a problem with the statute of limitations. Workers' compensation systems are driven by medical opinion, so there needs to be a physician's opinion that (at a minimum) the MSD was "more likely than not" caused or significantly aggravated by the job. The work-relatedness is commonly contested by the insurer. A study in New York found that 79% of diagnosed work-related carpal tunnel claims were contested, although 96% of those decided by the end of the study were ultimately awarded by the workers' compensation commission (although they averaged over a year to resolve) (Herbert, Janeway, & Schechter, 1999).

UNION CONTRACTS

Some union contracts have occupational health and safety provisions—most commonly provisions that the employer must provide a safe workplace and/or provisions for a union-management health and safety committee (some states also have statutes or workers' compensation incentives that require health and safety committees, such as Connecticut and Washington). Such language not only sets up a structure to deal with issues such as ergonomics but also makes health and safety conditions subject to a formal grievance procedure as a way to resolve differences between labor and management. Contracts may also be more specific, addressing specific problems such as requiring the employer to provide ergonomic workstations, lifting devices, or other prevention methods.

SUMMARY

MSD is a widespread occupational health problem, with severe consequences for the worker and the employer. While the reported problem is most common in manufacturing, there are also emerging problems in the service sector. It is possible to track MSDs for a workplace in order to prioritize ergonomic interventions, which are usually cost-effective and tend to decrease fatigue and improve productivity as well as reduce health problems. While OSHA does not have a specific standard on ergonomics, it does cite and fine companies with MSD problems based on the general duty clause and other provisions. There are useful voluntary guidelines that can reduce ergonomic risk factors, and there are ADA, workers' compensation, and union contract provisions that must be followed. Although it is certainly true that typically good ergonomics is also good economics, preventing MSDs is also crucial for good worker health.

REFERENCES

AFL-CIO. (2001). Workers' compensation and unemployment insurance under state laws, Jan. 1, 2001. Washington, DC: AFL-CIO.

Andreoni, D. (1986). The cost of occupational accidents and diseases (OSH Series #54). Geneva: International Labor Office.

Bureau of Labor Statistics. (1986). Record-keeping guidelines for occupational injuries and illnesses. Washington, DC: U.S. Dept. of Labor, Bureau of Labor Statistics (BLS).

Bureau of Labor Statistics. (2002). Industry injury and illness data, 2000. U.S. Bureau of Labor Statistics. Available: http://stats.bls.gov/iif/oshsum.htm [2002, August].

Boden, L. (2000). Workers' compensation. In B. Levy & D. H. Wegman (Eds.), *Occupational health.* Philadelphia, PA. Lippincott Williams and Wilkins.

CTDNews. (1997). Travelers takes dose of own ergo medicine. CTDNews, *6*(1), 2-4.

Dorman, P. (1996). Markets and mortality. New York, NY: Cambridge University Press.

General Accounting Office. (1997). Worker protection: Private sector ergonomics programs yield positive results (GAO/HEHS-97-163). Washington, DC: U.S. General Accounting Office (GAO).

Herbert, R., Janeway, K., & Schechter, C. (1999). Carpal tunnel syndrome and workers' compensation among an occupational clinic population in New York State. *American Journal of Industrial Medicine, 35*(4), 335-342.

Katz, J., Lew, R., Bessette, L., Punnett, L., Fossel, A., Mooney, N., et al. (1998). Prevalence and predictors of long-term work disability due to carpal tunnel syndrome. *American Journal of Industrial Medicine, 33,* 543-550.

Liss, G., Armstrong, C., Kusiak, R., & Gailitis, M. (1992). Use of provincial health insurance plan billing data to estimate carpal tunnel syndrome morbidity and surgery rates. *American Journal of Industrial Medicine, 22,* 395-409.

Maizlish, N., Rudolph, L., Dervin, K., & Sankaranarayan, M. (1995). Surveillance and prevention of work-related carpal tunnel syndrome: An application of the Sentinel Events Notification System for Occupational Risks. *American Journal of Industrial Medicine, 27*(5), 715-729.

McCaffrey, D. (1982). OSHA and the politics of health regulations. New York: Plenum Press.

Mont, D., Burton, J., Reno, V., & Thompson, C. (2002). Workers' compensation: Benefits, coverage and costs, 2000 new estimates. Washington, DC: National Academy of Social Insurance.

Morse, T., Punnett, L., Warren, N., Dillon, C., & Warren, A. (2003). The relationship of unions to prevalence and claim filing for work-related upper-extremity musculoskeletal disorders, *American Journal of Industrial Medicine,* in press, 2003.

Morse, T., Dillon, C., Warren, N., Hall, C., & Hovey, D. (2001). Capture-recapture estimation of unreported work-related musculoskeletal disorders in Connecticut. *American Journal of Industrial Medicine, 39*(6), 636-642.

Morse, T. F., Dillon, C., Warren, N., Levenstein, C., & Warren, A. (1998). The economic and social consequences of work-related musculoskeletal disorders: The Connecticut Upper-Extremity Surveillance Project (CUSP). *International Journal of Occupational and Environmental Health, 4*(4), 209-216.

Noble, C. (1986). *Liberalism at work: The rise and fall of OSHA.* Philadelphia: Temple University Press.

OSHA. (2001). Recording and reporting occupational injuries and illnesses, 29 CFR, Part 1904: U.S. Occupational Safety and Health Administration (OSHA).

Oxenburgh, M. (1997). Cost-benefit analysis of ergonomics programs. *American Industrial Hygiene Association Journal, 58,* 150-156.

Punnett, L. (1999). The costs of work-related musculoskeletal disorders in automotive manufacturing. *New Solutions, 9*(4), 403-426.

Silverstein, B. A., Stetson, D. S., Keyserling, W. M., & Fine, L. J. (1997). Work-related musculoskeletal disorders: comparison of data sources for surveillance. *American Journal of Industrial Medicine, 31*(5), 600-608.

Webster, B., & Snook, S. (1994). The cost of compensable upper extremity cumulative trauma disorders. *Journal of Occupational Medicine, 36*(7), 713-717.

Yassi, A., Sprout, J., & Tate, R. (1996). Upper limb repetitive strain injuries in Manitoba. *American Journal of Industrial Medicine, 30,* 461-472.

PART TWO

Conditions Related to MSDs: Diagnosis and Intervention

CHAPTER 5

Pathomechanics of MSDs

Susan V. Duff

The neuromuscular system is uniquely designed to withstand the stresses and strains of everyday life. Occasionally, the intrinsic and extrinsic demands placed on select structures exceed physiologic limits. The response of the body and nervous system to excessive demands can significantly influence one's participation in work, recreation, and self-care tasks. Musculoskeletal disorders (MSDs) or repetitive strain injuries (RSIs) are neuromuscular conditions that evolve secondary to low-intensity stresses applied gradually or repetitively (Piligian, Herbert, Hearns, et al., 2000). Disorders frequently attributed to MSDs include tendinitis/tendinosis, nerve compressions/entrapments, and focal hand dystonia. Related conditions include myofascial trigger points and bursitis. MSDs are explored in this chapter in terms of the mechanism of occurrence and anatomic and neural consequences. Evaluation and treatment of these disorders are reviewed in the next chapter.

NEUROMUSCULAR DISORDERS

Tendonopathies

Tendonopathies refer to acute and chronic neuromuscular disorders that can be linked to overuse in vulnerable structures (Maffulli, Khan, & Puddu, 1998). *Tendinitis* is regarded as an inflammatory condition of the muscle-tendon unit. If the involved tissues are not allowed to heal, *tendinosis* or degenerative changes can develop. To ensure full comprehension of these distinct disorders, tendon anatomy, biomechanics, and the histological features of pathology will be reviewed.

Regional Anatomy

Muscles attach to bone via tendons, and tendons attach to muscle at the myotendinous junction. Tension produced in skeletal muscle is transmitted through the myotendinous junction to the tendon and results in joint motion. Both the myotendinous junction and the tendon are uniquely designed to handle the forces encountered during contraction and resultant movement (Carlstedt & Nordin, 1989; Garrett, Nikolaou, Ribbeck, Glisson, & Seaber, 1988). Understanding tendon pathology first requires a review of anatomy and associated structures.

Tendon

The structure of tendons is well documented and pictured in Figure 5-1. Tendons are composed of 30% collagen and 2% elastin embedded within an extracellular matrix, 68% of which is water (Borynsenko & Beringer, 1989). Collagen resists tensile forces, whereas elastin increases tendon extensibility. Collagen fibrils, formed from fibroblasts, combine via cross-links to form microfibrils. The microfibrils are arranged in parallel, which enhances the tendon's ability to manage high unidirectional loads (Birk & Zycband, 1994; O'Brien, 1992). A sheath, called

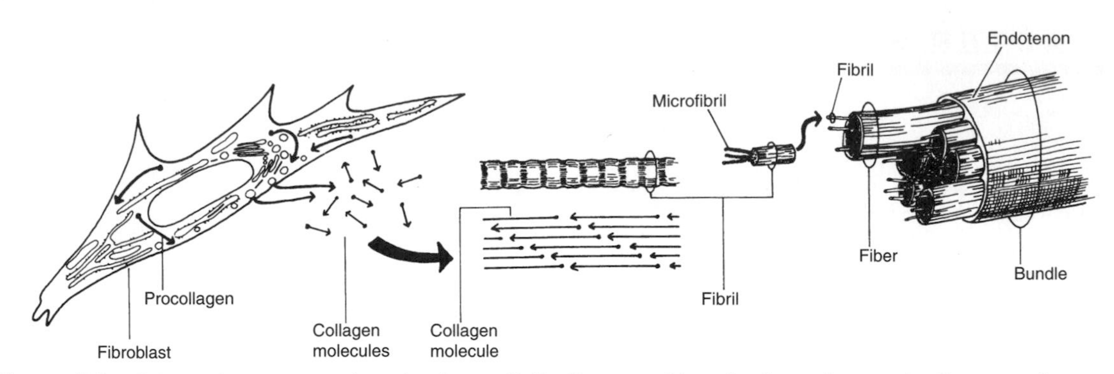

Figure 5-1 Schematic representation of collagen fibrils, fibers, and bundles in tendons and collagenous ligaments (not drawn to scale). Collagen molecules, triple helices of coiled polypeptide chains, are synthesized and secreted by the fibroblasts. These molecules (depicted with heads and tails to represent positive and negative polar charges) aggregate in the extracellular matrix in a parallel arrangement to form microfibrils and then fibrils. The staggered array of the molecules, in which each overlaps the other, gives a banded appearance to the collagen fibrils under the electron microscope. The fibrils aggregate further into fibers, which come together into densely packed bundles. (Reprinted with permission from Carlstedt, C. A. & Nordin, M. [1989]. Biomechanics of tendons and ligaments. In M. Nordin & V. H. Frankel [Eds.], *Basic biomechanics of the musculoskeletal system* [2nd ed.]. Philadelphia: Lea & Febiger.)

the *endotenon*, surrounds each myofibril bundle or fascicle. Nerves and blood vessels travel within this endotenon. Groups of fascicles are held together by a loose areolar tissue that has elastic and tensile properties and is called the *paratenon* or tenosynovium. The paratenon, which forms a protective sheath around the tendon and enhances gliding, may become inflamed secondary to repetitive movement across bony prominences or other structures (Thorson & Szabo, 1989). In regions of low friction, only the paratenon surrounds the tendon. In select areas of high friction, such as the long flexor tendons, a synovia-like membrane, called the *epitenon,* lies beneath the paratenon. This thin layer of epitenon surrounds several fiber bundles and adheres to the tendon surface. Lubricating fluid lies between the paratenon and epitenon in these select regions (Kasletic, Galeski, & Baer, 1978). At the insertion into bone, the endotenon continues as *Sharpey's fibers* and becomes continuous with the periosteum. Tendon composition at the insertion site is bonier and much less fibrous (Carlstedt & Nordin, 1989).

Myotendinous Junction

The myotendinous junction can be differentiated from tendon by its highly folded tissue. The multiple folds are set at extremely low angles to the force vectors that cross them. This unique structure increases the surface area for tension transfer 10- to 20-fold, enhancing the adhesive strength of the junction (O'Brien, 1992; Tidball, 1983). The sarcomeres near the myotendinous region are stiffer than are other muscle fibers, as evidenced by their shorter lengths when the muscle is loaded or stretched (Gordon, Huxley, & Julian, 1966). Despite its complex structure, the myotendinous junction is still viewed by some as the weakest link in the muscle-tendon unit.

Vascularity

Most tendons have extrinsic and intrinsic sources of vascularity (Gelberman, 1991). *Extrinsic* vascularity refers to blood supplied from an external source, whereas *intrinsic* vascularity refers to nutrition made available within the tendon. The extrinsic blood supply is divided among three tendon regions: the musculotendinous junction, the tendon length, and the tendon-bone junction. Tendon vessels that insert into cartilaginous regions are separated from those of bone (Woo et al., 1987). Tendons that insert into the periosteum or the diaphysis have an anastomosis between the tendon and bone (Curwin & Stanish, 1984; O'Brien, 1992). Small feeder vessels may branch from larger vessels, as exemplified by the vincula of the long finger flexor tendons.

Despite the reported extrinsic blood supply, tendons are relatively avascular, especially near the insertion sites, which is why they appear white (Fenwick, Hazleman, & Riley, 2002; Kahn, Cook, Bonar, Harcourt, & Astrom, 1999). In regions of excess force and pressure, the blood supply to tendons is variable. For instance, vessels are absent in regions in which the tendon must travel around a pulley. Because of this variable blood supply, the tendon must also rely on intrinsic blood flow. Diffusion of nutrients through synovial fluid diffusion during movement is one form of intrinsic blood supply (Fenwick et al., 2002). Tendons with a synovial sheath of epitenon, such as the long flexor tendons, receive some intrinsic nutrition in this manner (Lundborg & Rank, 1978). Although tendon injuries typically occur in regions with a reduced blood supply, Backman, Friden, and Widmark (1991) conclude that tendon degeneration cannot be attributed primarily to circulatory impairment. Thus, other factors such as tolerance to loads, friction, and repetitive motion contribute to tendon degeneration.

Nerve Innervation

Proprioceptive information from tendons is transduced by muscle spindles and Golgi tendon organs (GTOs), whereas pain information is picked up by nociceptors. Muscle spindles within the muscle belly and myotendinous junction are responsive to changes in muscle length and velocity. The spindles have both an afferent and efferent nerve supply. Variations in active muscle force (tension) are picked up by GTOs embedded in the myotendinous junction. Passive force, previously considered to be transduced through the GTOs, is now known to be transmitted primarily through surrounding connective tissue. The nerve fibers supplying the GTO receptors invaginate themselves between collagen fibers. As muscle tension is transferred to the tendon, collagen fibers compress the underlying nerve endings, producing a stream of nerve conduction. Although muscle spindles respond to alterations in muscle length and GTOs respond to muscle tension, they both provide feedback and feed-forward information necessary for adequate neuromotor control (Prochazka, Gillard, & Bennett, 1997a, 1997b; Rothwell, 1995). Myelinated and unmyelinated sensory nerve endings pick up noxious stimuli in the region of the tendon and myotendinous junction and carry them along either an A delta or C fiber to the spinal cord (Wolf, 1984). Pain information reaching the spinal cord connects with other regions of the central nervous system (CNS) and reaches a perceptual level once it makes a cortical connection.

Biomechanics of Tendons

Tendons are one type of connective tissue that respond to alterations in tensile load (stress) and length (strain). The strength of a tendon is correlated with its thickness and collagen content versus the maximal tension that its associated muscle can exert (Elliott, 1967; O'Brien, 1992). Both the size of a tendon and the demands placed on it will affect its biomechanical properties.

Stress-Strain Curve

As seen in Figure 10-1, the stress-strain curve demonstrates how loading affects tendons (Carlstedt, 1987; Curwin & Stanish, 1984). *Stress*, or load magnitude per unit area, is determined by dividing tensile load by the cross-sectional area perpendicular to the direction of the load. *Strain* is the percentage of tendon elongation (deformation) under a load relative to its resting length. The initial slow rise of the stress-strain curve (called the elastic range) refers to the initial response to loading or stretch, during which time the wavy collagen fibers straighten out. The linear rise in the curve represents the stiffening of the tendon in response to loading, which indicates that it takes a progressively greater force to generate elongation (plastic range). The peak in the curve refers to the maximum strength of the tendon. The normal range of length-tension in mammalian tendon is 49 to 98 N/m^2. If a tendon is loaded past this maximum point, usually it undergoes rapid failure. According to Elliott (1967), the maximum strength of a tendon is approximately twice the maximum isometric tension that can be generated in a tendon's muscle.

Viscoelasticity

Tendons display viscoelastic or rate-dependent (time-dependent) behavior with loads. At high rates of strain, tendons store more energy, require more force to rupture, and undergo greater elongation (Kennedy & Baxter-Willis, 1976). At high stress rates, tendons absorb less energy and are capable of moving heavy loads. At low stress rates, tendons absorb more energy and are less effective at moving heavy loads (Fyfe & Stanish, 1992). The creep test and the stress-relaxation test are two ways of measuring tendon viscoelasticity. *Creep* refers to the gradual lengthening of a tendon in response to a constant stress or load. During the creep test, the load is held safely below the linear portion of the stress-strain curve, and stress is held constant. If the load is altered cyclically instead of being held at a constant rate, the change in length is less pronounced. During the *stress-relaxation test,* strain (length) is held constant while the load is held below the linear region of the stress-strain curve. At a constant level of strain, tension in the tendon gradually decreases. Given cyclic alterations in strain, the reduction in stress is less significant (Carlstedt & Nordin, 1989).

Factors Affecting the Integrity of Tendons

Age and drugs can have a tremendous impact on the mechanical behavior of a tendon. The level of exercise and activity can also affect its integrity.

Aging

During early tendon maturation, collagen fibril diameter increases along with the number of cross-links, leading to maximum tendon strength between the third and sixth decade (Yamada, 1970). With aging, collagen stiffens, and the fibers shrink, thereby reducing tensile strength and increasing the potential for tearing (O'Brien, 1992). Furthermore, the metabolic activity is reduced in the aging tendon (Almekinders & Deol, 1999). By the seventh decade, strength has declined rapidly. However, Riley, Harrall, Constant, Cawston, & Hazleman, (1994) found no significant difference in content of the supraspinous tendon in individuals from 11 to 95 years of age. Instead, they postulated that changes in collagen content could be attributed to years of repeated injury that resulted in microtears, weakening of the tendon structure, and predisposition to injury.

Antiinflammatory Medications

The effect of antiinflammatory medications on tendon depends on whether they contain steroids. Nonsteroidal antiinflammatory drugs (NSAIDs) such as aspirin and indomethacin have been found to increase the rate of biomechanical restoration of tissue. Side effects from NSAIDs are minimal. Corticosteroid injections are also intended to reduce pain and inflammation. Despite their value, corticosteroids do have significant side effects that include a reduction in collagen and ground substance production. This reduction may lead to tendon atrophy and subsequent rupture after excessive physical activity (Carlstedt, Madsen, & Wredmark, 1986; Kennedy & Baxter-Willis, 1976; Nirschl, 1992; Ohkawa, 1982; Smith, Kosygan, Williams, & Newman, 1999; Vogel, 1977).

Mechanical Demands

Tendons remodel in response to mechanical demands, undergoing a continual process of resorption and repair. Despite this ability, they are less metabolically active than other human tissues. The rate of collagen turnover in tendons is between 50 and 100 days and is altered by exercise and disuse (Gerber, Gerber, & Altman,

1960; Langberg, Rosendal, & Kjaer, 2001). On the basis of animal studies, consistent exercise has been found to increase tendon tensile strength. This gain is accomplished through an increase in the number of collagen cross-links, water and ground substance content, and the size and number of collagen fibers (Woo, Matthews, Akenson, Amiel, & Convery, 1975). In contrast, disuse or immobilization results in decreased water and ground substance concentration and a decrease in metabolic enzymes. Inactivity also contributes to collagen degradation and resorption (Woo, 1982). These changes lead to a reduction in tensile strength.

Tendon Pathology

Disruptive Forces

Tension, compression, and shear are three forces that can disrupt the structure of normal tendons. Injury can occur when a force or load magnitude is too high, too frequent in occurrence, or both. Kastelic and Baer (1980) have suggested that tendons elongate secondary to slippage of the transverse bonds between collagen fibrils. Although these bonds are quite strong, after excessive or frequent force the proteoglycan matrix cannot hold them, resulting in inflammation and small microtears in the tendinous region. Individual collagen fibrils in tendons do lengthen in response to tensile stress, yet damage can occur even after an 8.5% elongation. Fast, eccentric contractions in weak or fatigued muscles may lead to injury (Kirkendall & Garrett, 2002). Muscles with a higher percentage of fast-twitch fibers are more likely to be involved in quick movements, which is why they may be the first muscles injured.

Vulnerable Anatomic Sites

Vulnerable sites for tendon injury include tendon attachment sites, the myotendinous junction, and segments in which the tendon must traverse a tunnel. Attachment sites are vulnerable because of their limited blood supply, which varies depending on whether the tendon inserts into bone or cartilage. The myotendinous junction is susceptible to injury because of its reduced sarcomere extensibility. This junction has been determined to be the most common place for rupture (Garrett, Nikolaou, Ribbeck, Glisson, & Seaber, 1988; Kvist et al., 1995). Given its two vulnerable conditions, the common extensor tendon near the elbow, which has a poor blood supply and whose attachment site lies close to the myotendinous junction, is highly susceptible to repetitive strain injury. Tunnels are a third vulnerable site. Gliding through tunnels may be restricted if the tendons or surrounding tissue have undergone partial trauma. For example, if, as a result of frequent high forces, the synovial sheaths of the long flexor tendons become inflamed within the carpal tunnel, the tendons and sheath may swell. The swollen tendons may not be able to glide freely and eventually could put undue pressure on the median nerve because of lack of space within the carpal canal (Pratt, 1991). When these vulnerable sites combine with conditions of risk, injury results.

Tendon Response to Injury

Overuse Terminology

A few key terms associated with tendon injuries are reviewed here and summarized in Table 5-1. *Tendinitis* is a general term that implies there has been a vascular disruption

Table 5-1
Definitions of Tendon Injuries

Tendinitis	Vascular disruption and small microtears to the tendon, induced by a high rate of stress or strain, resulting in an acute inflammation
Paratendinitis	An inflammation and thickening of the paratenon
Tenosynovitis	An inflammation of the synovial lining
Tendinosis	Chronic degenerative pathology of the tendon, caused by repetitive, low load, stress, and strain

Sources: Modified from Leadbetter, W. B. (1992). Cell-matrix response in tendon injury. *Clin Sports Med, 11,* 533–578; and Nirschl, R. P. (1992). Elbow tendinosis/tennis elbow. *Clin Sports Med, 11,* 851–869.

resulting in an acute inflammation induced by small tendon microtears. Acute tendinitis typically involves a high rate of elongation or strain that may resolve within a few months. *Paratendinitis* refers to an inflammation and thickening of the paratenon with resultant crepitus on examination. *Tenosynovitis* is used to describe an inflammation of the synovial lining; however, that term now falls under the category of paratendinitis. *Tendinosis* refers to chronic degenerative pathology of the tendon, caused by repetitive, low-load stress and strain (Leadbetter, 1992; Nirschl, 1992). With tendinosis there may not be clinical or histological signs of inflammation but degeneration is present (Maffulli et al., 1998).

Pathology

Tendon pathology can be divided into two general categories: macrotraumatic (i.e., acute tissue destruction) and microtraumatic (i.e., chronic abuse or load). The subacute phase refers to the stage in which the acute injury begins to subside and healing begins (Leadbetter, 1992). The pathology of these different forms of tendon injury differs in terms of histology and mechanism of occurrence.

Acute Conditions

Acute tendon injury results from quick eccentric movements made under heavy loads or high strain (Kirkendall & Garrett, 2002; Leadbetter, 1992). An acute injury sets up a cycle of regeneration and repair that begins with inflammation and progresses to collagen formation. If the stresses and strain on the tendon are alleviated and wound healing is allowed to progress, an acute injury should resolve quickly. Unfortunately, the typical sites for tendinitis are those vulnerable regions most subjected to repetitive forces by the light and heavy activities of daily living. As a result, many acute injuries go unresolved and may become chronic injuries affecting the integrity of the tissue itself. Animal models of chronic repetitive reach to grasp tasks (Barbe et al., 2003; Barr & Barbe, 2002) reveal that along with cellular and tissue changes including tendon fraying, motor skills began to deteriorate as early as the fifth and sixth week of repetitive use (4 reaches/minute, 2 hours/day, 3 days/week). Byl and Melnick (1997) have linked the deterioration in motor skills to repetitive movements that cause a degradation of sensory feedback and subsequent alteration in the somatosensory representation.

Chronic Conditions

In chronic conditions, the signs and symptoms of tendon injury last months or years without resolution. Unlike the acute stage, typical chronic injuries have an insidious onset caused by subthreshold, repetitive stresses or strains to vulnerable tendon regions (Leadbetter, 1992). If immature scar or unconditioned muscle tendon units are subjected to dynamic and cyclic overloading, degeneration results (Markison, 1992). Degenerative tendon pathology may stem from hypoxia, which eliminates the sequential progression of wound repair seen in acute injuries (Jozsa, Reffy, Kannus, Demel, & Elek, 1990). Specifically, it may signify a failure to repair the extracellular matrix after repetitive microinjury (Fenwick et al., 2001).

Chronic tendinitis has been referred to as *tendinosis* because histologic examination of chronic injuries often reveals the presence of atypical granulation-like tissue called *angiofibroblastic tendinosis* (Leadbetter, 1991; Nirschl, 1992). In chronically injured tendons, tissue degeneration has been reported on the basis of reduced and disorganized collagen fiber content, a gray, frail appearance of tendons, fibrosis at the insertion sites, and tendon calcification (Kahn et al., 1999; Riley et al., 1994). Tendons afflicted with tendinosis exhibit collagen bundle disorganization, scattered vascular ingrowth, occasional local necrosis, and calcification (Clancey, 1990; Mosier, Pomeroy, & Manoli, 1999; Puddu, Ippolito, & Postacchini, 1976). Although there is an absence of inflammatory cells in painful tendinosis (Jozsa et al., 1990; Leadbetter, 1992; Nirschl, 1992), high concentrations of lactate (Alfredson, Bjur, Thorsen,

Lorentzon, & Sandstrom, 2002) and glutamate (Alfredson & Lorentzon, 2002) have been found, perhaps as a result of the anaerobic conditions present in those conditions.

Conditions Related to Tendonopathies

Myofascial Trigger Points

A trigger point is a palpable, hyperirritable point within a nodule or taut band of muscle or its fascia (Meyer, 2002; Travell & Simons, 1983). It has been postulated that acute muscular strain may overload the contractile elements of the muscle (Travell & Simons, 1983). This strain may damage such muscle constituents as the sarcoplasmic reticulum and may cause release of calcium. If the sarcoplasmic reticulum is damaged, calcium cannot be restored to its original location after contraction. The normal energy source of adenosine triphosphate in combination with the excess calcium will cause a sustained contraction of the exposed muscle fibers. Uncontrolled metabolism in this region may cause local vasoconstriction and may lead to a trigger point–mediated reflex response via local sensory and sympathetic nerve fiber activation. As a result of local changes, muscle fibers in this region typically become shortened. In summary, a trigger point induced by excess stress or strain becomes the site of increased metabolism, reduced circulation, sensitized nerves, and shortened muscle fibers.

Once established, the trigger point can be palpated as a taut band or nodule. A twitch response may be produced on contraction of the taut band. Compression to the trigger point may induce local tenderness and *referred pain,* or pain perceived away from the site of origin. In addition, local tenderness with a palpable band of fibers will be noted on physical examination, and the muscle will be shortened and weak (Moran, 1994). Excess fatigue during repetitive contractions or repetitive contraction of a damaged region may exacerbate the condition and lead to chronic trigger points within a muscle region.

Bursitis

Bursitis is an inflammatory condition of the bursal lining or the synovial fluid encased within the bursa (Cyriax, 1982). Inflammation of any bursa can limit activity considerably. Inflammation of the synovial fluid may cause the bursa to enlarge. In the upper limb, the most commonly occurring bursitis is associated with the glenohumeral joint and the second most common is associated with the olecranon bursa of the elbow.

The glenohumeral joint bursa has two connected parts: the subdeltoid and the subacromial bursae; the terms are used interchangeably (Pratt, 1991). From this point on, the term *subacromial bursa* will be used (Figure 5-2). This bursa can be palpated with the humerus in passive extension, inferior to the acromion, and lateral to the bicipital groove. Because the inner wall of the subacromial bursa is the outer wall of the supraspinous tendon, bursitis often occurs in combination with supraspinous tendinitis (Cailliet, 1991). Bursitis in this region is also associated with impingement syndrome,

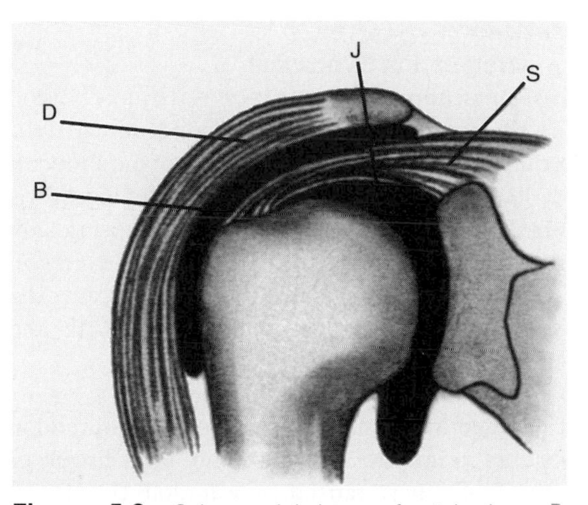

Figure 5-2 Subacromial bursa frontal view. *B,* Subacromial bursa; *D,* deltoid muscle; *J,* glenohumeral joint cavity; *S,* supraspinatous tendon. (Reprinted with permission from Mercier, L. R. [1995]. *Practical orthopedics* [4th ed., p. 55]. St. Louis: Mosby.)

described later in this chapter. Acute subacromial bursitis presents with a sudden onset of limited active abduction without any precipitating injury and with tenderness upon palpation. Typically, there is no capsular pattern or associated muscle spasm. In addition, pain is not elicited on resisted abduction. As the acute bursitis resolves, a painful arc emerges (a pain response elicited from 60 degrees to 120 degrees of active shoulder abduction). Recurrence is likely at intervals of 2 to 5 years. Typically, chronic bursitis has a gradual onset without a specific cause. With this condition, there is a painful arc of abduction but no pain with resisted movement. A calcified deposit may develop within the bursa (Cyriax, 1982).

Olecranon bursitis also may present as either an acute or chronic condition. With acute bursitis, the olecranon region is enlarged, limiting elbow extension and elbow weight bearing. The region is often tender to palpation. As the acute condition progresses to chronic, the olecranon region may remain engorged even though tenderness to touch is reduced. If elbow range of motion (ROM) is not preserved, limitations may persist after the initial inflammatory condition subsides (Cyriax, 1982).

Intersection Syndrome

Intersection syndrome is caused by an abrasion of the tendons within the second dorsal wrist compartment as the muscle bellies of the abductor pollicis longus (APL) and extensor pollicis brevis (EPB) cross over it during thumb and wrist flexion or repetitive wrist flexion and extension (Grundberg & Reagan, 1985). Specifically, the second compartment contains the ECRL and ECRB.

Trigger Finger (Thumb)

Triggering or snapping of a long flexor tendon occurs primarily in the thumb, long finger, or ring finger. It is caused by a nodule that forms on a long flexor tendon. This nodule often is located near the volar metacarpophalangeal (MP) joint and prevents smooth gliding under the A1 pulley located at the head of the metacarpal. The region of involvement, between the A1 and A2 pulleys, has been termed the *hypovascular watershed area* because of its limited vascular supply (Evans, Hunter, & Burkhalter, 1988; Littler, 1977). Occasionally, a trigger may form near the thumb interphalangeal (IP) joint, preventing smooth gliding during IP flexion and extension. Signs and symptoms of trigger thumb or finger range from stiffness in the affected digit to a painful snap on fist making or reextension; occasional locking may prevent either flexion or extension. Complications include intrinsic tightness with limited IP motion or a flexion contracture (Cailliet, 1991; Cyriax, 1982; Evans et al., 1988).

Focal Hand Dystonia

Repetitive, synchronous movements of the hands, as in musicians, can lead to an involuntary movement disorder often referred to as *focal hand dystonia* (Blake, Byl, & Merzenich, 2002). Byl and Merzenich (2002) report that the classic features of focal hand dystonia or occupational hand cramps are often linked to a specific target task. That target task usually demands precise movements, extremely repetitive fine-motor behavior, modulation via feedback, and goal-specific selective attention. Although writer's cramp is the most frequently reported, musicians and keyboard operators may present with symptoms. Individuals with this condition can present with motor control deficits without coexisting signs of tendinitis or nerve compression (Topp & Byl, 1999). However, subtle deficits such as excessive grip force employed during object manipulation (Odergren, Iwasaki, Borg, & Forssberg, 1996) may be evident. Byl and colleagues (Byl & Melnick, 1997; Byl & Merzenich, 2002) propose that focal hand dystonia may represent a form of learning or the result of negative neural adaptation to a target task. Changes in the somatosensory cortex associated with focal hand dystonia have been documented (Blake, Byl, Cheung, et al., 2002; Elbert, Candia, Altenmüller, et al., 1998). Elbert et al. (1998) proposed that a use-dependent susceptibility to fusion of digital representation may be partly responsible. However, it is not yet clear whether the changes in somatosensory representation are the cause or result of the disorder (Byl & Merzenich, 2002).

Peripheral Neurovascular Compressions and Entrapment Syndromes

Peripheral compression neuropathies and neurovascular entrapment syndromes frequently are linked to overuse. Typically, compressions are caused by anatomic abnormalities or adaptive shortening of tissues, which reduces the potential space in which the nerve travels. Over time, the nerve may become compromised because of inadequate space (Walsh, 1994). Entrapments are frequently caused by repetitive trauma to a nerve or its interfacing tissue, resulting initially in inflammation and which can lead to fibrosis (Sunderland, 1978). Compressions and entrapments may occur in combination. For example, a nerve may be vulnerable to compressive forces secondary to a reduction in travel space. Repetitive trauma within this reduced space may inflame the nerve or its surrounding tissue, leading to entrapment. A complete understanding of the implications of compressive neuropathies and entrapment conditions requires a review of physiology and pathology.

Nerve Anatomy and Physiology

Stimuli picked up by sensory receptors are coded by transducers into neural activity. Once transduced, the information is carried through peripheral nerves to the central nervous systems (CNS), where it eventually registers in the somatosensory cortex. Because processing of somatosensory and motor information occurs distributively throughout the nervous system (Shumway-Cook & Woollacott, 2001), both the peripheral nervous system (PNS) and the CNS, along with their associated connective tissues, are affected by nerve compressions and entrapments (Blake et al., 2002).

Connective Tissues

Continuity between the PNS and CNS is maintained through supportive connective tissues (Figure 5-3) (Matloub & Yousif, 1992; Sunderland, 1978). The central axon is surrounded by *endoneurium*. Groups of four or five axons, which form fascicles, are covered by a strong layer of *perineurium*. A bundle of fascicles is enveloped further in a loose layer of *epineurium*. The *mesoneurium* surrounds the entire nerve in a meshlike fashion, connecting it to nearby interfacing tissues. Most regions of the peripheral nerve contain all connective tissue layers, except for the nerve roots, which lie near the spinal cord. The lack of epineurium, in particular, significantly reduces the regeneration potential of nerve roots despite their close proximity to the cell bodies.

Vascularity

Nerves depend on an ongoing supply of oxygen and nutrients provided by a well-developed vascular network. Each connective tissue layer contains blood vessels with extensive anastomoses (Lundborg, 1979; Matloub & Yousif, 1992). A bidirectional perineurial *diffusion barrier* is the most external protective zone for the nerve. This perineurial barrier protects the endoneurium from the effects of proteins and edema. Epineurial blood vessels allow passage of small amounts of proteins, whereas the walls of the internal endoneurial capillaries provide a blood-nerve barrier. This endoneurial blood-nerve barrier, maintained by tight junctions of endothelial cells, protects the axon against the invasion of all proteins and from the ischemic effects of short-lasting epineurial edema (Olsson & Kristensson, 1971). Studies of animal models have determined that this blood-nerve barrier develops postnatally (Smith, Atchabahian, Mackinnon, & Hunter, 2001).

Transport of Axoplasm

The axon contains a viscouslike substance, axoplasm, which assists in the bidirectional flow of materials to and from the cell body. Axoplasm is considered thixotropic; therefore, movement is required to keep the viscosity low and to prevent gelling (Baker, Ladds, & Rubinson, 1977; Haak, Kleinhaus, & Ochs, 1976). Essential neural substances manufactured in the cell body are

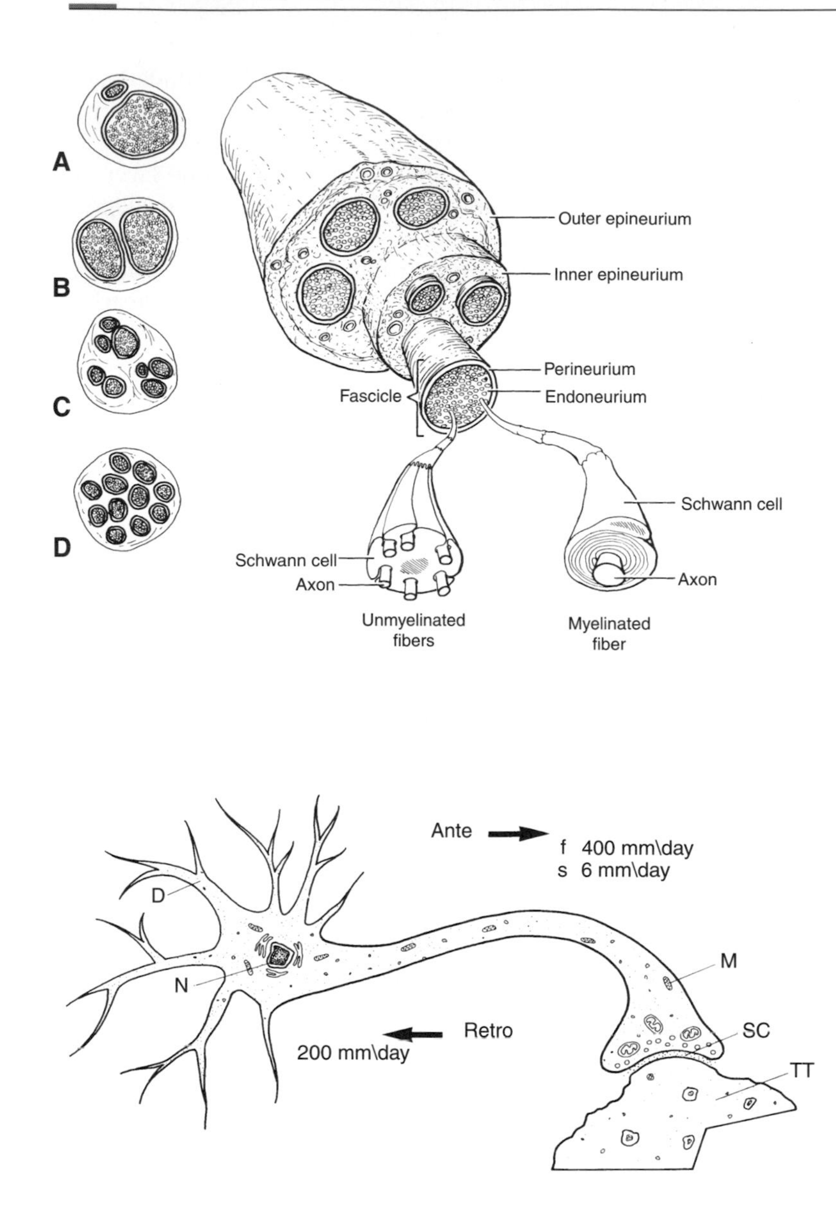

Figure 5-3 Connective tissues of peripheral nerves. Connective tissue elements consist of the endoneurium, the perineurium, and the inner and outer epineurium. Individual fascicles contain a heterogeneous mix of myelinated and unmyelinated fibers, but some fascicles demonstrate a preponderance of one type. Basic patterns of intraneural structure are demonstrated. A peripheral nerve is considered monofascicular if it holds one large fascicle **(A)** or oligofascicular for a few large fascicles **(B)**. Polyfascicular nerves consist of many fascicles, which may be grouped **(C)** or may exhibit no identifiable group patterns **(D)**. (Reprinted with permission from Terzis, J. K., & Smith, K. L. [1990]. *The peripheral nerve: Structure, function and reconstruction* [p. 16]. New York: Raven Press.)

Figure 5-4 Axoplasmic flow within a single neuron. *D,* Dendrite; *N,* nucleus; *M,* mitochondria; *SC,* synaptic cleft; *TT,* target tissue. (Reprinted with permission from Butler, D. S. [1991]. *Mobilisation of the nervous system* [p. 25]. New York: Churchill Livingstone.)

transported down the axon to the nerve terminal (synapse) via antegrade transport of axoplasm (Figure 5-4) (Dahlin & Lundborg, 1990; Droz, Rambourg, & Koenig, 1975; Grafstein & Forman, 1980). Translocation of materials from the nerve terminal is passed back through the axoplasm to the cell body via retrograde transport. Retrograde transport also informs the cell's body of the status of the axon, its terminals, and the nearby environment (Bisby & Keen, 1986).

The rate or velocity of axoplasmic flow is related to function (Grafstein & Forman, 1980). Slow antegrade transport replaces axoplasm along the length of the axon at a rate of 1 to 30 mm per day. Fast antegrade transport moves enzymes, neurotransmitters, vesicles, lipids, and glycoproteins at a velocity of 400 mm per day. Retrograde transport recycles vesicles from the nerve terminal and transports nerve growth factors to the cell body at a velocity ranging from

1 to 2 mm per day up to 300 mm per day. One role of nerve growth factors is to regulate select neuropeptides, such as substance P (Dahlin & Lundborg, 1990; Otten, 1984). Because axoplasmic flow enhances communication between the cell body, its axon, and its terminals, injury at one segment of the nerve may have an indirect impact on function at another segment (Upton & McComas, 1973).

Biomechanics of Peripheral Nerves

Response to Tension

Peripheral nerves initially respond to tension by straightening out fascicles. As a particular load increases, the nerve will elongate because of the elastic properties of its connective tissues (Bora, Richardson, & Black, 1980). It has been suggested that collagen, not elastin, may be responsible for the viscoelastic properties of the peripheral nerve, because elastin makes up only a small portion of the three connective tissues, being in greatest abundance within the perineurium (Tassler, Dellon, & Canoun, 1994). If mechanical deformation exceeds the nerve's ability to withstand a particular load, deterioration results.

Nerve Gliding

Peripheral nerves move in relation to their interfacing soft tissue (Figure 5-5). For example, during active motion, the median nerve glides 7 to 14 mm at the wrist level and 5 to 7 mm at the elbow level (Wilgis & Murphy, 1986). Internally, the interfascicular epineurium allows the nerve fascicles to glide against one another (Millesi, Zochy, & Rath, 1990; Rath & Millesi, 1990). Because peripheral nerves must have the ability to adapt passively and actively to different positions of the body, damage to the interfacing tissues or any nerve component will likely have a negative impact on nerve function (Millesi et al., 1990).

Pathology of Nerve Compressions

Disruptive Factors

Nerve compressions may arise from either ischemia, direct mechanical injury, or both. The initial cause of injury is often mechanical because of chronic low-pressure shear forces and excessive stretching (Dyck, Lais, Giannini, & Engelstand, 1990). Mechanical factors may induce ischemia and may affect microcirculation and vascular permeability. Mechanical factors include abnormal anatomy, postural deficits, trauma, and iatrogenic factors. After repetitive injury, the nerve may become entrapped (Walsh, 1994). After entrapment, the presence of edema and the formation of fibrosis begin to limit intraneural (internal) and extraneural (external) nerve mobility (Butler, 1991; Millesi et al., 1990). If the interfacing tissues become affected, nerve gliding may be reduced significantly.

Effect on Blood Flow

The maximum load a peripheral nerve can withstand depends on its course and composition. Although the connective tissues associated with a nerve can elongate, its blood vessels do not adapt to the same degree. Small alterations in length, pressure, or loading significantly affect nerves, and overstretching them may cause ischemia (Figure 5-6). The human median nerve can tolerate loads from 73 to 220 N, whereas the ulnar nerve can tolerate loads from 65 to 155 N without damage. Sunderland (1978) found the limit of nerve elongation to be between 11% and 17%, with structural failure occurring between 15% and 23% of resting length. Ogata and Naito (1986) found that average stretching of the sciatic nerve of more than 15.7% caused complete arrest of blood flow. Bora et al. (1980) found the maximal elongation of normal and operated nerves to be approximately 20%. Despite the ability to elongate, intraneural blood flow is altered when nerves are elongated more than 8% of their resting length, and blood flow ceases at 15% elongation (Lundborg & Rydevik, 1973). Clearly, nerves may sustain permanent damage from stretching.

Nerve compression of 20 to 30 mm Hg has been found to reduce venular blood flow in the epineurium. At pressures of 30 to 50 mm Hg, axonal transport may be inhibited and blood flow impaired (Rydevik, Lundborg, & Bagge,

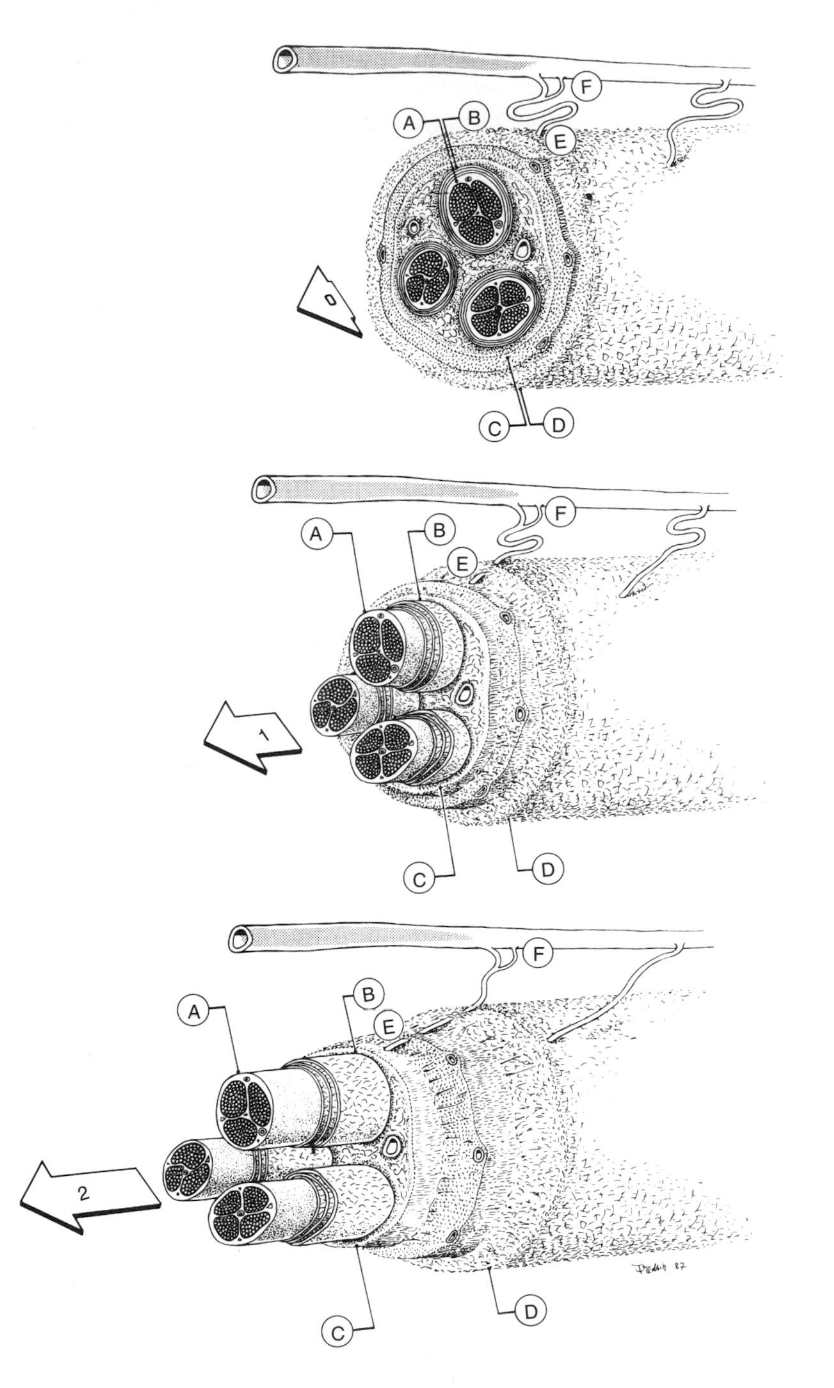

Figure 5-5 Gliding of inner connective tissues of peripheral nerves. *A,* Fascicle; *B,* perineurium; *C,* epineurium; *D,* adventitia; *E,* regional feeding vessel; *F,* extrinsic vessel. (Reprinted with permission from Lundborg, G. [1988]. *Nerve injury and repair* [p. 92]. New York: Churchill Livingstone.)

1981). Complete cessation of intraneural circulation has been observed with compression of 50 to 70 mm Hg or 60% to 70% mean arterial pressure (Ogata & Naito, 1986). Different postures influence compressive factors. For example, pronation of the forearm induces pressures greater than a neutral forearm position. Therefore, typists with suspected carpal tunnel

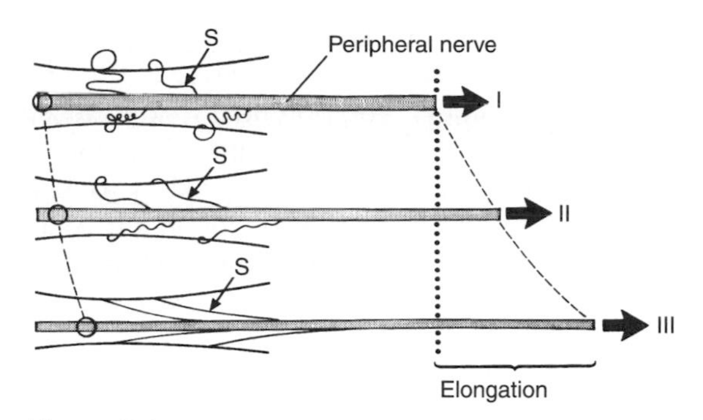

Figure 5-6 Nerve elongation and associated ischemia. Stage I: The segmental blood vessels *(S)* are normally coiled to allow for the physiologic movements of the nerve. Stage II: Under gradually increasing elongation, these regional vessels become stretched, and the blood flow within is impaired. Stage III: The cross-sectional area of the nerve (represented within the circle) is reduced during stretching, and the intraneural blood flow is further impaired. Complete cessation of all blood flow in the nerve usually occurs at approximately 15% elongation. (Reprinted with permission from Rydevik, B., Lundborg, G., & Skalak, R. [1989]. Biomechanics of peripheral nerves. In M. Nordin & V. H. Frankel [Eds.], *Basic biomechanics of the musculoskeletal system* [2nd ed., p. 81]. Philadelphia: Lea & Febiger.)

syndrome are advised to use "split keyboards," which encourages a neutral forearm position that reduces pressure within the carpal canal (Markison, 1990).

Effect on Axoplasmic Transport

Axoplasmic transport is affected by anoxia and ischemia because of its dependence on microvascular circulation. Alterations in transport may lead to morphologic and biochemical changes in the cell body. For instance, compression may alert the cell body through retrograde axonal transport to produce new Schwann cells (Lundborg & Dahlin, 1992). Changes in axonal flow or in the cell body also may make other parts of the nerve more susceptible to trauma (Dahlin & Lundborg, 1990). Nerves may experience double or multiple crush injuries, indicating that more than one region of the nerve may be impaired (MacKinnon, 1992; Osterman, 1988; Rydevik, McLean, Sjostrand, & Lundborg, 1990; Upton & McComas, 1973). Individuals with chronic compressive neuropathy may present with diffuse symptoms resulting from the presence of multiple segments of nerve damage (Anderson & Tichenor, 1994).

Neural Reorganization Secondary to Compression

Given alterations in sensory input secondary to peripheral nerve compressions, related regions of the CNS will reorganize (Lundborg, 2000; Merzenich & Jenkins, 1993). Through invasive animal studies, researchers have found that massive cortical reorganization occurs after sensory deafferentation (Byl & Melnick, 1997; Pearson, Arnold, Oladehin, Li, & Waters, 2001). Current hypotheses regarding mechanisms for reorganization in the somatosensory cortex can be divided into four categories.

1. There may be migration of cells that typically serve other parts of the body, into the deafferented region of the cortex (Allard, Clark, Jenkins, & Merzenich, 1991; Mogilner et al., 1993; Ramachandran, Rogers-Ramachandran, & Stewart, 1992). For example, the face may become more sensitive to light touch if the index finger has lost its sensibility.
2. Inhibitory controls in the affected region may be removed (Calford & Tweedale, 1991; Garraghty, Lachica, & Kaas, 1991; Rasmusson, Webster, & Dykes, 1992; Rothe et al., 1990; Turnbull & Rasmusson, 1990, 1991; Zarzecki, Witte, Smits, et al., 1993).
3. Existing subthreshold excitatory inputs and connections may be strengthened on the basis of experience postcompression (Beggs, Torsney, Drew, & Fitzgerald, 2002; Jenkins, Merzenich, & Raconzone, 1990; Merzenich & Sameshima, 1993; Pascual-Leone & Torres, 1993).
4. There may be subcortical reorganization, as in the basal ganglia, which project input to the cortex. (Garraghty et al., 1991; Merzenich, Kaas, Sur, & Lin, 1978; Pons, Garraghty, Ommaya, et al., 1991; Rasmusson et al., 1992).

Motor control is affected by the distorted or absent sensory input, as documented in clients with large-fiber neuropathy (Gordon, Ghilardi, &

Ghez, 1995; Sainburg, Poizner, & Ghez, 1993) and focal hand dystonia (Byl & Melnick, 1997). Diminished sensory input requires the use of adaptive strategies to maximize motor function. Because of the massive central reorganization after peripheral nerve injury, it is not surprising that individuals may have difficulty regaining full sensibility and motor control even with removal of compressive forces and regrowth of axons. Neural reorganization after injury is likely an activity-dependent process, so reduction or modification of exacerbating activities may in itself limit central reorganization (Beggs et al., 2002).

Classification of Nerve Injuries

Traditional Classification

Classification of nerve injuries enhances accurate communication among professionals. Seddon (1943) classified nerve injuries into three groups: neuropraxia, axonotmesis, and neurotmesis. Sunderland (1978) further separated nerve lesions into five categories. Both classifications are summarized in Figure 5-7. *Neuropraxia* (Sunderland I) is considered a conduction block induced by compression or stretching. *Axonotmesis* (Sunderland II) refers to an advanced nerve compression or traction injury. It suggests a loss of axonal continuity, with Wallerian degeneration and intact endoneurial tubes. Neurotmesis (Sunderland III-V) indicates loss of axonal continuity, with select loss of remaining elements of the nerve trunk. It refers also to cases of total nerve severance. Although this classification system is used widely, it is too extreme to sufficiently describe the subtle deficits found in mild compressive neuropathies.

Classification of Mild Compressions

A more useful classification of mild nerve compressions has been proposed by Butler (1991) (Table 5-2). The four general categories, which may occur in sequence, are: 1) the potential lesion, 2) physiologic pain, 3) the inflamed and irritated nerve, and 4) fibrosis of various areas. The *potential lesion* can be exemplified by edema in the carpal tunnel or blood around a nerve that induces *physiologic pain.* This pain may involve either the connective or neural tissue. Edema in the epineurial layer is the first sign of nerve injury. The potential lesion caused by edema may reduce blood flow. Irritation of the epineurium may develop secondary to mild compression or friction. A break in the perineurium may lead to persistent irritation or nerve pressure. If an irritation persists, intraneural or extraneural fibrosis may develop. Extraneural fibrosis may alter the ability of the nerve to glide against its surrounding tissues.

Acute Versus Chronic Conditions

Nerve compressions often are regarded as acute or chronic, with an intermediate subacute stage. The main difference between the two lies in the onset and progression of signs and symptoms.

As with tendinitis, injured nerves undergo an initial inflammatory response that will alter tissue integrity if the compressive forces or entrapping conditions are not alleviated. Secondary to compression or entrapment, nerves undergo focal slowing and display histologic signs of demyelinization and remyelinization (Nakano, 1991).

Long-standing peripheral nerve compression or entrapment may result in Wallerian degeneration. The components of Wallerian degeneration involve disintegration of the axon, shrinkage of the endoneurial tubes, breakdown of the myelin sheath, and disintegration of the end-organs. Degeneration may occur within select fascicles only and may not effect the entire nerve. Furthermore, even if the cell body reaction is minimal, reorganization of the somatosensory cortex is likely to occur (Wall, Xu, Wang, 2002). A reduction in proprioceptive feedback secondary to nerve compression will likely impact the recovery of motor control (Cope, Bonasera, & Nichols, 1994; Prochazka, Gillard, Bennett, 1997a, 1997b).

Major Upper-Limb Nerves with Potential Compression and Entrapment Sites

Cervicobrachial Region

The thoracic outlet (inlet) is a three-dimensional, triangular region that forms the

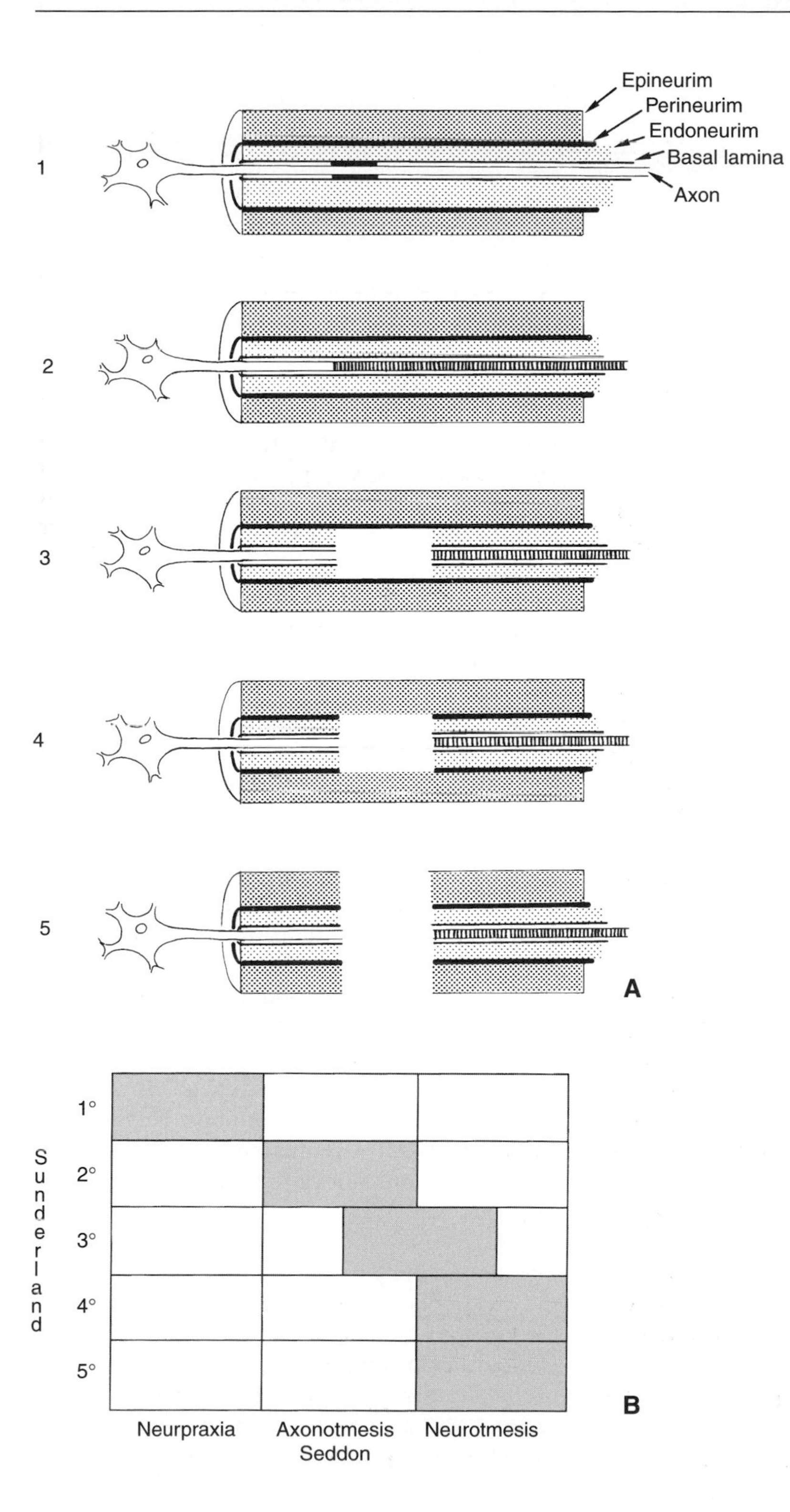

Figure 5.7 **A,** Classification of nerve injuries by Seddon and Sunderland. *1,* First-degree injury: local conduction blockade with minimal structural disruption. Prognosis: complete recovery within days to months. *2,* Second-degree injury: complete axonal disruption with wallerian degeneration; basal lamina remains intact. Prognosis: complete recovery within months. *3,* Third-degree injury: axonal and endoneurial disruption with interruption of the basal lamina. Prognosis: intrafascicular axonal admixture with regeneration yields mild to moderate reduction in function. *4,* Fourth-degree injury: axonal, endoneurial, and perineurial disruption. Prognosis: moderate to severe functional loss due to interfascicular axonal admixture; microsurgical manipulation can improve prognosis. *5,* Fifth-degree injury: complete structural disruption. Prognosis: No recovery without microsurgical manipulation. **B,** Comparison between Sunderland and Seddon's classifications. First-degree injuries correspond to neurapraxic injuries. Second-degree injuries are comparable to axonotmetric injuries. Third-degree injuries may be either axonotmetric or neurotmetric, and fourth- and fifth-degree injuries are neurotmetric. (Reprinted with permission from Terzis, J. K., & Smith, K. L. [1990]. *The peripheral nerve: Structure, function and reconstruction* [p. 40]. New York: Raven Press.)

Table 5-2
Pathophysiology of Mild Nerve Compressions

Potential Lesion	→ Physiologic Pain	→ Inflamed and Irritated Nerve	→ Fibrosis
Edema in carpal tunnel	Irritation of connective or neural tissue	Epineurial irritation; breach of perineurium with persistent irritation or nerve pressure	Intraneural or extraneural, which limits nerve gliding
Blood around a nerve	Reduced blood flow		

Source: Modified from D. S. Butler (1991). *Mobilisation of the nervous system.* New York: Churchill Livingstone.

superior opening of the thorax (Howell, 1991). Included in the medial wall of this triangle are the anterior scalene anteriorly, the middle scalene posteriorly, and the first rib inferiorly. The anterior-lateral wall extends from the second cervical vertebra to the clavicle and pectoralis minor. Finally, the posterior-lateral wall extends from the occiput to the attachments of the trapezius muscle (Pratt, 1991).

The subclavian artery and the brachial plexus, made up of spinal rami of C5, C6, C7, C8, and T1, travel together within the thoracic outlet, as seen in Figure 5-8 (Dawson, Hallett, & Millender, 1990; Pratt, 1991). After exiting the spinal cord, the spinal rami quickly combine into the upper, middle, and lower nerve trunks that, along with the subclavian artery, pass between the anterior and middle scalene musculature. All three trunks separate into posterior and anterior divisions before crossing over the first rib and beneath the clavicle in the region, termed the *costoclavicular interval*. As they travel beneath the pectoralis minor, the divisions combine to form the posterior, lateral, and medial cords. This region is termed the *axillary interval*. Within the axilla region, the cords eventually divide into terminal peripheral nerves.

The potential sites of compression or entrapment of the neurovascular structures that pass within this region include the interscalene triangle, the costoclavicular interval, and the axillary interval, as pictured in Figure 5-9 (Sanders & Haug, 1991; Walsh, 1994). Along with the listed sites, the presence of such anatomic anomalies as a cervical rib or a prefixed plexus (large C4 contribution) may exacerbate symptoms further.

Radial Nerve

The radial nerve is a continuation of the posterior cord of the brachial plexus (Pratt, 1991; Matloub & Yousif, 1992). As depicted in Figure 5-10, it courses through the axilla, then moves from medial to lateral on the posterior humerus in the spiral groove, where it innervates the triceps. The nerve then travels anteriorly at the elbow, where it innervates the brachioradialis, extensor carpi radialis longus (ECRL), and extensor carpi radialis brevis (ECRB). Distal to the elbow, it rests on the head of the radius, where it divides into a superficial and a deep branch. The deep branch (posterior interosseous nerve) travels beneath the edge of the ECRB. After it innervates and pierces the supinator muscle, it innervates the extensor carpi ulnaris, the extensor digitorum communis, the extensor digiti minimi, the abductor pollicis longus (APL), the extensor pollicis longus, the extensor pollicis brevis, and the extensor indicis. The superficial branch travels underneath the brachioradialis and emerges distally between the attachment of the brachioradialis and the ECRB, near the anatomic snuff-box. This sensory branch serves the cutaneous portion of the radial three and one-half digits, excluding the nail beds.

The potential sites of radial nerve entrapment include the axilla region between the heads of the triceps, the radial tunnel (region of supinator) between the tendons of the ECRL and brachioradialis in the forearm, and the region near the anatomic snuff-box (Rosenbaum, 1999; Szabo, 1989). The posterior interosseous branch may also become entrapped or compressed after

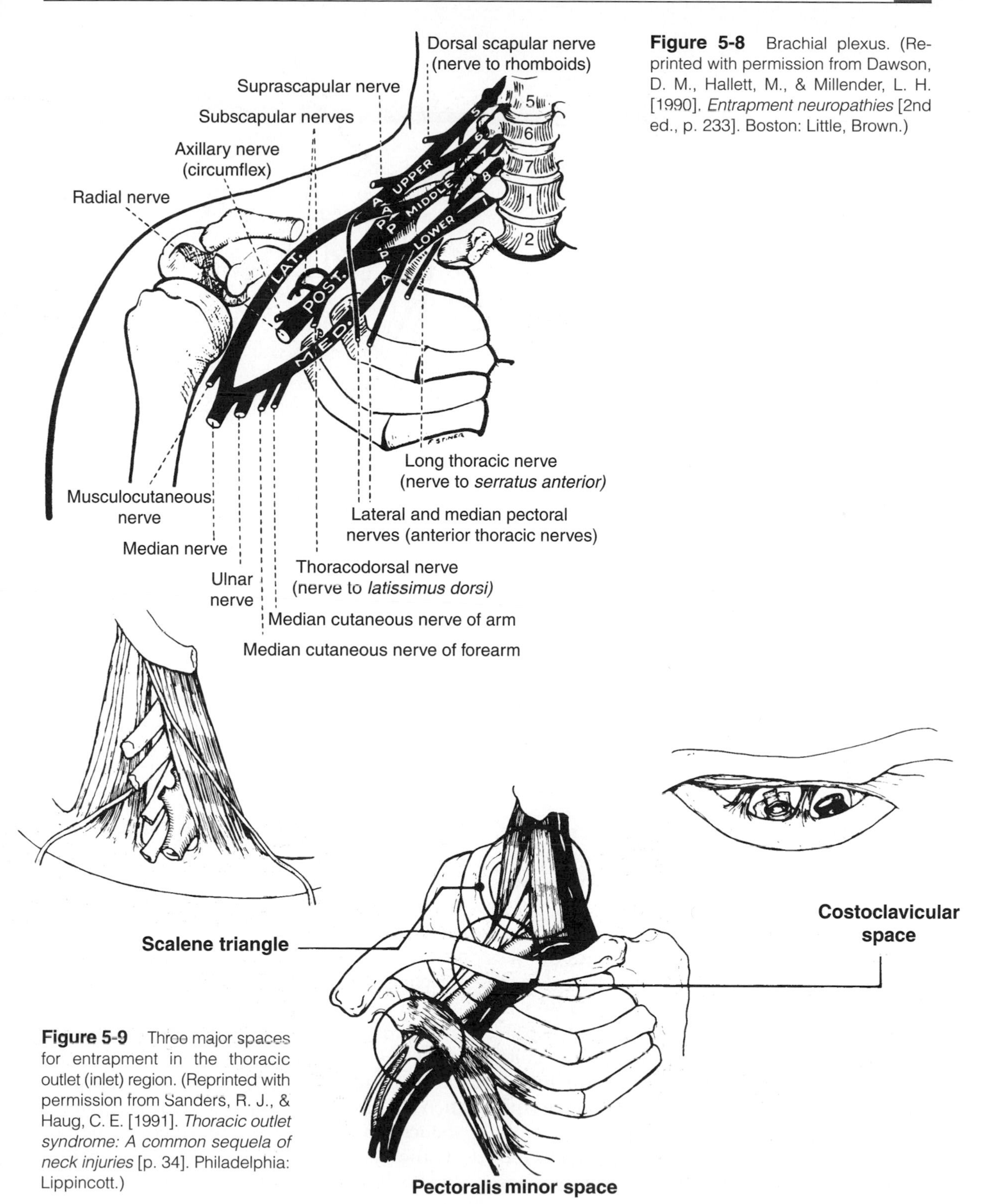

Figure 5-8 Brachial plexus. (Reprinted with permission from Dawson, D. M., Hallett, M., & Millender, L. H. [1990]. *Entrapment neuropathies* [2nd ed., p. 233]. Boston: Little, Brown.)

Figure 5-9 Three major spaces for entrapment in the thoracic outlet (inlet) region. (Reprinted with permission from Sanders, R. J., & Haug, C. E. [1991]. *Thoracic outlet syndrome: A common sequela of neck injuries* [p. 34]. Philadelphia: Lippincott.)

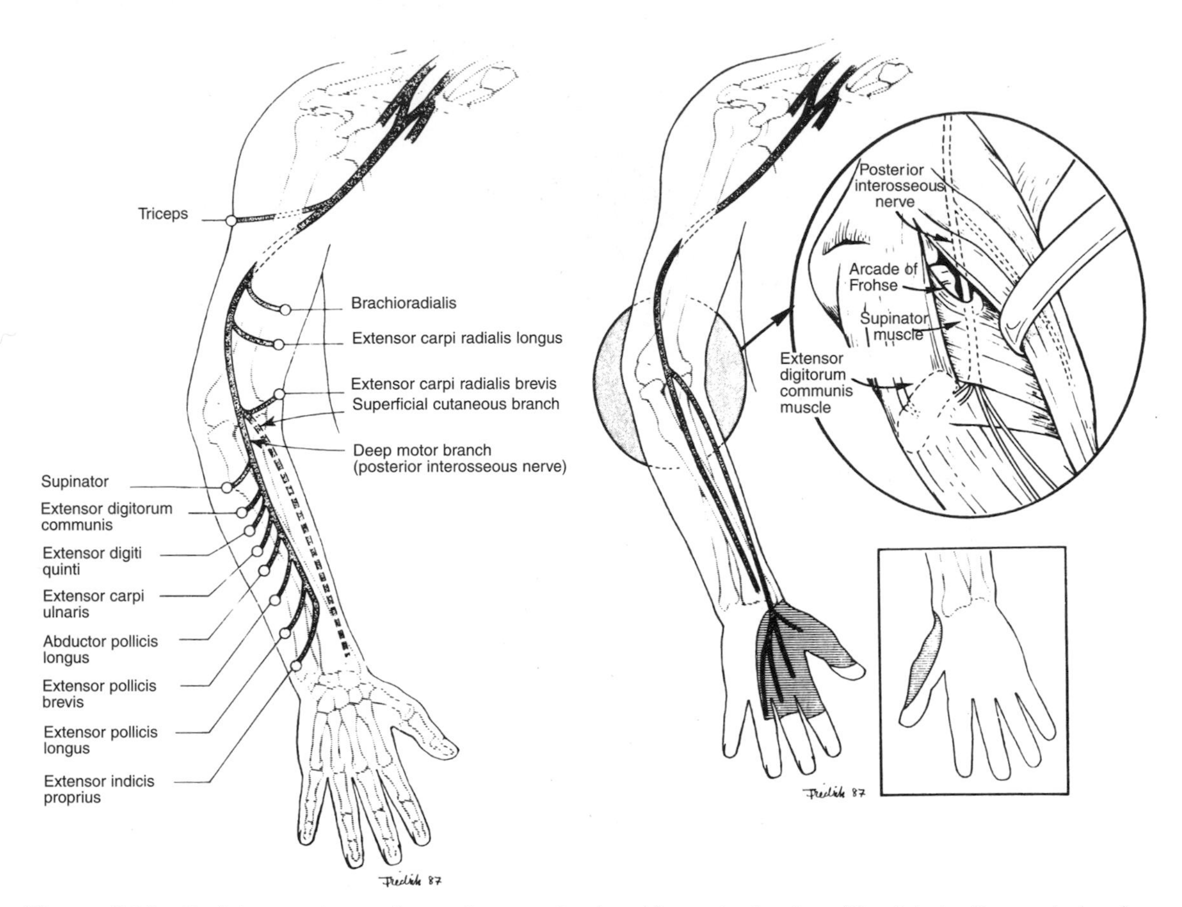

Figure 5-10 Radial nerve innervation patterns and vulnerable anatomic sites. (Reprinted with permission from Lundborg G. [1988]. *Nerve injury and repair* [p. 135]. New York: Churchill Livingstone.)

it branches off from the radial nerve. The supinator muscle region and the anatomic snuff-box region are the most vulnerable areas (see Figure 5-10).

Median Nerve

The median nerve receives branches off the lateral and medial cords of the brachial plexus, with spinal nerve contributions from C5, C6, C7, C8, and T1 (Matloub & Yousif, 1992; Pratt, 1991). The median nerve courses through the axilla and progresses medial to the humerus in the upper arm. Distally, it travels between the brachialis and the biceps until it passes beneath the ligament of Struthers. After this landmark, it begins to innervate the forearm muscles (Figure 5-11). In the cubital fossa, the nerve rests medial to the biceps tendon, then traverses under the bicipital aponeurosis. After passing through the two heads of the pronator teres, the median nerve plunges beneath the edge of the flexor digitorum superficialis (FDS). After traveling beneath the FDS in the forearm, the median nerve emerges 5 cm proximal to the carpal tunnel. It courses through the tunnel to serve the cutaneous portion of the radial three and one-half digits, lumbricals I and II, and the thenar muscle group: opponens pollicis, abductor pollicis brevis, and superficial portion of the flexor pollicis brevis. The palmar cutaneous branch, which serves the skin of the

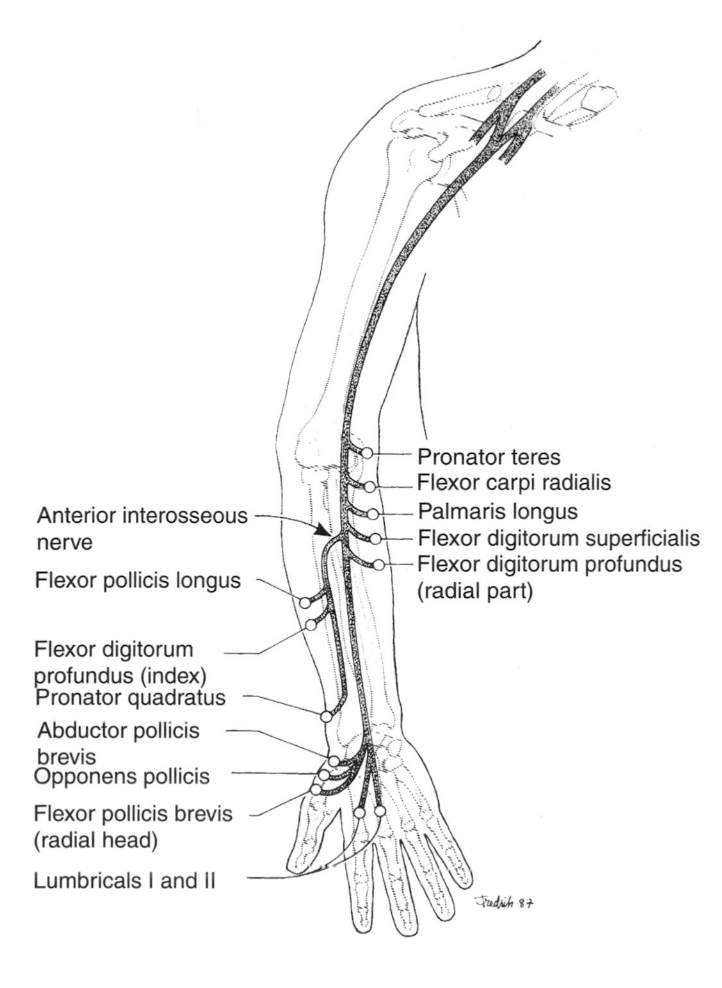

Figure 5-11 Median nerve innervation patterns. (Reprinted with permission from Lundborg G. [1988]. *Nerve injury and repair* [p. 113]. New York: Churchill Livingstone.)

thenar eminence, does not course through the carpal tunnel (Figure 5-12). The anterior interosseous nerve branches off from the median nerve approximately 5 cm distal to the medial epicondyle and innervates the flexor pollicis longus (FPL), the flexor digitorum profundus (FDP) to the index and long fingers, and the pronator teres.

Potential sites of entrapment (see Figure 5-12) are beneath the ligament of Struthers, the proximal forearm (location of pronator syndrome), and the carpal tunnel (Szabo, 1989). The anterior interosseous nerve may become compressed as it branches off from the median nerve.

Ulnar Nerve

The ulnar nerve is a continuation of the medial cord of the brachial plexus, with C8 and T1 spinal nerve contributions (Pratt, 1991; Matloub & Yousif, 1992). The ulnar nerve courses through the axilla medially to the triceps before moving posteriorly behind the medial epicondyle through the cubital tunnel. In the forearm, it traverses between the heads of the flexor carpi ulnaris and travels distally deep to this muscle. The muscles innervated by the ulnar nerve in the forearm include flexor carpi ulnaris and the FDP to the ring finger and small fingers (Figure 5-13). Approximately 2 cm proximal to the wrist, the nerve sends off a

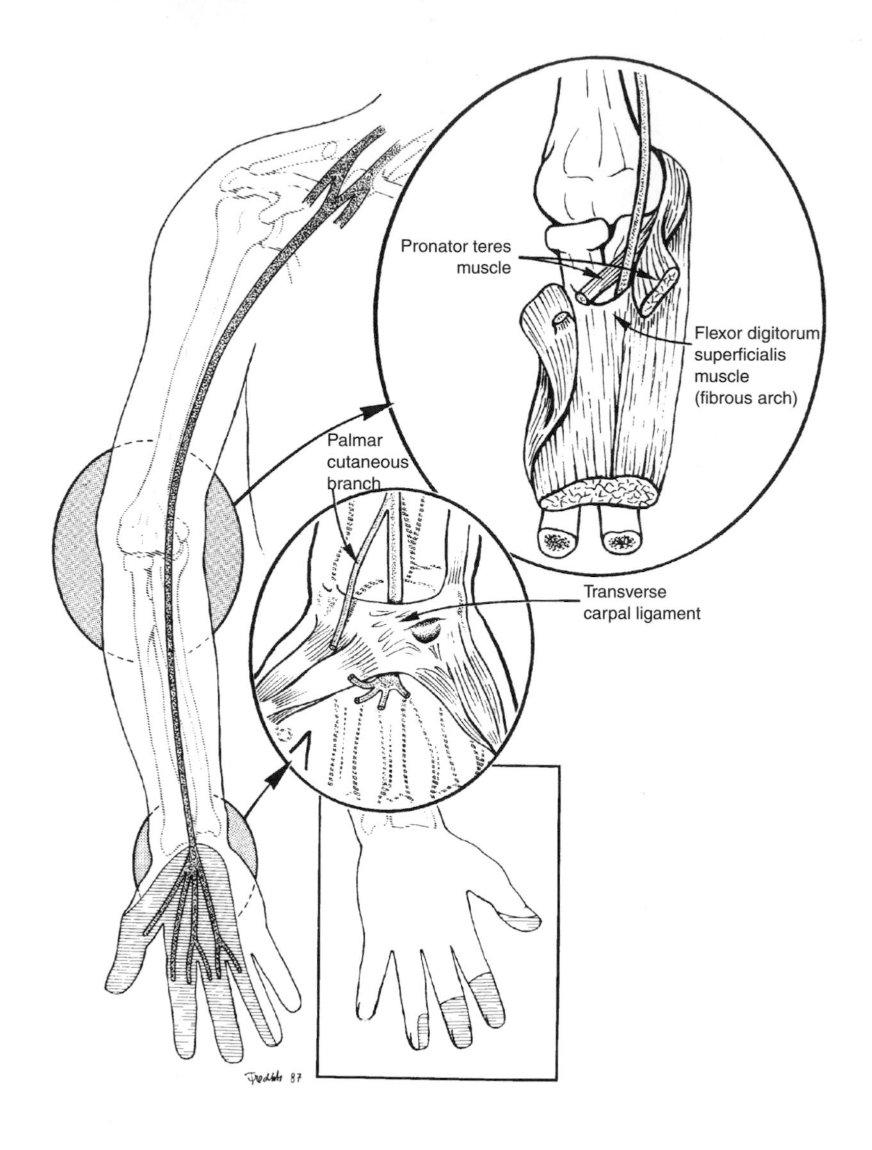

Figure 5-12 Median nerve cutaneous innervation and critical anatomic areas. (Reprinted with permission from Lundborg G. [1988]. *Nerve injury and repair* [p. 114]. New York: Churchill Livingstone.)

dorsal cutaneous branch to serve the dorsal one and one-half digits (Figure 5-14). The volar branch then continues its course through Guyon's tunnel. The ulnar nerve eventually innervates the ulnar side of the fifth digit and the ulnar half of the fourth digit. In the hand, it innervates the following muscles: flexor digiti minimi, adductor digiti minimi, opponens digiti minimi, dorsal and palmar interossei, lumbricals III and IV, the deep portion of the flexor pollicis brevis, and the adductor pollicis. Potential sites of entrapment or compression of the ulnar nerve include the cubital tunnel region and the region of Guyon's tunnel (see Figure 5-14) (Szabo, 1989).

Anastomosis

The median nerve may form connections with the ulnar nerve in the forearm. The most common is the Martin-Gruber anastomosis, a motor connection between the two in the proximal forearm (Amoiridis & Vlachonikolis, 2003; Matloub & Yousif, 1992). The anterior

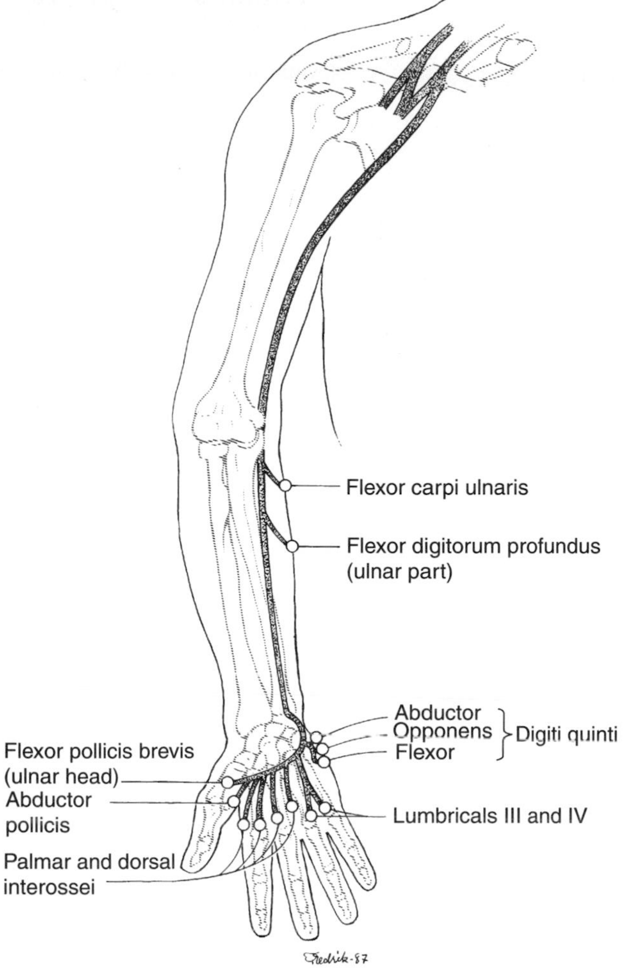

Figure 5-13 Ulnar nerve innervation patterns. (Reprinted with permission from Lundborg G. [1988]. *Nerve injury and repair* [p. 129]. New York: Churchill Livingstone.)

interosseous may also connect with the ulnar nerve more distally. Other less common anastomoses may be responsible for entrapment syndromes, causing symptoms that do not follow a logical pattern. Diagnosis of these unusual anastomoses is difficult. If symptoms are severe enough and impeding function, surgical intervention may be warranted.

SUMMARY

Musculoskeletal disorders often stem from overuse or repetitive injury to muscular or neural tissues. This chapter reviewed the anatomy and biomechanics associated with tendonopathies and nerve compressions or entrapments and their associated conditions. Understanding the anatomical and physiological complexities of these various disorders may provide the background needed to employ sensitive evaluation tools and search for treatment strategies that will enhance recovery. In the next chapter, evaluation strategies and methods of intervention for musculoskeletal disorders are reviewed.

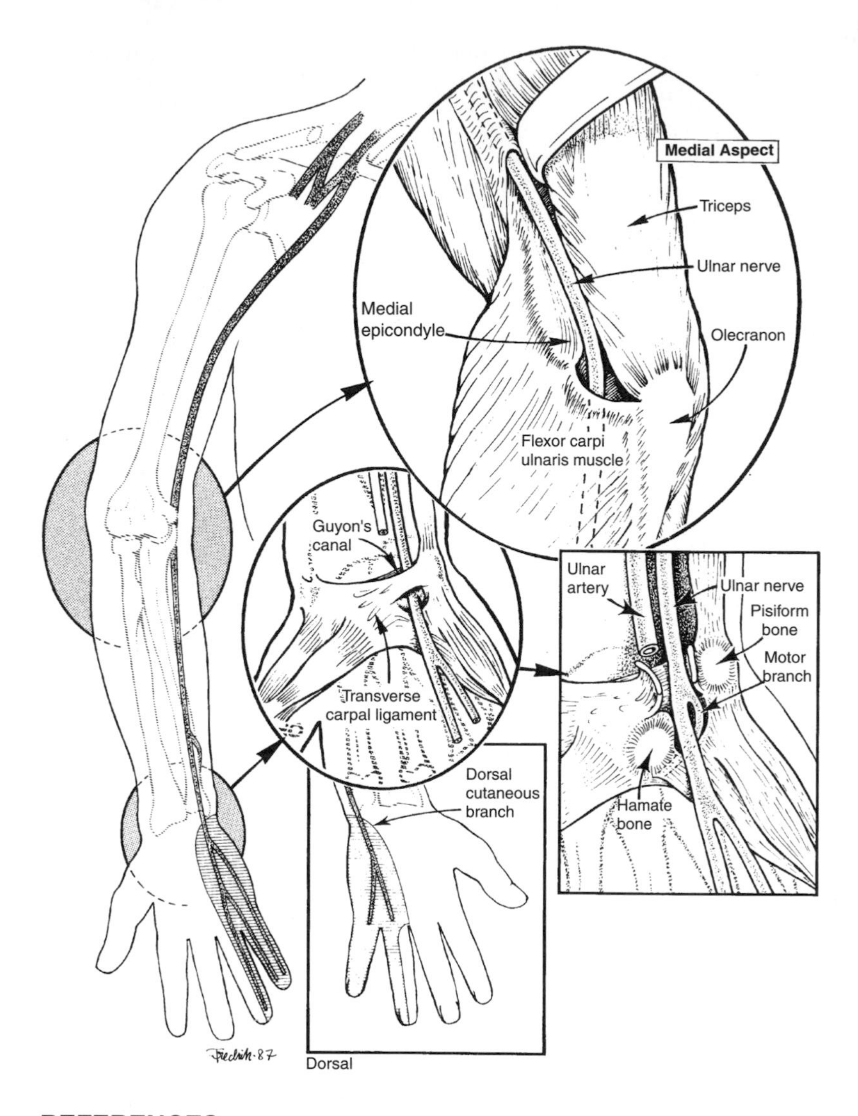

Figure 5-14 Ulnar nerve cutaneous innervation and critical anatomic area. (Reprinted with permission from Lundborg G. [1988]. *Nerve injury and repair* [p. 130]. New York: Churchill Livingstone.)

REFERENCES

Alfredson, H., Bjur, D., Thorsen, K., Lorentzon, R., & Sandstrom, P. (2002). High intratendinous lactate levels in painful chronic Achilles tendinosis. An investigation using microdialysis technique. *Journal of Orthopaedic Research, 20*(5), 934-938.

Alfredson, H., & Lorentzon, R. (2002). Chronic tendon pain: No signs of chemical inflammation but high concentrations of the neurotransmitter glutamate. Implications for treatment? *Current Drug Targets, 3*(1), 43-54.

Almekinders, L. C., & Deol, G. (1999). The effects of aging, anti-inflammatory drugs, and ultrasound on the vitro response of tendon tissue. *American Journal of Sports Medicine, 27*(4), 417-421.

Allard, T., Clark, S.A., Jenkins, W. M., & Merzenich, M. M. (1991). Reorganization of somatosensory area 3b representations in adult owl monkeys after digital syndactyly. *Journal of Neurophysiology, 66,* 1048-1058.

Amoiridis, G., & Vlachonikolis, I .G. (2003). Verification of the median-to-ulnar nerve motor fiber anastomosis in the forearm: An electrophysiological study. *Clinics in Neurophysiology, 14*(1), 94-98.

Anderson, M., & Tichenor, C J. (1994). A patient with de Quervain's tenosynovitis: A case report using an Australian approach to manual therapy. *Physical Therapy, 74,* 314-326.

Backman, C., Friden, J., & Widmark, A. (1991). Blood flow in chronic Achilles tendinosis. Radioactive microsphere study in rabbits. *Acta Orthopaedic of Scandanavia, 62,* 386-387.

Baker, P. F., Ladds, M., & Rubinson, K. A. (1977). Measurement of the flow properties of isolated axoplasm in a defined chemical environment. *Journal of Physiology (Lond), 269,* 10-11.

Barbe, M. F., Barr, A. E., Gorzelany, I., Amin, M., Gaughan, J. P., & Safadi, F. F. (2003). Chronic repetitive reaching and grasping results in decreased motor performance and widespread tissue responses in a rat model of MSD. *Journal of Orthopaedic Research, 21*(1), 167-176.

Barr, A. E., & Barbe, M. F. (2002). Pathophysiological tissue changes associated with repetitive movements: Review of the evidence. *Physical Therapy, 82*(2), 173-187.

Beggs, S., Torsney, C., Drew, L. J., & Fitzgerald, M. (2002). The postnatal reorganization of primary afferent input and dorsal horn cell receptive fields in the rat spinal cord is an activity-dependent process. *European Journal of Neuroscience 16*(7), 1249-1258.

Birk, D. E., & Zycband, E. (1994). Assembly of the tendon extracellular matrix during development. *Journal of Anatomy, 184,* 457-463.

Bisby, M.A., & Keen, P. (1986). Regeneration of primary afferent neurons containing substance P-like immunoreactivity. *Brain Research, 365,* 85-95.

Blake, D.T., Byl, N. N., Cheung, S., Bedenbaugh, P., Nagarajan, S., Lamb, M., & Merzenich, M. M. (2002). Sensory representation abnormalities that parallel focal hand dystonia in a primate model. *Somatosensory Motor Research, 19*(4), 347-357.

Blake, D.T., Byl, N. N., & Merzenich, M. M. (2002). Representation of the hand in the cerebral cortex. *Behavioral Brain Research, 135*(1-2), 179-184.

Bora, F.W., Richardson W., & Black J. (1980). The biomechanical responses to tension in a peripheral nerve. *Journal of Hand Surgery [Am], 5*(1), 21-25.

Borynsenko, M., & Beringer, T. (1989). *Functional histology* (3rd ed., pp. 105-112). Boston: Little, Brown.

Butler, D. S. (1991). *Mobilisation of the nervous system.* New York: Churchill Livingstone.

Byl, N. N., & Melnick, M. (1997). The neural consequences of repetition: Clinical implications of a learning hypothesis. *Journal of Hand Therapy, 10*(2), 160-174.

Byl, N. N., & Merzenich, M. M. (2002). Focal hand dystonia. In E. J. Mackin, A. D. Callahan, A. L. Osterman, T. M. Skirven, L. H. Schneider, & J. M. Hunter (Eds.), *Hunter-Mackin-Callahan Rehabilitation of the hand and upper extremity* (5th ed., pp. 2053-2075). St. Louis: Mosby.

Cailliet, R. (1991). *Shoulder pain* (3rd ed.). Philadelphia: Davis.

Calford, M. B., & Tweedale R. (1991). Immediate expansion of receptive fields of neurons in area 3b of macaque monkeys after digit denervation. *Somatosensory Motor Research, 8,* 249-260.

Carlstedt, C.A. (1987). Mechanical and chemical factors in tendon healing. Effects of indomethacin and surgery in the rabbit. *Acta Orthopaedics Scandinavian Supplement, 224,* 1-75.

Carlstedt, C.A., Madsen, K., & Wredmark, T. (1986). The influence of indomethacin on collagen synthesis during tendon healing in the rabbit. *Prostaglandins, 32,* 353.

Carlstedt, C.A., & Nordin, M. (1989). Biomechanics of tendons and ligaments. In M. Nordin & V. H. Frankel (Eds.), *Basic biomechanics of the musculoskeletal system* (2nd ed., pp. 59-74). Philadelphia: Lea & Febiger.

Clancy, W. G. (1990). Tendon trauma and overuse injuries. In W. B. Leadbetter, J. A. Buckwalter, & S. L. Gordon (Eds.), *Sports-induced inflammation: Clinical and basic science concepts* (p. 609). Park Ridge, IL: Academy of Orthopedic Surgeons.

Cope, T. C., Bonasera, S. J., & Nichols, T. R. (1994). Reinnervated muscles fail to produce stretch reflexes. *Journal of Neurophysiology, 71*(2), 817-820.

Curwin, S., & Stanish, W. D. (1984). *Tendinitis: Its etiology and treatment.* Lexington, MA: Collamore Press/DC Heath.

Cyriax, J. (1982). *Textbook of orthopaedic medicine, Vol 1: Diagnosis of soft-tissue lesions* (8th ed.). London: Bailliere Tindall.

Dahlin, L. B., & Lundborg, G. (1990). The neurone and its response to peripheral nerve compression. *Journal of Hand Surgery [Am], 15,* 5-10.

Dawson, D. M., Hallett, M., & Millender L. H. (1990). *Entrapment neuropathies* (2nd ed.). Boston: Little, Brown.

Droz, B., Rambourg, A., & Koenig, H. L. (1975). The smooth endoplasmic reticulum: Structure and role in the renewal of axonal membrane and synaptic vesicles by fast axonal transport. *Brain Research, 93,* 1-13.

Dyck, P. J., Lais, A. C., Giannini, C., & Engelstand, J. K. (1990). Structural alterations of nerve during cuff compression. *Proceedings from the National Academy of Science U S A, 87,* 9828-9832.

Elbert, T., Candia, V., Altenmüller, E., Rau, H., Sterr, A., Rockstroh, B. et al. (1998). Alteration of digital representations in somatosensory cortex in focal hand dystonia. *NeuroReport, 9,* 3571-3575.

Elliott, D. H. (1967). The biomechanical properties of tendon in relation to muscular strength. *Annals in Physical Medicine, 9,* 1.

Evans, R. B., Hunter, J. M., & Burkhalter, W. E, (1988). Conservative management of the trigger finger: A new approach. *Journal of Hand Therapy, 1*(2), 59-74.

Fenwick, S.A., Curry, V., Harrall, R. L., Hazleman, B. L., Hackney, R., & Riley, G. P. (2001). Expression of transforming growth factor-beta isoforms and their receptors in chronic tendinosis. *Journal of Anatomy, 199*(Pt 3), 231-240.

Fenwick, S.A., Hazleman, B. L., & Riley, G. P. (2002). The vasculature and its role in the damaged and healing tendon. *Arthritis Research, 4*(4), 252-260.

Fyfe, I., & Stanish, W. D. (1992). The use of eccentric training and stretching in the treatment and prevention of tendon injuries. *Clinics in Sports Medicine, 11,* 601-624.

Garraghty, P. E., Lachica, E.A., & Kaas, J. H. (1991). Injury-induced reorganization of somatosensory cortex is accompanied by reductions in GABA staining. *Somatosensory and Motor Research, 8,* 347-354.

Garrett, W. E. Jr., Nikolaou, P. K., Ribbeck, B. M., Glisson, R. R., & Seaber, A.V. (1988). The effect of muscle architecture on the biomechanical failure properties of skeletal muscle under passive tension. *American Journal of Sports Medicine, 16*(1), 7-12.

Gelberman, R. H. (1991). *Operative nerve repair and reconstruction,* Vols 1 & 2. Philadelphia: Lippincott.

Gerber, G., Gerber, G., & Altman, K. I. (1960). Studies on the metabolism of tissue proteins: I. Turnover of collagen labeled with proline-U-C14 in young rats. *Journal of Biology and Chemistry, 235,* 2653-2656.

Gordon, A. M., Huxley, A. F., & Julian, F. J. (1966). Tension development in highly stretched vertebrate muscle fibers. *Journal of Physiology, 184,* 143-169.

Gordon, J., Ghilardi, M. F., & Ghez, C. (1995). Impairments of reaching movements in patients without proprioception: I. Spatial errors. *Journal of Neurophysiology, 73,* 347-360.

Grafstein, B., & Forman, D. S. (1980). Intracellular transport in neurons. *Physiology Review, 60,* 1167.

Grundberg, A. B., & Reagan, D. S. (1985). Pathologic anatomy of the forearm: intersection syndrome. *Journal of Hand Surgery [Am], 10,* 299-305.

Haak, R.A., Kleinhaus, F.W., & Ochs, S. (1976). The viscosity of mammalian nerve axoplasm measured by electron spin resonance. *Journal of Physiology, 263,* 115-137.

Howell, J.W. (1991). Evaluation and management of thoracic outlet syndrome. In R. Donatelli (Ed.), *Physical Therapy of the Shoulder* (2nd ed., pp. 151-190). New York: Churchill Livingstone.

Jenkins, W. M., Merzanich, M. M., & Raconzone, G. (1990). Neocortical representational dynamics in adult primates. *Neuropsychologia, 28,* 573-584.

Jozsa, L., Reffy, A., Kannus, P., Demel, S., & Elek E. (1990). Pathological alterations in human tendons. *Archives of Orthopaedics and Trauma Surgery, 110,* 15-21.

Kahn, K. M., Cook, J. L., Bonar, F., Harcourt, P., & Astrom M. (1999). Histopathology of common tendinopathies. Update and implications for clinical management. *Sports, 27*(6), 393-408.

Kasletic, J., & Baer, E. (1980). Deformation in tendon collagen. *Symposium from the Society of Experimental Biology, 34,* 397-435.

Kasletic, J., Galeski, A., & Baer, E. (1978). The multicomposite structure of tendons. *Connective Tissue Research, 6,* 11-23.

Kennedy, J. C., & Baxter-Willis, R. (1976). The effects of local steroid injections on tendons: A biochemical and microscopic correlative study. *American Journal of Sports Medicine, 4,* 11-18.

Kirkendall, D.T., & Garrett, W. E. (2002). Clinical perspectives regarding eccentric muscle injury. *Clinics in Orthopaedics,* October (403 Suppl.), S81-89.

Kvist, M., Hurme, T., Kannus, P., Jarvinen, T., Maunu, V. M., Jozsa, L. et al. (1995). Vascular density at the myotendinous junction of the rat gastronemius muscle after immobilization and remobilization. *American Journal of Sports Medicine, 23*(3), 359-364.

Langberg, H., Rosendal, L., & Kjaer, M. (2001). Training-induced changes in peritendinous type I collagen turnover determined by microdialysis in humans. *Journal of Physiology, 534*(Pt 1), 297-302.

Leadbetter, W. B. (1991). Physiology of tissue repair. In *Athletic training and sports medicine*. Park Ridge, IL: American Academy of Orthopedic Surgeons.

Leadbetter, W. B. (1992). Cell-matrix response in tendon injury. *Clinics in Sports Medicine, 11,* 533-578.

Littler, J. W. (1977). Stenosing digital tendovaginitis. In J. M. Converse & J. W. Littler (Eds.), *Reconstructive plastic surgery, Vol 6: The hand and upper extremity* (pp. 3440-3443). New York: Saunders.

Lundborg, G. (1979). The intrinsic vascularization of human peripheral nerves: structural and functional aspects. *Journal of Hand Surgery, 4*(1), 34.

Lundborg, G. (2000). Brain plasticity and hand surgery: An overview. *Journal of Hand Surgery, 25*(3), 242-252.

Lundborg, G., & Dahlin, L. B. (1992). The pathophysiology of nerve compression. *Hand Clinics, 8,* 215-227.

Lundborg, G., & Rank, F. (1978). Experimental intrinsic healing of flexor tendons based on synovial fluid nutrition. *Journal of Hand Surgery [Am], 3,* 21-31.

Lundborg, G., & Rydevik, B. (1973). Effects of stretching the tibial nerve of the rabbit: A preliminary study of the intraneural circulation and the barrier function of the perineurium. *Journal Bone and Joint Surgery [Br], 55,* 390-401.

Mackinnon, S. E. (1992). Double and multiple entrapment neuropathies. *Hand Clinics, 8,* 369-390.

Maffulli, N., Khan, K. M., & Puddu, G. (1998). *Arthroscopy, 14*(8), 840-843.

Markison, R. E. (1990). Treatment of musical hands: Redesign of the interface. *Hand Clinics, 6,* 525-544.

Markison, R. E. (1992). Tendinitis and related inflammatory conditions seen in musicians. *Journal of Hand Therapy, 5*(2), 80-83.

Matloub, H. S., & Yousif, N. J. (1992). Peripheral nerve anatomy and innervation pattern. *Hand Clinics, 8,* 201-214.

Merzenich, M. M., & Jenkins, W. M. (1993). Reorganization of cortical representation of the hand following alterations of skin inputs induced by nerve injury, skin island transfers and experience. *Journal of Hand Therapy, 6*(2), 89-104.

Merzenich, M. M., Kaas, J. H., Sur, M., & Lin, C-S. (1978). Double representation of the body surface within cytoarchitectonic areas 3b and 1 in "S1" in the owl monkey (*Aotus trivirgatus*). *Journal of Comparative Neurology, 181,* 41-74.

Merzenich, M. M., & Sameshima, K. (1993). Cortical plasticity and memory. *Current Biology, 3,* 187-196.

Meyer, H. P. (2002). Myofascial pain syndrome and its suggested role in the pathogenesis and treatment of fibromyalgia syndrome. *Current Pain and Headache Report, 6*(4), 274-283.

Millesi, H., Zoch, G., & Rath, T. H. (1990). The gliding apparatus of peripheral nerve and its clinical significance. *Annals Hand Surgery, 9*(2), 87-97.

Mogilner, A., Grossman, J. A., Ribary, U., Joliot, M., Volkmann, J., Rapaport, D. et al. (1993). Somatosensory cortical plasticity in adult humans revealed by magnetoencephalography. *Proceedings of the National Academy of Science U S A, 90,* 3593-3597.

Moran, C. A. (1994). Using myofascial techniques to treat musicians. *Journal of Hand Therapy, 5*(2), 97-101.

Mosier, S. M., Pomeroy, G., & Manoli, A. II (1999). Pathoanatomy and etiology of posterior tibial tendon dysfunction. *Clinical Orthopedics and Related Research,* August (365), 12-22.

Nakano, K. K. (1991). Peripheral nerve entrapments, repetitive strain disorder, occupation-related syndromes, bursitis and tendonitis. *Current Opinion in Rheumatology, 3,* 226-239.

Nirschl, R. P. (1992). Elbow tendinosis/tennis elbow. *Clinics in Sports Medicine, 11,* 851-870.

O'Brien, M. (1992). Functional anatomy and physiology of tendons. *Clinics in Sports Medicine, 11,* 505-520.

Odergren, T., Iwasaki, N., Borg, J., & Forssberg, H. (1996). Impaired sensory-motor integration during grasping in writer's cramp. *Brain,* 119(Pt 2), 569-583.

Ogata, K., & Naito, M. (1986). Blood flow of peripheral nerve effects of dissection, stretching and compression. *Journal of Hand Surgery [Br], 11*(1), 10-14.

Ohkawa, S. (1982). Effects of orthodontic forces and anti-inflammatory drugs on the mechanical strength of the periodontium in the rat mandibular first molar. *American Journal of Orthodontics, 81,* 498.

Olsson, Y., & Kristennson, K. (1971). Permeability of blood vessels and connective tissue sheaths in the peripheral nervous system to exogenous proteins. *Acta Neuropathology, 5,* 61-69.

Osterman, A. L. (1988, January). The double crush syndrome. *Orthopedic Clinics of North America, 19,* 147-155.

Otten, U. (1984). Nerve growth factor and the peptidergic sensory neurons. *Trends in Pharmacology,* 7, 307-310.

Pascual-Leone, A., & Torres, F. (1993). Plasticity of the sensorimotor cortex representation of the reading finger in Braille readers. *Brain, 116,* 39-52.

Pearson, P. P., Arnold, P. B., Oladehin, A., Li, C. X., & Waters, R. S. (2001). Large-scale cortical reorganization following forelimb deafferentation in rat does not involve plasticity of intracortical connections. *Experimental Brain Research, 138*(1), 8-25.

Piligian, G., Herbert, R., Hearns, M., Dropkin, J., Landsbergis, P., & Cherniack, M. (2000). Evaluation and management of chronic work-related musculoskeletal disorders of the distal upper extremity. *American Journal of Industrial Medicine, 37*(1), 75-93.

Pons, T. P., Garraghty, P. E., Ommaya, A. K., Kaas, J. H., Taub, E., & Mishkin, M. (1991). Massive cortical reorganization after sensory deafferentation in adult macaques. *Science, 252,* 1857-1860.

Pratt, N.E. (1991). *Clinical musculoskeletal anatomy.* Philadelphia: Lippincott.

Prochazka, A., Gillard, D., & Bennett, D. J. (1997a). Implications of positive feedback in the control of movements. *Journal of Neurophysiology, 77*(6), 3237-3251.

Prochazka, A., Gillard, D., & Bennett, D. J. (1997b). Positive force feedback control of muscles. *Journal of Neurophysiology, 77*(6), 3226-3236.

Puddu, G., Ippolito, E., & Postacchini, P. (1976). A classification of achilles tendon disease. *American Journal of Sports Medicine, 4,* 145-150.

Ramachandran, V. S., Rogers-Ramachandran, D., & Stewart, M. (1992). Perceptual correlates of massive cortical reorganization. *Science, 258,* 1159-1160.

Rasmusson, D. D., Webster, H. H., & Dykes, R. W. (1992). Neuronal response properties within subregions of racoon somatosensory cortex 1 week after digit amputation. *Somatosensory and Motor Research, 9,* 279-289.

Rath, T., & Millesi, H. (1990). The gliding tissue of the median nerve in the carpal tunnel [German abstract]. *Handchirurgie Mikrochirurgie plastische Chirurgie, 22*(4), 203-205.

Riley, G. P., Harrall, R. L., Constant, C. R., Cawston, T. E., & Hazleman, B. L. (1994). Glycosaminoglycans of human rotator cuff tendons: Changes with age and in chronic rotator cuff tendinitis. *Annals of Rheumatological Disease, 53,* 367-376.

Rosenbaum, R. (1999). Disputed radial tunnel syndrome. *Muscle Nerve, 22,* 960.

Rothe, T., Hanisch, U. K., Krohn, K., Schliebs, R., Hartig, W., Webster, H. H. et al. (1990). Changes in choline acetyltransferase activity and high-affinity choline uptake, but not in acetylcholinesterase activity and muscarinic cholinergic receptors, in rat somatosensory cortex after sciatic nerve injury. *Somatosensory Motor Research, 7,* 435-446.

Rothwell, J. (1995). *Control of human voluntary movement* (pp. 86-126). New York: Chapman & Hall.

Rydevik, B., Lundborg, G., & Bagge, U. (1981). Effects of graded compression on intraneural blood flow. An in vivo study on rabbit tibial nerve. *Journal of Hand Surgery [Am], 6,* 3-12.

Rydevik, B., McLean, W.G., Sjostrand, J., & Lundborg, G. (1990). Blockage of axonal transport induced by acute, graded compression of the rabbit vagus nerve. *Journal of Neurology and Neurosurgery in Psychiatry, 43,* 690-698.

Sainburg, R. L., Poizner, H., & Ghez, C. (1993). Loss of proprioception produces deficits in interjoint coordination. *Journal of Neurophysiology, 70,* 2136-2147.

Sanders, R. J., & Haug, C. E. (1991). *Thoracic outlet syndrome: A common sequela of neck injuries* (p. 34). Philadelphia: Lippincott.

Seddon, H. (1943). Three types of nerve injury. *Brain, 66,* 237.

Shumway-Cook, A., & Woollacott, M. (2001). *Motor control: Theory and practical applications.* Baltimore: Williams & Wilkins.

Smith, A. G., Kosygan, K., Williams, H., & Newman, R. J. (1999). Common extensor tendon rupture following corticosteroid injection for lateral tendinosis of the elbow. *British Journal of Sports Medicine, 33*(6), 423-425.

Smith, C. E., Atchabahian, A., Mackinnon, S. E., & Hunter, D. A. (2001). Development of the blood-nerve barrier in neonatal rats. *Microsurgery, 21*(7), 290-297.

Sunderland, S. (1978). *Nerves and nerve injuries* (2nd ed.). London: Churchill Livingstone.

Szabo, R. M. (1989). *Nerve compression syndromes: Diagnosis and treatment.* Thorofare, NJ: Slack.

Tassler, P. L., Dellon, A. L., & Canoun, C. (1994). Identification of elastic fibres in the peripheral nerve. *Journal of Hand Surgery [Br], 19*(1), 48-54.

Thorson, E. P., & Szabo, R. M. (1989). Tendonitis of the wrist and elbow. In M. L. Kasdan (Ed.), *Occupational medicine: Occupational hand injuries* (pp. 419-431). Philadelphia: Hanley & Belfus, Inc.

Tidball, J. G. (1983). The geometry of actin filament-membrane associations can modify adhesive strength of the myotendinous junction. *Cell Motility and Cytoskeleton, 3,* 439-447.

Topp, K. S., & Byl, N. N. (1999). Movement dysfunction following repetitive hand opening and closing: anatomical analysis in Owl monkeys. *Movement Disorders, 14*(2), 295-306.

Travell, J. G., & Simons, D. G. (1983). *Myofascial pain and dysfunction, the trigger point manual, Vol 1: The upper extremities.* Baltimore: Williams & Wilkins.

Turnbull, B. G., & Rasmusson, D. D. (1990). Acute effects of total or partial digit denervation on racoon somatosensory cortex. *Somatosensensory Motor Research, 7,* 365-389.

Turnbull, B. G., & Rasmusson, D. D. (1991). Chronic effects of total or partial digit denervation on raccoon somatosensory cortex. *Somatosensensory and Motor Research, 8,* 201-213.

Upton, A. R. M., & McComas, A. J. (1973). The double crush in nerve entrapment syndromes. *Lancet, 2,* 359-362.

Vogel, H. C. (1977). Mechanical and chemical properties of various connective tissue organs in rats as influenced by non-steroidal antirheumatic drugs. *Connective Tissue Research, 5,* 91-95.

Wall, J. T., Xu, J., & Wang X. (2002). Human brain plasticity: an emerging view of the multiple substrates and mechanisms that cause cortical changes and related sensory dysfunctions after injuries of sensory inputs from the body. *Brain Research Reviews, 39*(2-3), 181-215.

Walsh, M. T. (1994). Therapist management of thoracic outlet syndrome. *Journal of Hand Therapy, 7*(2), 131-144.

Wilgis, S., & Murphy, R. (1986). The significance of longitudinal excursion in peripheral nerves. *Hand Clinics, 2,* 761.

Wolf, S. L. (1984). Neurophysiologic mechanisms in pain modulation: relevance to T.E.N.S. In J. S. Mannheimer & G. N. Lampe (Eds.), *Clinical transcutaneous electrical nerve stimulation* (pp. 41-55). Philadelphia: Davis.

Woo, S., Maynard, J., Butler, D., Lyon, R., Torzilli, P., Akeson, W. et al. (1987). Ligament, tendon, and joint capsule insertions to bone. In S. L-Y. Woo & J. A. Buckwalter (Eds.), *Injury and repair of the musculoskeletal soft tissues* (pp. 133-166). Park Ridge, IL: American Academy of Orthopedic Surgeons.

Woo, S. L-Y. (1982). Mechanical properties of tendons and ligaments: I. Quasi-static and nonlinear viscoelastic properties. *Biorheology, 19,* 385-396.

Woo, S. L-Y., Matthews, J. V., Akenson, W. H., Amiel, D., & Convery, F. R. (1975). Connective tissue response to immobility. Correlative study of biomechanical and biochemical measurements of normal and immobilized rabbit knees. *Arthritis and Rheumatism, 18*(3), 257-264.

Yamada, H. (1970). Strength of biological materials. In F. G. Evans (Ed.), *The biomechanical responses to tension in a peripheral nerve.* Baltimore: Williams & Wilkins.

Zarzecki, P., Witte, S., Smits, E., Gordon, D. C., Kirchberger, P., & Rasmusson, D. D. (1993). Synaptic mechanisms of cortical representational plasticity: Somatosensory and corticocortical EPSPs in reorganized raccoon SI cortex. *Journal of Neurophysiology, 69,* 1422-1432.

CHAPTER 6

Treatment of MSD and Related Conditions

Susan V. Duff

DIFFERENTIATING BETWEEN MUSCULOTENDONOUS OR NEURAL DISORDERS

In order to discern whether a musculoskeletal disorder is of neural or contractile tissue origin, a thorough evaluation is required. The information most useful to make this distinction includes an accurate history and findings from sensibility and resistance tests. The interpretation of test results for tendinitis/tendinosis and nerve compressions/entrapments are summarized in Table 6-1.

Table 6-1
Differentiating Tendinitis from Peripheral Nerve Compression or Entrapment

Finding	Tendinitis	Nerve Compression or Entrapment
Pain at rest	Possibly	Yes
Pain with resistive annual muscle test	Yes	Possibly
Weakness on manual muscle test	Possibly	Yes
Symptoms reproduced with provocative maneuvers	Yes	Yes
Abnormal sensibility tests	No	Yes
Abnormal electromyography/ nerve conduction velocity	No	Yes

Sources: Modified from Lundborg, G., & . Dahlin, L. B. (1992). The pathophysiology of nerve compression. *Hand Clin, 8,* 215–227; and Nirschl, R. P. (1992). Elbow tendinosis/tennis elbow. *Clin Sports Med, 11,* 851–870.

History and Subjective Assessment

Specific information regarding preexisting conditions and interventions as well as the impact of work, self-care, and leisure activity as related to the existing disorder may be obtained through an interview or a health history form (Kasch, 2002). The Canadian Occupational Performance Measure (COPM) is an outcome measure useful to document baseline and progressive, importance, performance, and satisfaction on client-identified issues pertinent to function (Law et al., 1990). This tool is rapidly gaining use in the clinical arena because of its ability to address and monitor "client-centered" goals.

Activity Tolerance

An accurate history enables one to begin differentiating tendinous conditions from those of neurogenic origin and to determine whether the disorder was insidious or traumatic in onset. Tasks or activities that exacerbate signs and symptoms should be highlighted. Specifically, one should ask for the location, duration, and description of symptoms. Nirschl (1992) outlined phases of tendon pathology on the basis of pain induced by specific activities. These phases can be translated into levels of recovery associated with either tendinosis or nerve compressions

(Table 6-2). For example, an individual may complain of pain in the lateral forearm after carrying a bag of groceries, a task that is categorized under level 2 as a "heavy activity of daily living." Lateral forearm pain may imply that there is compression of the radial nerve or a tendinosis of the common extensor tendon. As treatment continues, task simulation or verbal report can be used to assess tolerance to loads during performance or after a rest period. Thus, subjective reports associated with select activities aid treatment planning and evaluation of progress.

Pain Assessment

An objective measurement of pain provides a means of documenting subjective complaints, identifying the source(s), and establishing a baseline for treatment. Pain can be quantified through rating scales or questionnaires. Rating scales have been found to have good predictive validity and high concurrent validity in children (Bulloch & Tenenbein, 2002) and adults (Gallagher, Bijur, Latimer, & Silver, 2002). The visual analog scale (VAS) is one rating scale that documents the intensity or affective quality of pain (Fedorczyk & Barbe, 2002; Scott & Huskisson, 1979). Although there are variations, typically an unmarked 10-cm line is drawn vertically or horizontally on a sheet of paper with descriptive words placed at either end of the line. For example, if one wishes to measure pain intensity, the description at one end of the line might read "no pain," and the opposite description could read "intense pain." The individual is then asked to place a mark on the line between the two words to indicate the degree of pain he or she is experiencing. For an accurate interpretation, the 10-cm line is divided into 20 increments after the assessment, from which the distance from no pain to the mark can be measured and documented. The Faces Pain Rating Scale (Wong & Baker, 1988) resembles the VAS and can be used with children. Rating scales may be used in combination with questionnaires.

Table 6-2
Levels of Cumulative Trauma Based on Activity Tolerance and Associated Pain

Level	Cumulative Trauma
Level One	Constant pain (dull aching) and pain or paresthesia that disturbs sleep
	Intermittent pain or paresthesia at rest that does not disturb sleep
	Pain or paresthesia caused by light activities of daily living
Level Two	Pain or paresthesia caused by heavy activities of daily living
	Pain or paresthesia with exercise or activity that alters performance of the activity
	Pain or paresthesia with exercise or activity that does not alter performance of the activity
Level Three	Pain or paresthesia after activity that persists beyond 48 hours yet resolves with rest
	Mild pain or paresthesia after exercise or activity that resolves within 24 hours

Notes: Under each level are descriptors of activity tolerance, in decreasing order of severity. Level one represents the most restrictive level of activity. Reported symptoms may be compared against this list in order to plan for treatment by level.
Sources: Modified from Lindsay, M. (1993). Radial tunnel versus lateral epicondylitis. *Newsletter of the Section on Hand Rehabilitation of the American Physical Therapy Association, 10* (39),1; Nirschl, R. P. (1992). Elbow tendinosis/tennis elbow. *Clin Sports Med, 11,* 851–870.

One comprehensive tool is The McGill Pain Questionnaire (MPQ), which attempts to measure multiple aspects of pain in four parts (Melzack, 1975). In part one, descriptive words are divided into three main categories and 20 subcategories. The three main categories are sensory, evaluative, and affective components of pain. In each subcategory, there are six similar words that rank pain in descending order according to intensity. The individual is asked to circle one word from each applicable category and to leave blank any category that does not apply. Quantitative scoring involves the number of words chosen and a pain-rating index. Part two of the MPQ is the pain diagram. On a front and back diagram of the upper quadrant or whole body the individual marks the exact location and type of pain through designated symbols.

The therapist reviews the diagram with the individual after completion. In part three, the subject verbally describes the duration of pain and the activities that influence it. Part four asks the individual to rate pain on a 5-point scale, according to its intensity, to determine the present pain index. The scale is marked with descriptive terms: *mild, discomforting, distressing, horrible,* and *excruciating*. If all four parts of the MPQ are given, the test provides a more sensitive measure of pain than does the VAS alone. Regardless of the tool used, the reader is advised that cultural influences and expectations also play a role in pain but are difficult to measure.

Related History

It is important to obtain information regarding previous treatment and formal testing. For example, in cases of nerve compression or tendinosis, the physician may have injected the region with antiinflammatory medication. Although this may reduce inflammation and pain, multiple repeated injections may influence healing of the injured tissue (Nirschl, 1992; Smith, Kosygan, Williams, & Newman, 1999). Electromyography (EMG) and nerve conduction studies (NCSs) are formal tests frequently used by physicians in combination with other clinical tests to confirm or rule out nerve impairment. Although EMG and NCS results may guide early treatment, electrodiagnostic testing is not valuable the first 2 weeks after nerve injury, and specificity cannot be assumed. Because of the frequency of false-positive and false-negative results, electrodiagnostic test results are best interpreted against reported signs and symptoms and objective clinical findings (Tetro, Evanoff, Hollstien, & Gelberman, 1998).

Electromyography

Invasive EMG uses a needle electrode placed in muscle tissue to record electrical potentials produced by innervated and denervated muscle fibers (Brumback, Bobele, & Rayan, 1992). The needle of the EMG records activity from adjacent muscle fibers on insertion, during relaxation, and during minimal or strong contractions (Figure 6-1). Abnormal EMG findings include fibrillations and positive sharp waves, fasciculations, polyphasic motor units, and poor recruitment. Fibrillations are small-amplitude, short-duration, biphasic, or triphasic potentials with a discharge rate 13 to 15 times per second. Fibrillations are seen in cases of nerve disease and other conditions that may increase excitability of the nerve cell membrane. Positive sharp waves are similar to fibrillations, except that typically there is an initial positive deflection. Fasciculations are the visible twitching of muscle bundles as a result of spontaneous initiation of an action potential in a nerve axon branch. This activity eliminates the normal anterograde propagation. Instead, the propagation occurs in both directions: anterograde (toward the nerve terminal) and retrograde (toward the spinal cord). The size and duration of the motor unit as well as the number of phases may change in cases of nerve or muscle disease (see Chapter 9 for a complete discussion of surface EMGs).

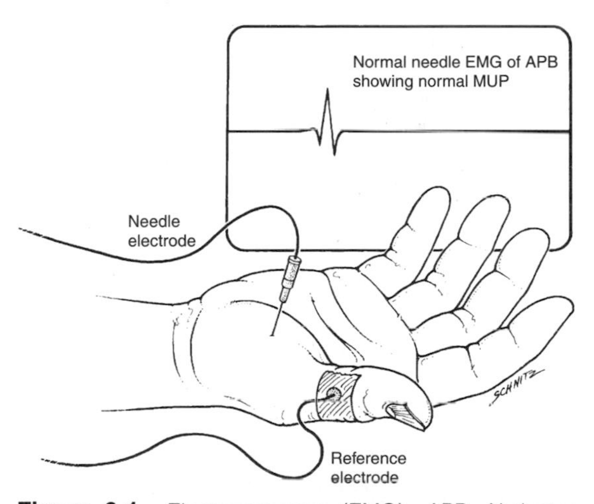

Figure 6-1 Electromyogram (EMG). *APB,* Abductor pollicis brevis; *MUP,* motor unit potentials. (Reprinted with permission from Hilburn, J. W. [1996]. General principles and use of electrodiagnostic studies in carpal and cubital tunnel syndromes: with special attention to pitfalls and interpretation. *Hand Clinics, 12,* 210.)

Nerve Conduction Studies

NCSs record the conduction velocity of nerve fiber action potentials by myelinated fibers (Figure 6-2). As a rule, conduction velocity is six times the diameter of a myelinated fiber (in micrometers per second, μm), and myelinated fiber diameter varies between 1 and 20 μm (Brumback et al., 1992). Thus, the largest myelinated fiber can conduct up to 120 μm per second. Nerve conduction velocity for an individual with suspected nerve compression is often evaluated against the noninvolved extremity because there is a large age variance among normative data.

Objective Clinical Assessments

After an accurate history and activity tolerance screen are obtained, a physical assessment should be done. This portion of the evaluation may begin with visual inspection and progress to range-of-motion (ROM) and strength testing. In some instances, it may be necessary to conduct an upper-quadrant screen, as outlined in Box 6-1. To discriminate between a disorder of neurogenic or tendinous orgin, sensibility and adverse neural tension tests should be done. Findings may be further supported with tissue palpation and observation of prehension patterns during select tasks. Each portion of the assessment provides important clues about the tissue involved and the activities that provoke signs and symptoms.

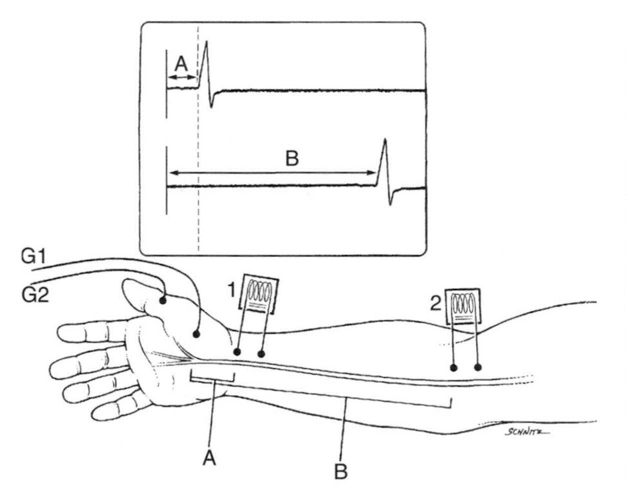

Figure 6-2 Median nerve conduction study. *A,* Distal motor latency; *B,* proximal motor latency; *G1,* active point; G*2,* reference point; *1,* distal stimulation site; *2,* proximal stimulation site. (Reprinted with permission from Hilburn, J. W. (1996). General principles and use of electrodiagnostic studies in carpal and cubital tunnel syndromes: with special attention to pitfalls and interpretation. *Hand Clinics, 12,* 212.)

Visual Inspection

Before the initiation of any physical tests, it is wise to survey the reported region of involvement. With long-standing tendon or neural pathology, there may be observable signs of muscle atrophy when comparing the involved side to the noninvolved side. Visual inspection of the involved extremity may also reveal sites of biomechanical deformity, edema, skin discoloration, or burns that should be further examined.

Range-of-Motion Tests

Extensibility of the muscle-tendon unit is assessed through active and passive ROM tests (Clarkson & Gilewich, 2000). Because tendons are contractile, pain may be elicited with passive stretching of the injured tissues. To assess muscle-tendon units that cross two or more joints, it is necessary to induce a stretch across all the joints involved simultaneously before documenting passive motion at one or more joints. For example, the finger flexors cross the wrist and digits. To assess them at maximum length, the fingers and wrist must be extended simultaneously. In this position, wrist extension can be measured to document changes in tissue extensibility with treatment. Active ROM measures the ability to move through the range without resistance.

Strength Assessment

In the clinic, the tools used to assess strength are manual muscle tests, grip-pinch dynamometers, and isokinetic dynamometers. When performing manual muscle tests it should be specified

BOX 6-1
Upper-Quadrant Screen

Observation and Inspection
Body build: endomorph, ectomorph, or mesomorph
Weight: _______ Height: ________ (unusual features)
Assistive devices or orthotics
General mobility and static limb posture (on entrance into clinic or during interview)
Alterations in skin (e.g., scars, edema)
Reported functional use
Static posture (lateral, posterior, and anterior)
- Scapular position (elevated, abducted, etc.)
- Head position (forward head posture, tilted)
- Pelvic position (anterior or posterior pelvic tilt, lateral tilts, or rotations)
- Position of arm and shoulder
- Asymmetries

Function Tests
Cervical spine (rule out pathology related to cervical spine): degree and quality of motion, pain location and severity recorded
- Active cervical motion followed by overpressure (e.g., forward bend, backbend, rotations, and lateral flexion)
- Axial compression and distraction (performed manually)

Neurologic evaluation via a quick manual muscle test to check for weakness: therapist positioned behind patient and giving resistance bilaterally
Motor:
- C2: axial flexion
- C3-C4: shoulder shrug
- C5: shoulder abduction at 90 degrees
- C6: elbow flexion
- C7: elbow extension
- C8: wrist extension
- T1: finger abduction

Sensory:
- Dizziness: yes or no
- Tinnitus: yes or no
- Light touch (may use monofilaments): tested via dermatome mapping and recorded
  - C4: top of shoulder
  - C5: deltoid area
  - C6: lateral arm to thumb
  - C7: middle finger
  - C8: ulnar aspect of hand
  - T1: medial upper arm
- Reflex (hammer):
  - C5-C6: biceps tendon
  - C7: triceps tendon
- Provocative thoracic outlet tests (see text)

Source: Reprinted from Moran, C., & Saunders, S. R. (1991). Evaluation of the shoulder: a sequential approach. In R. A. Donnatelli (Ed.), *Physical therapy of the shoulder* (2nd ed, pp. 19–62). New York: Churchill-Livingstone.

whether the test measured an isometric or an isotonic contraction (Clarkson & Gilewich, 2000). Active contraction of the muscle-tendon unit against resistance may elicit pain or weakness (Cyriax, 1982). Response to resistance done in the midrange or throughout the range may be interpreted according to a scale used by Cyriax (Table 6-3). Weakness or poor endurance is often discovered in cases of nerve compression. Grip strength testing using a dynamometer has been found to be a reliable tool when used in conjunction with pain measures (Smidt, van der Windt, Assendelft, et al., 2002). As pain subsides and the injured tissue is allowed to recover or as the nerve compression is lifted, strength measures should improve.

In cases of mild tendinitis or nerve compressions, task simulation can be used to assess functional limitations. Task simulation and subsequent analysis may reveal whether the injury is acute or chronic and help determine the best method of treatment to promote full healing of the involved tissue(s). In cases of acute tendinitis, pain during select task simulations may be induced secondary to small microtears and subsequent inflammation. In chronic conditions, tissue shortening may be noted, and the individual may be unable to sustain loads in the involved limb without significant pain or weakness. The strength, biomechanics, and function of distant areas of the kinetic chain might be altered secondary to injury elsewhere and affect performance (Burkart & Post, 2002; Kibler, Chandler, & Pace, 1992). For instance, the proximal shoulder girdle may present with weakness in the case of distal nerve compression.

Table 6-3
Interpretation of Resistive Tests

Response to Resistance	Interpretation
Painless	Muscle-tendon unit may be normal
Painful on repetition of resistance	Questionable neurovascular disorder
Strong and painful	Minor lesion of muscle-tendon unit
Weak and painful	Partial rupture of tendon (if passive joint range is normal)
Weak and painless	Complete rupture of muscle-tendon unit or nerve involvement

Source: Modified from Cyriax, J. (1982). *Textbook of Orthopaedic Medicine, Vol 1: Diagnosis of Soft-Tissue Lesions* (8th ed). London: Bailliere Tindall.

Adverse Neural Tension Assessment

Adverse neural tensions are those abnormal physiologic and mechanical responses produced by neural structures when their extensibility and range is tested (Butler & Guth, 1993). *Assessment* of adverse neural tension is important, especially if a neurogenic disorder is suspected (Butler, 1991; Elvey, Quintner, & Thomas, 1986). Elvey and Butler advise putting tension into the nervous system through selective passive placement techniques to reproduce the signs and symptoms that the individual frequently experiences. The ROM available at one or more select joints, while tension is placed on the system, provides an objective measure of tolerance to tension. Figure 6-3 is an example of a sequential upper-limb tension test 1 for the median nerve. It requires passive depression of the scapula in steps 1 and 2, followed by wrist extension and shoulder external rotation in steps 3 and 4. At this point, the tension is now directed at the elbow. When elbow extension begins to create a pins-and-needles sensation or other neurogenic sign, the clinician should stop the stretch and measure the degree of passive elbow extension.

Sensibility Tests

Sensibility is the conscious appreciation and interpretation of a stimulus that produces sensation. Both academic and functional sensibility tests may be used to identify the extent of nerve damage and to document return. *Academic sensibility* involves interpretation of passive tactile stimuli. It may be assessed through threshold tests, innervation density tests, provocative tests, and tests of sympathetic function. *Functional sensibility* refers to the use of tactile information for active exploration in daily activities and work (Bowden, 1954; Seddon, 1954; Zachary, 1954). It is often measured by using specific functional or dexterity tests. After nerve injury, it is possible to achieve recovery of academic sensibility with minimal recovery of functional sensibility (Moberg, 1962). The reader is referred to Stone (1992) for a summary of test administration and scoring of common sensibility tests discussed.

Threshold Tests

Threshold tests help determine the minimal tactile stimulus perceived by an individual with vision occluded (Callahan, 2002). Threshold testing can be used to track gradual or progressive changes after nerve compression (Szabo & Gelberman, 1987). Classic threshold tests include those used to measure pain, temperature, touch-pressure, and vibratory sensibility. The most reliable and repeatable clinical tool used is the Semmes-Weinstein monofilaments test, which is a test of light touch (Bell-Krotoski & Buford, 1997). The Semmes-Weinstein monofilaments (Figure 6-4) bend when they reach a peak force ($\log_{10}$ F g) and maintain a constant force until recovery. The monofilaments require frequent calibration to ensure accurate length and diameter. The Weinstein enhanced sensory test (WEST) has been introduced as an alternative test of light touch (Weinstein, 1993). The surface area of the contacting tip of the WEST monofilament is textured to prevent slippage and is hemispheric in shape rather than smooth

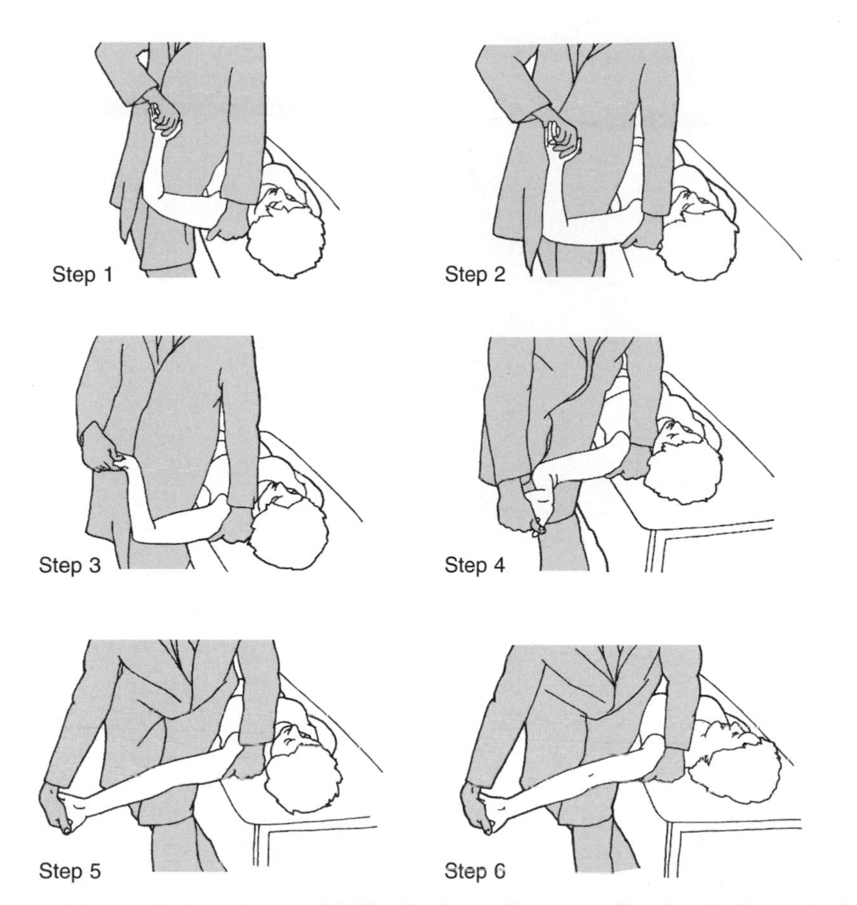

Figure 6-3 Sequential upper-limb tension test (ULTT) 1 for the median nerve. (Reprinted with permission from Butler, D. S. [1991]. *Mobilisation of the nervous system* [p. 149]. New York: Churchill Livingstone.)

and flat, like the monofilaments. On bending of the WEST filaments, the same surface area of the tip remains in contact with the skin. To make the results easier to interpret, the forces (in milligrams) used to bend the monofilaments are printed on the device itself (Weinstein, 1993). Studies to establish normal values for the WEST have been conducted (Schultz, Bohannon, & Morgan, 1998). Both the Semmes-Weinstein and the WEST are available in 5-filament, pocket-sized versions of the larger 20-filament tests. These two monofilaments tests are the only handheld instruments that have some control of force if calibrated.

Innervation Density Tests

Tests of innervation density are based on a select region of nerve innervation and its cortical representation. The most widely used density tests assess static (Weber, 1835) and moving two-point discrimination (Dellon, 1978). Weber's test originally required that two compass points be moved inward until the subject could no longer detect two points; this was modified to touching the individual with either one point or two. Although the two-point discrimination test has frequently been referred to as a strong measure of tactile gnosis, it is considered to have only fair reliability and validity because of the

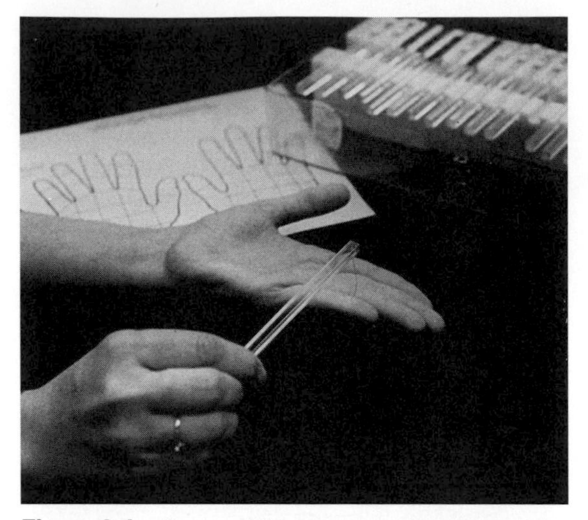

Figure 6-4 Semmes-Weinstein monofilaments used to measure sensibility threshold for light touch.

variation in force application of the handheld test device (Bell-Krotoski & Buford, 1997). Moving two-point discrimination varies in both rate and force of application, further compromising its reliability and validity. Despite the caution, Dellon, MacKinnon, and Crosby (1987) demonstrated better reliability in testing two-point discrimination by using the "Disk-Criminator" with a specific protocol. The reader should be cognizant of the concerns addressed when interpreting the results of two-point discrimination tests (Aszmann & Dellon, 1998; Jerosch-Herold, 2000; Rozental, Beredjiklian, Guyette, & Weiland, 2000). A tuning fork or biothesiometer is another instrument that some have found to be a sensitive tool for vibration testing (Sorman & Edwall, 2002), whereas others believe the application force is not well controlled (Bell-Krotoski & Buford, 1997).

Provocative Tests

Provocative tests are screening tools that invoke a signal or sign of sensation or lack of sensation on the basis of response to a specific movement. Common provocative tests are those of nerve percussion, nerve compression, and stress testing. Nerve percussion was introduced by Tinel (1915) and involves tapping over the nerve (at either a superficial location or the location to which the nerve end has regenerated). A positive result induces tingling or paresthesias in the distal nerve distribution. Tinel's sign has become a popular method of detecting the presence of axons and serves as an indication of regeneration. Compression tests are used to provoke signs of nerve involvement by placing the involved region in compromising positions (Callahan, 2002). One well-known test is Phalen's (1966) wrist flexion test, which "squeezes" the median nerve between the flexor tendons, the radius, and the transverse carpal ligament. The subject is requested to hold the forearms vertically, leaning on the elbows and allowing both hands to drop into complete flexion. The subject is asked to hold this position for 1 minute. Phalen's test may induce feelings of numbness and paresthesias if the median nerve already is partially compressed.

Because some nerve compressions and cases of tendinitis are caused by repetitive motion over a period of time, it may be necessary to replicate the cause of symptoms through job simulation, provocative activities, or stress tests (Callahan, 2002). Initially, baseline measurements, including sensibility, pain, and edema (volume) are taken, then job simulation is conducted or the provocative activity is introduced. For example, to provoke the symptoms associated with radial tunnel or pronator syndrome, often found in cashiers, the individual may be requested to perform repetitive forearm rotation by turning over cards to simulate scanning in a checkout line. After simulating the provocative-activity, post-test measures are taken. A comparison between the baseline and post-test may implicate structures affected by repetitive activity that can be addressed through treatment or activity modification.

Sympathetic Signs of Nerve Injury

Sympathetic signs of nerve injury may be highlighted by select objective tests. Four categories of sympathetic testing include vasomotor tests of skin color or temperature; sudomotor or sweat tests; tests for pilomotor (or gooseflesh response); and tests for trophic changes, such as alterations in skin texture, soft-tissue atrophy, nail changes, hair growth, and rate of healing. Two tests, the sweat test and the wrinkle test, are commonly used. The Ninhydrin sweat test of sudomotor (sweat) function was introduced by Guttman in 1940 and modified by Moberg in 1954 (Moran & Callahan, 1983). The O'Riain (1973) wrinkle test was based on O'Riain's observation that the skin of denervated tissue did not wrinkle when immersed in water. Of the two tests, the Ninhydrin sweat test has been used most frequently with children and in cases of malingering to verify nerve injury.

Functional Sensibility Tests

Functional sensibility (or tactile gnosis) is defined as the quality of cutaneous sensibility needed for a precision sensory grip or "seeing" with the fingers (Moberg, 1960). Stereognosis tests are the primary measure of tactile gnosis, whereas dexterity tests measure manual or finger dexterity (Apfel & Carranza, 1992; Dellon & Kallman, 1983; Ng, Ho, & Chow, 1999; Stone, 1992). While most stereognosis tests require in-hand manipulation (Exner, 1990) to ease object identification, the Byl Cheney-Boczai Sensory Discriminator Test (BCBI) (Byl, Leano, & Cheney, 2002) does not require it. The BCBI requires matching of designs embedded on a plastic cube to the designs on an answer sheet. Dexterity and functional tests differ as to required tool use and grasp patterns; thus, a combination of tests may help to correlate individual prehensile skill and the status of the nerve. Common dexterity tests include the Purdue pegboard test, the Crawford small parts test, the Moberg pick-up test, the nine-hole peg test, and the Minnesota rate of manipulation test. Specific functional tests include the Jebsen-Taylor hand function test (Jebsen, Taylor, Trieschmann, Trotter, & Howard, 1969), the modified Moberg pick-up test, the Sollerman grip and function test, and the Apfel 19-item pick-up test. For accurate verification of one's functional status, more comprehensive tests with up-to-date functional tasks may need to be designed.

Dellon (1993) has proposed a grading scale of peripheral nerve function. Scores on a hierarchical 0-10 scale of mutually exclusive categories for motor and sensory function could be calculated on the basis of findings from a clinical assessment. A score of 0 would be equated with findings in the normal range. A score of 10 would be given for severe atrophy and severely limited sensibility test findings. Although this scale has yet to be validated, it may enhance communication among professionals regarding findings from multiple sources of assessment.

Palpation

Because palpation is the least reliable method of determining the nature of the disorder and may introduce bias, it should be the last item performed in a physical examination (Cyriax, 1982; Rodineau, 1991). Palpation of the involved region may induce pain or reveal alterations in tissue integrity (including atrophy). Tenderness over select sites may reveal the source of pain or indicate an area of referred pain. Trigger points and sites of specific tendon or nerve irritation may be localized. For example, in cases of tennis elbow, the lateral epicondyle may be particularly sensitive to touch pressure.

Adaptive Changes in Nearby Tissue

Adaptive changes in the musculature and joints both distal and proximal to the affected area may influence the effectiveness of rehabilitation if not evaluated and addressed. Such alterations may involve muscle strength, tissue flexibility, joint integrity, and biomechanics. For instance, shoulder weakness and inflexibility in the individual with lateral epicondylitis may delay healing because the shoulder musculature may not contribute fully during upper-limb resistive tasks. Therefore, excess stress may be imparted to the vulnerable common extensor tendon, the bony attachment of which lies very close to the myotendinous junction.

THERAPEUTIC INTERVENTION

Therapeutic intervention for musculoskeletal disorders requires careful consideration of tissue involvement and its condition. Recovery from injury can resemble the stages of wound healing. These stages are reviewed along with corresponding treatment. Separate sections will address select intervention strategies for tendinosis and nerve compressions and entrapments.

Stages of Wound Healing

The three phases of wound healing—inflammation, proliferation, and remodeling—although distinct, overlap. For example, there may be some inflammatory cells present in a healing wound as it begins to proliferate new fibroblasts (Fyfe & Stanish, 1992). *Acute* injuries follow a relatively sequential process of wound healing in the absence of further stress. However, *chronic* injuries typically do not follow this course, and healing is often halted at one phase or another. While conservative treatment for chronic injuries may promote sequential wound repair, if it is unsuccessful, surgical intervention may be needed to remove degenerative or compressive tissue and to induce tissue repair.

Inflammatory Phase (Acute)

The postinjury inflammatory phase lasts approximately 5 to 7 days (Peacock, 1965). The cardinal signs of inflammation (redness, pain, heat, swelling) are induced by an enzymatically driven sequence, led by the production of arachidonic acid, phospholipids, and other metabolites (Rubin & Faber, 1988). In this phase, the vascular disruption initiates platelet activation and a clotting mechanism. A fibrin clot is formed when fibronectin or adhesive molecules cross-link with collagen. During this phase, any tissue damaged in the initial trauma is removed from the region. In addition, endothelial sites and fibroblasts are recruited and stimulated to divide (Martens, Wouters, Burssens, & Mulier, 1982).

Proliferation (Subacute)

The subacute phase, which can last from 3 days to as long as 6 to 8 weeks, has been termed *fibroplasia*. This phase begins with the production of collagen by the third day. The relative hypoxia within the wound and the increase in lactate levels are the critical operating forces (Hunt & Hussain, 1992). During this stage, vascularity is increased, and by day 12, there is a significant reduction in inflammatory cells. The teknocyte is the reparative cell or the source of collagen production, protein mediators, and matrix proteoglycans. The mobile macrophage directs the sequence of events leading to wound repair (Martens et al., 1982; Rubin & Faber, 1988). It is able to release growth factors, chemoattractants, and proteolytic enzymes when needed, to activate fibroblasts or tendon repair. If the provocative activity causing the injury is modified or avoided during this phase, the tissue should mature and recondition.

Remodeling

This stage of healing continues throughout life. However, 17 to 28 days after injury, the collagen content is weaker than normal (Peacock, 1965). During this period, cellularity and synthetic activity are decreased. There is an increase in extracellular matrix organization and normalization of the biochemical profile (Laurent, 1987). Longitudinal tension induced through select activity aids remodeling. If the tissue is allowed to progress through this phase, collagen matures, and linear realignment of fibers is noted by 2 months.

Intervention for Tendonopathies and Related Conditions

Treatment of tendinitis or tendinosis may follow a conservative nonsurgical course. The overall goal of nonsurgical treatment is to promote revascularization and collagen repair, allowing the formation of a strong yet mobile scar that can withstand the loads sustained during functional activity and recreation (Cyriax, 1982). Treatment level is based on clinical findings.

Generally, tendinitis or tendinosis can be treated at all three levels after the phases of wound healing. General goals and methods for conservative treatment are listed in Table 6-4. Restriction of the provocative activity is the most effective mode of intervention. Key restrictions for most types of upper-limb tendonopathies are listed in Table 6-5.

Table 6-4

Management of Tendinitis and Tendinosis

Goal	Method
Level One	
Protect and rest affected regions	Restrict provocative activities
	Splint affected areas
	Provide ergonomic equipment
	Encourage frequent breaks
Reduce pain and inflammation	Rest and support affected areas
	Ice
	Transcutaneous electrical nerve stimulation
	Phonophoresis or pulsed ultrasound
	Iontophoresis
Level Two	
Increase mobility and length of the involved tissue	Superficial heat modalities
	Continuous low-level ultrasound
	Massage
	Myofascial release techniques
	Active range of motion with stretching
Increase knowledge of cause and prevention of tendinitis	Perform task analysis
	Educate
Level Three	
Increase tolerance to controlled stress	Graded strengthening
Enhance motor control in work-related and sports tasks and activities of daily living	Practice
Promote return to premorbid function	Task simulation

Note: At all levels, it is important to monitor pain associated with activity.

Management of tendinous disorders and related conditions can be complicated because injury often occurs in those muscles of the upper limb that are frequently used to accomplish daily activities. Thus, it may be difficult to advance an individual through the phases of wound healing in a sequential manner.

If signs and symptoms persist or are severe enough over a prescribed course of time, surgical intervention may be warranted. The primary goal of surgical treatment is to remove degenerated tissue and to promote a renewed cycle of wound repair so as to alter the cell matrix of the tendon (Leadbetter, 1991). Goals after surgical treatment resemble those for nonsurgical treatment, with the additional goal of postoperative scar management.

Intervention for Nerve Compressions and Entrapments

Most of the research regarding regeneration has been done on nerve lacerations and repairs. In terms of compressions, inferences often are made because there is much variation in terms of recovery. Recovery can begin when the compressive forces or entrapping structures have

Table 6-5

Key Restrictions in Upper-Limb Tendinitis

Disorder	Restriction
Rotator cuff tendinitis	Overhead activities
Bicipital tendinitis	Resisted elbow flexion and shoulder flexion with elbow extended
Lateral epicondylitis	Resisted gripping, wrist extension, and excessive elbow motion
Medial epicondylitis	Resisted wrist flexion, pronation, and excessive elbow motion
Intersection syndrome	Thumb and wrist flexion
Flexor paratendinitis (tenosynovitis)	Resisted gripping
de Quervain's disease	Resisted pinching
Trigger thumb or finger	Resisted thumb or finger flexion

been removed. Decompression may involve removal of causative factors, such as edema or fibrosis. As with tendon pathology, conservative management of nerve compressions involves limiting the provocative activity. If the nerve compression is not relieved with removal of the presumed cause or provocative activity, surgical decompression may be necessary. Once decompressed, the nerve may follow the course of wound repair. However, it is vital that regeneration of the damaged axons occurs in order for nerve integrity to improve.

Anatomic Considerations in Nerve Regeneration

Ideally, regeneration results in a reversal of changes that may have occurred during the period of compression. The type and location of the peripheral nerve compression determines the outcome of the reinnervation. Proximal lesions have a better chance of full return than do distal lesions, because of their proximity to the cell body. The number and types of axons that establish functional connections with cutaneous receptors will determine recovery of sensation. In addition, changes in the encoding properties of regenerated fibers and the response of the somatosensory cortex to deprivation of input also will affect return (Braune & Schady, 1993). The number and type of reconnections to the end organs serving the muscles will determine motor function. In compressions, there is a strong possibility that some endoneurial tubes were left intact. With the tube intact, the axon has a better chance of regrowing toward the correct receptor or muscle fiber (Brandenburg & Mann, 1989).

Regeneration after nerve lacerations and repair typically is preceded by a 2- to 3-week latency period. Following this latency period, the nerve has been found to regrow at a rate of 1 mm per day or greater (Chan, Smith, & Snyder, 1989). Insidious onset of nerve compression alters this typical concept of nerve regeneration. Instead of the entire nerve, only one axon or fascicle may have suffered damage. Intraneural fibrosis will effect the ability of the axon to regrow. After a period of compression, the regenerating nerve may also undergo a latency period before regeneration secondary to the effects of fibrosis (Braune & Schady, 1993). As research continues, one explanation may prove more valid than the others may.

Factors Affecting Regeneration

Successful nerve regeneration requires that the following specific conditions be in place.

1. The central neuron must survive.
2. The environment must be able to support axonal sprouting and growth.
3. The regenerated axon must make appropriate distal contact with receptors.
4. The CNS must integrate the signals from the PNS appropriately.

Axon regeneration is encouraged through contact guidance and neurotropism. In studies of nerve lacerations, factors within the distal nerve stump seem to be associated with regrowth of the proximal segments. Humoral, cellular, and molecular factors may serve to guide the regenerating axon. In addition, cell bodies of regenerating nerves send out chemical messengers that make their way down the axon by traveling within the axoplasm (see Figure 5-4), directed by the distal segment (Lundborg, Dahlin, Danielson, & Nachemason, 1986; Mackinnon, Dellon, Lundborg, Hudson, & Hunter, 1986). Because some component of the connective tissue surrounding the axon is often intact in compression injuries, it is hypothesized that regeneration guided through neurotropism is achieved with greater success.

Enhancement of the environment surrounding the axon is currently being researched. Investigations regarding local drug application to nerve sites damaged by crush injuries or lacerations have begun. In animal studies, Kanje, Lundborg, and Edstrom (1988) injected a regenerating sciatic nerve encased in a silicone tube. The authors found the rate of regeneration to be on the order of 3.5 mm per day, which followed an initial delay of 1.6 days. They further supported the notion that proliferation and protein synthesis of cells around the affected axon were required for regeneration. Fortunately, in compression there is often some continuity of connective tissue structures that allows for the regeneration without the need for such intervention. However, future research may prove the benefit of drug injection to be the enhancement of the environment surrounding the nerve.

Given the conditions outlined earlier, a damaged nerve will eventually grow back into its former location. Unfortunately, nerve regeneration is often delayed and unpredictable. The complications to regeneration include shrinkage of the endoneurial tubes; mismatching of motor, sensory, and sympathetic nervous system fibers; degeneration of end receptors; the presence of scarring at the injury site; and ineffective central reorganization.

Promoting Regeneration

Clinicians are always looking for conservative methods to improve function (see Table 6-6). Treatment methods frequently employed are splinting and sensory reeducation. Splints can be used for support or to reduce the effects of muscle imbalances caused by nerve injury. Sensory reeducation may enhance the recovery of sensibility. Individuals can follow *protective sensory programs* as they progress from absent sensation to the return of light touch. Once the finger exhibits protective sensation (as detected by a 4.31-gauge filament from the Semmes-Weinstein monofilament test) (Bell-Krotoski, 2002) a *sensory reeducation program* is initiated. Although touch pressure thresholds cannot be improved by means of reeducation or functional use, sensory reeducation may enhance central reorganization (Pascual-Leone & Torres, 1993). Enhancement of central reorganization may result in an increase in the receptive field representation for the involved nerve or an increase in the number of central regions recruited during select tasks.

What can be done to promote quicker and more accurate regeneration of peripheral nerves?

Table 6-6

Management of Nerve Compression or Entrapment

Goal	Method
Level One	
Protect and rest affected regions	Restrict provocative activities Splint affected areas Provide ergonomic equipment Encourage frequent breaks
Reduce pain and inflammation	Rest and support affected areas Ice Transcutaneous electrical nerve stimulation Phonophoresis or pulsed ultrasound Iontophoresis
Reduce pressure	Viscoelastic inserts, ergonomic tools
Level Two	
Increase circulation	Active range-of-motion exercises Thermal modalities (monitor decreased sensation) Avoid caffeine and nicotine Aerobic exercises
Promote soft-tissue mobility	Massage Myofascial release techniques Stretching, range of motion
Enhance nerve gliding	Nerve-gliding techniques (passive and active) Myofacial release techniques
Level Three	
Enhance motor control and function	Task simulation Work-site evaluation

Note: At all levels, it is important to monitor edema, sensitivity, motor recovery, and strength.

Various studies have examined the use of pulsed electromagnetic fields (PEMF) (Longo et al., 1999; Walker et al., 1994), functional neuromuscular stimulation (FNS) (Zealear, Billante, Chongkolwatana, & Herzon, 2000), extracorporeal shockwave therapy (Daecke, Kusnierczak, & Loew, 2002), and exogenous delivery of neurotrophins (Funakoshi et al., 1998) to promote nerve regeneration. Lundborg (2000) discussed that despite the advances in experimental biological models of regeneration, few are currently in clinical use. As research on neural plasticity expands, the important role activities and function in context play in the rehabilitation of nerve injuries will likely expand (Beggs, Torsney, Drew, & Fitzgerald, 2002).

Treatment by Levels

Although many have divided treatment into acute and chronic phases, this chapter uses the concept of treatment levels described by Lindsay (1994). Designation by levels allows guidance through sequential treatment while monitoring pain and activity tolerance. Although there is a distinct difference between treatment of tendinous and neurogenic disorders, there are enough similarities to warrant discussion of the available treatment strategies in a combined fashion.

Level 1: Inflammatory Phase

The primary goals of conservative treatment at this level are to reduce pain and inflammation and to prevent further injury, whether neurogenic or tendinous. It is also important to protect and monitor the acute condition.

Activity Modification

During this phase, it is best to avoid activities or tasks that provoke or exacerbate signs and symptoms. This avoidance may be accomplished via supportive splinting or activity modification. Static splinting may be indicated to protect the affected area from repetitive trauma or compressive forces and to reduce inflammation or edema. The afflicted individual should appreciate all tasks that may interfere with tendon or nerve healing. Because of the negative effects of immobilization, maintenance of ROM at uninvolved regions and nerve mobilization away from the injured site should be encouraged. According to Butler (1991), nerve mobilization at this level requires taking up slack in the neural system away from the site of pain and mobilizing the neural system for brief intervals (e.g., 1-second pressure on, 1-second pressure off, for a total of 20 seconds).

Modalities

Pain and inflammation may be reduced via steroids or nonsteroidal antiinflammatory drugs (NSAIDs), phonophoresis, cryotherapy techniques, pulsed ultrasound, transcutaneous electrical nerve stimulation (TENS) and rest (Fedorczyk, 1997).

Antiinflammatory Medication

Local injections are one method used to reduce inflammation in cases of tendinitis and inflammation surrounding a nerve. In select cases, a mixture of anesthetic and water-soluble corticosteroid is used. For cases of tenosynovitis, corticosteroids work by interacting with the synovial fluid; thus, they should be injected into the tendon sheath. To avoid negative side effects, the number of injections is frequently limited to three, with a 6-week interval between injections (Warhold, Osterman, & Skirven, 1993). Rupture of the common extensor tendon has been reported following corticosteroid injections (Smith et al., 1999). It has been postulated that postinjection ultrasound might enhance the benefits of the injected corticosteroid (Newman, Kill, & Frampton, 1958).

To avoid the effects of needle injection, ultrasound may be used to drive antiinflammatory medication through the skin to the involved tendon or nerve region—a process termed *phonophoresis* (Byl, 1995; Kahn, 1991; Michlovitz, 2002). Theorctically, the molecular transmission across the skin occurs because of changes in tissue permeability with ultrasound heating and because the radiation pressure of the ultrasound beam forces the medication away from the transducer. Although hydrocortisone and dexamethasone are commonly used, lidocaine and zinc oxide are also suitable molecules for phonophoresis. The strength of medication that should be used is controversial. In the case of hydrocortisone, some recommend that at least 10% strength be used, but others report no difference in penetration between 5% and 10% hydrocortisone (Davick, Martin, & Albright, 1988). Despite the use of a coupling agent, the amount of medication that penetrates the tissue via ultrasound is minimal because of the entrapment of air at a microscopic level, which serves as a blocking mechanism. To enhance the effects of transmission, some have advocated massaging the medication into the site first and then applying the ultrasound, using a coupling gel (Byl, McKenzie, Halliday, Wong, & O'Connell, 1993; Kahn, 1991). Further research is warranted to examine the efficacy of phonophoresis and to specify ultrasound parameters for the most efficient drug diffusion (Byl, 1995).

Iontophoresis (or ion transfer) involves the use of low-voltage direct current to drive medication into the affected area (Kahn, 1994). The process uses the physics principle: *Like charges repel*. The desired antiinflammatory medication is repelled from beneath an electrode with an identical charge into the skin subdermally. Although the medication penetrates to a depth of less than 1 mm, deeper absorption occurs through transmembrane transport and capillary circulation. Therapeutic compounds are formed as the ions recombine with ions and radicals in the bloodstream. The ionic charge of the medication and the pathology determine whether the positive (anode) or negative (cathode) electrode should be used. For example, hydrocortisone contains positive ions, so the positive electrode is used; dexamethasone contains negative ions, so the negative electrode is used. The anode (+) produces a weak hydrochloric acid, is sclerotic or tends to harden tissue, and serves as an analgesic on the basis of the local release of oxygen. The cathode (-) releases hydrogen and is sclerotic, tending to soften tissue. The cathode is considered ideal for use as the active electrode, but it can lead to chemical burns due to the formation of sodium hydroxide at the electrode site. Other complications from iontophoresis include heat burns from excess tissue resistance, sensitivities, and allergic reactions. Units designed exclusively for use with iontophoresis have made the modality easier and safer to use, thus more popular during the acute condition. An example of the setup of iontophoresis to treat lateral epicondylitis is pictured in Figure 6-5.

Other Modalities

Cryotherapy, or the use of cold agents, can be used effectively to reduce pain and decrease inflammation (Michlovitz, 1996). In addition, cold alters the synaptic activity and conduction velocity of peripheral nerves. Popular clinical methods of cryotherapy include cold packs, ice massage, and vapocoolant sprays. The location and size of the body part to be treated determines the best method. If commercial cold packs are used, a moist towel interface between the cold pack and the skin will eliminate much of the air interface and will facilitate energy transfer. Typically, ice massage is done over small areas, such as tendons, using water frozen in a paper cup. Ice massage will produce four separate sensations: intense cold, burning, aching, and analgesia. Vapocoolant sprays are often used to inactivate trigger points and to increase passive ROM of the muscle-tendon unit. The *stretch-and-spray technique* first places the muscle on stretch, and then the muscle is sprayed from proximal to distal attachment 2 to 3 times over the region of referred pain in parallel unidirectional sweeps. The spray is angled at approximately 30 degrees, 18 inches from the skin, and is moved at

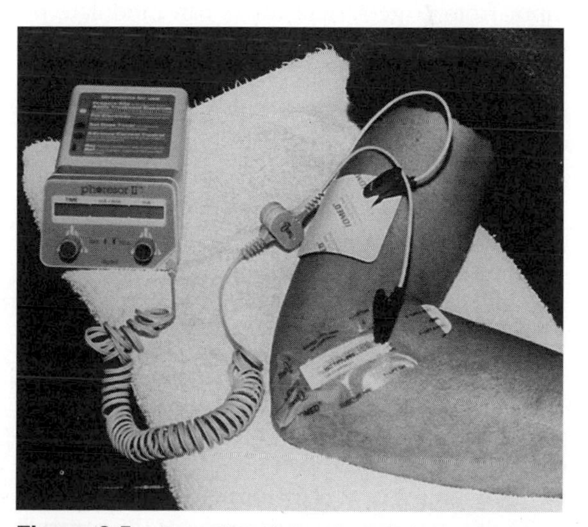

Figure 6-5 Example of iontophoresis in the treatment of lateral epicondylitis.

a rate of 10 cm per second (Travell & Simons, 1983). Cryotherapy is contraindicated with cold insensitivity (e.g., Raynaud's phenomenon). Local hypersensitivity is indicated by wheals (small regions with erythematous raised borders and blanched centers). Cold treatment should be used cautiously in hypertensive individuals and in the early stage of wound healing because of its effect on blood flow.

A pulsed mode of ultrasound at 20% or 50% without medication can be used to treat tendinitis successfully on the basis of its nonthermal effects (Michlovitz, 2002). Within the pulsed mode, it is advisable to extend the application period to allow for maximal penetration of the sound waves. To penetrate superficial structures less than 2 cm in depth (finger flexor tendons) a frequency of 3 MHz is recommended (Michlovitz, 2002). A frequency of 1 MHz can penetrate to tissue depths of 5 cm (shoulder joint capsule).

Transcutaneous Electrical Nerve Stimulation (TENS) can also be used to reduce pain (Mannheimer & Lampe, 1984). Two theories that attempt to explain the positive effect of TENS are the *gate theory* by Melzack and Wall (1965) and the *endorphin concept* (Adler, 1982; Sjolund & Eriksson, 1979). The gate theory (Melzack & Wall, 1965) proposes that pressure or touch input from large A beta fibers can modulate or gate the specific or diffuse pain signals sent by small A delta or C fibers. Originally, T-cells or second-order neurons within lamina II in the dorsal horn of the spinal cord (substantia gelatinosa) were considered to be the primary transmission sites for nerve fibers carrying the sensation of pain to the thalamus. However, because of recent research findings other brain regions must also be considered as transmission sites. Therefore, a reduction in large A beta fiber input at a transmission junction decreases presynaptic control, opening the gate and allowing pain sensations carried over small fibers to reach the thalamus. If transmission sites are activated through large A beta-fiber input (touch, pressure, or TENS), there is greater presynaptic control, and the gate is closed, reducing the pain sensation. The second theory describes how endorphins, or morphinelike molecules produced by the body, serve as endogenous analgesics to pain. Levels of endorphins increase in the blood when afferent brain signals indicate pain. Low-frequency TENS of 1 to 4 Hz have been found to increase endorphin production. Therefore, for those with chronic tendinitis and pain caused by nerve compressions and entrapments, low-rate TENS may provide the most pain relief (Wolf, 1984).

Level 2: Proliferative Phase

During the proliferative phase, the primary goals are to increase mobility and length of the involved tissue while preventing recurrence of the injury and resultant inflammation.

Superficial or deep heating may increase blood flow prior to massage, stretching, myofascial release techniques, or active exercise. Because of its vasodilation effect, heat is best used after the threat of inflammation has subsided sufficiently. Superficial heat penetrates to depths of 1 cm. Methods include hot packs, paraffin wax, or "fluidotherapy." Deeper heating may be obtained with continuous ultrasound at a frequency of 1 MHz, which can penetrate tissues 3 to 5 cm in depth (Michlovitz, 2002). In addition to increasing blood flow, low-intensity ultrasound may induce tissue growth in involved structures (Dyson, Pond, Joseph, & Warwick, 1968). It has been postulated that acoustic streaming, a nonthermal effect of ultrasound, may alter ion fluxes across tissue membranes, thereby facilitating repair.

In cases of tendinitis, deep-friction (cross-fiber) massage theoretically breaks up adhesions that typically form during healing of small tendon tears (Cyriax, 1982). Soft-tissue massage and isometrics increase blood flow in the region of the myotendinous junction and tendon, wherein blood flow typically is much less than that of the muscle belly. Forcing blood into the undernourished myotendinous-tendon regions may be achieved by massaging from the muscle belly toward the tendon. This technique would be followed by a stretch, to the involved muscle-tendon unit.

Myofascial release is another method of intervention that addresses restrictions within the loose connective tissue associated with the muscle-tendon unit and peripheral nerves. Several techniques may be used, including *unwinding* and *cross stretch*. In cases of peripheral nerve compression, it may be advantageous to first perform adverse neural tension tests, and then to perform myofascial release techniques to address the interfacing tissues associated with the nerve.

Researchers have found that isometric warm-up with follow-up stretching gives the muscle greater toleration of force before failure (Safran, Garrett, & Seaber, 1988). If isometrics or nonresisted eccentric-concentric loading induces pain, it may be best to follow the treatment with ice. An ideal sequence of treatment may involve a heat modality over the involved region, then massage followed by stretching or myofascial release, initiation of isometrics or nonresisted eccentric-concentric loading, and ending with ice. When the individual does not have pain with simple stretching or moderate loading, it may be safe to reintroduce the activity or task that typically caused the most pain.

During level 2, active exercise should be included in the program to restore range of motion and to strengthen uninvolved muscles. Active and passive nerve mobilization at the site of compression may also be performed as long as it does not provoke symptoms. If symptoms are provoked nerve mobilization should be initiated in a remote region of the nervous system (away from the irritated nerve) (Walsh, 2002). Myofascial release techniques may also be used to enhance nerve gliding via its reported effect on the loose connective tissue. The client should be asked to report any neurogenic signs during the treatment phase. In select cases, it may be necessary to continue protection of the involved site and to avoid the provocative activity. Ongoing evaluation should coincide with treatment, especially as compressive forces are alleviated and nerve function begins to increase.

Level 3: Recovery Stage

During level 3 treatment, the primary goals are to increase tolerance to controlled stress of involved regions and to enhance motor control within work, sports, and activities of daily living. In addition, it is important to educate the individual as to the cause of injury and methods of prevention.

Healing tendon and myotendinous regions requires a controlled loading stimulus to form an organized scar. Weak tissue with a poorly organized scar may be at risk for reinjury if repetitive forceful activity is resumed prematurely. Strengthening the involved areas should begin first with isometrics, as in level 2, and progress through eccentric work and general progressive resistive exercise. Controlled loading should be introduced and progressed. In addition, strengthening of proximal regions may reduce distal signs and symptoms significantly. Curwin and Stanish (1984) outlined in detail the components of an eccentric exercise program for tendinitis. Their program highlighted key features: length, load, and speed of contraction. In sequence, the program involves stretch, eccentric exercise, and stretch again, then ice. Interestingly, Almekinders and Almekinders (1994) found that neither activity modification nor nonsteroidal antiinflammatory drugs (NSAIDs) with stretching and strengthening was associated with healing and conditioning of an injured tendon unit on the basis of a questionnaire. This may suggest that further clinical research is needed to verify the efficacy of treatment interventions.

During the phase of recovery from nerve injury, regeneration should be monitored in terms of motor, sensory, and sympathetic function. In some cases, relearning of movement and prehension patterns must be addressed. Sensory reeducation may be indicated to promote desensitization and to enhance protective and discriminative sensibility through cortical reorganization. It may be necessary to incorporate postural concepts and ergonomics as they pertain to causative factors. Aerobic exercise and proper breathing strategies may further enhance the recovery of function.

Finally, preparation for return to regular occupations, including work and recreation, are indicated. Enhancing motor control and the timing of muscle recruitment may be the key to promoting carryover of any rehabilitation procedures. In preparing an individual to return to work or sports activity, simulation of the related tasks is vital. In addition, it may be necessary to evaluate the size and weight of tools or sports implements used, and to redesign the work and recreation space, because the setup of the workplace itself may be perpetuating injury. These issues are addressed in later chapters.

Because research into effective treatment methodology for musculoskeletal disorders is somewhat controversial, it is essential that a problem-solving approach be used and each case examined individually. The next section provides suggestions for intervention for disorders of musculature and neurogenic origin by body region, which may be used to guide individual treatment(s).

Interventions for Common Upper-Limb Cumulative Trauma Disorders

Cervicobrachial Region

Thoracic Outlet Syndrome

Typically, signs and symptoms of thoracic outlet syndrome (TOS) fall under a larger category termed *neurovascular entrapment syndromes of the upper quadrant* (Edgelow, 1995). Edgelow (1995) emphasizes that TOS is actually a problem of reversible or irreversible stenosis or rigid narrowing from acquired or congenital conditions. Figure 5-9 highlights common regions of stenosis. Despite Edgelow's clear distinction of TOS as a problem of stenosis, others continue to separate TOS into either a compressive or an entrapment disorder.

Findings from cervical x-rays and other diagnostic tests should be obtained before a physical examination is conducted. In addition, history and pain reports may provide insight into the disorder. In compressions, pain is often nocturnal or activity-related. Because of its location, the lower plexus (including nerve fibers from C8 to T1) is at a greater risk of compression. However, it is possible that any region of the plexus may be implicated (Kelly, 1979; Szabo, 1989). Entrapments often have some association with cervical-shoulder trauma, an anatomic abnormality or long-standing repetitive stress (Walsh, 1994). Figure 6-6 exemplifies the severe damage that may ensue from long-standing plexus entrapment, in this case from a cervical rib. Pain associated with entrapments can be divided into nerve trunk pain and dysesthetic pain. Nerve trunk pain occurs secondary to increased activity in the nociceptive endings of the nerve nervorum (sheath). Dysesthetic pain occurs by virtue of impulses from damaged or regenerating afferent fibers (Asbury & Fields, 1984).

Confirmation of TOS should include assessment of static and active posture, shoulder-cervical spine active ROM, grip and pinch strength, sensibility, provocative testing, and endurance testing (see Box 6-2). Postural deficits may perpetuate signs and symptoms induced

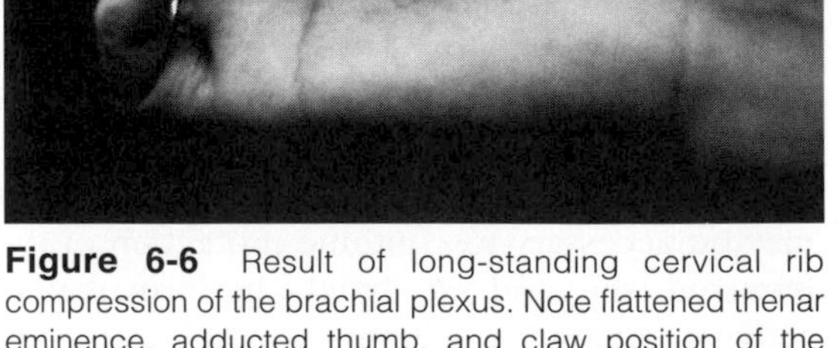

Figure 6-6 Result of long-standing cervical rib compression of the brachial plexus. Note flattened thenar eminence, adducted thumb, and claw position of the fingers as this woman attempts to make a fist.

BOX 6-2
Cervicobrachial Syndromes: Subjective and Objective Findings

Thoracic Outlet Syndrome
- Pain, paresthesias, and numbness in an ulnar nerve distribution
- Occasional transitory ischemia and edema
- Burning pain over select dermatomal regions
- Progressive sensory and motor loss in distal sites
- Possible positive findings with provocative maneuvers

Cervical Radiculopathy
- Neck pain and referred pain of a dermatomal nature rather than a diffuse one
- Symptoms of cervical disc protrusion *reproduced* with neck bending to the opposite side
- Spinal stenosis symptoms *relieved* with neck bending to the opposite side
- Often, muscle group weakness (rhomboids, trapezius) and abnormal tendon reflexes
- Symptoms from cervical disc and stenosis relieved with cervical traction and exacerbated with compression
- Provocative thoracic outlet syndrome tests negative
- Possible coexistent cervical nerve compression and distal site of compression

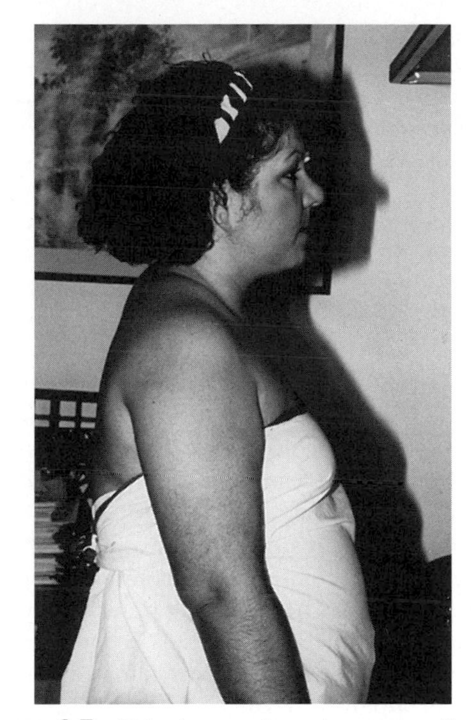

Figure 6-7 Side-view posture of woman with suspected thoracic outlet syndrome. Note her rounded shoulders, dowager's hump, and forward head posture.

from repetitive strain disorders. For example, the individual pictured from the side in Figure 6-7 presented with neurogenic signs and subtle postural deficits, such as a dowager's hump, rounded shoulders, abducted scapulas, and slight forward head posture. These postural deficits may be related to TOS signs and symptoms.

Provocative tests should be used cautiously because they can produce a high incidence of false-positive results. Adson's (1951) maneuver tests for nerve compression within the scalene triangle. It requires a 30-second palpation of the radial artery while the individual takes a deep breath, elevates the chin, and rotates the head first in the direction of pain, then in the opposite direction. A positive test involves a reduction in palpable pulse rate or exacerbation of symptoms during extremes of movement. This test supposedly induces upper-trunk symptoms versus those of the lower trunk. Wright's maneuver requires neck rotation to the opposite side and passive abduction above 90 degrees while changes in the radial pulse and neurogenic symptoms are monitored (Walsh, 1994; Wright, 1945). This maneuver tests for nerve compression beneath the pectoralis minor muscle at less than 90 degrees humeral abduction and compression between the clavicle and first rib at more than 90 degrees. The costoclavicular compression test attempts to rule out compression between the first rib and the clavicle. With the arms at the side, an individual actively retracts and depresses the scapula while the radial pulse and symptoms are monitored. Harris (1994) recommended that endurance be tested through timed grasping of a 10-lb gripper (normal: 5 minutes) and the Roos (1966) elevated stress test. The Roos test, or the 3-minute elevated-arm stress test, is the most reliable provocative test for evaluating for TOS. In the "surrender" position (arms abducted and externally rotated to 90 degrees with the forearms pronated), the subject is asked to open and close the hands once every 2 seconds and to describe symptoms during the 3-minute test. This position accentuates the abnormal compressions affecting the brachial plexus and vessels. It narrows the costoclavicular space and tenses the neck and shoulder muscles. In most positive tests, the individual cannot complete 3 minutes without reproduction of symptoms. With positive TOS, there are complaints of heaviness or fatigue in the involved extremity. Feelings of pins and needles or numbness may follow, along with a progressive ache.

Within level 1, treatment may involve restriction of aggravating activities, such as humeral hyperabduction, static neck flexion, and repetitive overhead shoulder flexion. It is recommended that pressure on the plexus be minimized through elbow propping, avoidance of carrying or lifting, and the use of a backpack or pull cart rather than a shoulder bag. Muscular and nerve inflammation as well as edema may be addressed via NSAIDs, ice, or TENS. Edgelow (1995) stressed the importance of relaxing the scalene muscle(s) (or other related musculature) if inflamed or enlarged. Although nerve gliding away from the involved region may be introduced at this level, myofascial release may relieve compression and thus promote relief of symptoms.

By level 2, the inflammatory phase has typically subsided, and heat and stretch techniques, along with myofascial release strategies, may be used to enhance circulation and tissue extensibility. Postural deficits such as rounded shoulders and forward head posture can be addressed through correctional exercises. This activity may involve the lengthening of shortened tissues and the strengthening of weakened muscles. For example, the pectoralis major may be lengthened and the middle and lower trapezius may be strengthened. Nerve gliding in the involved region may be done by simulating the median nerve tension test (see Figures 6-3 and 6-8).

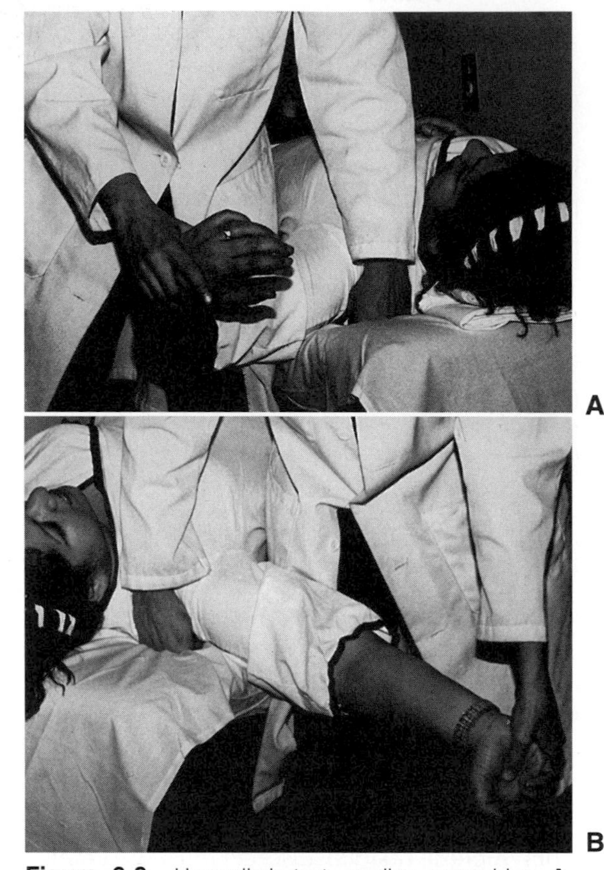

Figure 6-8 Upper-limb test, median nerve bias. **A,** Initial position. Note therapist's fisted hand and her arm depressing the shoulder while she begins to passively externally rotate the patient's shoulder and extend the wrist. **B,** Final position. Note elbow extension. The therapist's hand remains in neutral secondary to the patient's low tolerance to lateral side bending.

By level 3, modality treatment should be discontinued. General conditioning through aerobic exercise may be used. Given the high incidence of work-related TOS, posture and ergonomics related to occupational tasks should be emphasized. Work-site evaluations and subsequent modifications may be required to ensure adequate carryover of the treatment program.

Cervical Disc and Foraminal Stenosis

At the cervical level, nerve roots may be irritated secondary to entrapment within the foramen, cervical disc herniation, cervical spondylosis, or posttraumatic subluxation (Cailliet, 1991). Cervical root involvement may mimic signs of brachial plexopathy or distal peripheral nerve compressions.

It is possible to differentiate cervical disc-foraminal stenosis from more distal disorders through an upper-quadrant screen (see Box 6-1). Suspected findings may include neck pain and referred pain of a dermatomal rather than diffuse nature. Dermatomal symptoms of numbness, tingling, and pain may be reproduced by bending the neck to the opposite side in cases of cervical disc protrusion. Alternatively, bending the neck to the opposite side may relieve spinal stenosis symptoms. In addition, abnormal neurologic signs may be reflected as muscle group tenderness or weakness or abnormal tendon reflexes (Cailliet, 1991). For example, there may be tenderness through the rhomboids or the trapezius. In both types of disorders, symptoms are relieved with cervical traction and exacerbated with compression. Provocative TOS tests will be negative. Although it is important to differentiate between the presence of cervical and distal nerve involvement, it also is possible to have a proximal (cervical) nerve compression coexist with a distal site of compression (Osterman, 1988).

Treatment may progress through all three levels (see Table 6-4). Treatment at level 1 typically involves providing relief from symptoms through the use of thermal agent modalities or cervical traction, if indicated. Some clinicians prefer to treat via joint mobilization from day 1 (Maitland, 1991). At level 1, it is important to address posture and avoidance of provocative positions. Once the individual begins to feel relief, he or she may be ready for simple cervical ROM exercises and postural correctional exercises typical of level 2 treatment. Myofascial release strategies and soft-tissue mobilization techniques may be preceded by heat modalities or TENS to prepare the tissue and reduce pain. This level of treatment may continue for some time until the individual is ready for level 3. Once the pain no longer limits activity or if it resolves within 24 hours, afflicted individuals are ready to tolerate upper-body conditioning if needed and work-simulation activities. Level 3 treatment for those with cervical radiculopathy will vary widely.

Shoulder Region

Typical injuries that occur within the shoulder region, secondary to overuse, include rotator cuff tendinitis and bicipital tendinitis (Box 6-3). Associated conditions include trigger points and bursitis. Risk factors associated with shoulder overuse include awkward or static postures, direct load bearing, overhead work, heavy work, repetitive movements, and lack of rest (Burkart & Post, 2002; Sommerich, McGlothlin, & Marrar, 1993).

Rotator Cuff Tendinitis

Tendinitis of the rotator cuff has been linked to impingement of structures within the supra-

BOX 6-3

Shoulder Disorders in Tendinitis: Subjective and Objective Findings

Rotator Cuff Tendinitis (Tendinosis)

Supraspinous
- A painful arc of abduction
- Pain with resisted abduction and internal rotation combined
- Pain with full passive elevation
- Pain on palpation to tendon (lateral to acromion or anterior humeral head given position of humeral extension)
- Positive impingement test (passive flexion with internal rotation)

Infraspinous
- Pain with resisted external rotation
- Pain on tendon palpation (lateral humeral head given position of horizontal adduction)

Bicipital Tendinitis (Tendinosis)
- Pain with isotonic shoulder flexion, which increases with resistance
- Pain with resisted elbow flexion and forearm supination
- Painless passive movement
- Possible tenderness to touch over proximal biceps tendon

Source: Modified from Cyriax, J. (1982). *Textbook of orthopaedic medicine, Vol 1: Diagnosis of soft-tissue lesions* (8th ed). London: Baillere Tindall.

humeral (subacromial) space. This tight space lies between the head of the humerus and the coracoacromial arch. The arch is formed by the coracoid process, the acromion, and the coracoacromial ligament. Superiorly to inferiorly, this space contains the subacromial (subdeltoid) bursa, the supraspinous muscle and tendon, the superior part of the shoulder joint capsule, the tendon of the long head of the biceps brachii, and, possibly, the anterior portion of the infraspinous tendon (Neer & Welsh, 1982; Pratt, 1991). The subacromial space may narrow secondary to posterior joint capsule tightness, congenital malformation of the acromion into a downward arc, spur development beneath the acromion, or humeral head elevation relative to the glenoid fossa. If the muscular depressors of the humeral head are weaker than the elevators, the humeral head may tend to ride in an elevated position within the glenoid fossa, predisposing the suprahumeral space to compression. The depressors of the humeral head are the long head of the biceps muscle, the infraspinous, the latissimus dorsi, and the teres minor and major muscles. The elevators are the deltoid and the supraspinous muscles.

Neer and Welsh (1982) devised a classification system for impingement, as outlined in Table 6-7. Impingement of subacromial structures typically occurs in those individuals who engage in overhead activities such as are required in baseball pitching, swimming, tennis, and painting. In the presence of impingement, nutrition to the distal end of the tendon may be restricted. Given this restriction of blood supply, an injured supraspinous tendon may heal slowly. In elderly individuals, tendon degeneration may occur secondary to repeated bouts of tendon microtrauma producing a defect in the tendon rather than a true tear (Schmelzeisen, 1990).

Impingement syndrome may be associated with tendinitis or tears to the cuff's related tendons (Kelly, 2002). Typically, the supraspinous tendon is implicated, although the

Table 6-7
Classification of Subacromial Impingement

Stage	Anatomic Changes	Primary Complaint	Signs and Symptoms
Stage I	Edema and hemorrhage	Anterior shoulder ache	Painful arc 70-120 degrees abduction
		Occasional radiation to posterior capsule and pain following activity	Positive impingement sign
Stage II	Subacromial (subdeltoid) bursa involved	Pain during and after activity	Weakness
	Fibrosis and thickening of rotator cuff		Painful abduction arc
			Positive impingement sign
Stage III	Permanent thickness of rotator cuff	Pain during and after activity	Persistent weakness
	Spurring of acromion		Painful abduction arc
	Calcification of rotator cuff and biceps tendon		Positive impingement sign
	1-cm tears in rotator cuff		
Stage IV	Muscle atrophy	Pain during and after light activities of daily living	Severe weakness
	Rotator cuff tears >1 cm		Minimal active range of motion against gravity
	Bicep tears, partial or full		May develop adhesive capsulitis

Source: Modified from Neer, C. S. & Walsh, R. P. (1982). The shoulder in sports. *Orthopedic Clinics of North America, 8,* 439.

infraspinous tendon may be involved. The signs and symptoms of supraspinous tendon impingement include a painful arc of abduction, pain with combined resistance to abduction and internal rotation, pain with full passive elevation, and pain on palpation. The impingement test reported by Hawkins and Kennedy (1980) notes that symptoms can be reproduced from a position of 90 degrees of humeral flexion with forceful passive internal rotation, which causes the humeral head to drive the rotator cuff underneath the coracoacromial ligament. However, some suggest that this test is not a valid predictor of outcome following surgical decompression (Kirkley, Litchfield, Jackowski, & Lo, 2002). The supraspinous tendon may be palpated in its superior position on the humeral head lateral to the acromion process or from a position of shoulder extension. If involved, the supraspinous tendon may be tender to palpation. Complete rupture of the supraspinous tendon is indicated by an inability to maintain humeral abduction after passive placement of the arm in this position (drop-arm test). If one suspects involvement of the supraspinous tendon but there is not a painful arc or pain with passive elevation, the myotendinous junction may be implicated (Cyriax, 1982).

Treatment for supraspinous tendinitis (partial tear) may be approached in levels, as outlined previously (also see Burkart & Post, 2002). At level 1, overhead activities are restricted, and inflammation may be reduced by use of NSAIDs or physical agent modalities such as iontophoresis, phonophoresis, or pulsed ultrasound. At level 2, cross-fiber massage may reduce adhesions and massage from the supraspinous muscle belly toward the tendon may enhance blood flow. To enhance mobility of the muscle-tendon unit, stretching into shoulder adduction after massage is recommended. Isometrics may be initiated at this treatment level. Postural correctional exercises are initiated as indicated. Isotonic resistive loading of the rotator cuff is begun at level 3. Eccentric activities generally are not used for supraspinous tendinitis. Instead, training of scapular depressors and retractors is used to strengthen and balance the scapulothoracic and glenohumeral musculature. Once the tendon shows signs of tolerance to resistance, conditioning of the supraspinous muscle itself can be undertaken. Because supraspinous tendinitis is often induced by overhead work, job or task simulation should be incorporated into the treatment program. Ergonomic redesign of work tasks may be necessary to avoid recurrence.

Infraspinous tendinitis is associated with pain on resisted external rotation. The posteriorly located infraspinous tendon can be palpated over the humeral head if the humerus is horizontally adducted. This tendon may be tender to palpation if involved. Treatment may be followed as above, with the replacement of external rotation for abduction at levels 2 and 3.

Bicipital Tendinitis

Bicipital tendinitis involves the long head of the biceps tendon in the proximal anterior humeral region. The long head of the biceps might become inflamed as it is recruited during resisted shoulder flexion and elbow flexion.

Signs and symptoms include pain elicited on resisted elbow flexion and forearm supination as well as on isotonic shoulder flexion (see Figure 6-9). Passive movement is typically painless (Cyriax, 1982). The region over the proximal biceps tendon may be tender to touch.

During level 1 treatment for bicipital tendinitis, the provocative activity must be avoided. However, because of the large number of movements for which the long head of the biceps is recruited, it may be difficult to determine which activity is implicated. To reduce inflammation, methods such as NSAIDs, phonophoresis, iontophoresis, pulsed ultrasound, and ice may be used. An injection of corticosteroid also may be given. At treatment level 2, cross-friction massage over the tendon may assist in reducing adhesions, and massage from the muscle belly proximally toward the tendon can help to increase blood flow. It is best to stretch the biceps tendon immediately after these therapeutic

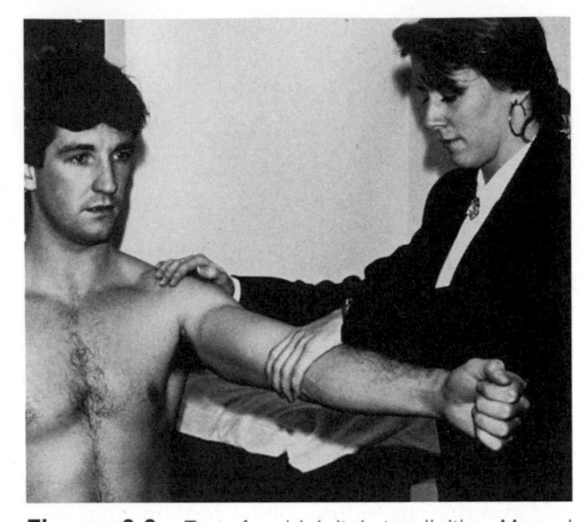

Figure 6-9 Test for bicipital tendinitis. Manual resistance during isotonic shoulder flexion. Positive test reproduces pain in the region of the biceps tendon or referred areas.

interventions to take advantage of the increased blood flow. The stretch may be accomplished by extending the elbow and shoulder in forearm pronation. During treatment level 3, conditioning may ensue once symptoms have subsided. Treatment should include eccentric training because eccentric activities often are the cause of bicipital tendinitis. Reconditioning for work or recreational tasks should be incorporated into level 3 activities.

Myofascial Trigger Points

To deactivate the trigger points, treatment should be directed at the muscle itself. The stretch-and-spray technique involves stretch of the muscle followed by the application of a vapocoolant spray (Travell & Simons, 1983). Ischemic compression or firm digital pressure to the trigger point causes ischemia with hypoxia and may be followed by a reactive hyperemia. Other modalities such as TENS, laser, or acupuncture may prove very effective at treating trigger points. Acupuncture involves injection of a dry needle, saline, or local anesthetic. As stated earlier, some centers advocate using pulsed ultrasound for three consecutive days after injection of trigger points (Nagler, 1995). Ultrasound applied at low intensities over a sustained period may inactivate the trigger point through thermal and nonthermal effects.

After trigger point inactivation, the muscle and its fascia should be addressed. Moist heat may be used, followed by myofascial release strategies. As one progresses into treatment levels 2 and 3, reconditioning of the involved muscle as well as retraining should be undertaken to enhance muscle balancing during activities of daily living and work activities.

Subacromial Bursitis

Goals for treatment of subacromial bursitis include reducing pain and inflammation, preventing further injury, increasing active and passive ROM, increasing strength, enhancing motor control, and returning the client to work and functional activities. The methods for reaching these goals are similar to those prescribed for tendinitis secondary to impingement.

The primary method of treatment for acute or chronic bursitis is protection from further injury through avoidance of provocative activities or, in the case of olecranon bursitis, use of a padded elbow sleeve. A physician may prescribe antiinflammatory agents and/or cortisone injections. Some physicians opt to drain the bursa. Pulsed ultrasound, iontophoresis, or phonophoresis can be used during the acute inflammatory period. Some individuals with chronic bursitis develop calcium deposits, which also may be resolved with ultrasound (Cyriax, 1982). Once the initial pain and inflammation subsides, the individual may tolerate simple active ROM exercises against gravity, progressing to general conditioning as needed. The reader is referred to the previous section on rotator cuff tendinitis for conditioning strategies applicable to bursitis in the glenohumeral joint region because of its association with impingement.

Elbow-Forearm Region

Most upper-limb movements involve elbow structures, and so the region is susceptible to many forms of tendinous and neurogenic cumulative trauma including cubital tunnel syndrome, lateral epicondylitis, radial tunnel syndrome, medial epicondylitis, pronator syndrome, and anterior interosseous syndrome.

The two typical forms of tendinitis occurring within the elbow-forearm region are lateral epicondylitis (tennis elbow) and medial epicondylitis (golfer's elbow). These two repetitive injuries stem from different provocative activities and implicate separate anatomic regions. The frequency with which medial epicondylitis occurs is approximately 10% to 20% that of lateral epicondylitis (Powell & Burke, 1991).

Common nerve compressions in this region involve three distinct peripheral nerves: radial, median, and ulnar. Because of the close proximity of structures and the similarity of causative activities, some conditions may have both a tendinous and a neurogenic component, both of which must be evaluated and treated. It may be necessary to treat the neurogenic signs first and then to treat the tendon injury (Lindsay, 1993).

Cubital Tunnel Syndrome

The cubital tunnel lies between the medial epicondyle of the humerus and the olecranon process of the ulna. The floor of the tunnel consists of the medial collateral ligament of the elbow (Pratt, 1991). The two heads of the flexor carpi ulnaris make up the sides, and the triangular arcuate ligament composes the roof. In full elbow extension, the triangular arcuate ligament is slack, whereas at 90 degrees of elbow flexion this ligament is taut and the medial collateral ligament bulges, raising the tunnel floor, while the medial triceps pushes the ulnar nerve anteromedially. Because of their superficial position beneath the arcuate ligament, the motor fibers to the intrinsic hand muscles and the cutaneous sensory fibers to the hand are vulnerable to external compression (Szabo, 1989). Although the cubital tunnel region is frequently implicated, there are other potential sites of ulnar nerve compression around the elbow, as pictured in Figure 6-10.

Signs and symptoms of ulnar nerve compression in this region (listed in Box 6-4) include a numbness or tingling in the volar and dorsal small finger and half of the ring finger as well as the ulnar side of the palm. There may be weakness in the muscles innervated by the ulnar nerve below the elbow. Diminished innervation or denervation will limit wrist ulnar

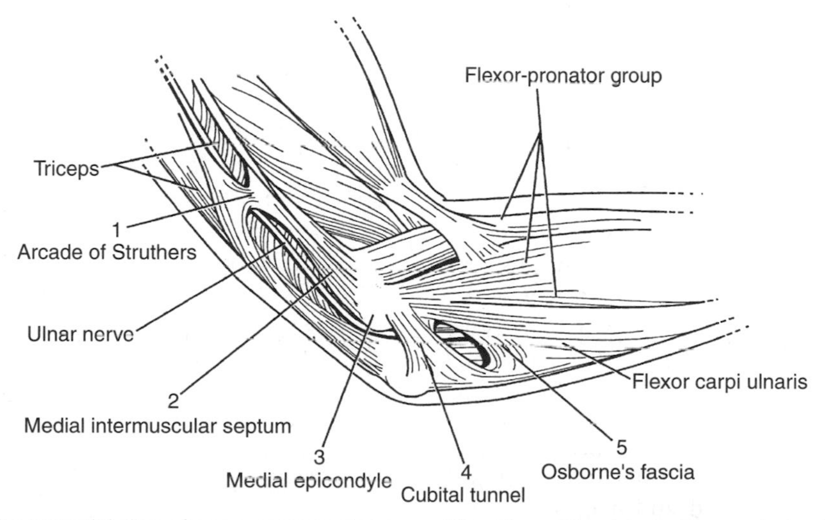

Figure 6-10 Five potential sites of nerve compression around the elbow. (Reprinted with permission from Osterman, A .L., & Davis, C. A. [1996]. Subcutaneous transposition of the ulnar nerve for treatment of cubital tunnel syndrome. *Hand Clinics, 12* , 422.)

BOX 6-4
Ulnar Nerve Compressions: Subjective and Objective Findings

Cubital Tunnel Syndrome

- Sharp or aching pain in medial-proximal forearm, with possible proximal or distal radiation exacerbated by elbow flexion and extension
- Sensibility diminished through dorsal and volar regions of the hand in the ulnar one and a half digits
- Numbness and tingling in an ulnar nerve distribution
- Weakness in intrinsics of hand, possibly causing:
  - Altered grip and pinch strength
  - Slight atrophy of hypothenar eminence
  - Hyperextension of fourth and fifth metacarpophalangeal joints
- Weakness of flexor carpi ulnaris and flexor digitorum profundus to small and ring fingers
- Altered nerve conduction
- Tinel's sign in cubital tunnel
- Froment's sign (excess flexion of thumb interphalangeal joint secondary to weak adductor pollicis noted on lateral pinch)
- Wartenberg's sign (excess small-finger abduction secondary to overpull of the extensor digiti minimi and weak dorsal interossei muscles)
- Jeneau's sign

Guyon's Tunnel Syndrome

- Diminished sensibility of volar cutaneous distribution of fifth digit and half of the fourth digit (dorsal cutaneous branch spared as it originates 5 cm proximal to Guyon's tunnel)
- Strong flexor digitorum profundus to fourth and fifth digits and flexor carpi ulnaris
- Weakness in intrinsics of hand, possibly causing:
  - Altered grip and pinch strength
  - Atrophy of hypothenar eminence
  - Hyperextension of fourth and fifth metacarpophalangeal joints (less prominent than cubital tunnel)
- Tinel's sign near Guyon's tunnel
- Froment's sign (excess flexion of thumb interphalangeal joint secondary to weak adductor pollicis during lateral pinch)
- Wartenberg's sign (excess small-finger abduction secondary to overpull of the extensor digiti minimi and weak dorsal interossei muscles)

Source: Modified from Rayan, G. M. (1992). Proximal ulnar nerve compression. Cubital tunnel syndrome. *Hand Clin, 8,* 325–336.

deviation and flexion; distal flexion of the distal interphalangeal joint (DIP) of the fourth and fifth digits; finger abduction; finger-thumb adduction; flexion of the metacarpophalangeal joint (MP) of the thumb, ring, and small fingers; and small-finger abduction and opposition. In general, gross grasp and prehensile functions such as lateral pinch and handwriting may be affected. Sensibility in the ulnar distribution will be diminished. On physical examination, a positive Tinel's sign will be found, and symptoms will be reproduced with the sustained elbow flexion test (wrists extended), which increases pressure within the cubital tunnel. The test position of elbow flexion is held for 1 minute while the subject reports any symptoms (Szabo, 1989).

Treatment during level 1 involves reducing the nerve compression and avoiding provocative activities. Typically, to reduce the compression and rest the region, a long arm splint is fabricated (Figure 6-11). Some authors advocate a position of 45 degrees of elbow flexion when splinting because this puts minimal pressure on the ulnar nerve within the cubital tunnel. The 90-degrees position may also be recommended. NSAIDs or other modalities can be used to reduce pain, inflammation, and edema. In addition, associated regions of involvement

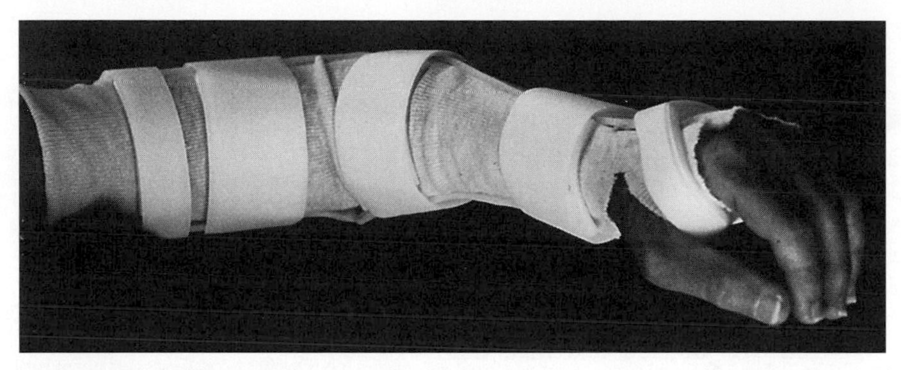

Figure 6-11 Long arm splint. Often used in cases of cubital tunnel or severe cases of lateral epicondylitis.

may require attention at level 1. For example, the distal medial triceps may be tender and show signs of edema or enlargement. Nerve mobilization away from the site of injury may be used.

Once the inflammation has subsided and the significant signs of paresthesia have diminished, heat treatments and massage may be used at level 2. The client may be able to tolerate a "heelbo" or soft splint (Figure 6-12), which prevents direct elbow pressure yet allows greater mobility than a plastic splint. Nerve mobilization and myofascial release techniques may be used near the site of injury and throughout the site of the involved region.

Level 3 treatment including aerobic and muscular conditioning can begin once the client's activity tolerance begins to increase. The primary precaution is avoidance of excessive or repetitive elbow flexion and extension. As stated previously, the final rehabilitative phase should include task simulation and work-site evaluation, as needed, to avoid recurrence of signs and symptoms. If conservative treatment is unsuccessful, the individual may require surgical decompression. One common form of decompression is an ulnar nerve transposition, which typically involves relocating the ulnar nerve to a more protected anterior position. Treatment after surgical intervention resembles the treatment by levels as just outlined.

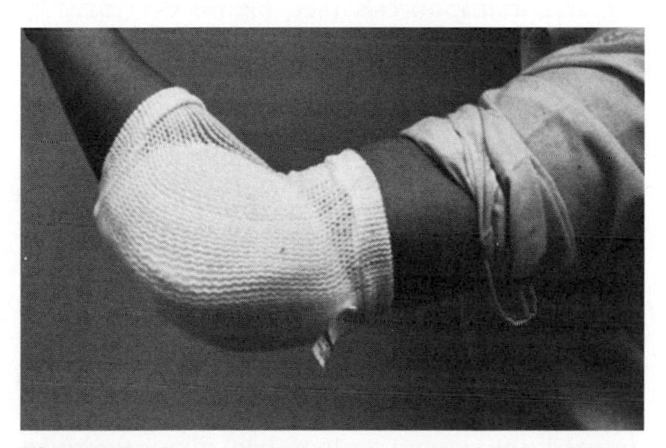

Figure 6-12 "Heelbo," which cushions the elbow in cases of cubital tunnel and olecranon bursitis or provides neutral warmth in cases of lateral or medial epicondylitis.

Olecranon Bursitis

Olecranon bursitis has been described by Cyriax (1982). If the bursa has not been drained, the primary goal at level 1 is to protect the bursa from further insult. This may be accomplished by use of a long arm splint with a cutout for the enlarged elbow or by use of a heelbo if a small enough size is available. If the excess fluid is not absorbed by the system, the bursa may need to be drained or surgically treated. As the pain subsides, level 2 strategies of ROM exercises and gentle forearm and upper-arm conditioning exercises may be done. Level 3 treatment may not be indicated.

Lateral Epicondylitis

The lateral epicondyle serves as the attachment site for the common extensor tendon and includes the extensor carpi radialis longus (ECRL) and brevis (ECRB), extensor digitorum (ED), and extensor digiti minimi (EDM) (Pratt, 1991). Microrupture and subsequent fibrosis of the ECRB and the common extensor tendon of the lateral epicondyle are considered primary pathologic causes of tennis elbow, as first noted by Cyriax (1936) and later confirmed by Nirschl and Pettrone (1979) through histologic evidence of pathologic alteration of the ECRB muscle tissue. The anterior extensor digitorum and the ECRL typically are affected less than the ECRB. The work of Nirschl and Pettrone (1979) supported the belief that tennis elbow was a degenerative process; these researchers labeled the condition *angiofibroblastic tendinosis*.

Lateral epicondylitis is often found in less accomplished tennis players who exhibit poor backhand mechanics, in which eccentric forces cause a lesion to the wrist extensors. However, lateral epicondylitis is not isolated to tennis players; activities unrelated to sports, including repetitive assembly work, gardening, and typing, have also been implicated as causes (Powell & Burke, 1991).

Among the key signs and symptoms of lateral epicondylitis are pain and weakness experienced with excessive gripping and resisted wrist extension, point tenderness on the lateral epicondyle, and pain with stretching of the wrist extensors (Fedorczyk, 2002; Powell & Burke, 1991) (Box 6-5). Maudsley's test or the long-finger extension test may be positive due to the influence of the extensor digitorum (Fairbank & Corlett, 2002). Symptoms will be reproduced with wrist extension and radial deviation and with elbow extension and finger flexion. Pain also may occur with resisted supination and wrist extension. Because of the close proximity of the lateral epicondyle to the radial nerve, impingement of the radial nerve in the proximal forearm must be ruled out, as must cervical nerve involvement.

Treatment at level 1 may include rest within a wrist splint or counterforce brace with a clasp or cuff placed over the origin of the ECRB (common extensor tendon). Counterforce bracing serves to reduce pain and control tendon overload. It also constrains the involved muscle groups and maintains muscle balance. Groppel and Nirschl (1986) reported that counterforce bracing of the elbow decreased angular acceleration of the elbow and reduced EMG activity in the wrist extensors (Figure 6-13). In conditions that are resistant to low-level immobilization, a long arm splint may be used. Antiinflammatory medication, ice, phonophoresis, and iontophoresis (see Figure 6-5) may be used to reduce inflammation.

At level 2, extensibility of the tissue should be emphasized. Cross-friction massage may help to restore mobility between tissue interfaces. With the client's elbow flexed and the forearm supinated, the therapist uses his or her index or long finger or thumb to massage perpendicular to the ECRB tendon for 6 to 12 minutes (Cyriax, 1982). Because the common extensor tendon has a limited blood supply and lacks a synovial sheath, massage from the muscle belly (ECRB) toward the lateral epicondyle may effectively increase blood flow. Stretching of the common extensor tendon is best achieved with "alphabet

BOX 6-5
Elbow Tendon Disorders: Subjective and Objective Findings

Lateral Epicondylitis
- Pain and weakness experienced with excessive gripping and resisted wrist extension
- Point tenderness over lateral epicondyle
- Pain with stretching of wrist extensors, given elbow extension and finger flexion (may have extrinsic shortening)
- Must rule out impingement of the radial nerve in the region of the radial tunnel due to its close proximity to the extensor carpi radialis brevis

Medial Epicondylitis
- Pain with resisted wrist flexion and finger flexion and, possibly, resisted pronation
- Pain with passive elbow, wrist, and finger extension
- On supination with the elbow extended, possible replication of symptoms secondary to stretch of the pronator teres
- Point tenderness over medial epicondyle

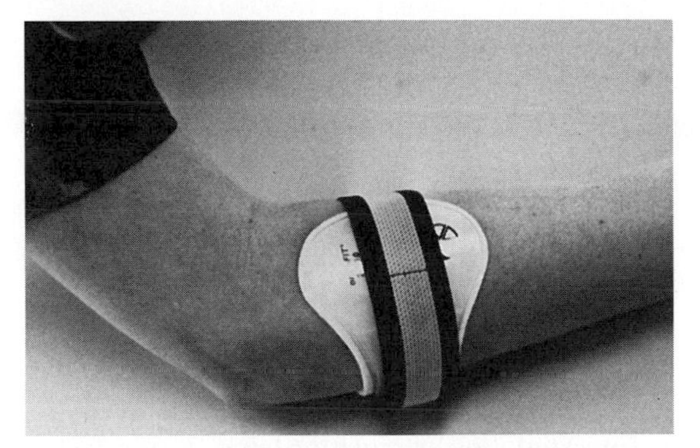

Figure 6-13 Counterforce brace used to treat lateral epicondylitis. Theoretically, the clasp acts as an alternative attachment site from which the muscle can pull, thus allowing for tendon healing.

exercises": To complete these exercises, the individual draws the capital letters of the alphabet with his or her index finger, moving the wrist into flexion and extension while the finger joints are maintained in extension, the shoulder is flexed to 90 degrees, and the elbow extended.

At level 3, conditioning of the extensor region follows the concept of isometric to eccentric loading (Fyfe & Stanish, 1992). Wrist extension with the elbow flexed as well as extended should be emphasized. Because strong gripping is a common cause of pain, sustained grip activities should be included in the conditioning program. It may be necessary to use a semi-mobile wrist splint during select tasks (Figure 6-14) to allow use of the extensor muscle group in a modified wrist ROM. Finally, the program should be completed with job or recreational simulation and follow-up work-site analysis, as needed.

Radial Tunnel Syndrome

The radial tunnel region extends from the elbow to the insertion of the posterior interosseous nerve into the supinator. It involves compression of the deep motor or posterior interosseous branch of the radial nerve, induced primarily through repetitive forearm rotation (Peimer & Wheeler, 1989; Pratt, 1991). One activity that may induce this disorder is repetitive supination and pronation, performed routinely by checkout clerks who scan items.

Radial tunnel syndrome may be differentiated from lateral epicondylitis by physical examination. In cases of lateral epicondylitis, resistance specific to the ECRL and ECRB may invoke pain. Palpation of the lateral epicondyle will be painful, and, at rest, the pain will be localized to the epicondyle region. Signs and symptoms of radial tunnel syndrome include pain in the

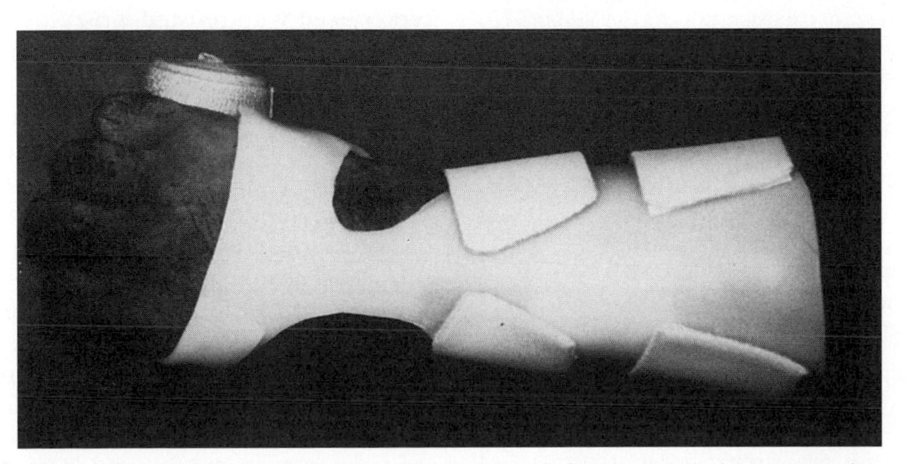

Figure 6-14 Semimobile wrist splint allows use of wrist extensors in functional tasks in a protected range of motion. Note that a 1-inch bar at the wrist allows for some movement.

proximal-dorsal forearm that increases with daytime rotational activities or pain at night (Box 6-6). On physical examination, symptoms will be reproduced with resisted supination and resisted middle-finger extension with the wrist flexed or extended (ECRB). Pressure on the supinator or between the brachioradialis and ECRB may reproduce symptoms in the dorsal radial nerve distribution (Peimer & Wheeler, 1989).

At level 1, the treatment strategies for radial tunnel syndrome include restriction of forearm supination and extension, possible provision of a dorsal or volar wrist cock-up splint to restrict extension of the wrist and to provide external support, NSAIDs, and modalities to reduce inflammation (e.g., ice, phonophoresis, iontophoresis). Pulsed ultrasound may be initiated. Myofascial release strategies also might be effective. Nerve gliding should be performed away from the site of pain.

BOX 6-6
Radial Nerve Compressions: Subjective and Objective Findings

Radial Tunnel Syndrome
- Pain at rest over the mobile extensor muscle mass, which increases with activity
- Pain with resisted third-finger extension if elbow and wrist are extended secondary to contraction of extensor carpi radialis brevis
- Pain with wrist extension and supination
- Pain with wrist flexion and pronation secondary to stretching over the extensor carpi radialis brevis and supinator
- Functional loss secondary to weakened supination, thumb abduction, and wrist, finger, and thumb extension
- Restriction in proximal-dorsal forearm, given adverse neural tension testing of the radial nerve
- No sensory deficits

Superficial Radial Nerve Compression
- Pain over the dorsal radial aspect of the hand
- Pain on writing or sustained grip
- Sensory loss over the distribution of the radial nerve
- Positive Tinel's sign over the nerve near the snuff-box
- Positive Finkelstein's test
- No pain with thumb extension and no tenderness over the first dorsal compartment

Once the individual progresses to level 2, local radial nerve-gliding technique may be used while myofascial release strategies are continued. Massage may be done according to the client's tolerance, followed by active stretching of the proximal-dorsal forearm musculature.

At level 3, reconditioning of the weakened extensors and supinator may be undertaken. If tolerated, job simulation and a work-site evaluation can be conducted.

Medial Epicondylitis

The medial epicondyle serves as the attachment site of the pronator teres, flexor carpi radialis, flexor carpi ulnaris, FDS, and palmaris longus muscles (Pratt, 1991). Medial epicondylitis is frequently caused by overuse of the wrist flexors or pronator teres muscle-tendon units that attach to the medial epicondyle. Powerful forehand strokes, golfing, and typing are examples of activities that can contribute to this disorder. This form of tendinitis may be induced by acute forceful injury more often than is lateral epicondylitis. Nerve compression of the ulnar nerve and, occasionally, of the median nerve will need to be ruled out because of the similarities in symptomatology.

On physical examination, pain is often reproduced with resisted wrist flexion, resisted finger flexion and, possibly, resisted pronation (see Box 6-5). Passive stretching into elbow, wrist, and finger extension also may induce pain secondary to an extreme muscle stretch. Supination with the elbow extended may replicate symptoms secondary to stretching of the pronator teres; therefore, it is important to rule out pronator syndrome.

Treatment for medial epicondylitis is similar to that listed for lateral epicondylitis, with a few exceptions. Counterforce bracing typically is unsuccessful in medial epicondylitis. In some conditions, a soft elbow support may provide the necessary cushioning and neutral warmth during levels 1 and 2 and might help to enhance blood flow for healing of involved tissues once the inflammatory phase resolves. At level 2, heat and massage from the flexor-pronator muscle group toward the medial epicondyle may be an effective preparation for myofascial release strategies and gentle stretching. Reconditioning of the tissue in this region through treatment levels 2 and 3 should be carried out cautiously. It is advisable to avoid full-range stretching into elbow extension unless pain is minimal. In addition, strengthening should be done in a slow, graded fashion to avoid reinjury. Because of the vulnerability of the affected site, medial epicondylitis may take a long time to heal fully but, once reconditioning is successful, retraining for job and recreational tasks may be undertaken.

Pronator Syndrome

The median nerve can become compressed by the lacertus fibrosus between the two heads of the pronator teres and underneath the proximal arch to the FDS (Rehak, 2001). Signs and symptoms of pronator syndrome (Box 6-7) include numbness or paresthesias in the radial three and a half digits, weakness in grip and pinch during repetitive writing or related tasks, and pain in the volar forearm that increases with activity. On physical examination, findings may include firmness with tenderness to palpation over the enlarged pronator teres, a positive Tinel's sign over the distal margin of the pronator teres, and a negative Phalen's test. Symptoms may be reproduced with the following: 1) resisted pronation (and will increase with movement from flexion to extension, implicating the pronator teres); 2) isolated flexion of the long and ring proximal interphalangeal (PIP) joints (indicating entrapment at the FDS), 3) active elbow flexion with supination (indicating entrapment by the lacertus fibrosus), and 4) resisted elbow flexion past 120 degrees (indicating entrapment by the ligament of Struthers). Rarely is a conduction defect found on electrodiagnostic testing.

Treatment at level 1 includes strategies to reduce inflammation such as NSAIDs and other

BOX 6-7
Median Nerve Compressions: Subjective and Objective Findings

Pronator Syndrome

- Numbness or paresthesias in the radial three and a half digits
- Weakness in grip and pinch during repetitive writing or related task
- Firmness and tenderness to palpation over enlarged pronator teres
- Positive Tinel's sign over distal margin of the pronator teres
- Negative Phalen's test
- Symptoms reproduced with the following resisted movements:
  - Pronation (increases with movement from flexion to extension, implicating pronator teres)
  - Isolated flexion of long and ring proximal interphalangeal joints (flexor digitorum superficialis), indicating entrapment at the flexor digitorum superficialis
  - Elbow flexion with supination, indicating entrapment by the lacertus fibrosus of the biceps brachii
- Rarely, conduction defect on electrodiagnostic testing

Anterior Interosseous Syndrome

- Weakness: possible denervation seen on electromyographic studies of flexor pollicis longus, index and long flexor digitorum profundus, and pronator quadratus
- Abnormal pinch patterns with decreased dexterity
- Elbow pain with resisted pronation (elbow flexed to isolate the pronator quadratus)
- No cutaneous deficits
- Negative nerve conduction studies

Carpal Tunnel Syndrome

- Intermittent paresthesias or pain
- Numbness, particularly nocturnal burning pain
- Inability to sustain grip on objects, with thenar atrophy, weak abductor pollicis brevis, and strong flexor pollicis longus and flexor digitorum profundus
- Positive Tinel's sign and Phalen's test
- Abnormal sensibility in median nerve distribution, with diminished sudomotor activity (normal sensibility in proximal palm)
- Abnormal electromyographic and nerve conduction studies in median nerve distribution

modalities (e.g., ice, phonophoresis, iontophoresis, and pulsed ultrasound). TENS may assist in pain reduction. Avoidance of provocative activities may require task modification and supportive splinting. At this treatment level, nerve mobilization should be performed away from the injury site. However, myofascial release techniques may be done within the affected region.

By level 2, continuous ultrasound may be substituted for pulsed ultrasound to induce a heating effect. Massage may be used to enhance muscle blood flow before stretching in a direction of supination and elbow flexion. (Elbow flexion may remain tender for an extended period.) Isometrics may be initiated.

By level 3, the client should be ready to advance from isometrics to isotonic resistive exercises. Reconditioning for work or recreational tasks that require forearm rotation should be undertaken. Surgical decompression may need to be performed if conservative treatment is ineffective.

Anterior Interosseous Syndrome

The anterior interosseous nerve branches off the median nerve approximately 5 cm distal to the medial epicondyle. It innervates the FPL, the pronator quadratus, and the FDP to the index and long finger. Although such compressions are uncommon, this nerve may be compressed by the deep head of the pronator teres, the origin of the FDS, the origin of the flexor carpi radialis, and accessory muscles from the FDS to the FDP, including Gantzer's muscle (FPL) (Spinner, 1970). Other causes of the anterior interosseous syndrome include trauma and vascular insufficiency. The onset of this entrapment syndrome is often insidious.

In approximately one-third of reported cases, there is an insidious onset of proximal forearm pain followed by several hours of weakness or paralysis to the affected muscles. In the other two-thirds of reported cases, individuals often recall a bout of strenuous or repetitive forearm activity, prolonged forearm pressure, or trauma. Some individuals report having difficulty only with handwriting. On further examination, thumb interphalangeal (IP) flexion is weak or absent (Chidgey & Szabo, 1989). Index DIP flexion may or may not be affected. The characteristic pinch deformity involves collapse of the thumb IP joint and index DIP joint into extension. There may be a positive Tinel's sign over the proximal forearm with distal radiation toward the pronator quadratus. Proximal forearm pain may be reproduced by the Mills' test, which involves wrist and finger flexion with the forearm hyperpronated or elbow extension from a flexed position (see Box 6-7). The differential diagnosis for anterior interosseous syndrome includes partial lesion of the median nerve or lateral cord.

Treatment at level 1 primarily involves avoidance of provocative activities, particularly forearm rotation. The use of TENS and other modalities may be required to reduce inflammation, edema, and pain. Myofascial release techniques may be tolerated.

When the initial symptoms have subsided, treatment level 2 may be initiated. This involves heat application, such as a hot pack or continuous ultrasound, followed by anterior forearm massage and light ROM.

Progression to level 3 involves reconditioning of palmar pinch and forearm pronation. During this level of treatment, one must be alert for recurrence of signs and symptoms. The individual who tolerates reconditioning well should be ready to perform job simulation tasks, such as handwriting. If conservative treatment fails or EMG and NCSs indicate an unresolvable entrapment, surgical intervention may be warranted.

Wrist and Hand Regions

Common injuries of the wrist and hand region include flexor peritendinitis (tenosynovitis) that may precede carpal tunnel syndrome, Guyon's tunnel syndrome, intersection syndrome, de Quervain's disease, and trigger finger or thumb.

Flexor Tenosynovitis

Flexor peritendinitis (tenosynovitis) is an inflammation of the flexor tendon synovial sheaths from repetitive use or frequent high force when engaged in such prehensile activities as typing and playing musical instruments. Inflammation may lead to edema and fibrotic changes in the tissue itself. Because the flexor tendons lie in the carpal tunnel, edema may reduce the available room in the canal (Butler, 1991). With pressure in this region, the median nerve can become compressed because it is soft and lies close to the volar transverse carpal ligament (Pratt, 1991).

The site of pain varies along the length of the tendons and may be present at rest or may increase with resistive/sustained grip activities. There often is point tenderness along the volar palm in a select region of the flexor tendons. Box 6-8 lists most symptoms.

At level 1, rest is best accomplished with avoidance of provocative activities and splinting. Tendon-gliding exercises, exemplified by hook fisting, may prevent formation of adhesions. Strategies such as phonophoresis or iontophoresis may be used to reduce inflammation. As the individual progresses, stretching and reconditioning strategies, as advocated at treatment levels 2 and 3, may be used.

BOX 6-8
Wrist Tendon Disorders: Subjective and Objective Findings

Flexor Tenosynovitis
- Pain with sustained grip activities
- Pain with resisted finger flexion
- Tenderness over the flexor tendons in the palm
- Possible edema in the region of the palm or carpal tunnel (may be a precursor to carpal tunnel syndrome)

Intersection Syndrome
- Pain, tenderness, swelling, and crepitus over the radial-dorsal aspect of the distal forearm 4-8 cm proximal to Lister's tubercle

Possible Symptoms with Resisted Thumb Extension and Finkelstein's Test
- Differentiated from de Quervain's as the palpable point of tenderness is more proximal
- Provocative tests: resisted wrist radial deviation and resisted wrist extension with rotation

Carpal Tunnel Syndrome

An arch of carpal bones forms the floor of the carpal tunnel. It is covered in the volar aspect by the transverse carpal ligament that attaches in the ulnar aspect to the pisiform bone and hook of the hamate bone and radially to the scaphoid tubercle and trapezium (Pratt, 1991). The median nerve traverses the carpal tunnel along with the eight long finger flexor tendons and the FPL. The palmar cutaneous branch to the thenar region does not traverse the carpal canal; rather it courses above it.

Causes of carpal tunnel syndrome include inflammatory and metabolic disorders, repetitive trauma, tumors, and developmental disorders. To confirm carpal tunnel syndrome, the differential diagnosis includes testing for diabetic neuropathy, cervical root impingement, pronator syndrome, and anterior interosseous syndrome.

Signs and symptoms of carpal tunnel syndrome (see Box 6-7) include: 1) numbness or nocturnal burning pain through the radial-volar side of the hand, 2) pain and paresthesias in the median nerve distribution of the hand that occasionally radiate proximally, and 3) reports of dropping objects or an inability to sustain grip of objects. On physical examination, there may be thenar atrophy with weakness of the abductor pollicis brevis, diminished sensibility within the median nerve distribution of the hand, a positive Phalen's test, a positive Tinel's sign, and diminished sudomotor activity. The FPL and FDP will be strong. Sensibility will be normal in the proximal palm. Diagnostic confirmation may be accomplished using EMG or NCSs. Using a regression model, Szabo, Slater, Farver, et al. (1999) found CTS could be diagnosed with 86% probability given specific tests results. These tests included: an abnormal hand diagram, diminished sensibility based on the Semmes-Weinstein Monofilament Test (in wrist neutral), a positive Durkan's compression guage (Wainner, Boninger, Balu, et al., 2000), and night pain.

Initial conservative treatment includes dorsal or volar cock-up splinting to hold the wrist in neutral to 10 degrees of extension. Methods to reduce inflammation may include the use of NSAIDs or corticosteroid injections and avoidance of pinching, gripping, or repetitive wrist motions. Some have advocated the use of phonophoresis or iontophoresis instead of injections. Symptoms might be reduced and gliding of the nerve promoted through myofascial release or nerve-gliding techniques. Tendon-gliding exercises for the long finger flexors should be done. If symptoms begin to resolve, therapy may progress through levels 2 and 3, including ROM exercises and reconditioning with theraputty and resistive grip tasks. If the signs and symptoms progress, however, surgical decompression may be indicated through either direct or endoscopic technique. In either case, workplace modifications and proper hand use should be addressed to avoid further problems with the disease.

Guyon's Tunnel Syndrome

Guyon's tunnel is located between the hook of the hamate and the pisiform bone. The transverse carpal ligament makes up the floor and the pisohamate ligament makes up the roof of this tunnel. In addition to the volar sensory ulnar nerve and the deep motor branch, Guyon's tunnel contains the ulnar artery and vein (Pratt, 1991). Activities that can induce nerve compression include long-distance cycling, use of the palm as a hammer, and pressure from the head of a screwdriver or pliers.

Signs and symptoms include paresthesias and diminished sensibility in the ulnar nerve distribution on the volar side only (see Box 6-4), and weak finger abduction and adduction, weak fourth and fifth MP flexion, weak small-finger opposition, and thumb adduction. Froment's sign, which is exaggerated thumb IP flexion with attempted thumb adduction, may be present. Grip strength and lateral pinch strength will be significantly reduced.

Treatment at level 1 includes avoidance of provocative activities, splinting of the wrist in neutral, and the application of inflammation-reducing methods such as NSAIDs, cortisone injections, or other modalities. Progression to level 2 may involve ulnar nerve-gliding techniques and easy prehensile tasks. As tolerance increases, level 3 resistive tasks (e.g., theraputty and sustained grip tasks) should be incorporated into treatment. Job simulation may be undertaken according to the client's tolerance. If conservative treatment is not successful, surgical decompression might be attempted. Treatment after decompression is similar to the presurgical conservative treatment plan.

Dorsal Radial Sensory Nerve Compression and Entrapment

The dorsal radial sensory nerve (DRSN) passes between the dense fascia of the forearm and the tendons of the brachioradialis and ECRL muscles before it becomes superficial at the anatomic snuff-box. In this superficial position, it is vulnerable to radial-side injury, compressive forces, and neuritis. More proximally, forearm pronation may squeeze the DRSN between the tendons of the brachioradialis and ECRL. The resultant tethering of the distal segment of the nerve can lead to entrapment, known as *Wartenberg's syndrome* (Ehrlich, 1986).

Signs and symptoms of entrapment include pain over the dorsal and radial aspect of the hand that is exacerbated by writing or sustained grip tasks (see Box 6-6). If the DRSN is irritated, as in neuritis, tingling or burning pain may be distributed over the dorsal and radial aspect of the thumb. On examination, sensitivity over the distribution of the radial nerve may be diminished, and there may be a positive Tinel's sign near the attachment of the brachioradialis. Finkelstein's test will be positive. This test involves a stretch into forearm hyperpronation with ulnar deviation and thumb flexion, which may provoke symptoms significantly. It is important to differentiate nerve involvement from de Quervain's disease. The absence of pain with thumb flexion and wrist ulnar deviation and the absence of tenderness over the first dorsal compartment are indicative of nerve entrapment.

Treatment at level 1 for superficial radial nerve compression includes rest and avoidance

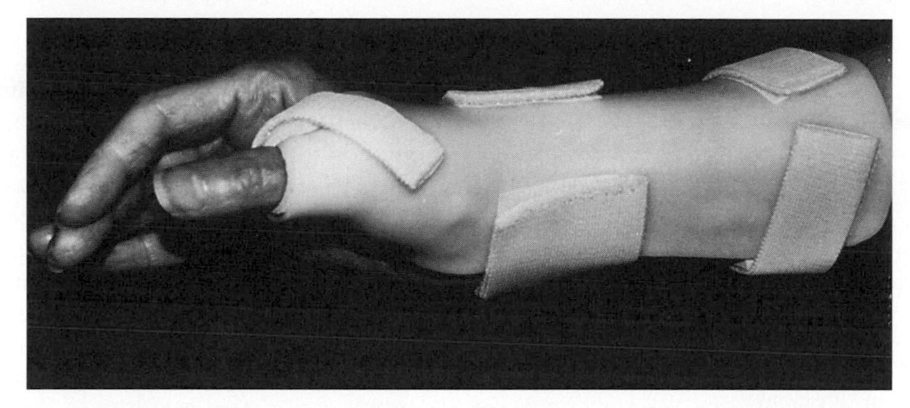

Figure 6-15 Thumb spica splint used in cases of de Quervain's disease, intersection syndrome, and dorsal radial sensory nerve irritation and compression.

of the provocative activity; a thumb spica splint should be worn (Figure 6-15). Care should be taken that the edges of the splint do not put pressure on the superficial radial nerve. NSAIDs or other modalities may be used to reduce inflammation. Ice and TENS work well if the radial nerve is irritated or compressed. However, other modalities may also be useful, including iontophoresis or phonophoresis. As symptoms subside, the client may be able to engage in gentle reconditioning through treatment levels 2 and 3. Wearing of the thumb spica at night through levels 2 and 3 is advisable to promote full recovery. If conservative treatment is not effective, surgical decompression may be necessary.

de Quervain's Disease

de Quervain's disease affects the extensor pollicis brevis (EPB) and abductor pollicis longus (APL) within the first dorsal compartment of the wrist. It is caused by an abrasion of the tendons and their sheath as they angle around the radial styloid process during simultaneous pinch and wrist motions. Increased active or passive tension of the EPB and APL induces pain. Muckart (1964) found that a firm gross grasp with radial wrist deviation creates the greatest stress on the structures of the first dorsal compartment. This position causes the taut APL tendon to apply a tensile force to the fibrous extensor retinaculum. The extensor retinaculum thickens to resist the strain, resulting in more pain and pressure.

Signs and symptoms of de Quervain's disease (Box 6-9) include localized tenderness and swelling in the region of the radial styloid and radial wrist pain radiating proximally into the forearm and distally into the thumb (Anderson & Tichenor, 1994; Cailliet, 1975). Finkelstein's (1930) test stretches the tendons in the first dorsal compartment; the test requires that the thumb be held in flexion by the fingers during wrist ulnar deviation, which increases symptoms if positive. Resisted thumb abduction or extension may also reproduce symptoms. Active thumb abduction may be decreased at the carpometacarpal (CMC) joint. Palpable thickening of the extensor sheath and the tendons distal to the first dorsal compartment may occur secondary to reduced vascularity and edema. Crepitus is rare. It is important to rule out DRSN irritation, extensor pollicis longus tenosynovitis, and CMC arthritis.

Conservative treatment at level 1 consists primarily of resting the wrist and thumb in a thumb spica splint (see Figure 6-15). This may be coupled with antiinflammatory treatment via phonophoresis, iontophoresis, or physician-administered cortisone injection. In addition, massage may be done along the length of the

BOX 6-9
Hand Tendon Disorders: Subjective and Objective Findings

de Quervain's Disease

- Pain with resisted thumb abduction or extension
- Positive Finkelstein's test (thumb flexion with wrist ulnar deviation), pain induced
- Pain when performing specific tasks such as writing
- Possible palpable pain near tendons of first dorsal compartment (near snuff-box)
- Might be confused with irritation of dorsal radial sensory nerve; latter must be ruled out

Trigger Finger (Thumb)

- Either locking in flexion of "catch" and "snap" to release on attempted extension
- Possible palpable nodule at volar base of metacarpophalangeal joint
- Possible weakness and pain when performing sustained grip or pinch tasks

tendon (longitudinally). As the inflammation subsides, levels 2 and 3 may be initiated through active motion and conditioning with light resistance (theraputty). de Quervain's disease is easily exacerbated. Therapists are cautioned against quick progression through the treatment program and encouraged to educate clients about the disease process. If conservative treatment fails, surgical release of the first dorsal compartment may be indicated.

Intersection Syndrome

The signs and symptoms (see Box 6-8) include pain, tenderness, swelling, and crepitus over the radial-dorsal aspect of the distal forearm 4 to 8 cm proximal to Lister's tubercle, which is where the first compartment crosses over the second (Grundberg & Reagan, 1985). Provocative tests include resisted wrist radial deviation and resisted wrist extension with rotation. Intersection syndrome is frequently misdiagnosed as de Quervain's disease because resistive thumb extension and Finkelstein's test may reproduce symptoms in either condition. However, the two are differentiated by the more proximal location of the palpable point of tenderness in intersection syndrome (as described previously).

Treatment during level 1 may include rest in a thumb spica and avoidance of the provocative activity. In addition, antiinflammatory medications, injections, ice, iontophoresis, or phonophoresis may be used. The affected area often is very tender in the acute stages, making massage intolerable. At level 2, tendon gliding may be done as tolerated. Flexibility and strength reconditioning may be undertaken as symptoms subside, per level 3. If conservative treatment is not effective, some surgeons perform a synovectomy to the APL muscle (Wulle, 1993).

Trigger Finger (Thumb)

Conservative treatment of this disorder, at level 1, typically includes injection with local steroid, NSAIDs, splinting, and tendon gliding. Phonophoresis or iontophoresis may be also used to reduce inflammation. It often is advisable to avoid the use of resistive devices or sustained grip tasks because those are usually the activities that cause the trigger to form (Cailliet, 1975; Cyriax, 1982; Evans, Hunter, & Burkhalter, 1988). Again, avoidance or modification of the provocative activity is advised. For example, a trigger may be induced through use of assistive devices such as a cane with a small-handle diameter. Altering the cane to incorporate a wider handle may help to resolve the problem. Once the trigger has resolved, it is best to guide the individual gradually into normal activities at level 2.

Progression to level 3 involves conditioning with resistive activities. If conservative treatment fails, surgical resection of the A1 pulley is performed.

Evans et al. (1988) advocate conservative management of trigger finger that alters the mechanical pressures of the proximal pulley systems and encourages differential tendon gilding between the flexor digitorum superficialis and profundus. Under this protocol (Evans et al., 1988) the individual makes use of an MP block splint that prevents MP flexion but allows PIP and DIP flexion (Figure 6-16). This protocol may be considered to be a progression

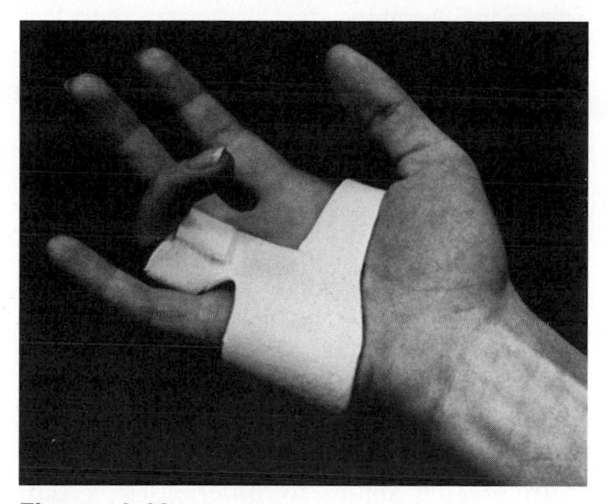

Figure 6-16 Single-finger block splint used to promote tendon gliding within the trigger finger protocol.

through levels 1 and 2 only because resistive activities such as theraputty are not advocated because the tendon may be degenerated and thus susceptible to further injury as well as to rupture. The authors conducted a prospective study of 54 digits with triggering in 38 (nonrheumatoid) individuals managed with this 3- to 6-week treatment protocol. In 52% of the reported cases, there was an excellent result or resolution of the trigger at an average follow-up of 8.8 months. The treatment protocol followed in the study is now widely used clinically (Box 6-10).

Treatment of a trigger at the thumb IP joint may involve rest in a small IP block splint (Figure 6-17), which prevents IP motion and redirects the muscle force toward MP joint motion. Treatment also may involve progression from pulsed to continuous ultrasound over a longer time period. Longitudinal massage along the thumb may follow ultrasound and precede active ROM exercises. Active movement should begin through a small range and increase as tolerated. Unfortunately, this type of trigger often recurs because the provocative activity (resisted thumb IP flexion) is difficult to avoid because of occupational and ADL requirements.

BOX 6-10
Trigger Finger Protocol

1. Provocative activities requiring repetitive grasping or acute flexion are avoided.
2. A hand-based static splint is used to immobilize the involved metacarpophalangeal joints at 0 degrees, allowing full interphalangeal flexion. Within this splint, the individual is instructed to make a "hook fist" and to repeat this maneuver 20 times every 2 hours. The splint is to be worn during waking hours for at least 3 weeks (up to 6). (Theoretically, this splint encourages maximal differential tendon gliding of the superficialis and profundus tendons and promotes circulation of the synovial fluid within the tendon sheath.) Flexion contractures at the proximal interphalangeal joints are managed with finger-based volar static extension splints worn at night.
3. Every 2 hours, the splint is removed for place-and-hold full-fist exercises and massage. Longitudinal massage of the digit is performed to soften the pulley area and increase circulation.
4. After 3 weeks, the finger is checked for triggering. If triggering persists, the protocol may be continued for another 6 weeks.

Source: Modified from Evans, R. B., Hunter, J. M., & Burkhalter, W. E. (1988). Conservative management of the trigger finger: a new approach. *J Hand Ther, 1*(2),56–74.

Focal Hand Dystonia

Evaluation for occupational hand cramps or focal hand dystonia requires a thorough history and activity analysis (Byl & Merzenich, 2002). Along with subtle yet progressive signs and symptoms the individual may have sustained an acute trauma, which may have quickly exacerbated the condition. The key to an accurate diagnosis is the inability of the individual to perform the provocative activity without exhibiting cramping or stereotypical tonic posturing (Fahn, Marsden, & Calne, 1987). Dystonia can be quite disabling to a performing musician, since the provocative activity (practice and performances) is directly related to the condition.

Somatosensory representation can be degraded with repetitive rapid stereotypical movements (Byl, Merzenich, & Jenkins, 1996). Along with

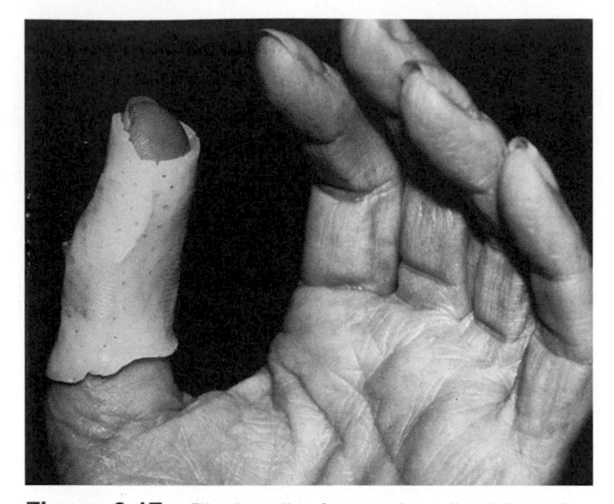

Figure 6-17 Block splint for treating distal interphalangeal joint trigger of the thumb.

a complete neurological examination, an important part of the evaluation encompasses cortical sensory discrimination testing such as stereognosis and graphesthesia (Ayres, 1989). A complete task analysis is necessary with attention to specific movements and motor control (Byl & Merzenich, 2002).

Treatment for focal hand dystonia involves the administration of botulinum toxin, desensitization and sensory discriminative training, conditioning, and education on ergonomics and performance of the target task or occupation (see Byl & Merzenich, 2002). Although botulinum toxin is a common modality, it only addresses the overactive muscle tissue involved and not the underlying cause of the disorder. Therefore, nonpharmacologic strategies must be used in conjunction with or instead of pharmaceuticals. Along with the methods listed above, Candia et al. (1999) used the paradigm of constraint-induced movement therapy for 2 weeks in an attempt to improve performance with reported success. Because of the disabling nature of this condition, evaluation and treatment requires one to recognize the impact of cortical reorganization in etiology as well as recovery.

FUTURE TRENDS

Musculoskeletal disorders are being diagnosed and referred for treatment more frequently than ever before. As the public becomes better educated about the types of activities that may lead to work-related musculoskeletal disorders, the incidence may subside. Currently, the key components to a quick recovery are early diagnosis, avoidance of the provocative activities, promotion of recovery or regeneration, and adequate reconditioning. If acute injuries are treated early, the problems associated with chronic conditions may also be avoided. Also, with greater ability to differentiate clearly between a disorder of tendinous or neurogenic origin, treatment may be better directed and more effective from the outset.

The research on reorganization of the cortex following functional use and peripheral nerve injury is exciting and has tremendous implications for recovery from musculoskeletal disorders. Clinicians who use sensory reeducation strategies have already taken advantage of the plasticity within the nervous system to promote recovery from nerve injury. Knowledge of the importance of functional use to aid reorganization should motivate therapists working with individuals with MSDs to ensure that their clinic and home treatment programs are rich in sensorimotor exploration and meaningful tasks. As the medical community and neuroscience further explore healing processes and neural changes associated with musculoskeletal disorders, greater variations in treatment can be expected.

REFERENCES

Adler, M.W. (1982). Endorphins, enkephalins and neurotransmitters. *Medical Times, 110,* 32.

Adson, A.W. (1951). Cervical ribs: Symptoms, differential diagnosis and indications for section of the insertion of the scalenus anticus muscle. *The Journal of the International College of Surgeons, 16,* 546-559.

Almekinders, L. C., & Almekinders, S.V. (1994). Outcome in the treatment of chronic overuse sports injuries: a retrospective study. *Journal of Orthopedic and Sports Physical Therapy, 19*(3), 157-161.

Anderson, M., & Tichenor, C. J. (1994). A patient with de Quervain's tenosynovitis: A case report using an Australian approach to manual therapy. *Physical Therapy, 74,* 314-326.

Apfel, E. R., & Carranza, J. (1992). Dexterity. In J.S. Cassanova (Ed). *Clinical assessment recommendations* (2nd ed., pp. 85-94). Chicago: American Society of Hand Therapists.

Asbury, A., & Fields, H. (1984). Pain due to peripheral nerve damage—a hypothesis. *Neurology, 34,* 1587-1590.

Aszmann, O. C., & Dellon, A. L. (1998). Relationship between cutaneous pressure threshold and two-point discrimination. *Journal of Reconstructive Microsurgery, 14*(6), 417-421.

Ayres, A. J. (1989). *Sensory integration and praxis tests.* Torrence CA: Sensory Integration International.

Beggs, S., Torsney, C., Drew, L. J., & Fitzgerald, M. (2002). The postnatal reorganization of primary afferent input and dorsal horn cell receptive fields in the rat spinal cord is an activity-dependent process. *European Journal of Neuroscience, 16*(7), 1249-1258.

Bell-Krotoski, J. A. (2002). Sensibility testing with the Semmes-Weinstein monofilaments. In E. M. Mackin, A. D. Callahan, T. M. Skirven, L. H. Schneider, & A. L. Osterman, (Eds.), *Hunter, Macklin, & Callahan's rehabilitation of the hand and upper extremity* (5th ed., pp. 194-213). St. Louis: Mosby.

Bell-Krotoski, J. A., & Buford, W. L. (1997). The force/time relationship of clinically used sensory testing instruments. *Journal of Hand Therapy, 10*(4), 297-309.

Bowden, R. E. M. (1954). Factors influencing functional recovery. In H. J. Seddon (Ed.), *Peripheral nerve injuries* (pp. 298-353). London: Her Majesty's Stationery Office.

Brandenburg, G. A., & Mann, M. D. (1989). Sensory nerve crush and regeneration and the receptive fields and response properties of neurons in the primary somatosensory cerebral cortex of cats. *Experimental Neurology, 103*(3), 256-266.

Braune, S., & Schady, W. (1993). Changes in sensation after nerve injury or amputation: The role of central factors. *Journal of Neurology and Neurosurgery in Psychiatry, 56,* 393-399.

Brumback, R. A., Bobele, G. B., & Rayan, G. M. (1992). Electrodiagnosis of compressive nerve lesions. *Hand Clinics, 8,* 241-254.

Bulloch, B., & Tenenbein, M. (2002). Validation of 2 pain scales for use in the pediatric emergency department. *Pediatrics, 110*(3), 33.

Burkart, S. L., & Post, W. R. (2002). A functionally based neuromechanical approach to shoulder rehabilitation. In E. J. Mackin, A. D. Callahan, T. M. Skirven, L. S. Schneider, & A. L. Osterman (Eds.), *Hunter, Mackin, & Callahan's rehabilitation of the hand and upper extremity* (5th ed., pp. 1351-1393). St. Louis: Mosby.

Butler D. S. (1991). *Mobilisation of the nervous system.* New York: Churchill Livingstone.

Butler, D. S., & Guth, B. P. (1993, May). *Mobilization of the nervous system.* Course sponsored by Summit Physical Therapy, PC. Syracuse, NY.

Byl, N. N. (1995). The use of ultrasound as an enhancer for transcutaneous drug delivery: phonophoresis. *Physical Therapy, 75*(6), 539-553.

Byl, N., Leano, J., & Cheney, L. K. (2002). The Byl-Cheney-Boczai Sensory Discriminator: Reliability, validity, and responsiveness for testing stereognosis. *Journal of Hand Therapy, 15*(4), 315-330.

Byl, N. N., McKenzie, A., Halliday, B., Wong, T., & O'Connell, J. (1993). The effects of phonophoresis with corticosteroids: A controlled pilot study. *Journal of Orthopedic and Sports Physical Therapy, 18*(5), 590-600.

Byl, N. N., & Merzenich, M. M. (2002). Focal hand dystonia. In E. J. Mackin., A. D. Callahan, T. M. Skirven, L. S. Schneider, & A. L. Osterman (Eds.), *Hunter, Mackin, & Callahan's rehabilitation of the hand and upper extremity* (5th ed., pp. 2053-2075). St. Louis: Mosby.

Byl, N. N., Merzenich, M. M., & Jenkins, W. M. (1996). A primate genesis model of focal dystonia and repetitive strain injury: I. Learning-induced dedifferentiation of the representation of the hand in the primary somatosensory cortex in adult monkeys. *Neurology, 47*(2), 508-520.

Cailliet, R. (1975). *Hand pain and impairment* (2nd ed.). Philadelphia: Davis.

Cailliet, R. (1991). *Shoulder pain* (3rd ed.). Philadelphia: Davis.

Callahan, A. D. (2002). Sensibility assessment for nerve lesions-in continuity and nerve lacerations. In E. J. Mackin, A. D. Callahan, T. M. Skirven, L. S. Schneider, & A. L. Osterman (Eds.), *Hunter, Mackin, & Callahan's rehabilitation of the hand and upper extremity* (5th ed., pp. 214-239). St. Louis: Mosby.

Candia, V., Elbert, T., Altenmuller, E., Rau, H., Schafer, T., & Taub, E. (1999). Constraint-induced movement therapy for focal hand dystonia in musicians. *Lancet, 353*(9160), 1273-1274.

Chan, H., Smith, R. S., & Snyder, R. E. (1989). Junction between parent and daughter axons in regenerating myelinated nerve: Properties of structure and rapid axonal transport. *Journal of Comparative Neurology, 28*(3), 391-404.

Chidgey, L. K., & Szabo, R. M. (1989). Anterior interosseous nerve palsy. In R. M. Szabo (Ed.), *Nerve compression syndromes: Diagnosis and treatment* (pp. 153-162). Thorofare, NJ: Slack, Inc.

Clarkson, H. M., & Gilewich, G. B. (2000). *Musculoskeletal assessment: Joint range-of-motion and manual muscle strength* (2nd ed.). Baltimore, MD: Williams & Wilkins.

Curwin, S., & Stanish, W. D. (1984). *Tendinitis: Its etiology and treatment.* Lexington, MA: Collamore Press/DC Heath.

Cyriax, J. (1982). *Textbook of orthopaedic medicine, Vol 1: Diagnosis of soft-tissue lesions* (8th ed.). London: Bailliere Tindall.

Cyriax, J. H. (1936). The pathology and treatment of tennis elbow. *Journal of Bone and Joint Surgery [Am], 18,* 921-940.

Daecke, W., Kusnierczak, D., & Loew, M. (2002). Extracorporeal shockwave therapy (ESWT) in tendinosis calcarea of the rotator cuff. Long-term results and efficacy [German]. *Orthopade, 31*(7), 645-651.

Davick, J. P., Martin, R. K., & Albright, J. P. (1988). Distribution and deposition of tritiated cortisol using phonophoresis. *Physical Therapy, 68,* 1672-1675.

Dellon, A. L. (1978). The moving two point discrimination test: clinical evaluation of the quickly adapting fiber/receptor system. *Journal of Hand Surgery [Am], 3,* 474-481.

Dellon, A. L. (1993). A numerical grading scale for peripheral nerve function. *Journal of Hand Therapy, 6*(2), 152-160.

Dellon, A. L., & Kallman, C. H. (1983). Evaluation of functional sensation in the hand. *Journal of Hand Surgery [Am], 8,* 865-870.

Dellon, A. L., MacKinnon, S. E., & Crosby, P. M. (1987). Reliability of two point discrimination measurements. *Journal of Hand Surgery [Am], 12,* 693-696.

Dyson, M., Pond, J. B., Joseph, J., & Warwick, R. (1968). The stimulation of tissue regeneration by means of ultrasound. *Clinical Science, 35,* 273-285.

Edgelow, P. I. (1995, February). *Thoracic outlet syndrome: Thoughts on cause and correction.* Presented at the American Physical Therapy Association's Combined Section Meeting, Reno, NV.

Ehrlich, W. (1986). Cheiralgia paresthetica (entrapment of the radial sensory nerve). *Journal of Hand Surgery [Am], 11,* 196.

Elvey, R. L., Quintner, J. L., & Thomas, A. N. (1986). A clinical study of RSI. *Australian Family Physician, 15,* 1314-1322.

Evans, R. B., Hunter, J. M., & Burkhalter, W. E. (1988). Conservative management of the trigger finger: a new approach. *Journal of Hand Therapy, 1*(2), 59-74.

Exner, C. (1990). Content validity of the In-hand Manipulation Test. *American Journal of Occupational Therapy, 47*(6), 505-513.

Fahn, S., Marsden, C. D., & Calne, D. (1987). Classification and investigation of dystonia. In C. D. Marsden & S. Fahn (Eds.), *Movement disorders, Vol 2.* London: Butterworth-Heinemann.

Fairbank, S., & Corlett, R. (2002). The role of the extensor digitorum communis muscle in lateral epicondylitis. *Journal of Hand Surgery [Br], 27*(5), 405.

Fedorczyk, J. (2002). Therapist's management of elbow tendonitis. In E. J. Mackin, A. D. Callahan, T. M. Skirven, L. S. Schneider, & A. L. Osterman (Eds.), *Hunter, Mackin, & Callahan's rehabilitation of the hand and upper extremity* (5th ed., pp. 1271-1281). St. Louis: Mosby.

Fedorczyk, J. (1997). The role of physical agents in modulating pain. *Journal of Hand Therapy, 10,* 110.

Fedorczyk, J. M., & Barbe M. F. (2002). Pain management: principles of therapists' intervention. In E. J. Mackin, A. D. Callahan, T. M. Skirven, L. S. Schneider, & A. L. Osterman (Eds.), *Hunter, Mackin, & Callahan's rehabilitation of the hand and upper extremity* (5th ed., pp. 1725-1741). St. Louis: Mosby.

Finkelstein, H. (1930). Stenosing tendovaginitis at the radial styloid process. *Journal of Bone and Joint Surgery, 12,* 509.

Funakoshi, H., Risling, M., Carlstedt, T., Lendahl, U., Timmusk, T., Metsis, M. et al. (1998). Targeted expression of a multifunctional chimeric neurotrophin in the lesioned sciatic nerve accelerates regeneration of sensory and motor axons. *Proceedings from the National Academy of Science, 95*(9), 5269-5274.

Fyfe, I., & Stanish, W. D. (1992). The use of eccentric training and stretching in the treatment and prevention of tendon injuries. *Clinics in Sports Medicine, 11,* 601-624.

Gallagher, E. J., Bijur, P. E., Latimer, C., & Silver, W. (2002). Reliability and validity of a visual analog scale for acute abdominal pain in the ED. *American Journal of Emergency Medicine, 20*(4), 287-290.

Groppel, J. L., & Nirschl, R. P. (1986). A mechanical and electromyographical analysis of the effects of various joint counter force braces on the tennis player. *American Journal of Sports Medicine, 14*(3), 195-200.

Grundberg, A. B., & Reagan, D. S. (1985). Pathologic anatomy of the forearm: Intersection syndrome. *Journal of Hand Surgery [Am], 10,* 299-305.

Harris, L. (1994, August). *Treating thoracic outlet syndrome.* Lecture given at the conference, Current Topics in Hand Rehabilitation, sponsored by the Section on Hand Rehabilitation of the American Physical Therapy Association. New Orleans, LA.

Hawkins, R., & Kennedy, J. (1980). Impingement syndrome in athletes. *American Journal of Sports Medicine, 8,* 151-157.

Hunt, T. K., & Hussain, Z. (1992). Wound micro environment. In I. K. Cohen, R. F. Diegelmann, & W. J. Lindblad (Eds.), *Wound healing* (p. 274). Philadelphia: Saunders.

Jebsen, R. H., Taylor, N., Trieschmann, R. B., Trotter, M. J., & Howard, L. A. (1969). An objective and standardized test of hand function. *Archives in Physical Medicine and Rehabilitation, 50,* 311-319.

Jerosch-Herold, C. (2000). Should sensory function after median nerve injury and repair be quantified using two-point discrimination as the critical measure? *Scandinavian Journal of Plastic and Reconstructive Surgery, 34*(4), 339-343.

Kahn, J. (1991). Response to N. T. Edwards' "Phonophoresis ... let me count the ways." *Physical Therapy Forum,* August 7.

Kahn, J. (1994). *Principles and practice of electrotherapy* (3rd ed.). New York: Churchill Livingstone.

Kanje, M., Lundborg, G., & Edstrom, A. (1988). A new method for studies of the effects of locally applied drugs on peripheral nerve regeneration in vivo. *Brain Research, 439,* 116–121.

Kasch, M. C. (2002). Therapist's evaluation and treatment of upper extremity cumulative trauma disorders. In E. J. Mackin, A. D. Callahan, T. M. Skirven, L. S. Schneider, & A. L. Osterman (Eds.), *Hunter, Mackin, & Callahan's rehabilitation of the hand and upper extremity* (5th ed., pp. 1005–1018). St. Louis: Mosby.

Kelly, M. (2002). Clinical evaluation of the shoulder. In E. J. Mackin, A. D. Callahan, T. M. Skirven, L. S. Schneider, & A. L. Osterman (Eds.), *Hunter, Mackin, & Callahan's rehabilitation of the hand and upper extremity* (5th ed., pp. 1311–1350). St. Louis: Mosby.

Kelly, T. (1979). Thoracic outlet syndrome: current concepts of treatment. *Annals in Surgery, 190,* 657–662.

Kibler, W. B., Chandler, T. J., & Pace, B. K. (1992). Principles of rehabilitation after chronic tendon injuries. *Clinics in Sports Medicine, 11,* 661–670.

Kirkley, A., Litchfield, R. B., Jackowski, D. M., & Lo, I. K. (2002). The use of the impingement test as a predictor of outcome following subacromial decompression for rotator cuff tendinosis. *Arthroscopy, 18*(1), 8–15.

Laurent, T. C. (1987). Structure, function and turnover of the extracellular matrix. *Advances in Microcirculation, 13,* 15–34.

Law, M., Baptiste, S., McColl, M., Opzoomer, A., Polatajko, H., & Pollock, N. (1990). The Canadian occupational performance measure: An outcome measure for occupational therapy. *Canadian Journal of Occupational Therapy, 57*(2), 82–87.

Leadbetter, W. (1991). Physiology of tissue repair. In *Athletic training and sports medicine*. Park Ridge, IL: American Academy of Orthopedic Surgeons.

Lindsay, M. (1993, November). Radial tunnel versus lateral epicondylitis. *Newsletter of the Section on Hand Rehabilitation of the American Physical Therapy Association, 10*(39), 1.

Lindsay, M. (1994, June). Evaluation and management of elbow disorders. Presented at the *American Society of Hand Therapists' Upper Extremity Expo*, Atlanta, GA.

Longo, F. M., Yang, T., Hamilton, S., Hyde, J. F., Walker, J., Jennes, L. et al. (1999). Electromagnetic fields influence NGF activity and levels following sciatic nerve transection. *Journal of Neuroscience Research, 55*(2), 230–237.

Lundborg, G. (2000). A 25-year perspective of peripheral nerve surgery: evolving neuroscientific concepts and clinical significance. *Journal of Hand Surgery, 25*(3), 391–414.

Lundborg, G., Dahlin, L. B., Danielsen, N., & Nachemason, A. K. (1986). Tissue specificity in nerve regeneration. *Scandinavian Journal of Plastic and Reconstructive Surgery and Hand Surgery, 20,* 279–283.

Mackinnon, S. E., Dellon, A. L., Lundborg, G., Hudson, A. R., & Hunter, D. A. (1986). A study of neurotropism in a primate model. *Journal of Hand Surgery [Am], 6,* 888–894.

Maitland, G. D. (1991). *Peripheral mobilization* (3rd ed.). Boston: Butterworth-Heinemann.

Mannheimer, J. S., & Lampe, G. N. (1984). *Clinical Transcutaneous Electrical Nerve Stimulation.* Philadelphia: F.A. Davis Co.

Martens, M., Wouters, P., Burssens, A., & Mulier, J. C. (1982). Patellar tendinitis: Pathology and results of treatment. *Acta Orthopaedics Scandinavia, 53,* 445.

Melzack, R. (1975). The McGill Pain Questionnaire: Major properties and scoring methods. *Pain, 1,* 277.

Melzack, R., & Wall, P. D. (1965). Pain mechanisms: A new theory. *Science, 150,* 971.

Michlovitz, S. L. (1996). Cryotherapy: The use of cold as a therapeutic agent. In S. L. Michlovitz (Ed.), *Thermal agents in rehabilitation* (3rd ed.). Philadelphia: Davis.

Michlovitz, S. L. (2002). Ultrasound and selected physical agent modalities in upper extremity rehabilitation. In E. J. Mackin, A. D. Callahan, T. M. Skirven, L. S. Schneider, & A. L. Osterman (Eds.), *Hunter, Mackin, & Callahan's rehabilitation of the hand and upper extremity* (5th ed., pp. 1745–1763). St. Louis: Mosby.

Moberg, E. (1960). Evaluation of sensibility in the hand. *Surgical Clinics of North American, 40,* 357–361.

Moberg, E. (1962). Criticism and study of methods for examining sensibility of the hand. *Neurology, 12,* 8–9.

Moran, C. A., & Callahan, A. D. (1983). Sensibility measurement and management. In C. A. Moran (Ed.), *Hand rehabilitation* (pp. 45–68). New York: Churchill Livingstone.

Muckart, R. D. (1964). Stenosing tendovaginitis of abductor pollicis longus and extensor pollicis brevis at the radial styloid (de Quervain's disease). *Clinics in Orthopaedics, 33,* 201–208.

Nagler, W. (1995). Personal communication. New York Hospital, Rehabilitation Department.

Neer, C. S., & Welsh, R. P. (1982). The shoulder in sports. *Orthopaedic Clinics of North America, 8,* 439.

Newman, M. K., Kill, M., & Frampton, G. (1958). Effects of ultrasound alone and combined with hydrocortisone injections by needle or hydrospray. *American Journal of Physical Medicine, 37,* 206.

Ng, C. L., Ho, D. D., & Chow, S. P. (1999). The Moberg pickup test: results of testing with a standard protocol. *Journal of Hand Therapy, 12*(4), 309-312.

Nirschl, R. P. (1992). Elbow tendinosis/tennis elbow. *Clinics in Sports Medicine, 11 ,* 851–870.

Nirschl, R. P., & Pettrone, F. A. (1979). Tennis elbow: the surgical treatment of lateral epicondylitis. *Journal of Bone and Joint Surgery [Am], 61,* 832–839.

O'Riain, S. (1973). New and simple test of nerve function in the hand. *British Medical Journal, 3,* 615–616.

Osterman, A. L. (1988, January). The double crush syndrome. *Orthopaedic Clinics of North America, 19,* 147–155.

Pascual-Leone, A., & Torres, F. (1993). Plasticity of the sensorimotor cortex representation of the reading finger in Braille readers. *Brain, 116,* 39–52.

Peacock, E. E. (1965). Biological principles in the healing of long tendons. *Surgical Clinics of North America, 45,* 461.

Peimer, C. A., & Wheeler, D. R. (1989). Radial tunnel syndrome (posterior interosseous nerve compression). In R. M. Szabo (Ed.), *Nerve compression syndromes: Diagnosis and treatment.* (pp. 177–192). Thorofare, NJ: Slack, Inc.

Phalen, G. S. (1966). The carpal tunnel syndrome: Seventeen years' experience in diagnosis and treatment of six hundred fifty four hands. *Journal of Bone and Joint Surgery [Am], 48,* 211–228.

Powell, S. G., & Burke, A. L. (1991). Surgical and therapeutic management of tennis elbow. An update. *Journal of Hand Therapy, 4,* 64–68.

Pratt, N. E. (1991). *Clinical musculoskeletal anatomy.* Philadelphia: Lippincott.

Rehak, D. C. (2001). Pronator syndrome. *Clinics in Sports Medicine, 20*(3), 531–540.

Rodineau, J. (1991). Tendinitis and tenosynovitis of the wrist [French abstract]. *Rev Praticien, 41,* 2699–2706.

Roos, D. B. (1966). Experience with first rib resection for thoracic outlet syndrome. *Annals of Surgery, 163,* 354–358.

Rozental, T. D., Beredjiklian, P. K., Guyette, T. M., & Weiland, A. J. (2000). Intra- and interobserver reliability of sensibility testing in asymptomatic individuals. *Annals of Plastic Surgery, 44*(6), 605–609.

Rubin, E., & Faber, J. L. (1988). *Pathology.* Philadelphia: Lippincott.

Safran, M. R., Garrett, W. E., & Seaber, A. V. (1988). The role of warm-up in muscular injury prevention. *American Journal of Sports Medicine, 16*(2), 123–129.

Schmelzeisen, H. (1990). Evaluating histologic findings of the rotator cuff of the shoulder [German abstract]. *Aktuelle Traumatol, 20*(3), 48–51.

Schultz, L. A., Bohannon, R. W., & Morgan, W. J. (1998 Normal digit values for the Weinstein Enhanced Sensory Test. *Journal of Hand Therapy, 11*(3), 200–205.

Scott, J., & Huskisson, E. C. (1979). Vertical and horizontal analog scales. *Annals of Rheumatologic Disease, 38,* 560.

Seddon, H. J. (1954). *Peripheral nerve injuries* (pp. 1–15). London: Her Majesty's Stationery Office.

Sjolund, B. H., & Eriksson, M. B. E. (1979). Endorphins, analgesia produced by peripheral conditioning stimulation. In J. J. Bonica (Ed.), *Advances in pain research and therapy,* (Vol. 3, p. 587). New York: Raven Press.

Smidt, N., van der Windt, D. A., Assendelft, W. J., Mourits, A. J., Deville, W. L., de Winter, A. F. et al. (2002). Interobserver reproducibility of the assessment of severity of complaints, grip strength, and pressure pain threshold in patients with lateral epicondylitis. *Archives in Physical Medicine and Rehabilitation, 83*(8), 1145–1150.

Smith, A. G., Kosygan, K., Williams, H., & Newman, R. J. (1999). Common extensor tendon rupture following corticosteroid injection for lateral tendinosis of the elbow. *British Journal of Sports Medicine, 33*(6), 423–425.

Sommerich, C. M., McGlothlin, J. D., & Marrar, W. S. (1993). Occupational risk factors associated with soft tissue disorders of the shoulder: a review of recent investigations in the literature. *Ergonomics, 36,* 697–717.

Sorman, E., & Edwall, L. L. (2002). [Examination of peripheral sensibility. Vibration test is more sensitive than monofilament test]. *Lakartidningen, 99*(12), 1339-1340.

Spinner, M. (1970). The anterior interosseous nerve syndrome. With special attention to its variations. *Journal of Bone and Joint Surgery [Am], 52,* 84.

Stone, J. H. (1992). Sensibility. In J. Casanova (Ed.), *Clinical assessment recommendations* (2nd ed., pp. 71–94). Chicago: American Society of Hand Therapists.

Szabo, R. M. (1989). *Nerve compression syndromes: Diagnosis and treatment.* Thorofare, NJ: Slack.

Szabo, R. M., & Gelberman, R. H. (1987). The pathophysiology of nerve entrapment syndromes. *Journal of Hand Surgery [Am], 12,* 881–884.

Szabo, R. M., Slater, R. R. Jr, Farver, T. B., Stanton, D. B., & Sharman, W. K. (1999). The value of diagnostic testing in carpal tunnel syndrome. *Journal of Hand Surgery [Am], 24*(4), 704–714.

Tetro, A. M., Evanoff, B. A., Hollstien, S. B., & Gelberman, R. H. (1998). A new provocative test for carpal tunnel syndrome. Assessment of wrist flexion and nerve compression. *Journal of Bone and Joint Surgery [Br], 80*(3), 493–498.

Tinel, J. (1915). Le signe du "fourmillement" dans les lesions des nerfs peripheriques [the "tingling" sign in peripheral nerve lesions]. (E. B. Kaplan, Transl.) *Presse Medicale, 23,* 388–389. In M. Spinner (1978). *Injuries to the Major Branches of Peripheral Nerves of the Forearm* (2nd ed.). Philadelphia: Saunders.

Travell, J. G., & Simons, D. G. (1983). *Myofascial pain and dysfunction, the trigger point manual, Vol 1: The upper extremities.* Baltimore: Williams & Wilkins.

Wainner, R. S., Boninger, M. L., Balu, G., Burdett, R., & Helkowski, W. (2000). Durkan gauge and carpal compression test: an accuracy and diagnostic test properties. *Journal of Orthopedic Sports Physical Therapy, 30*(11), 676–682.

Walker, J. L., Evans, J. M., Resig, P., Guarneri, S., Meade, P., & Sisken, B. S. (1994). Enhancement of functional recovery following a crush lesion to the rat sciatic nerve by exposure to pulsed electromagnetic fields. *Experimental Neurology, 125,* 302–305.

Walsh, M.T. (1994). Therapist management of thoracic outlet syndrome. *Journal of Hand Therapy, 7*(2), 131-144.

Walsh, M.T. (2002). Rationale and indications for the use of nerve mobilization and nerve gilding as a treatment approach. In E. J. Mackin, A. D. Callahan, T. M. Skirven, L. S. Schneider, & A. L. Osterman (Eds.), *Hunter, Mackin, & Callahan's rehabilitation of the hand and upper extremity* (5th ed., pp. 762-775). St. Louis: Mosby.

Warhold, L. G., Osterman, A. L., & Skirven, T. (1993). Lateral epicondylitis: how to treat it and prevent recurrence. *Journal of Musculoskeletal Medicine, 10*(6), 55-73.

Weber, E. H. (1835). Ueber den Tastsinn. *Arch Anat Physiol Wissen Med Muller's Arch, 1,* 152-159.

Weinstein, S. (1993). Fifty years of somatosensory research: from the Semmes-Weinstein monofilaments to the Weinstein enhanced sensory test. *Journal of Hand Therapy, 6*(1), 11-22.

Wolf, S. L. (1984). Neurophysiologic mechanisms in pain modulation: relevance to T.E.N.S. In J. S. Mannheimer & G. N. Lampe (Eds.), *Clinical transcutaneous electrical nerve stimulation* (pp. 41-55). Philadelphia: Davis.

Wong, D., & Baker, C. (1988). Pain in children: Comparison of assessment scales. *Pediatric Nursing, 14*(1), 9-17.

Wright, I. S. (1945). The neurovascular syndrome produced by hyperabduction of the arms. The immediate changes produced in 150 normal controls, and the effects on some persons of prolonged hyperabduction of the arms, as in sleeping, and in certain occupations. *American Heart Journal, 29,* 1.

Wulle, C. (1993). Intersection syndrome [German abstract]. *Handchirurgie Mikrochirurgie plastsche Chirurgie, 25*(1), 48-50.

Zachary, R. B. (1954). Results of nerve suture. In H. J. Seddon (Ed.), *Peripheral nerve injuries* (pp. 354-388). London: Her Majesty's Stationery Office.

Zealear, D. L., Billante, C. L., Chongkolwatana, C., & Herzon, G. D. (2000). The effects of chronic electrical stimulation on laryngeal muscle reinnervation. *ORL; Journal for Oto-rhino-laryngology and its Related Specialties, 62*(2), 87-95.

CHAPTER 7

Joint Injury and Arthritis in the Spectrum of Workplace MSDs

Charles F. Dillon[1]

INTRODUCTION

Musculoskeletal disorders (MSDs) are traditionally considered "soft tissue" injuries. The synovial joints are key functional components of the musculoskeletal system, but in the medical literature they are not given any serious consideration as contributing to the overall MSD problem. Save for isolated examples such as wrist ganglion cysts or "gamekeeper's thumb," major MSD reviews usually do not mention joints. In actuality, bony articulations are not impervious to harm, and considerable evidence exists that joint pathology results from persistently applied workplace biomechanical forces. Further, many traditional MSDs such as tendinitis and carpal tunnel syndrome are powerfully influenced by joint mechanics.

Work-related joint MSDs and arthritis are important because they are widely prevalent and frequently lead to disability. Practitioners who routinely treat nonoccupational arthritis and joint disorders often overlook work-related diagnoses simply because the possibility of occupational causation is not routinely considered. Also, most practitioners do not ordinarily perform joint exams in the MSD context. Further, many practitioners don't possess the clinical skills necessary to perform detailed upper-extremity joint exams. Such circumstances leave many MSD patients undiagnosed, untreated, and at risk for continuing injury. The purpose of this chapter is to improve this situation by providing a general review of upper-extremity joint MSDs, their pathoanatomy, clinical evaluation, and risk factors.

JOINT DESIGN AND INJURY PATTERNS

Anatomic Design

The anatomic function of upper-extremity joints is to organize and direct motion. Muscular energy is projected into dimensional space, while providing dynamic stabilization for the production of applied forces. The joints are the dynamic framework upon which muscle-tendon units operate, orienting and stiffening to provide rigid support for the local application of forces. The generic design of joints provides a typology of structures that may be susceptible to injuries from repetitive use.

A joint is the union of two bones, the ends covered with a cushion of smooth, shock-absorbent hyaline cartilage. Normally, bony joint surfaces never come into direct contact, although the subchondral bone bears loads transmitted through its cartilage coating. Joint load-bearing surfaces may be reinforced by intraarticular fibrocartilage discs or plates (e.g., the ulnar border of the wrist and the acromioclavicular joint). Externally, the joint capsule and synovial

[1]Dr. Charles Dillon authored this work in his private capacity. No official support or endorsement by the CDC or the Federal Government is intended or should be inferred.

membrane define the joint margins (Neumann, 1999). Clinically, each of these structures can be injured with repetitive loading.

Collateral and intraarticular ligaments are joint stabilizing structures that resist translational or shear forces perpendicular to the axis of joint action. They also function as the initial stabilizer in instantaneous joint loading, yet have sufficient laxity to permit normal joint play. Typically, collateral ligaments are placed in pairwise fashion at the medial and lateral aspects of a joint, but they may occur at other positions or even circumferentially. The perception of joint pain and position sense arises from nerve endings that supply the ligaments, joint capsule, and adjacent muscles; articular cartilage is not pain sensitive (Klippel, Weyand, & Wortmann, 1997).

Joint stability is achieved through both active and passive mechanisms. Bony anatomy can passively stabilize joints. For example, at the terminally limiting (close packed) position, the olecranon limits elbow extension; in the radiocarpal joint, the ellipsoid shape of the scaphoid and lunate constrain free joint range of motion (Kapandji, 1982). The periarticular muscles provide an active stabilizing envelope or sheath. This accepts significant compressive loading that may exceed that borne by internal joint contact surfaces. Deficits in periarticular muscle strength therefore increase internal joint loading, leading to joint damage. Generally, as joint range of motion increases, the importance of periarticular musculature tone in joint alignment also increases.

If ligamentous and muscular stabilizers fail, the joint capsule provides some passive support resisting translational stress. More importantly, the synovial membrane and joint capsule provide a closed physiological system producing negative internal joint pressure. This functions to bind joint surfaces together. Synovial fluid also creates an adhesive seal permitting sliding movement between joint surfaces but resisting distracting forces (Klippel et al., 1997).

JOINT MSD INJURY PATTERNS

A variety of MSD joint injury patterns exist, ranging from simple repetitive strains to frank osteoarthritis (Box 7-1). These disorders are also well known to result from acute trauma or nonoccupational disease (Klippel et al., 1997). For clinical purposes, joint injuries may be classified as derangements of either compressive loading or joint stabilization structures. This is a useful, but not exhaustive, didactic classification; other injury mechanisms occur in special instances, and in complex joints a variety of mechanisms may simultaneously contribute to injury.

Compressive Loading Injuries

Some level of continued compressive loading is a prerequisite to maintaining healthy joint cartilage (Sokoloff, 1987). Extreme loading may result in injury. Loading injuries cause local joint inflammation, and mild synovitis or effusion. Injuries include focal articular cartilage disruption

BOX 7-1
The Types of Joint-Related MSDs

Chronic MSD Joint Injuries
Articular (hyaline) cartilage injury:
fibrillation, tears (flaps), erosions
Osteochondral loose bodies
Articular disc or plate tear
Avascular necrosis of bone (Kienbock disease)
Bursitis (periarticular)
Collateral and intraarticular ligament strain, tear
Joint instability, subluxation
Contracture of periarticular musculature
Ganglion cyst
Joint impingement syndromes

MSD Osteoarthritis and Degenerative Changes
Joint space narrowing
Subchondral bone sclerosis
Bone (synovial) cyst
Mucous cysts
Osteophytes
(Carpal) boss
Joint erosions
Bony hypertrophy, deformity
Joint angulation

(fissures, chondral flaps) or loss of a cartilage segment. Cartilaginous loose bodies may form and float freely in the joint fluid, causing joint locking and inflammation. Subchondral bone cysts occur from transmission of intraarticular pressure through cartilage surface defects into the marrow spaces of subchondral bone. Compressive strain may cause degeneration of intraarticular ligaments, joint subluxation, and ganglion cyst formation. Injury to intraarticular plates or discs results from compressive loading or rotational stress, causing joint pain, swelling, and clicking.

Injuries to Joint Stabilizing Structures

Some translational play is a normal feature of joint kinematics. The collateral ligaments resist pathologic extremes of joint translation. These are pain-sensitive structures, and both acute trauma and degeneration from repetitive use can cause debilitating symptoms. Collateral ligament injuries from repetitive translational stresses occur in a spectrum: Grade I injuries (simple strains) are minimal tears, Grade II injuries are partial tears, and Grade III injuries are complete tears with joint instability. Grade III tears require surgical repair because they cause joint subluxation, abnormal joint wear, and degeneration.

Myofascial Responses to Joint Injury

Physiologic responses of muscles to joint injury are considered adaptive but may prove harmful in the long run (O'Reilly, Jones, & Doherty, 1997). Joint injury induces selective change in muscle fiber type. A decreased ratio of Type II to Type I muscle fibers stiffens periarticular muscle but may in turn increase internal joint loading. Arthrokinetic inhibition is a neurally mediated inhibition of periarticular muscle activity in response to joint pathology. These physiologic responses can combine with pain-mediated reduction in joint use to cause secondary complications such as muscle and joint capsule contracture.

UPPER-EXTREMITY ARTHRITIS AS AN MSD

The importance of arthritis as a work-related MSD is its link to permanent impairment and disability, as opposed to shorter-term, occasionally reversible joint injuries. The arthritis subtype most likely related to cumulative biomechanical stresses is osteoarthritis (OA), the commonest form of arthritis among adults. Osteoarthritis is a severe form of articular cartilage loss leading to "bone-on-bone" joint contact, with deteriorating joint structure and function. OA biochemical and microscopic pathology causing localized joint cartilage degeneration has been extensively investigated (Allan, 1998; Klippel et al., 1997). Radiologic hallmarks of OA include joint space narrowing caused by loss of articular cartilage. This can be seen directly in radiographs or measured by indices such as "carpal height." Characteristic radiologic sclerosis (scarring) of subchondral bone is seen at points of maximal joint pressure. In advanced OA, reactive bony overgrowths, or osteophytes, form. Initially, this is a physiologic response to increase available load-bearing joint surfaces, but ultimately osteophytes lead to restricted joint motion.

Evaluation of occupational risks for arthritis is a clearly stated priority in consensus statements on arthritis research needs (Brandt, Mankin, & Shulman, 1986) and a priority for surveillance, epidemiology, and prevention research in the U.S. National Arthritis Action Plan (Arthritis Foundation, 1999). Currently, there is convincing evidence that occupational physical factors are causal in OA of lower-extremity weight-bearing joints such as the hip and knee (Croft, Coggon, Cruddas, & Cooper, 1992; Felson, 1990; Vingard, 1996; Vingard, Alfredsson, Goldie, & Hogstedt, 1991). There is considerable evidence that the same is true for upper-extremity OA. The conceptual basis for biomechanical risks and work-related ergonomic exposures leading to upper-extremity OA has been extensively reviewed (Allan, 1998; Felson, 1994; Genti, 1989;

Peyron, 1986; Radin, Burr, Caterson, Fyhrie, Brown, & Boyd, 1991; Sokoloff, 1987).

Epidemiologic Data for Upper-Extremity Osteoarthritis

The association between OA and occupation has been extensively reviewed (Felson, 1994, 1999; Jensen, Boggild, & Johansen, 1999). There are a variety of general findings that support a causal role of biomechanical risks for upper-extremity OA, which include the following.

1. Hand-wrist OA prevalence is significantly increased in joints that from an anatomical point of view have the highest compressive loading. For example, OA prevalence is greatest at sites of maximal loading on the radial side of the hand at the thumb carpometacarpal joint, and the index finger distal interphalangeal joints (Radin, Parker, & Paul, 1971).
2. General hand-use patterns are associated with OA distribution. Major population-based surveys have shown generally increased prevalence and severity of OA in the joints of the right hand (Egger, Cooper, Hart, Doyle, Coggon & Spector, 1995) as well as in a person's dominant major hand (Acheson, Chan, & Clemett, 1970; Hadler, Gillings, Imbus, Levitin, Makuc, Utsinger et al., 1978).
3. OA is rare in the absence of biomechanical exposures. For example, the joints of paralyzed limbs are rarely affected by OA (Glyn, Sutherland, Walker, & Young, 1966; Goldberg, Zulman, & Genant, 1980; Segal, Avrahami, Lebdinski, Habut, Leibovitz, Gil et al., 1998; Stecher & Karnosh, 1947).
4. There is a significant general association between power grip strength and hand OA incidence in prospective studies (Chaisson, Zhang, Sharma, Kannel & Felson, 1999).
5. Both compressive and translational loading of joints are identified in a number of studies as principal pertinent biomechanical risks for hand-wrist OA (Felson, 1994, 1999; Neumann 1999; Turner, 1989, 1991).
6. In workers, OA often occurs at sites that are uncommonly affected in the general population. For example, OA of the metacarpophalangeal joints, the elbow, and glenohumeral joint in manual laborers (Felson, 1998; 1999).
7. Characteristic, at times virtually unique, patterns of OA joint involvement occur relating to specific biomechanical work tasks (Bard, Sylvester, & Dussault, 1984; Ferreiro, Gomez, Ibanez, & Formigo, 1997; Turner, 1989).
8. Population-based epidemiologic studies of hand-wrist arthritis have demonstrated significant associations with specific occupations and industry sectors (Bergenudd, Lindgarde, & Nilsson, 1989; Dillon, Petersen, & Tanaka, 2002; Engel & Burch, 1966, 1967). These findings are summarized in Box 7-2.
9. Dose-response relationships have been demonstrated between hand-wrist arthritis and cumulative years of hand-wrist bending at work (Dillon et al., 2002).

BOX 7-2
Industries and Occupations Associated with Hand-Wrist Arthritis

Industry Sectors
Agriculture, forestry, fisheries
Business and repair services
Construction
Manufacturing
Mining

Occupational Categories
Craftsmen (carpenters, electricians, plumbers, and so on)
Farmers, foresters, fishery workers
Laborers, handlers, helpers
Machine operators, assemblers
Miners
Precision production workers

Professional Specialties
Repairmen-repairwomen
Technicians
Transportation and material movers

UPPER-EXTREMITY JOINT DIAGNOSTICS

The physical examination of upper-extremity joints has been reviewed in detail (American Society for Surgery of the Hand, 1990; Hoppenfeld & Hutton, 1976; McGee, 1992; Skirven, 1996; Watson & Weinzweig, 1997; Wilk & Andrews, 1993). A systematic upper-extremity joint examination is important to verify a patient's problem and to reproduce the chief complaint. The physical examination also identifies articular problems that were not initially obvious either to the patient or clinician. There are six generic examination components that should be applied to every joint: visual inspection, joint landmark identification, axial loading tests, translational stability testing, range-of-motion tests, and periarticular muscle-tendon unit assessment.

Visual Inspection

Joint physical examination is principally a tactile skill. Although visual inspection is helpful to identify extreme instances of joint pathology (for example, gross misalignment, swelling, or deformity such as Heberden's or Bouchard's nodes), a normal visual impression is deceptive. The great majority of joint MSDs appear entirely normal on initial inspection. Conclusions about joint normality should not be drawn until the physical examination and diagnostic studies are complete.

Identifying Joint Landmarks

Each "joint-line" needs to be precisely located. This is the external rim of the junction between the two adjacent bones in joint. Pain-sensitive structures are located at the joint rim, including the joint capsule, the synovial membrane, and collateral ligaments. The technique of "opening" a joint by placing it in flexion is a useful aid to palpation and is especially valuable in smaller joints. Once located, one can "walk" the fingers around the joint line, palpating for abnormalities.

Axial (Compression) Loading

The hyaline cartilage joint contact surfaces are not directly palpable. Classically, physical examination tests, such as pain on passive joint motion or the presence of joint crepitation, are used to assess the integrity of the joint contact surfaces. Beyond these, applying a compression force in the line of the joint axis is a useful and more sensitive test for joint injury; it can elicit joint symptoms even when patients are unaware of problems. It is also specific, since axial loading does not elicit pain in normal joints. Examples of axial loading tests are the thumb carpometacarpal (CMC) grind test (Hoppenfeld & Hutton, 1976) and the distal radioulnar joint (DRUJ) press test (Lester, Halbrecht, Levy, & Gaudinez, 1995). Axial loading tests are classically recommended for only a few joints, but the technique should be applied generically as a screening maneuver.

Translational Stability Testing

Translational injury is collateral ligament pain or instability. Collateral ligament examination is performed by securing the bones adjacent to the joint, one in each hand, and stabilizing the uninjured side with the thumbs, then carefully pulling the bones back from the uninjured side to assess the degree of joint opening. Interpretation of joint stability should consider normal variations in joint laxity and prior trauma history. MSDs are characterized by localized, asymmetric painful instability, correlated with the ergonomic history. Joint instability defines a patient subset prone to joint degeneration and arthritis.

Range-of-Motion Evaluation

Normal ranges of motion (ROM) for upper-extremity joints are described in detail (American Medical Association, 1993). Some examiners perform ROM evaluation as a screening test, with the idea that if ROM testing is normal, serious joint abnormality is unlikely. ROM testing is not infallible in this sense, but ROM abnormalities are often seen in patients who appear normal to visual inspection. ROM deficits can be caused simply by joint pain or swelling, by internal joint derangement or joint capsule contracture. Pain and crepitation on passive motion of a joint are hallmarks of degenerative osteoarthritis.

Periarticular Muscle-Tendon Unit Assessment

Periarticular muscle-tendon unit contracture is traditionally thought to be a late complication of major joint injury. This isn't the case. Such disorders exist as a spectrum from mild to moderate changes. For example, the shoulder is especially susceptible to pathologic combinations of lengthening and contracture in its stabilizer muscle groups. Periarticular muscle-tendon unit contracture may also simply result from the restricted envelope of habitual postures normally assumed by an individual. This situation is readily amenable to treatment.

REVIEW OF SELECTED UPPER-EXTREMITY JOINT MSDS

This section reviews selected upper-extremity MSD joint diagnoses by anatomical area, outlining pathology, physical exam tests, and biomechanical risk factors (Table 7-1).

The Finger Interphalangeal Joints

The distal and proximal interphalangeal (DIP, PIP) and thumb interphalangeal (IP) joints are simple hinge-type joints. These are commonly injured, especially at the thumb and index finger. DIP and PIP strains occur from compressive loads in repetitive tip-pinch (Radin et al., 1971), although hand power grip may affect PIP joint injury (Chaisson et al., 1999). Because of force distributions in tip-pinch, DIP joint strain prevalence is greater than PIP joint strains. Once a DIP joint is injured, however, the PIP joint in the same ray may be secondarily injured as a part of the same kinetic chain.

DIP and PIP joint strain symptoms are local pain and a sensation of grating, snapping, or locking with joint use. In simple strains, visual inspection is typically normal, but gross deformity is the rule in OA (DIP joint Heberden's nodes and PIP joint Bouchard's nodes). Joint line identification can be difficult because of the small joint size. Compression loading while putting the joint through its range of motion will elicit pain or grating. In simple DIP joint strains translational stability testing is typically normal; however, in established OA translational deformity (joint angulation) it is common. Translational loading in specific work tasks leads to collateral ligament failure, joint instability, and DIP OA (Turner, 1989). Neumann (1999) reviews specific mechanisms in DIP OA translational joint injury.

DIP and PIP joint OA is common in the general population, but studies clearly link DIP and PIP OA to specific occupations. Work requiring fine pincer grip (tip-pinch) is a significant risk for DIP joint OA (Hadler et al., 1978; Lehto, Ronnemaa, Aalto, & Helenius, 1990; Nakamura, Horii, Imaeda, Nakao, & Watanabe, 1993; Tsujita, Kido, Fukuda, & Onoyama, 1989). For example, increased DIP and PIP OA risk is seen among men and women with repetitive work requiring finger dexterity, including occupation as a typist (Elsner, Nienhaus, & Beck, 1995). In English cotton mills, an increase in severe radiologic DIP and PIP OA was found in male spinners (Lawrence, 1961). In female American textile workers, significant increases in DIP OA and PIP finger malalignment were found among textile spinners and burlers, whose work requires precision or pincer grip with the second and third fingers (Hadler et al., 1978).

Further, there is increased incidence of DIP OA and deformity with heavy general physical job demands (Bergenudd et al., 1989). Increased DIP OA is also demonstrated in cooks and food service workers (Nakamura et al., 1993) and in paper mill workers (Tsujita et al., 1989). DIP and metacarpophalangeal OA is also described in pianists, associated with a unique syndrome of axial rotation of the third, fourth, and fifth digits, and sclerosis and flattening of the distal pha-

Table 7-1
Clinical Evaluation and Biomechanical Risk Factors for Selected Upper-Extremity Joint MSDs

Joint Location	Visual Inspection	Joint Opening Maneuvers	Axial Compression Testing	Translational Stability Testing	ROM Testing	Contracture Assessment	Biomechanical Risk Factors for Injury
DIP joint	Heberden's nodes	DIP flexion	Manual compression	Medial-lateral stress	Decreased flexion	Retinacular test	Tip pinch
PIP joint	Bouchard's nodes	PIP flexion	Manual compression	Medial-lateral stress	Decreased flexion	Littler-Bunnell test	Tip pinch, power grip
MCP joint	Joint hypertrophy	MCP flexion	Manual compression	Medial-lateral and anterior-posterior stress testing	Decreased flexion		Power grip
1st CMC joint	Joint squaring, subluxation; thumb adduction	Wrist ulnar deviation and thumb adduction	CMC grind test	Instability in radioulnar plane	Decreased thumb extension, abduction	Thumb adduction contracture	Thumb opposition, power grip, lateral pinch
Scapho-lunate interval	Dorsal wrist swelling; ganglion cyst	Wrist flexion	Finger extension test	Scaphoid shift maneuver and others (see Watson & Weinzweig, 1997)	Decreased wrist flexion		Wrist twisting, extension, radially loaded wrist compression (pushing), high-frequency impact vibration
TFCC	Local swelling ulnar border of the wrist	Wrist radial deviation	Push-off test, press test, ulnocarpal stress test	Anterior-posterior instability	Restricted ulnar deviation	NA	Loaded pronation-supination; ulnar wrist compression or distraction (stretching)
DRUJ	NA	Neutral position	Radioulnar compression test (see text)	Piano key test	Supination lag (decreased supination)	Pronator teres and quadratus contracture	Loaded pronation-supination maneuvers
Elbow	Flexion contracture; increased carry angle	NA (large joint); forearm rotation for radio-humeral joint	Manual axial loading	Valgus stress (MLLC), posterior to anterior loading (annular ligament injury)	Decreased flexion, end-range extension pain (posterior impingement)	Elbow flexion contracture	Valgus extension stress (MLLC); close-packed excursions (PI); high-impact, low-frequency vibration (OA); pronation-supination tasks (RH)

Table 7-1
Clinical Evaluation and Biomechanical Risk Factors for Selected Upper-Extremity Joint MSDs—cont'd

Joint Location	Visual Inspection	Joint Opening Maneuvers	Axial Compression Testing	Translational Stability Testing	ROM Testing	Contracture Assessment	Biomechanical Risk Factors for Injury
AC joint	Hypertrophy of joint (OA); joint step-off (subluxation)	Palpate along distal clavicle to locate joint line	Shoulder adduction	Depression of the acromion vs. the clavicle	Joint ROM is minimal	Decreased shoulder adduction	Arm adduction; forward; (bench) press; lifting, arms extended below the waist (AC separation)
Gleno-humeral joint	Sulcus sign	Abduction, external rotation	Axial loading with arm elevation	Apprehension test	Decreases in flexion, extension abduction, internal-external rotation; impingement signs	Decreases in flexion, extension abduction, internal-external rotation; frozen shoulder	Arm loading in shoulder abduction, elevation; high-impact, low-frequency vibration

See text for references to syndromes, exam tests, and injury risk factors.
AC, Acromioclavicular joint; *DIP,* finger distal interphalangeal joint; *DRUJ,* distal radioulnar joint; *1st CMC,* thumb carpometacarpal joint; *MCP,* metacarpophalangeal joint; *MLLC,* medial laxity, lateral compression syndrome; *PI,* elbow posterior impingement; *PIP,* finger proximal interphalangeal joint; *RH,* radiohumeral joint; *SLAC,* scapho-lunate advanced collapse, *TFCC,* wrist triangular fibrocartilaginous complex.

langeal tufts (Bard et al., 1984). In musicians, fingertip percussion forces may also lead to selective phalangeal tuft fracture (Young, Bryk, & Ratner, 1977).

The Metacarpophalangeal Joints

Simple strains of the finger metacarpophalangeal (MCP) joints and the metacarpophalangeal (MP) joint of the thumb are common but underdiagnosed. They have a radial bias, occurring often at the index and middle fingers. Biomechanically, MCP strains are associated with power grip maneuvers. MCP pain is often poorly localized, and joint line palpation is essential to verify the diagnosis. Inexperienced examiners often confuse the metacarpal heads (the "knuckles") for the MCP joint line, but it is actually located distal to the metacarpal heads. Flexing the MCP joints open before palpating is the best means of identifying the joint line.

MCP joint visual inspection is typically uninformative, and even OA joint deformity can be difficult to assess. Compression loading while putting the joint through its normal range of motion will elicit pain and reproduce the patient's symptoms. MCP joint instability is more common than usually supposed and should be routinely assessed. The classic example of MCP joint collateral ligament injury caused by repetitively applied translational stress is rupture of the ulnar collateral ligament of the thumb MP joint ("gamekeeper's thumb"). At the thumb MP joint, various degrees of painful collateral ligament instability can be seen prior to actual ligament rupture.

OA of the MCP joints is relatively uncommon in the general population, but it has higher prevalence in men (Caspi, Flusser, Farber, Ribak, Leibovitz, Habot, et al., 2001). Numerous studies indicate high MCP OA prevalence in manual laborers, and hand power grip is the chief biomechanical exposure. Also, in prospective studies, there is a significant general association between power grip strength and the incidence of MCP OA (Chaisson et al., 1999). MCP OA has been especially noted in agricultural workers and other manual laborers but also in professional musicians (Bard et al., 1984; Fam & Kolin 1986; McDonald & Marino, 1990; Schmid, Dreier, Muff, Allgayer, & Schlumpf, 1999; Ulreich & Klein, 1991; Williams, Cope, Gaunt, Adelstein, Hoyt, & Singh et al., 1987). The MCP arthritis is often noted to have increased severity in the dominant hand.

The Thumb Carpometacarpal Joint

The carpometacarpal joint of the thumb is also called the 1st CMC joint, the trapeziometacarpal joint, or the thumb basal joint. It is a highly mobile joint with an especially vital function in thumb opposition. The first CMC joint is among the most commonly injured joints in the body, both with respect to simple mechanical strains and degenerative arthritis. Both types of 1st CMC joint MSDs result from repetitive occupational power grip and lateral pinch maneuvers.

Physical examination of the first CMC joint requires care. Visual examination is not helpful, except for frank joint subluxation or the "squaring" of end-stage bony hypertrophy. Joint landmarks are difficult to identify: the most useful "joint-opening" maneuver is wrist ulnar deviation and thumb adduction. The CMC joint "grind" test (Hoppenfeld & Hutton, 1976) is a sensitive axial loading test. Translational abnormalities are common on examination. Thumb adduction contracture is also common in first CMC joint derangement. Often reversible in its early stages, it becomes irreversible when chronic translation deformity is established.

Longitudinal studies show a significant association between power grip strength and first CMC joint OA in men (Chaisson et al., 1999). It is significant that first CMC OA is principally localized at a small trapezial contact area where the volar metacarpal lodges during routine opposition of the thumb (Marzke, 1992). Occupational studies demonstrate increased first CMC OA in cotton mill workers (Lawrence, 1961) and carpenters (Staxler, Nisell, Vingard, & Nylen, 1994). In certain occupations, translational joint loading may lead to first CMC joint OA (Turner, 1991).

The Region of the Radiocarpal Joint

It is estimated that in neutral position, 80% of force transmission across the wrist is at the radiocarpal joint (Berger, 1996). The percentage loading increases with radial deviation and decreases with ulnar deviation of the wrist. Further, within the radiocarpal joint approximately 45% of forces are transmitted at the radioscaphoid joint, and 35% at the radiolunate. A radial compression loading bias is consistent with the known relatively higher prevalence of MSDs at the radial aspect of the wrist and hand. This pattern is also seen with degenerative OA (Egger et al., 1995).

Compressive loading commonly causes subchondral bone cysts in the radius and lunate of jackhammer operators (Harrington, Lichtman, & Brockmole, 1987) and in the scaphoid, lunate, and triquetrum of chainsaw operators (Kumlin, Wiikeri, & Sumari, 1973; Suzuki, Takahashi, & Nakagawa, 1978). High-frequency impact vibration from handheld tools is primarily attenuated by the hand and wrist, causing injury at those locations (Kihlberg & Hagberg, 1997). Bone cysts are commonly asymptomatic but may become painful and progress to severe OA (Rifkin & Levine, 1985). Repeated compressive trauma is also thought to result in avascular necrosis of the lunate (An, 1997), a disabling syndrome prevalent among carpenters, pneumatic tool and wrench users, spot welders, sheet metal workers, farmers, and factory workers (Fredericks, Fernandez, & Pirela-Cruz, 1997a, 1997b).

The scapholunate (SL) interval, adjacent to the radiocarpal joint, is a special focus of biomechanical loading, and hence pathology. It is a well-known site of injury in acute trauma and degenerative injury in repetitive use. The finger extension test is the most useful compression technique. Wrist flexion palpating proximally from the dorsal third metacarpal is the most helpful "joint-opening" maneuver (Watson & Weinzweig, 1997). Dorsal wrist ganglion cysts are thought to most frequently arise from degeneration of the SL ligament. The "dorsal wrist syndrome" is subluxation, instability, and local synovitis resulting from SL ligament failure (Watson, Weinzweig, & Zeppieri, 1997). Continued loading results in SL advanced collapse (SLAC), a severe localized degenerative arthritis (Watson & Ryu, 1986; Watson et al., 1997). This particular MSD is of great antiquity: severe bilateral SLAC lesions developing on a chronic basis are described in a prehistoric stone tool user (Masmejean, Dutour, Touram, & Oberlin, 1997). In special circumstances, wrist subluxation and degeneration caused by eccentric loading may occur, as in tree fellers and stonemasons, whose jobs require heavy lifting with the arms held in extension (Kern, Zlatkin, & Dalinka, 1988).

The Carpal Boss

The carpal boss presents as a mass evident on the dorsum of the wrist. It is a bony eminence at the base of the second or third metacarpal, sometimes expanding to the trapezoid and capitate bones. Carpal bosses can spontaneously occur as asymptomatic, bilateral accessory ossicles (Cuono & Watson, 1979). Asymmetric carpal boss caused by localized degenerative arthritis can, however, result from recurrent occupational strain (Hazlett, 1992). Work requiring loaded wrist flexion-extension maneuvers is a primary risk factor for degenerative arthritis of these joints.

The Wrist Triangular Fibrocartilaginous Complex

The triangular fibrocartilaginous complex (TFCC) is an intraarticular disc at the ulnar aspect of the wrist. Anatomically, the TFCC occupies the potential space between the distal ulna and triquetrum, which is designed to allow ulnar deviation of the wrist. The TFCC accepts ulnar compression loads and also stabilizes the distal radioulnar joint. Positive ulnar variance in relation to the distal radius is considered a principal risk factor for TFCC disorders (Boulas & Milek, 1990). Also, positive variance may be dynamic rather than fixed because forceful grip and pronation increase ulnar variance (Friedman, Palmer, Short, Levinsohn, & Halperin, 1993; LaStayo & Weiss, 2001; Tomaino, 1998).

TFCC MSDs typically result from repetitive loading of the ulnar aspect of the wrist associated with either ulnar deviation or pronation-supination maneuvers—the "ulnar impaction syndrome" (Friedman & Palmer, 1991). TFCC tears may also be distraction injuries caused by chronic stretching in pulling tasks. TFCC tears cause pain at the ulnar border of the wrist. Examination is by axial loading testing holding the wrist in ulnar deviation and moving it through flexion and extension. This elicits pain and clicking. Alternate tests are the "press" or "push-off" maneuver (Lester et. al., 1995) or the "ulnocarpal stress test" (Nakamura et al., 1997).

The Wrist Pisiform-Triquetral Joint

Pain and tenderness in the palm at its proximal, ulnar aspect can be due to tendinitis of the flexor carpi ulnaris, vascular injury (hypothenar hammer syndrome), or to disease of the pisiform-triquetral (P-T) joint. This small joint is also a common site of OA caused by repetitive use and acute trauma (Paley, McMurtry, & Cruickshank, 1987). P-T joint disorders may cause secondary ulnar nerve paresthesias. The pisiform contributes to ulnar wrist stability; it holds the triquetrum in position, preventing subluxation and also transduces forearm muscular forces to the hand (Beckers & Koebke, 1998). On physical examination with the wrist positioned in ulnar deviation, there is characteristic pain with resisted wrist flexion (Saffar & Duek, 2002). In P-T joint injury, inspection of the palm is typically normal. Special radiologic views are mandatory. Pisiform excision maintaining flexor carpi ulnaris continuity is the accepted therapy for disabling P-T joint OA (Saffar & Duek, 2002), although some think that the long-term biomechanical effects of this procedure need to be further evaluated (Beckers & Koebke, 1998).

The Distal Radioulnar Joint

The DRUJ is located between the distal radius and ulna, just proximal to the wrist (Jaffe, Chidgey, & LaStayo, 1996; Skirven, 1996). This unique cylindrical joint mediates forearm and hand rotation. The DRUJ is readily examined and is frequently a site of MSDs yet is one of the areas most often overlooked. It is a relatively recent evolutionary acquisition and is frequently injured as a result of repeated loaded pronation-supination tasks, as with production workers who repetitively lift and turn parts on an assembly line. DRUJ strains have also been seen in pianists, and DRUJ OA is documented in chain saw operators (Horvath & Kakosy, 1979; Suzuki et al., 1978).

Axial compression testing of the DRUJ is achieved by holding the distal radius and ulna in the hand and squeezing. Instability testing is performed using the "piano key" maneuver—stabilizing the distal radius with one hand and the distal ulna with the other, then attempting to translate the radius and ulna past each other (Jaffe et al., 1996). Standard wrist radiographs only partly visualize the DRUJ, and, as a rule, radiologists typically do not comment on DRUJ status. Nevertheless, DRUJ sclerosis or degeneration is a frequent finding in standard wrist films of symptomatic patients. Special radiographic views are needed for proper imaging.

The Elbow

The elbow permits forearm flexion-extension and assists in forearm pronation-supination. The joint line is readily palpated without joint opening maneuvers. Stress testing for translational instability is important because abnormalities are not visually evident. The lateral collateral ligament is most often injured. Posterolateral rotatory and annular ligament instability are rare in adults, but testing for the latter should be performed when patients have antecubital fossa pain, or routinely perform repetitive pronation-supination tasks (O'Driscoll, 1999). In established elbow joint injury, flexion contractures are common. This is especially true in manual laborers (Sakakibara, Suzuki, Momoi, & Yamada, 1993).

Elbow joint MSDs are a biomechanical result of repeated excursions to extremes of end-range joint extension, repetitively applied translational forces, or repetitive, low-frequency, high-amplitude compression (impact) forces. The "posterior impingement syndrome" is an example of repetitive end-range excursion injury. This is classically described in professional pitchers (Wilson, Andrews, Blackburn, & McCluskey, 1983) and pneumatic drillers (Burke, Fear, & Wright, 1977). Here, there is impingement on the articular wall of the olecranon fossa, creating a local area of chondromalacia. Posterior osteophytes form, leading to painful mechanical joint impingement.

Chronic elbow instability and degeneration also result from translational stresses applied to the humeroulnar-radial joint axis. The elbow "medial-laxity, lateral-compression" (MLLC) syndrome exists in a spectrum from mild to severe cases. Extreme examples are found in professional throwing athletes (Lee, Rooney, & Sturrock, 1974; Oka, 1999) and in foundry workers who routinely use mechanical tongs for lifting and twisting hot metal rods (Mintz & Fraga, 1973). Here, valgus stresses inherent in the twisting or throwing maneuver cause repetitive microinjury to the anterior portion of the medial collateral ligament at the humeroulnar joint. With repetitive use, the integrity of the medial collateral ligament as a stabilizing structure is lost. A valgus deformity of the elbow results, which leads to chronic compression and degeneration at the humeroradial joint (Bennet & Tullos, 1985). In advanced MLLC, osteochondritis dessicans of the capitellum and radial head may occur, resulting in cartilaginous loose bodies that may cause painful joint locking. Long-standing cases may result in humeroradial joint OA. MLLC, or in fact any humeroradial joint pain, may mimic that of lateral epicondylitis.

Clinically symptomatic elbow OA is a distinctly rare disorder in the general population. Nevertheless, elbow OA caused by compressive loading has been described in a number of work settings (Hagberg, 2002). Vibrating handheld tool uses, especially repetitive shocks of low-frequency, high-magnitude vibration, are considered elbow and shoulder OA risk factors (Kihlberg & Hagberg, 1997). Studies of jackhammer and pneumatic tool operators find that 5% to 10% of workers have clinically evident elbow OA (Felson, 1999; Malchaire, Maldague, Huberlant, & Croquet, 1986). Significant increases in radiographic elbow OA related to vibratory tool operation is found in stone quarry workers (Sakakibara et al., 1993) and in chainsaw operators (Une, Kondo, & Goto, 1985). Elbow OA also occurs with increased prevalence in dockworkers (Partridge & Duthie, 1968), steelworkers, boilermakers, miners (Lawrence, 1987), chipping and grinding tool operators (Bovenzi, Fiorito, & Volpe, 1987; Gemne & Saraste, 1987), and resin-tappers (Jurgens, Ristow, & Pernack, 1990).

The Acromioclavicular Joint

The small acromioclavicular (AC) joint of the shoulder represents the sole bony articulation of the shoulder and arm with the axial skeleton. It is therefore an extremely common site for MSDs, acute injuries, and arthritis. Paradoxically, it is one of the least frequently examined joints in the body. The AC joint has an intraarticular cartilaginous plate to resist compression stress. The acromioclavicular ligaments are weak but structurally reinforced by the conoid and trapezoid ligaments that prevent medial scapular displacement. These latter are the primary ligaments disrupted in ordinary shoulder separations.

The AC joint line is palpated by "walking" the fingers along the clavicle to find the opening. A useful compression test is adduction of the arm across the chest. The AC joint has minimal ROM, so instability is readily apparent. Instability can be tested by palpating the joint while pulling the subject's arm downward. In complete joint separation, there is a characteristic "step-off" appearance. In advanced OA, AC joint hypertrophy is also visually obvious.

The AC joint cartilaginous plate is typically injured by repetitive compressive loading (pushing or lifting) during arm elevation. Symptoms and signs are local joint pain, clicking, and swelling. Degeneration of the trapezoid and conoid ligaments may occur from repetitive lifting below shoulder height, especially with downward extended arms, resulting in AC joint instability or separation. Arthritis is especially common at the AC joint, including posttraumatic, rheumatoid arthritis, and OA. It is also a common site for work-related OA (Hagberg, 2002; Mahowald, 2001; Stenlund, 1993; Stenlund, Goldie, Hagberg, Hogstedt, & Marions, 1992).

The Glenohumeral Joint

Visual inspection of the glenohumeral joint is not usually helpful but may reveal a step-off consistent with joint subluxation or moderate to severe degrees of joint effusion and synovitis. The joint is readily palpated. A useful compression test is asking the patient to horizontally abduct the upper arm and then push against an adjacent wall. The joint is highly mobile, and shoulder ROM testing is therefore a critical means of screening for pathology. Although supporting ligaments contribute, the shoulder's complex periscapular muscle groups are preeminent in maintaining shoulder stability. Anterior shoulder instability is the most common and is assessed by the "apprehension test" (Hoppenfeld & Hutton, 1976). Instability may also be multidirectional (Wilk & Andrews, 1993). Shoulder instability may result from acute trauma or inherent joint laxity. In MSD treatment, instability occurs secondary to deconditioning in neck or shoulder injury.

The primary risk factor for shoulder MSDs is work at or above shoulder height. Work combining shoulder abduction and forward flexion is associated with rotator cuff tendinitis and shoulder impingement syndrome (Muggleton, Allen, & Chappell, 1999). Loaded arm movements may also contribute to glenoid labral tears. Shoulder bursitis and impingement syndromes are reviewed in Chapters 5 and 6. Glenohumeral OA is uncommon in the general population except as a sequel of major trauma such as fracture. Specific occupational groups are nevertheless at high risk, including miners (Kellgren & Lawrence, 1952; Schlomka, Schroter, & Ochernal, 1955), construction workers (Mahowald, 2001), cotton operatives (Lawrence, 1961), and dentists (Katevuo, Aitasalo, Lehtinen, & Pietila, 1985). For dentists, shoulder OA appears to result from repetitive light static loading of the glenohumeral joint. The typical work posture, with the shoulders mildly abducted and elevated, functions to maximize glenohumeral joint surface contact. Glenohumeral OA in miners is associated with extremes of shoulder elevation and abduction, with greater mechanical loading.

ARTICULAR MSD MEDICAL MANAGEMENT

Ergonomic workplace intervention is the most important treatment modality for occupational MSDs. Control of preventable biomechanical risks can provide patients with substantial alleviation of symptoms as well as the possibility of joint injury healing. Even for patients with irreversible arthritis, the clinical course can be significantly impacted. Current practice in the clinical management of nonarthritic joint disorders has been extensively reviewed (Mackin, Callahan, Osterman, Skirven, Schneider & Hunter, 2002; Melvin & Jensen, 1998; Wilk & Andrews, 1993). Standard therapeutic regimens include selective short-term splinting; treatment of ligamentous, capsular, and muscle contracture; restoration of joint ROM; and strengthening muscle groups contributing to joint stabilization. Standards for the therapy of established osteoarthritis are surveyed by a number of authors (Ehrlich, 1986; Kelley & Ramsey, 2000; Robbins, Burckhardt, Hannan, & DeHoratius, 2001). Therapy includes many techniques used for nonarthritic joint disorders, as well as functional retraining and joint protection programs.

It is important to be aware of the rheumatologic differential diagnosis for articular conditions and to accurately identify nonoccupational arthritis cases that may require systemic treatment (Klippel et al., 1997). The possibility that ergonomic stresses from off-work activities contribute to a specific patient's presentation should always be considered. These need to be identified and controlled for effective therapy to proceed.

WORK-RELATEDNESS OF JOINT MSDs

Work-relatedness of joint injury and arthritis are typically determined on a case-by-case basis. The following general guidelines expand on the work of Turner (1991). The probability of work-relatedness is increased when the following conditions are present.

1. An ergonomic workplace assessment demonstrates that the affected joint(s) are functionally active in the patient's occupation.
2. Ergonomic job assessment indicates that affected joints are overloaded or subject to other significant risks such as static or translational stress.
3. The occupational history and workplace ergonomic assessment indicate that biomechanical exposures are greater than those that would normally occur.
4. The occupational history shows sufficient exposure time for the disease to develop.
5. There is an unusual pathologic pattern of joint injury that can be related to functional job tasks or particularly severe asymmetric localized disease correlated with ergonomic stresses.

Work-relatedness should be strongly considered in special circumstances: the onset of significant arthritis in much younger age groups than normally expected, the disease present in joints not usually affected in ordinary OA, or multiple employees with a specific job afflicted with similar MSDs. For all cases, preexisting or nonoccupational disease should be excluded. In many jurisdictions, however, a permanent work-aggravation of nonoccupational conditions can be considered compensable in the workers' compensation system.

SUMMARY

Work-related articular MSDs include a broad spectrum of conditions, ranging from minor localized joint injury to degenerative arthritis. Further, the occurrence of traditional soft-tissue MSDs such as tendinitis and carpal tunnel syndrome closely parallels joint location and mechanics. The joints exist in a structured, musculotendinous, neurologic environment. Joint injury frequently implies injury to periarticular structures, and vice versa.

It is well known, both in clinical practice and in epidemiologic studies, that many symptomatic MSD patients go undiagnosed. Joint-related diagnoses explain many such cases. An articular focus thus significantly enlarges the scope of the traditional definition of MSDs as "cumulative trauma disorders" and helps dispel some of the enigma surrounding these conditions. At the same time, a more complete view of the overall impact of ergonomic and biomechanical risk factors is provided. An expanded definition and prevalence of MSDs therefore provides not only a more comprehensive perspective but also organizing focus for MSD interpretative models and research.

REFERENCES

Acheson, R. M., Chan, Y. K., & Clemett, A. R. (1970). New Haven survey of joint diseases XII: Distribution and symptoms of osteoarthritis in the hands with reference to handedness. *Annals of Rheumatic Disease, 29*, 275-286.

Allan, D. A. (1998). Structure and physiology of joints and their relationship to repetitive strain injuries. *Clinical Orthopedics and Related Research, 351*, 32-38.

American Medical Association. (1993). *Guidelines to the evaluation of permanent impairment* (4th ed.). Chicago: American Medical Association.

American Society for Surgery of the Hand. (1990). *The hand: Examination and diagnosis* (3rd ed.). New York: Churchill-Livingstone.

An, K. N. (1997). Biomechanics of the Wrist and Hand. In M. Nordin, G. B. J. Andersson, & M. H. Pope (Eds.), *Musculoskeletal disorders in the workplace: Principles and practice* (pp. 431-436). St. Louis: Mosby.

Arthritis Foundation, Association of State and Territorial Health Officials, & Centers for Disease Control and Prevention. (1999). *National arthritis action plan: A public health strategy.* Atlanta: Centers for Disease Control and Prevention.

Bard, C. C., Sylvester, J. J., & Dussault, R. G. (1984). Hand osteoarthropathy in pianists. *Journal of the Canadian Association of Radiology, 35*, 154-158.

Beckers, A, & Koebke, J. (1998). Mechanical strain at the pisotriquetral joint. *Clinical Anatomy, 11*, 320-326.

Bennett, J. D., & Tullos, H. S. (1985). Ligamentous and articular injuries in the athlete. In B. F. Morrey (Ed.), *The elbow and its disorders* (pp. 502-520). Philadelphia: W.B. Saunders.

Bergenudd, H., Lindgarde, F., & Nilsson, B. (1989). Prevalence and coincidence of degenerative changes of the hands and feet in middle age and their relationship to occupational work load, intelligence and social background. *Clinical Orthopedics and Related Research, 239*, 306-310.

Berger, R. (1996). The anatomy and basic biomechanics of the wrist joint. *Journal of Hand Therapy, 9*, 84-93.

Boulas, H. J., & Milek, M. A. (1990) Ulnar shortening for tears of the triangular fibrocartilagenous complex. *Journal of Hand Surgery [Am], 15,* 415-420.

Bovenzi, M., Fiorito, A., & Volpe, C. (1987). Bone and joint disorders in the upper extremities of chipping and grinding operators. *International Archives of Occupational and Environmental Health, 59,* 189-198.

Brandt, K. D., Mankin, H. J., & Shulman, L. E. (1986). Workshop on etiopathogenesis of osteoarthritis. *The Journal of Rheumatology, 13,* 1126-1160.

Burke, B. J., Fear, E. C., & Wright, V. (1977). Bone and joint changes in pneumatic drillers. *Annals of Rheumatic Diseases, 36,* 276-279.

Caspi, D., Flusser, G., Farber, I., Ribak, J., Leibovitz, A., Habot, B. et al (2001). Clinical radiologic, demographic, and occupational aspects of hand osteoarthritis in the elderly. *Seminars in Arthritis and Rheumatism, 30,* 321-331.

Chaisson, C. E., Zhang, Y., Sharma, L., Kannel, W., & Felson, D. T. (1999). Grip strength and the risk of developing radiographic hand osteoarthritis: Results from the Framingham Study. *Arthritis and Rheumatism, 42,* 33-38.

Croft, P., Coggon, D., Cruddas, M., & Cooper, C. (1992). Osteoarthritis of the hip: An occupational disease in farmers. *British Medical Journal, 304*(6837), 1269-1272.

Cuono, C. B., & Watson, H. K. (1979). The carpal boss: Surgical treatment and etiological considerations. *Plastic and Reconstructive Surgery, 63,* 88-93.

Dillon, C. F., Petersen, M., & Tanaka, S. (2002). Self-reported hand and wrist arthritis and occupation: Data from the U.S. National Health Interview Survey-Occupational Health Supplement. *American Journal of Industrial Medicine, 42,* 318-327.

Egger, P., Cooper, C., Hart, D. J., Doyle, D. V., Coggon, D., & Spector, T. D. (1995). Patterns of joint involvement in osteoarthritis of the hand: The Chingford Study. *Journal of Rheumatology, 22,* 1509-1513.

Ehrlich, G. E. (1986). *Rehabilitation management of rheumatic conditions* (2nd ed.). Baltimore: Williams & Wilkins.

Elsner, G., Nienhaus, A., & Beck, W. (1995). Arthroses of the finger joints and thumb saddle joint and occupationally related factors. *Gesundheitswesen, 57,* 786-791.

Engel, A., & Burch, T. A. (1966). Osteoarthritis in adults by selected demographic characteristics 1960-1962. *Vital and Health Statistics, 11,* 1-27.

Engel, A., & Burch, T. A. (1967). Chronic arthritis in the United States Health Examination Survey. *Arthritis and Rheumatism, 10,* 61-62.

Fam, A. G., & Kolin, A. (1986). Unusual metacarpophalangeal osteoarthritis in a jackhammer operator. *Arthritis and Rheumatism, 29,* 1284-1289.

Felson, D. T. (1990). The epidemiology of knee osteoarthritis: results from the Framingham Osteoarthritis Study. *Seminars in Arthritis and Rheumatism 20*(3 Suppl 1), 42-50.

Felson, D. T. (1994). Do occupation-related physical factors contribute to arthritis? *Baillière's Clinical Rheumatology, 8,* 63-77.

Felson, D. T. (1998). Epidemiology of osteoarthritis. In K. D. Brandt, M. Doherty & L. S. Lohmander (Eds.), *Osteoarthritis* (pp. 13-22). New York: Oxford University Press.

Felson, D. T. (1999). Occupation related physical factors and osteoarthritis. In L. D. Kaufman & J. Varga (Eds.), *Rheumatic diseases and the environment* (pp. 189-195). London: Arnold and Oxford University Press.

Ferreiro, S. J. L., Gomez, R. N., Ibanez, R. J., & Formigo, R. E. (1997). Hand arthropathy of professional origin: Milking man hand. *Medicina Clínica, 109,* 667-668.

Fredericks, T. K., Fernandez, J. E., & Pirela-Cruz, M. A. (1997a). Kienbock's disease. I. Anatomy and Etiology. *International Journal of Occupational Medicine and Environmental Health, 10,* 11-7.

Fredericks, T. K., Fernandez, J. E., & Pirela-Cruz, M. A. (1997b). Kienbock's disease. II. Risk factors, diagnosis, and ergonomic interventions. *International Journal of Occupational Medicine and Environmental Health, 10,* 147-157.

Friedman, S. L., & Palmer, A. K. (1991). The ulnar impaction syndrome. *Hand Clinics, 7,* 295-310.

Friedman, S. L., Palmer, A. K., Short, W. H., Levinsohn, E. M., & Halperin, L. S. (1993). The change in ulnar variance with grip. *Journal of Hand Surgery [Am], 18,* 713-716.

Gemne, G., & Saraste, H. (1987). Bone and joint pathology in workers using hand-held vibrating tools. An overview. *Scandinavian Journal of Work and Environmental Health, 13,* 290-300.

Genti, G. (1989). Occupation and osteoarthritis. *Baillière's Clinical Rheumatology, 3,* 193-204.

Glyn, J. H., Sutherland, I., Walker, G. F., & Young, A. C. (1966). Low incidence of osteoarthritis in hip and knee after anterior poliomyelitis: A late review. *British Medical Journal, 2,* 739-742.

Goldberg, R. P., Zulman, J. I., & Genant, H. K. (1980). Unilateral primary osteoarthritis of the hand in monoplegia. *Radiology, 135,* 65-66.

Hadler, N. M., Gillings, D. B., Imbus, H. R., Levitin, P. M., Makuc, D., Utsinger, P.D. et al. (1978). Hand structure and function in an industrial setting. *Arthritis and Rheumatism 21,* 210-220.

Hagberg, M. (2002). Clinical assessment of musculoskeletal disorders in workers exposed to hand-arm vibration. *International Archives of Occupational and Environmental Health, 75,* 97-105.

Harrington, R. H., Lichtman , D. M., & Brockmole, D. M. (1987). Common pathways of degenerative arthritis of the wrist. *Hand Clinics, 3,* 507-527.

Hazlett, J. W. (1992). The third metacarpal boss. *International Orthopedics, 16,* 369-371.

Hoppenfeld, S., & Hutton, R. (1976). *Physical examination of the spine and extremities*. New York: Appleton-Century-Crofts.

Horvath, F., & Kakosy, T. (1979). Arthrosis of the distal radio-ulnar joint in workers using motorized saws. RöFo. *Fortschritte auf dem Gebiete der Röntgenstrahlen und der Nuklearmedizin, 131,* 54-59.

Jaffe, R., Chidgey, L. K., & LaStayo, P. C. (1996). The distal radioulnar joint: Anatomy and management of disorders. *Journal of Hand Therapy, 9,* 129-138.

Jensen, V., Boggild, H., & Johansen, J.P. (1999). Occupational use of precision grip and forceful gripping, and arthrosis of finger joints: A literature review. *Occupational Medicine (London), 49,* 383-388.

Jurgens, W. W., Ristow, B., & Pernack, E. F. (1990). Effect of physically hard labor on the locomotor system—results of an epidemiological cross-sectional study of resin tappers. *Zeitschrift für die gesamte Hygiene und ihre Grenzgebiete, 36,* 155-158.

Kapandji, I. A. (1982). *The physiology of the joints.* New York: Churchill-Livingstone.

Katevuo, K., Aitasalo, K., Lehtinen, R., & Pietila, J. (1985). Skeletal changes in dentists and farmers in Finland. *Community Dentistry and Oral Epidemiology, 13,* 23–25.

Kelley, M. J., & Ramsey, M. L. (2000). Osteoarthritis and traumatic arthritis of the shoulder. *Journal of Hand Therapy, 13,* 148–162.

Kellgren, J. H., & Lawrence, J. S. (1952). Rheumatism in miners. Part II. X-ray study. *British Journal of Industrial Medicine, 9,* 197–207.

Kern, D., Zlatkin, M. B., & Dalinka, M. K. (1988). Occupational and post-traumatic arthritis. *Radiologic Clinics of North America, 26,* 1349–1358.

Kihlberg, S., & Hagberg, M. (1997). Hand-arm symptoms related to impact and nonimpact hand-held power tools. *International Archives of Occupational and Environmental Health, 4,* 282–288.

Klippel, J. H., Weyand, C. M., & Wortmann, R. (Eds.). (1997). *Primer on the rheumatic diseases* (11th ed.). Atlanta: The Arthritis Foundation.

Kumlin, T., Wiikeri, M., & Sumari, P. (1973). Radiologic changes in the carpal and metacarpal bones and phalanges caused by chain saw vibration. *British Journal of Industrial Medicine, 30,* 71–73.

LaStayo, P., & Weiss, S. (2001). The GRIT: A quantitative measure of ulnar impaction syndrome. *Journal of Hand Therapy, 14,* 173–179.

Lawrence, J. S. (1961). Rheumatism in cotton operatives. *British Journal of Industrial Medicine, 18,* 270–276.

Lawrence, J. S. (1987). The epidemiology of degenerative joint disease: Occupational and ergonomic aspects. In H. J. Helminen, I. Kiviranta, A-M. Saamanen, M. Tammi, K. Paukkonen, & J. Jurvelin (Eds.), *Joint loading: Biology and health of articular structures* (pp. 316–251). Bristol: Wright Publishing.

Lee, P., Rooney, P. J., & Sturrock, R. D. (1974). Aetiology and pathogenesis of OA. *Seminars in Arthritis and Rheumatism, 3,* 189–218.

Lehto, T. U., Ronnemaa, T. E., Aalto, T. V., & Helenius, H. Y. (1990). Roentgenological arthrosis of the hand in dentists with reference to manual function. *Community Dentistry and Oral Epidemiology, 18,* 37–41.

Lester, B., Halbrecht, J., Levy, I. M., & Gaudinez, R. (1995). "Press test" for office diagnosis of triangular fibrocartilage complex tears of the wrist. *Annals of Plastic Surgery, 35,* 41–45.

Mackin, E.J., Callahan, A.D., Osterman, A.L., Skirven, T.M., Schneider, L.H., & Hunter, J.M. (Eds.). (2002). *Rehabilitation of the hand: Surgery and therapy* (5th ed.). St. Louis: Mosby.

Mahowald, M. L. (2001). Shoulder disorders and treatments. In L. Robbins, C.S. Burckhardt, M.T. Hannan, & R. J. DeHoratius (Eds.), *Clinical care in the rheumatic diseases* (2nd ed., pp. 231–238). Atlanta: Association of Rheumatology Health Professionals.

Malchaire, J., Maldague, B., Huberlant, J. M., & Croquet, F. (1986). Bone and joint changes in the wrists and elbows and their association with hand and arm vibration exposure. *Annals of Occupational Hygiene, 30,* 461–468.

Marzke, M. W. (1992). Evolutionary development of the human thumb. *Hand Clinics, 8*(1), 1–8.

Masmejean, E., Dutour O., Touram, C., & Oberlin, C. (1997). Bilateral SLAC (scapholunate advanced collapse) wrist: An unusual entity. Apropos of a 7000-year-old prehistoric case. *Annales De Chirurgie De La Main Et Du Membre Superieur (Paris), 16,* 207–214.

McDonald, E., & Marino, C. (1990). Manual labor metacarpophalangeal arthropathy in a baker. *New York State Journal of Medicine, 90,* 268–269.

McGee, D. J. (1992). *Orthopedic physical assessment.* Philadelphia: W.B. Saunders.

Melvin, J. & Jensen, G. (1998). *Rheumatologic rehabilitation series: Assessment and management.* Bethesda, MD: The American Occupational Therapy Association, Inc.

Mintz, G., & Fraga, A. (1973). Severe osteoarthritis of the elbow in foundry workers: an occupational hazard. *Archives of Environmental Health, 27,* 78–80.

Muggleton, J. M., Allen, R., & Chappell, P. H. (1999). Hand and arm injuries associated with repetitive manual work in industry: A review of disorders, risk factors and preventive measures. *Ergonomics, 42,* 714–739.

Nakamura, R., Horii, E., Imaeda, T., Nakao, E., & Watanabe, K. (1997). The ulnocarpal stress test in the diagnosis of ulnar-sided wrist pain. *Journal of Hand Surgery [Br], 22,* 719–723.

Neumann, D.A. (1999). Joint deformity and dysfunction: A basic review of underlying mechanisms. *Arthritis Care and Research, 12,* 139–151.

O'Driscoll, S.W. (2000). Classification and evaluation of recurrent instability of the elbow. *Clinical Orthopaedics and Related Research, 370,* 34–43.

Oka, Y. (1999). Debridement for osteoarthritis of the elbow in athletes. *International Orthopedics, 23,* 91–94.

O'Reilly, S., Jones, A., & Doherty, M. (1997). Muscle weakness in osteoarthritis. *Current Opinion in Rheumatology, 9,* 259–262.

Paley, D., McMurtry, R.Y., & Cruickshank, B. (1987). Pathologic conditions of the pisiform and pisotriquetral joint. *Journal of Hand Surgery [Am], 12,* 110–119.

Partridge, R. E., & Duthie, J. J. (1968). Rheumatism in dockers and civil servants: A comparison of heavy manual and sedentary workers. *Annals of Rheumatic Disease, 27,* 559–568.

Peyron, J. G. (1986). Review of the main epidemiologic-etiologic evidence that implies mechanical forces as factors in osteoarthritis. *Engineering in Medicine, 15,* 77–79.

Radin, E. L, Burr, D. B., Caterson, B., Fyhrie, D., Brown, T. D., & Boyd, R. D. (1991). Mechanical determinants of osteoarthritis. *Seminars in Arthritis and Rheumatism, 21*(3 Suppl 2), 12-21.

Radin, E. L., Parker, H. G., & Paul, I. L. (1971). Pattern of degenerative arthritis. Preferential involvement of distal finger-joints. *Lancet, 1*(7695), 377-379.

Rifkin, M. D., & Levine, R. B. (1985). Driller's wrist (vibratory arthropathy). *Skeletal Radiology, 13,* 59-61.

Robbins, L., Burckhardt, C. S., Hannan, M.T., & DeHoratius, R. J. (2001). *Clinical care in the rheumatic diseases* (2nd ed.). Atlanta: Association of Rheumatology Health Professionals.

Saffar, P., & Duek, C. (2002). Piso-triquetral osteoarthritis. Thirteen case reports and review of the literature. *Chirurgie De La Main, 21,* 107-112.

Sakakibara, H., Suzuki, H., Momoi, Y., & Yamada, S. (1993). Elbow joint disorders in relation to vibration exposure and age in stone quarry workers. *International Archives of Occupational and Environmental Health, 65,* 9-12.

Schlomka, G., Schroter, G., & Ochernal, A. (1955). Uber die bedeutung des beruflichen belastung fur die entstehung der degenerativen gelenkleiden. *Zeitschrift für Innere Medizin, 10,* 993-999.

Schmid, L., Dreier, D., Muff, B., Allgayer, B., & Schlumpf, U. (1999). Lifelong heavy agricultural work and development of arthrosis of the hand—a case study. *Zeitschrift für Rheumatologie, 58,* 345-350.

Segal, R., Avrahami, E., Lebdinski, E., Habut, B., Leibovitz, A., Gil, I. et al. (1998). The impact of hemiparalysis on the expression of osteoarthritis. *Arthritis and Rheumatism, 41,* 2249-2256.

Skirven, T. (1996). Clinical examination of the wrist. *Journal of Hand Therapy, 9,* 96-107.

Sokoloff, L. (1987) Loading and motion in relation to aging and degeneration of joints: Implications for prevention and treatment of osteoarthritis. In H. J. Helminen, I. Kiviranta, A-M. Saamanen, M. Tammi, K. Paukkonen, & J. Jurvelin (Eds.), *Joint loading: Biology and health of articular structures* (pp. 412-424). Bristol: Wright Publishing.

Staxler, L., Nisell, R., Vingard, E., & Nylen, S. (1994). CMC I arthrosis in two carpenters with excessive stress on the thumb. *Lakartidningen, 91,* 2248-2249.

Stecher, R. M., & Karnosh, L. J. (1947). Heberden's nodes. The effect of nerve injury upon the formation of degenerative joint disease of the fingers. *American Journal of Medical Science, 213,* 181-191.

Stenlund, B. (1993). Shoulder tendinitis and osteoarthrosis of the acromioclavicular joint and their relation to sports. *British Journal of Sports Medicine, 27,* 125-130.

Stenlund, B., Goldie, I., Hagberg, M., Hogstedt, C., & Marions, O. (1992). Radiographic osteoarthrosis in the acromioclavicular joint resulting from manual work or exposure to vibration. *British Journal of Industrial Medicine, 49,* 588-593.

Suzuki, K., Takahashi, S., & Nakagawa, T. (1978). Radiologic changes of the wrist joint among chain saw operating lumberjacks of Japan. *Acta Orthopaedica Scandinavica, 49,* 464-468.

Tomaino, M. M. (1998). Ulnar impaction in the ulnar negative and neutral wrist. Diagnosis and pathoanatomy. *Journal of Hand Surgery [Br], 23,* 754-757.

Tsujita, Y., Kido, M., Fukuda, T., & Onoyama, Y. (1989). Deformity of the fingers among women workers at a papermaking mill. *Sangyo Igaku, 31,* 70-76.

Turner, W. E. (1989). Occupational osteoarthritis-Landmark ACC decision. *New Zealand Medical Journal, 102*(877), 540.

Turner, W. E. (1991). Pricer's thumb. *New Zealand Medical Journal, 104* (924), 501-502.

Ulreich, A., & Klein, E. (1991). A rare arthrosis of the metacarpophalangeal joints—a degenerative disease in heavy manual labor. *Zeitschrift für Rheumatologie, 50,* 6-9.

Une, H., Kondo, S., & Goto, M. (1985). Radiographical changes in the elbow joints of chainsaw operators. *Sangyo Igaku, 27,* 152-157.

Vingard, E., Alfredsson, L., Goldie, I., & Hogstedt, C. (1991). Occupation and osteoarthrosis of the hip and knee: A register-based cohort study. *International Journal of Epidemiology, 20,* 1025-1031.

Vingard, E. (1996). Osteoarthrosis of the knee and physical load from occupation. *Annals of Rheumatic Disease, 55,* 677-679.

Watson, H. K., & Ryu, J. (1986). Evolution of arthritis of the wrist. *Clinical Orthopedics and Related Research, 202,* 57-67.

Watson, H. K., & Weinzweig, J. (1997). Physical examination of the wrist. *Hand Clinics, 13,* 17-37.

Watson, H. K., Weinzweig, J., & Zeppieri, J. (1997). The natural progression of scaphoid instability. *Hand Clinics, 13,* 39-49.

Wilk K. E., & Andrews, J. R. (Eds.). (1993). *The athlete's shoulder.* New York: Churchill-Livingstone.

Williams, W.V., Cope, R., Gaunt, W. D., Adelstein, E. H., Hoyt, T. S., Singh, A. et al. (1987). Metacarpophalangeal arthropathy associated with manual labor (Missouri metacarpal syndrome). Clinical radiographic, and pathologic characteristics of an unusual degeneration process. *Arthritis and Rheumatism, 30,* 1362-1371.

Wilson, F. D., Andrews, J. R., Blackburn, T. A., & McClusky, G. (1983). Valgus extension overload in the pitching elbow. *American Journal of Sports Medicine, 11,* 83-88.

Young, R. S., Bryk, D., & Ratner, H. (1977). Selective phalangeal tuft fractures in a guitar player. *British Journal of Radiology, 50,* 147-148.

PART THREE

Ergonomic Risk Factors Related to MSDs in Business and Industry

CHAPTER 8

The Expanded Definition of Ergonomics

Nick Warren

Despite the recent intense battles about an ergonomic standard, occupational medicine practitioners and much of the business community agree in principal that ergonomic interventions can be cost-effective ways of reducing injury and improving productivity. However, experience shows that some intervention techniques and strategies are more effective than others and that proven ergonomic changes that improve one workplace may be ineffective or even detrimental in another. These contradictions suggest that our understanding of ergonomic risk factors is incomplete and that researchers and practitioners should expand identification of ergonomic risk factors to develop consistently and optimally effective interventions. At base, this requires an expanded definition of ergonomics itself. This chapter develops an expanded definition and examines its implications for understanding the etiology and prevention of MSDs (musculoskeletal disorders) in the following sections.

1. Generally accepted derivation and meaning of the science of ergonomics
2. Outline of the elements needed in an expanded definition of ergonomics
3. Models of MSD etiology that incorporate an expanded definition of ergonomics
4. Difficulties in identifying risk factors and implications of a multifactoral causal model
5. Interaction of personal risk factors and capacity with external risk factors

ORIGINS OF ERGONOMICS

All ergonomics textbooks begin with the Greek derivation of the word *ergonomics*, which comes from *ergon* ("work") and *nomos* ("natural law"). The working definition of ergonomics, used by occupational health practitioners, is simple: It is the study of how to fit work to the worker. More generally, in everyday parlance, ergonomics has come to mean the design of tools and equipment, in both work and nonwork settings, to reduce the risk factors for musculoskeletal disorders (MSDs). Although many consumer products are now touted as being ergonomically designed (often with no understanding of the word and certainly with no regulatory oversight as to truth in advertising), this chapter will address ergonomics in its occupational health context only. It presents an expanded definition of ergonomics that looks beyond physical risk factors to a much more comprehensive examination of the fit between work and the worker. This broader framework for ergonomics has important implications for effective intervention strategies and programs to control MSD incidence.

Historically, the study of ergonomics evolved from the study of human performance, in particular from human factors. Human factors is the science of designing the interface between operator and machine (broadly interpreted to include not just manufacturing machines but computers, vehicles, and even the workpiece) to improve the exchange of information and control and to reduce errors. Although this volume does not address this aspect of the fit between work and the worker, human factors are related to physical ergonomics. Do this simple thought experiment: Imagine trying to find the correct knob for a burner on an unfamiliar stove top or trying to operate a faucet whose handles turn in directions opposite from what you are used to. We have all experienced these dilemmas, but imagine making these decisions when the quality of an expensive product or the safety of oneself and one's coworkers depends on rapid choice. It immediately becomes apparent that the intuitive design of displays and controls is a crucial factor in reducing errors. Further, poorly designed controls and displays may increase physical risk factors for MSDs by requiring extra movements, awkward postures, increased forces, and higher levels of work stress.

THE EXPANDED DEFINITION OF ERGONOMICS

To understand the complexity of identifying and controlling MSD risk factors, it is necessary to understand ergonomics more broadly than the usual definitions allow. Traditionally, ergonomics has focused on analysis and reduction of MSD risk factors at the job level: tool and workstation characteristics, attributes of the work piece, work flow, and the fit of these aspects of work to individual worker characteristics. Figure 8-1 embeds these individual-level aspects in the larger picture of the workplace, the work organization, and the company. The physical and psychosocial characteristics of the job are the result of work organization: the way workers, raw materials, workstations, tools, and techniques are brought together to produce a product or a service. (For simplicity, this chapter uses terminology related to manufacturing. But the principles, with appropriate changes in terminology, are also applicable to the service sector, the knowledge industry, and other nonmanufacturing types of work.) This work organization is itself the logical creation of company-level characteristics: the technology chosen to produce the product or service, the organizational structure, its relationships with suppliers and customers, and the organizational culture. Finally, this multilevel, dynamic set of relationships is itself embedded in local, national and global economic, political, regulatory, and cultural determinants—the macro-work environment.

In assessing these deeper roots of MSD risk, it becomes evident that the physical (biomechanical) risk factors associated with work at the individual level do not represent the full spectrum of possible risks. The macro- and organization-level risk factors in the diagram underlie not only the physical but also psychosocial job characteristics, both determined in large part by the way work is organized. Thus, ergonomic interventions designed to reduce the incidence of MSDs should ideally analyze and control the combination of physical and psychosocial risk factors on the "shop floor." And to be fully effective interventions should have a multilevel component that addresses as much as possible the underlying work organization and the company-level risk factors that determine levels of "shop-floor" risk. In identifying and controlling these MSD risk factors, ergonomics, the science of fitting work to the worker, becomes a much broader field than one focused on biomechanical risk control at the job level alone. In fact, from a practical point of view, interventions focused solely on biomechanical job change may even increase psychosocial risk factors (e.g., if employee input is not solicited in the risk factor identification and job redesign).

MODELS OF MSD ETIOLOGY

As a beginning, it is important to understand that the various types of tissue damage discussed in previous chapters are, to a degree, unavoidable. Any physical activity, even at low

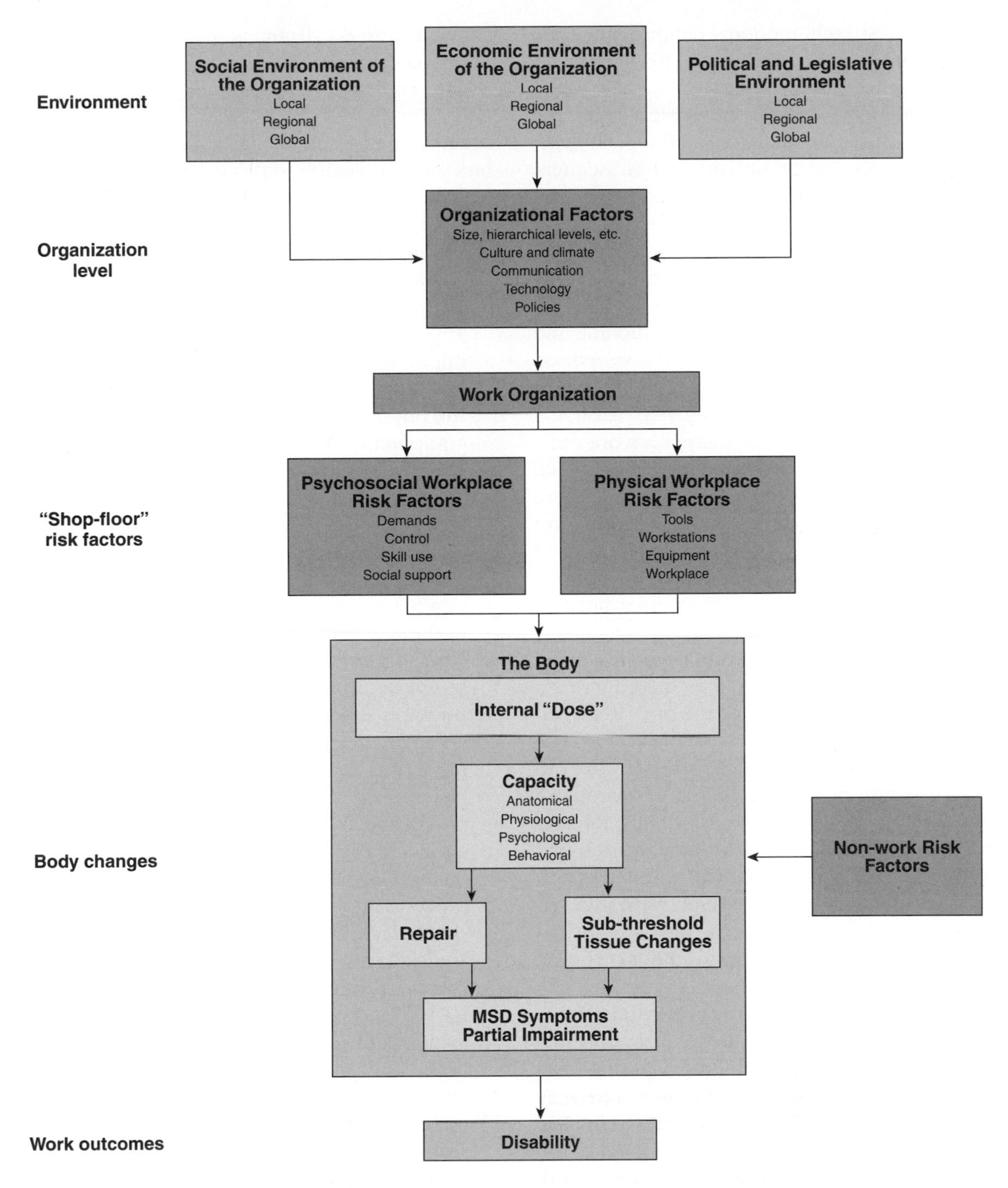

Figure 8-1 Expanded model of ergonomics: multilevel MSD risk factors and internal disease process.

levels, can stretch tendons, compress nerves, injure muscle fibers, and so on. In many cases these so-called microtraumas are actually examples of failure by design (the "design" being the result of natural selection). Minor damage, resultant pain and/or fatigue, and subsequent behavioral change help the organism avoid more serious tissue injury. The body has remarkable reparative mechanisms, and given enough recovery time, these microtraumas can easily be repaired. Indeed, muscle damage and subsequent repair are the basis for conditioning and strengthening regimes. The operative phrase "given enough recovery time" is often the key to an effective intervention: Simply increase the ratio of recovery time to activity in a work cycle or over the workday. There are more subtle mechanisms involved in some MSDs, and more sophisticated models of MSD etiology are available, but as a first overview, the concept of injury rate exceeding rate of repair is helpful in understanding how normal processes become pathologic.

Armstrong et al. (1993) proposed a model of the MSD disease process that incorporates a staged series of challenges to the body as well as the body's responses to these challenges. The body's response to a particular stressor dose can itself generate new physiological or anatomical stressors. For instance, overuse of the forearm flexor tendons can result in inflammation and swelling of the synovial sheaths through which the tendons pass. This natural reparative response can then compress the median nerve in the carpal tunnel, leading to the neurologic symptoms of carpal tunnel syndrome. The effectiveness of the body's response to both the external stressors and these new, internal stressors also depends partly on individual capacity. Although this model addressed only biomechanical risk factors at the individual level, it can easily be extended to incorporate the effects of psychosocial risk factors—work stress—and can be embedded in the larger organizational and societal context outlined above. Figure 8-1 diagrams this larger definition of ergonomics

The central box in Figure 8-1, entitled "The Body," represents the internal processes of the Armstrong et al. model just discussed. The single box of "Physical Workplace Risk Factors" represents the domain of conventional ergonomics. The expanded view of ergonomics adds the following extra pieces to the etiological model.

1. *Expanded analysis of local external stressors.* In particular, research over the last 15 years has demonstrated the central importance of psychosocial risk factors in MSD etiology. Interventions that change only the physical aspects of workstations, equipment, tools, and so forth often fail to identify and address low levels of worker control, reduced opportunities for learning and skill use, excessive psychological demands, reduced job security, compromised or negative levels of social support from coworkers or supervisors, and other deficits in the workplace social system.
2. *Work organization.* Both local physical and psychosocial risk factors are themselves primarily determined by the way the company organizes work. Companies make numerous and continuing decisions that result in altered levels of physical and psychosocial risk factors. For instance, the choice to organize work along an assembly-line model has implications for constrained postures and rates of repetition (physical risk factors) and employees' level of control and skill use (psychosocial risk factors).
3. *Organizational characteristics.* The choices for how to organize work, and the resultant local risk factors and resultant body changes in the individual, are rooted in the defining characteristics of the organization. These include basic organizational demographics: size, number of hierarchical levels, "flat" versus centralized structure, labor sources (e.g., temporary vs. permanent), and so on. More complex organizational characteristics

include the company culture and climate, the technology chosen for production, company policies and procedures, and so on.

4. *Organizational environment.* The organizational characteristics are themselves rooted in and affected by the larger social, economic, political, and legislative aspects of the local, national, and international environments. It has been a characteristic of the globalization of capital markets and business ownership that these high-level forces have become more important in their effect on "shop-floor" risks.

Note that this is not a static model. The realities of the twenty-first-century work environment include increasing levels of uncertainty and change, which themselves can contribute to increased physical and psychosocial risk factors. However, with proper intervention, justification, and carefully employed political power, this flexibility presents opportunities for positive (i.e., toward a healthier workplace) change as well.

Thus, if practitioners and researchers take literally the task of ergonomics—fitting work to the worker—it is imperative to take these different types and different levels of risk factors into account. It is obviously not possible to control all risk factors, particularly those at the macroergonomic level of the regional, national, and international political economy. But awareness of their influence on the "shop-floor" risk factors studied by traditional ergonomics allows interventions to more fully address the complexity of MSD reduction. Integrated, multifactoral, and multilevel interventions are much more likely to be effective.

DIFFICULTIES IN THE IDENTIFICATION OF RISK FACTORS: MULTIFACTORAL ETIOLOGY OF MSDs

With the preceding model in mind, this chapter and subsequent chapters examine methods for evaluating work and identifying this broader conceptualization of "risk factors" as well as the problems inherent in this identification.

In estimating the relative strength of MSD risk factors, identifying probable causes of MSDs, and determining proper control strategies and tactics, practitioners are hampered by the multifactoral nature of MSD etiology. This term should be understood to have at least the following four interconnected meanings: multiple risk factors present in the workplace, occupational and nonoccupational risk factors, combination of physical (biomechanical) and psychosocial risk factors, and multilevel risk factors.

MSDs usually result from exposure to multiple risk factors (Bernard, 1997; Kourinka & Fourcier, 1995; Putz-Anderson, 1988), with the possible exception of vibration-related disorders. The various types of risk factors discussed in this volume are usually present in an often daunting array of intensity, duration, and temporal distribution over the course of the worker's day, week, year, and entire career. It is difficult to estimate the relative contribution of a single risk factor because its effect is often modified by the level of another risk factor. For instance, most workers can lift a 1-lb weight every 5 minutes for a full workday. But if the repetition rate is increased to once every 2 seconds, this safe level of force becomes risky. This type of multifactoral causation makes it very difficult to estimate a safe level of any one risk factor. This is in contrast to chemical exposures, for which research can determine, in theory, a TLV (Threshold Limit Value) or PEL (Permissible Exposure Limit) around which to build regulations.

Despite these multifactoral difficulties, the American Conference of Governmental Hygienists has recently used a broad array of evidence to develop the TLV concept for hand, wrist, and forearm MSD risk: the HAL Voluntary Standard, establishing permissible combinations of force and average hand activity level (HAL) (ACGIH, 2001). (See Chapters 4 and 10 for further discussion.)

Further, the present state of knowledge does not allow a clear determination of whether these multiple risk factors act additively or synergistically (i.e., in a true, multiplicative interaction) within the workplace, although some studies suggest the latter (e.g., Silverstein, Fine, & Armstrong, 1986, 1987). One of the best-known examples of a multiplicative exposure-outcome relationship is the combined lung cancer risk from smoking and asbestos exposure. The risk of combined exposure is greater than the sum of lung cancer risk from smoking or asbestos individually. There is a synergistic mechanism, through which the effect of one risk factor is potentiated by the presence of the other.

This combination of multifactoral causation, lack of knowledge about interaction, and the unavoidable difficulty of studying risk factors in isolation makes it difficult to determine the effect of a given type of biomechanical exposure. A more practical approach, accepting the intricate interplay of risk factors in MSD causation, may be to simultaneously assess all the risk factors in a given workplace. Punnett (1998) has demonstrated the effectiveness of predicting MSD prevalence using an exposure index that combines assessment of multiple risk factors: work pace, grip force, postural stressors, contact (compressive) stress, vibration, and machine-pacing of work. This research found that the prevalence of MSDs (whether defined by symptom reports or physical examination) increased markedly as the number of risk factors contributing to the index increased. The obvious corollary is that multifactoral interventions will reduce MSD incidence more effectively than interventions targeting only a single risk factor or a small subset of the risk factors actually present in the workplace.

Figure 8-1 also notes the influence of nonwork risk factors in MSD etiology. The risk factors presented in this volume are not encountered solely in the work environment; MSD risk does not stop at the plant or office door. Nonwork activities also incorporate their own levels and distributions of physical and psychosocial risk factors that may contribute to disease causation. (See Chapters 18 to 20 for further discussion.) The undisputed existence and contribution of nonoccupational risk factors is often used to argue that a particular MSD or symptom is not work-related, generally by those with the most to lose if work-relatedness is established (e.g., owners, insurers, and some academics). However, with some exceptions (e.g., individuals training for and performing high-level sports activities), most nonwork activities are not performed with the duration, intensity, or time constraints characteristic of occupational exposures.

In addition, certain industries, such as meatpacking (OSHA, 1990), demonstrate disease clusters and rates of disease that are substantially above population background rates and rates found in other industries. Franklin, Haug, Heyer, Checkoway, and Peck et al. (1991) reviewed Washington workers' compensation claims from 1984 to 1988. These investigators found that, compared to industry-wide carpal tunnel syndrome (CTS) incidence rates, oyster and crab packers demonstrated a relative risk (RR) of 14.8 (95% CI: 11.2-19.5) and the meat and poultry industries had an RR of 13.8 (95% CI: 11.6-16.4). The 1998 NAS report (National Academy of Sciences, 1998) concludes, "There is a higher incidence of reported pain, injury, loss of work, and disability among individuals who are employed in occupations where there is a high level of exposure to physical loading than for those employed in occupations with lower levels of exposure." The existence of these elevated rates, despite the random distribution of nonwork risk factors experienced by employees in all industries, suggests the primacy of workplace risks in MSD causation.

As noted previously, research has begun to uncover the role of psychosocial risk factors in the etiology of MSDs. As with purely physical risk factors, the additive or multiplicative nature of combined biomechanical and psychosocial risk factors is complicated and the subject of ongoing research. Estimating relative independent and combined effects of these two risk factor classes is complicated by the fact that biomechanical risk factors, in general, act locally on the tissues directly involved in the work activity. In contrast, psychosocial risk factors act on the central nervous system and associated physiological pathways to produce more general effects that may predispose tissues to physical injury.

As noted previously and in Figure 8-1, the combination of biomechanical and psychosocial risk factors is the direct or indirect outcome of the ways in which the company organizes work and the company characteristics and environmental roots that affect these choices of work organization. Thus, a full estimation of risk factors must also consider these roots of the task-level stressors, the department-, facility-, and company-level characteristics that create or protect against disease and that are an appropriate target of ergonomic control programs.

PERSONAL RISK FACTORS

Estimating the relative effect of the various classes and types of risk factors outlined previously is further complicated by the variability in individual characteristics of the worker. These characteristics, including preexisting disease, are clearly implicated in MSD development and recovery as factors that modify the body's response to external risk factor exposure and its ability to recover from such exposures. The physiologic effects of the risk factors and modifiers presented in this volume are themselves modified by the worker's individual capacity to absorb or repair the damage caused. This capacity may be likened to the ability of the body to process a chemical exposure. Depending on the body's defenses, a given atmospheric concentration of toxin will result in cells and tissues receiving a particular dose of the toxin. Over time, this dose, modified by the body's capacity to detoxify or clear the substance and its metabolites, will result in a measurable body burden.

Although the analogy is simplistic and other disease mechanisms are probable, it is possible to visualize certain effects of MSD risk factors through this model. An exposure to a biomechanical or psychosocial risk factor of given intensity, duration, and temporal profile can result in an internal dose that makes demands on the body's reparative capacity for detoxification of the dose. This cumulative trauma model suggests that the resultant body burden may be seen as partly the result of exposure and individual repair capacity, as proposed by the Armstrong et al. (1993) model. Likewise, preexisting or underlying disease can also compromise reparative capacity as well as predisposing tissues to further injury.

The components of individual reparative capacity include genetic factors, acquired characteristics, and work techniques and skill level. Genetic factors include basic inherited characteristics of the individual, such as body dimensions (anthropometry), physiological and structural variables, and gender. Genetically based personal differences include variation in bone length and tendon attachment points (which affect the mechanical advantage of a muscle in a given posture), muscle mass and distribution of fiber types, laxity of ligaments, intervertebral disk cross-sectional area and nucleus fluidity, tendon size, and carpal tunnel size (Radwin & Lavender, 1998). To the degree that future research determines the genetic basis of personality, it is likely that individual workers vary in their ability to repair the psychologic and physical effects of work stress.

Gender may be seen partly as representing anatomical and physiological differences among workers (see summary in Faucett & Werner, 1998). Women's anthropometry may not fit many jobs designed originally for the average male. It is important to understand that gender is also a surrogate for a large complex of social and economic differences among workers as well as gender-based differences in exposure between males and females. Many of these differences influence patterns of disease and recovery

(Messing, Chatigny, & Courville, 1998; Messing, Tissot, Saurel-Cubizolles, Kaminski & Bourgine 1998).

Acquired characteristics include physical conditioning, other lifestyle factors (alcohol and tobacco use, weight, psychological resilience, etc.), previous or concurrent disease status, and the effects of aging. The aging process itself is strongly influenced by both genetic and acquired characteristics. Acquired characteristics can modify other genetically based characteristics—for example, type and intensity of exercise can alter muscle mass and fiber type distribution. Likewise, a worker's level of skill and work habits can substantially affect the impact of biomechanical stressors on body tissues.

Acquired personal characteristics also include the employee's work technique and skill level. In some situations, the predominant factors influencing MSDs are individual anatomy, work style, posture, and technique. For example, the well-recognized upper-extremity disorders of sign language interpreters (Feuerstein & Fitzgerald, 1992) or the hand problems of musicians (Amadio & Russoti, 1990; Fry, 1986) are usually remediated through retraining and movement modification, because the potential for tool modification is limited or nonexistent. It also seems likely that some differences in individual susceptibility to MSDs in industry are related to technique. In particular, the higher incidence of MSDs in new hires may relate to the lack of time or proper training that would enable new workers to develop more economical, less stressful patterns of motion and microbreak schedules.

Other work situations cannot be easily addressed by technique modification and retraining. For example, the vascular and neurologic problems produced by hand-arm vibration occur with such high attack rates and predictability that an effective control strategy must address the tool rather than individual susceptibility (Bovenzi, Petronio, & Di Marino, 1980; Pyykko 1986). In some industries, such as meatpacking, hand and wrist problems have been so prevalent and associated so strongly with particular tasks that identifying the cause is unambiguous, and focusing the intervention on tools and the work process is clearly required (Masear, Hayes, & Hyde, 1986; Schottland, Kirschberg, Fillingim, Davis, Hogg, 1991).

In still other settings, the multidimensional pattern of personal risk factors, nonwork risk factors, and external, work-related risk factors complicates etiology characterization and may require interventions aimed at tool redesign, technique modification, and even home risk factor reduction.

It is important to recognize that the effects of risk factors and modifiers found in the work environment are modified at the individual level by these personal factors. But their presence in the etiological model does not remove the primary necessity to identify and control external, workplace-based risk factors. Although "work-hardening," skill improvement, and even individually oriented stress management approaches may have an impact on increased personal capacity, most personal characteristics are difficult or impossible to change. Interventions focused solely in modifying personal characteristics are seldom of long-term use. In fact, the psychosocial impact of person-oriented interventions can be quite negative if employees perceive that management does not take seriously the very real presence of environmental physical and psychosocial risk factors.

REFERENCES

American Conference of Government Industrial Hygienists (ACGIH) (2001). Hand Activity Level—DRAFT.

Amadio, P. C., & Russoti, G. M. (1990). Evaluation and treatment of hand and wrist disorders in musicians. *Hand Clinics, 6,* 405–416.

Armstrong, T. J., Buckle, P., Fine, L. J., Hagberg, M., Jonsson, B., Kilbom, A. et al (1993). A conceptual model for work-related neck and upper-limb musculoskeletal disorders. *Scandinavian Journal of Work, Environment and Health, 19,* 73–84.

Bernard, B. (Ed.). (1997). *Musculoskeletal disorders and workplace factors*. Cincinnati, OH: U.S. Department of Health and Human Services, Public Health Service, Centers for Disease Control, National Institute for

Occupational Safety and Health. DHHS (NIOSH) Publication #97-141.

Bovenzi, M., Petronio, L., & Di Marino, F. (1980). Epidemiological survey of shipyard workers exposed to hand-arm vibration. *International Archive of Occupational Environmental Health, 46,* 251-266.

Faucett, J., & Werner, R.A. (1998). Non-biomechanical factors potentially affecting musculoskeletal disorders. In *National academy of sciences. Work-related musculoskeletal disorders: The research base*. Washington, DC: National Academy Press.

Feuerstein, M., & Fitzgerald, T. (1992). Biomechanical factors affecting upper extremity cumulative trauma disorders in sign language interpreters. *Journal of Occupational Medicine, 34,* 257-264.

Franklin, G. M., Haug, J., Heyer, N., Checkoway, H., & Peck, N. (1991). Occupational carpal tunnel syndrome in Washington State, 1984-1988. *American Journal of Public Health, 81*(6), 741-746.

Fry, H.J.H. (1986). Overuse syndrome of the upper limb in musicians. *Medical Journal of Australia, 144,* 182-185.

Kourinka, I., & Forcier, L. (Eds.). (1995). *Work related musculoskeletal disorders (WMSDs): A reference book for prevention*. London: Taylor & Francis.

Masear, V. R., Hayes, J. M., & Hyde, A. G. (1986). An industrial cause of carpal tunnel syndrome. *Journal of Hand Surgery, 11A,* 222-227.

Messing, K., Chatigny, C., & Courville, J. (1998). "Light" and "heavy" work in the housekeeping service of a hospital. *Applied Ergonomics, 29*(6), 451-459.

Messing, K., Tissot, F., Saurel-Cubizolles, M. J., Kaminski, M., & Bourgine, M. (1998). Sex as a variable can be a surrogate for some working conditions: Factors associated with sickness absence. *Journal of Occupational and Environmental Medicine, 40*(3), 250-260.

National Academy of Sciences (1998). *Work-related musculoskeletal disorders: A review of the evidence*. Washington, DC: National Academy Press.

Occupational Safety and Health Administration (OSHA) (1990). *Ergonomics program guidelines for meatpacking plants*. U.S. Department of Labor. OSHA Publication #3123.

Punnett, L. (1998). Ergonomic stressors and upper extremity disorders in vehicle manufacturing: Cross sectional exposure-response trends. *Occupational and Environmental Medicine, 55,* 414-420.

Putz-Anderson, V. (Ed.). (1988). *Cumulative trauma disorders: A manual for musculoskeletal diseases of the upper limbs.* New York: Taylor & Francis.

Pyykko, I. (1986). Clinical aspects of the hand-arm vibration syndrome: A review. *Scandinavian Journal of Work, Environment and Health, 12,* 439-447.

Radwin, R. G., & Lavender, S. A. (1998). Work factors, personal factors, and internal loads: Biomechanics of work stressors. In *National academy of sciences. Work-related musculoskeletal disorders: The research base*. Washington, DC: National Academy Press.

Schottland, J. R., Kirschberg, G. J., Fillingim, R., Davis, V. P., & Hogg, F. (1991). Median nerve latencies in poultry processing workers: an approach to resolving the role of industrial "cumulative trauma" in the development of carpal tunnel syndrome. *Journal of Occupational Medicine, 33,* 627-631.

Silverstein, B. A., Fine, L. J., & Armstrong, T. J. (1986). Hand wrist cumulative trauma disorders in industry. *British Journal of Environmental Medicine, 43,* 779-784.

Silverstein, B. A., Fine, L. J., & Armstrong, T. J. (1987). Occupational factors and the carpal tunnel syndrome. *American Journal of Industrial Medicine, 11,* 343-358.

CHAPTER 9

Physiologic Risk Factors

Barbara J. Headley

The current dilemma presented by musculoskeletal disorders (MSDs) posits that despite addressing workplace risk factors and providing solutions, in many cases these corrections have not solved the problem. The mechanisms that underlie muscle fatigue and neural changes have been identified as critical in establishing risk, severity, and recovery from most MSDs and thus represent a significant area of concern. We require a better understanding of workplace and physiologic risk factors to enhance our ability to address early physiologic changes that lead to functional loss and impairment.

This chapter discusses factors affecting the development of surface electromyography (sEMG) within the physiologic function of the neural muscular systems. Muscle fatigue plays a significant role in the determination of who develops MSDs by its profound influence on employees' abilities to function. Understanding muscle fatigue, both the localized and central types, can affect both prevention and intervention by targeting the problem early, allowing specific intervention to meet the employees' needs, and measuring the effects of various interventions. By having an influence on all stages of prevention, treatment, and outcome parameters, the use of sEMG to study muscle fatigue has taken a lead in the industry's quest to reduce expenses, lost time from work, pain, and suffering associated with MSDs in the workplace. The use of sEMG opens the door to understanding the types of dysfunction that occur in the neural input to recruitment of a given muscle, and demonstrating that changing neural input provides more lasting results than treatment directed only at the muscle. A phone line full of static or satellite potholes in cell phones can lead to misinterpretation of the message to the end receiver. Likewise, a muscle cannot fire appropriately if the message to activate it is firing too fast (demonstrating disorganized motor unit action potential [MUAP]) or so slow the muscle cannot be recruited. All of these factors, and others found at the neural muscular level, influence how and which muscles fire, and therefore how appropriately one moves. Compensatory movement adds stress to soft tissue; normal movement eliminates symptoms of musculoskeletal origin. The ability to take sEMG into the workplace and study the user interfacing with a workstation enables a therapist to alter physiologic risk factors long before they become symptomatic or to find the cause of current symptoms and allow alteration of the situation without progression of injury. Some terms related to sEMG and neural muscular function that will be used in this chapter are defined in Table 9-1.

sEMG is not new; it was first used to treat a reporter who suffered from migraine headaches in the late 1960s and has since progressed to assist in the treatment of a large number of disorders. Once the secrets of the power spectral

Table 9-1
Terminology

Term	Definition
Amplitude	Sum of the motor unit action potentials within the sampling area of the surface electrodes. Measured in microvolts (μVs) and displayed on biofeedback and surface EMG equipment.
Motoneuron	The junction of a nerve and the fibers within a specific muscle that it innervates. The muscle fibers share similar characteristics—that is, fast or slow twitch. If the nerve is sending faulty transmission to the muscle, muscle dysfunction is often the result. To remain healthy, a muscle must have healthy innervation signals.
Rate coding	The speed at which the active motor units are firing. This determines whether slow or fast twitch fibers are activated as adaptation occurs with progress fatigue.
Load sharing	The rotation of several healthy MCSs to alternate the muscle fiber bundles (motor units) or muscles used when performing a task. This allows a work-rest cycle.
Overflow	When a muscle is progressing from task-specific to global inhibition, the central drive mechanism in the brain must create excessive activation of effort, activating more muscles than the one in inhibition. Facilitation to a greater brain area creates electrical activity to the contralateral muscle and, at times, other nearby muscles.
Motor control strategy	A "software program" in the brain that designates which muscles fire in what order, speed, through what range of motion, and with which other muscles. Brushing the teeth and writing are two common motor tasks performed unilaterally due to the complex MCS built to perform the task, which is done automatically, with little conscious effort.
Muscle spasm vs. inhibition	Both clinically present as muscles that are hard upon palpation, are resistant to stretch, and painful with motion. Inhibition shows no EMG activity, whereas spasm shows very high levels of involuntary EMG activity even when the muscle should be resting.
Hyperresponsivity	MU's threshold is lowered, so that motor units fire with less stimulation/input, in greater number, and to stimuli that would otherwise not activate the MUs. Stimuli not usually noxious are activated and non-nociceptive (nonpainful) stimuli become painful.
Static load	A constant level of muscle contraction, often when the muscle should be resting or showing minigaps as part of load-sharing in performing a task. The static load decreases the rest time and increases the rate of fatigue onset.
Minigaps	Minute breaks in EMG activity from the motor unit action potential collection site of an electrode, showing MU silence for brief milliseconds. These provide a break in contraction and restoration of energy resources needed to continue working. Been shown to slow rate of fatigue onset.
Selective fatigue	Recruitment of appropriate slow twitch MUs for low-load work without compensatory fast twitch use creates fatigue of only slow twitch fibers. The muscle is then capable of power tasks but not continued static low-level tasks because of the selective fatigue. Load sharing should ideally be among various slow twitch MUs to continue performance of static or repetitive low-load task.
Proprioceptive wandering	A change in recruitment seen after loss of sensory input caused by invasive procedures or extreme fatigue with inhibition of prime movers, the lack of input regarding the effect or appropriateness of the choice of muscles recruited decreases the ability to continue using proper muscles. Each repetition can be seen to have a different physiologic profile, meaning different muscles are used each time the task is performed, adding to stress or strain of soft tissue.

EMG, Electromyography; *MU*, motor unit.

analysis using complex multivariate analysis methods were identified, it was found to be useful at the complex level of MSDs, failed low-back syndromes, and other dilemmas facing the therapist in the workplace.

A NEW FRONTIER

Fatigue and failure to recover have been the hidden invaders of MSDs. The fatigue is selective to certain motoneurons such as those needed to meet the unique workload demands of static and other long-term endurance tasks and is limited within the muscle to motoneurons with specific characteristics. Every muscle has some ratio of fast and slow twitch fibers, decided first by our genetic code and second by adaptation for the tasks one chooses to perform for lengthy periods of time. The muscle as a whole seldom contracts because activation is dependent on the kind of task at hand, so fibers bundled by the nerve that innervates similar types of fiber can be used for long periods of time during which the rest of the muscle does not fire. Therefore, fatigue selectivity of fiber bundles needed to meet the workload demands is limited within the muscle to motoneurons with specific characteristics.

The traditional medical workup of these employees, including x-ray, magnetic resonance imaging, electromyography (EMG), diagnostic testing, and blood work sheds no light on the inability of these individuals to perform their job tasks. Surface electromyography (sEMG) examination of fatigue and neural activity initiating contraction is providing insight and validation for many of these employees. Jensen's work on motor unit (MU) recruitment and rate coding has helped clarify this issue, along with selective fatigue, central changes (Jensen, Laursen, & Sjogaard, 2000), and other work on biomechanics and environmental stressors (Middaugh, Kee, & Nicholson, 1994) as well as changes in afferent threshold changes at the peripheral and central level (Mense, Simons, & Russell, 2001; Yaksh, 1996).

Using the standard of perceived exertion during work tasks has been a subjective way to determine how the subject feels after a given job demand. (Refer to Chapter 10 for further discussion.) The subjective reports have often appeared out of proportion to their ability to perform other tasks, such as the perceived exertion of a task when task-specific muscle fatigue was being studied. In one study, the subjects reported exertion being "close to exhaustion" during the recovery period when two shoulder muscles showed signs of localized muscle fatigue (Jensen, Pilegaard, & Sjogaard, 2000). In a study comparing proprioceptive (e.g., holding a weight) versus visual (pushing against a force transducer) feedback, the rating of perceived exertion was higher when proprioceptive feedback was used (Sjogaard, Jorgensen, Ekner, & Sogaard, 2000). Larger amplitudes had been collected during the proprioceptive feedback portion than during the visual feedback portion of the study. The authors concluded that the method of feedback may determine the extent of fatigue and recovery. Headley's work in progress on automated multivariate analysis of many parameters allows observance of changes that occur as clinical fatigue increases in severity.

These new insights on fatigue and fatigue failure help explain how one worker among hundreds develops an MSD. Findings focus assessment of the physical needs of the employees rather than question validity of complaints, including how an employee interacts with the workstation (Middaugh et al., 1994). Work-related musculoskeletal disorders have high incidence and prevalence among workers who are exposed to manual handling, repetitive and static work, vibrations, and unhealthy psychologic and social conditions (Kilbom et al., 1996). Exploration of the physiologic factors related to the resultant fatigue and to the failure of muscles to recover from fatigue is now providing answers into the inability of employees to perform tasks that they often appear capable of doing. The extensive research being done on fatigue is providing valuable information on the functionality of muscle(s) under extended low-level demands once thought to never create fatigue. Research includes perpetuating faults that extend localized muscle fatigue in a single trigger point to a full "spider web" of factors that create fatigue, spread it, and increase its severity. The afferent changes in neural input may be a significant contributing fault to increase nociceptive activity with several sites being altered. Afferent sprouting, spontaneous activity, and central facilitation all represent contributing factors (Yaksh, 1996). Here, it seems, lie many answers to MSD and open new possibilities to prevention and treatment.

MUSCLE ACTIVATION: BEGINNING MOVEMENT

Muscle recruitment patterns and their effect on pain or functional limitations have been studied by numerous authors (Middaugh, & Kee, 1987; Wolf, Basmajian, Russe, & Kutner, 1979). In a review of 31 studies, Jensen et al. (2000) stress that control mechanisms underlying the recruitment and gradation of muscle activity in complex multiple muscle systems during various voluntary exertions is still not fully understood. Load-sharing principles apply, influenced by such factors as demand, fatigue, and metabolic factors. Shoulder muscles appear to have a fairly consistent load-sharing pattern at low-load levels but are not immune to failure under certain conditions. Work-related symptoms may be due in part to the failure of load sharing, reducing of muscle activation rotation, and increasing singular motoneuron demands. Work by other researchers provides insight into what can be gained from further evaluation and intervention with employees in industry (Christensen, 1986; Hagberg, 1981; Hagberg & Kvarnstrom, 1984; Kilbom, 1988; Westgaard, 1988).

The work of these early pioneers provides a strong foundation to which new technology can add insight from combining technology. Vast numbers of subject databases, automated and standardized evaluation of thousands of parameters in cluster analysis, and stabilization of the data in ways that have been impossible have opened new levels of understanding. MSD clients have new chances to regain function, return to work, and live with a better quality of life.

sEMG: THE GUIDE TO UNDERSTANDING MSD

The capability of sEMG for examining muscle activity offers quantification of fatigue at multiple sites, and fatigue presents as the most valuable key in understanding MSDs. Surface electrodes are applied to the skin and collect a summation of MUAPs beneath the sampling area. Precise electrode placement using well-defined anatomic landmarks and carefully measured interelectrode distances provide valuable information about recruitment patterns. Dynamic movements based on electrode activity at each site can now be studied with parameters offering far more information than just amplitude. Although amplitude offers easy interpretation of dynamic activity, raw data must be used to obtain an sEMG power spectrum (sEMG-PS).

Amplitude represents the sample of MUs under the electrode and is affected by adipose, skin resistance, distance separating the electrodes, and motion of muscles under the electrodes. By using power spectrum data, information is available on the function and health of the nerve going to the muscle, such as the firing pattern of the nerve, its speed, and more. Although no single parameter is discriminatory in identifying high dysfunctional parameters, multivariate analysis of several parameters can be exceptional at targeting dysfunction in tissue.

The use of amplitude sEMG values to assess muscle fatigue has several potential drawbacks. First, careful consideration should be given to the collection methodology before conclusions are drawn when dealing with amplitude measures. Second, amplitude observations over only a short period may provide misleading clues regarding the degree of fatigue in a given muscle. Using parameters beyond amplitude (i.e., the sEMG-PS) enhances sEMG's ability to examine fatigue. Third, sEMG amplitude is of limited value as an objective method of localized muscle fatigue (LMF) assessment.

Wheras force and amplitude have a near-linear relationship in healthy muscle, in muscle with this form of hyporesponsivity the amplitude is high, but the force generation is low. When the normal curvilinear relationship is absent, force generation is minimal in the presence of amplitude. The fatigued MUs can no longer produce the expected levels of force, as shown in Figure 9-1. In this case, the wrist extensors show fatigue-induced inhibition and the wrist flexors show neural distress, with the muscle firing inappropriately (hyper-responsivity).

The sEMG-PS analysis in examination of LMF (Nyland, 1993), examined through fast Fourier transformation of the raw EMG signal from the time domain to the frequency domain, is an example (Figure 9-2). The analysis of the sEMG signal in the frequency domain involves measurements and parameters that describe specific aspects of the frequency spectrum of the signal (Basmajian & DeLuca, 1985). Headley has reported using multivariate analysis techniques to further stabilize the changes found in sEMG fatigue measurement. In addition, Headley has correlated changes in the MU firing pattern with clinical changes in muscle activation timing, force production, and amplitude capability in the muscle (Headley & Hocking, Unpublished). sEMG is helpful in identifying LMF although not always the exact location of its source.

The power spectrum histogram typically shifts to the left with fatigue, as shown in Figure 9-3. Tissue filtering effect determines the shape of the MU action potential's composite (Basmajian & DeLuca, 1985; Nyland, 1993). Peripheral factors that have also been reported to alter the sEMG-PS distribution include muscle force level, muscle length, muscle fiber composition and distribution, skin and tissue impedance, electrode properties and geometry, muscle thickness, muscle fiber diameter, cross-talk between muscle, and various metabolic factors (Nyland, 1993). Yaksh and Mense et al. add research on

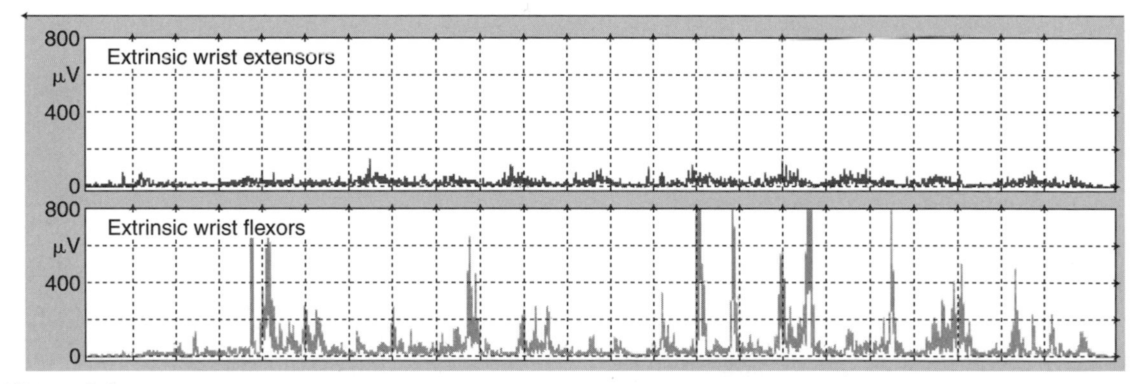

Figure 9-1 The forearm flexor site is not producing much activity while typing, and the spikes seen represent the use of the index finger on the mouse. The amplitude is much higher than the force being produced, demonstrating a loss of muscle skill in the forearm flexors where force is not appropriately reflected in amplitude. The extrinsic forearm extensor site, however, should be stabilizing the wrist and some cocontraction activity should be seen during typing as wrist extension and finger flexion occur. The lack of the long extrinsic wrist extensors to provide a stabilizing function for the flexors is a result of active MTrPs and fatigue-induced inhibition. The inhibition is task specific, the same electrode site showing activity with non-work–related tasks.

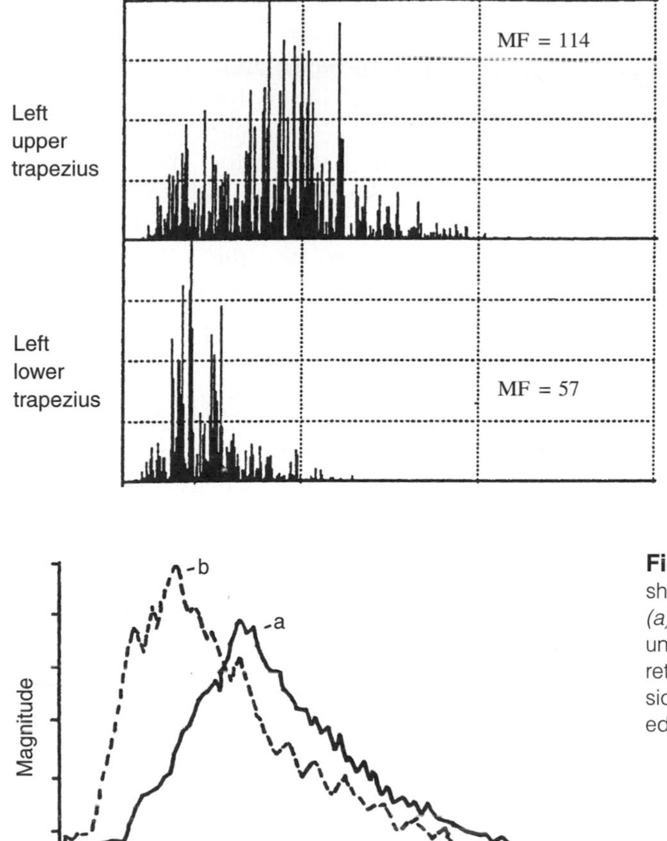

Figure 9-2 Median frequency (MF) values are calculated from the raw electromyographic data during a sustained isometric contraction. MF values are shown for the upper and lower trapezius muscles.

Figure 9-3 The median frequency in this case is shown before and after fatigue. The prefatigue value *(a)* is contrasted to the slower firing rate of the motor units after fatigue *(b)*. This shift in the power spectrum returns to normal after rest. (Reprinted with permission from Basmajian, J. V. [1985]. *Muscles alive* [5th ed., p. 205]. Baltimore: Williams & Wilkins.)

altered neural activity as perpetuating muscle dysfunction (Mense et al., 2001; Yaksh, 1996). There were noted changes in the recruitment pattern of MUs with fatigue development. The tendency of recruitment to gradually decrease dominated the results. The constant force was sustained by the mechanisms of space coding (recruitment of additional MUs). Some recruitment patterns for additional MU activation during holding phases were found when muscle force was constant (Christova & Kossev, 2001), suggesting the use of load sharing by rotation of MUs.

Although sEMG cannot examine individual MU activity, therapists seek to improve function and must consider how an individual maintains force or task demands and when a task is terminated because of increased muscle dysfunction secondary to some type of fatigue failure. Examination of raw data during sustained contraction shows deterioration of MUAPs as a group with fatigue. Recruitment is difficult to sustain if innervation patterns fail. Comparison of innervation activation pattern at 1.5 second versus 9 second of a 10-second isometric hold shows significant deterioration of the MU pattern, with a large increase in median frequency despite sustained amplitude levels. In this case, amplitude hides the aberrant neural input that prohibits sustaining proper output and muscle dysfunction. Headley verifies multiple examples of amplitude decrease related to changes in innervation activity to the sample of MUs, supporting the possibility that muscle dysfunction can in some cases be secondary to neural distress (Headley & Hocking, Unpublished).

Changes in neural activity are predictive of muscle recovery from fatigue and inhibition. Multivariate analysis of sEMG-PS parameters can establish what load demands the muscle can now tolerate. Headley describes a four-phase clinical recovery stage through which neural changes result in concordant improvement in muscle activation patterns, fatigue, and endurance (Headley & Hocking, Unpublished).

For the therapist using this fatigue model, a symptomatic employee can be evaluated at an ergonomically correct workstation by collecting 40 parameters to determine how persistent muscle dysfunction is perpetuating the employee's inability to tolerate job demands. Observation of muscle inhibition no longer has an "assumed" cause, but via multiplex analysis, data provides a precise determination of cause, stage of severity, types of fault perpetuators, and steps needed for intervention to achieve recovery (Headley, 1997).

Dynamic functional muscle testing using sEMG has provided insight into the muscle dysfunction and symptom complaints of static, low-load MSD problems. Standard protocols have been developed by the author, including testing of active, resisted, static, repetitive, and loaded tasks. In addition, a fatigue-testing format combines isometric testing of fatigue before the protocol, a dynamic movement protocol, and repeat fatigue isometric testing on completion of the protocol and after a standardized rest period. The Functional Analysis of Movement with Electromyography (FAME) evaluation format produces not only an automated report, Physiological Analysis Compilation (PAC), which is based on a continually growing database. It quantifies the interpretation of more parameters than could be done manually, allowing for a more stable, in-depth analysis that therapists have not been able to report on a reliable basis. FAME has been instrumental in establishing the deficit stages of MSD and other soft-tissue problems and the means by which to isolate intervention needs. Its results must take into consideration the other factors about the client that are not known by the software: the clinician's full history and evaluation (Headley, 1997). Muscles are not the only aspect of physiologic risk factors (PRF) that determine the development of MSD, its course of development, and the outcome of any changes made to the workstation, rest breaks, or treatment. To appreciate and understand the full scope of MSD, one must take into consideration higher-level systems. Only then can treatment that is effective in the early stages be developed; changes that can keep the employee at work doing repetitive or static jobs. Progression of MSD to the last state (refer to Table 9-2, the deficit stage of Adaptive Failure) finds the employee unable to recover sufficiently to return to the job demands. Impairment is much higher and only partially reversible.

FAULTS INITIATE PHYSIOLOGIC RISK FACTORS

Physiologic Risk Factors (PRF) cannot be narrowed down to one single element. PRF is an umbrella for the plethora of factors that can, if they progress, lead to one or more stages of Movement Adaptation Syndrome (MAS). The relationships of these stages and the stages of MSD are shown in Table 9-2. The key element, if not prevention, is early understanding of the progression, identifying the perpetuating faults and therefore the recovery intervention stage to begin treatment. sEMG has taken a lead role as a tool that can provide vast insight into the MSD dilemma. When deficits identifying location and type of abnormal activity are found and can be matched into the stages of MSDs, understanding leads to appropriate intervention.

Although rehabilitation has had protocols to follow, many lack validation, a way to determine

Table 9-2
MSD Stages as They Relate to Physiologic Risk Factors

Neural-Kinetic Fault Stages	As They Correspond with MSD Symptoms
Stage 1: Hyper-responsivity	Loss of skill. Muscle fires at higher amplitude than necessary and the amplitude pattern is more erratic. The higher amplitude does not coincide with increased force as in healthy muscle.
A. Trigger Points (primary muscles based on progression of MSD).	Lower trapezius (LTR), upper trapezius (UTR).
B. Fatigue Characteristics	Mild delay (2-3x normal) in recovery from fatigue.
	Pain between shoulder blades, UTR area; possible soreness when leaving work at end of day; no problem performing leisure activities; seldom recognized as an evolving MSD problem.
	Posture plays a role in rate of progression, adding soft tissue stress and strain.
Stage 2: Neural Distress	Neural signs may include facilitation of nerve root, erratic firing pattern, sympathetic nervous system involvement, autonomic dysregulation, "proprioceptive wanderer" activation pattern.
A. Trigger Points	LTR, UTR, levator, cervical paraspinals, infraspinatus, serratus posterior superior, scalenes.
B. Muscle Dysfunction	Proximal scapular stabilization is compromised.
C. Fatigue Characteristics	Moderate delay (4-6x normal) in recovery from fatigue; fatigue failure is specific (i.e., limited to low-load fibers, static load levels, latency to rest, and neural tension dysfunctions).
D. Functional and System Complaints	Pattern of direction of MSD is taking form (e.g., carpal tunnel, TMJ, migraines, or tendonitis).
Stage 3: Overload	Reduction of amplitude with increased demand or with multiple repetitions.
	The amplitude is below expected levels and fast twitch fibers are being used to achieve activation when slow twitch would be the appropriate response.
A. Trigger Points	LTR, UTR, levator, cervical paraspinals, infraspinatus, serratus posterior superior, scalene, teres minor, posterior deltoid, FA flexors.
B. Muscle Dysfunction	Muscle dysfunction is present with decreased LTR, FA flexors, and FA extensors and SCM showing either high or low activity. Increased activity in scalenes.
	Dysfunction is present not just at job task but is generalized to other tasks as well.
C. Fatigue Characteristics	Severe delay (8-12 hr) in recovery from fatigue; fatigue failure more generalized, involving entire muscle(s) as demands increase in speed, duration without breaks and loss of job rotation or breaks.
	Increasing fatigue during week; reported need by midweek to continue working; use of weekend and holidays to recover, great difficulty maintaining a static work task.
Stage 4: Task-Specific Inhibition without Compensation	Task-specific lack of muscle firing; muscle works fine in other tasks; some also having pattern of task-specific inhibition caused by how and why each muscle fatigues.
A. Trigger Points	LTR, UTR, cervical paraspinals, levator, infraspinatus, serratus posterior superior, scalene, teres minor, posterior deltoid, FA flexors and extensors, SCM, deep cervical flexors.
B. Muscle Dysfunction	Decreased activity in LTR, UTR, scalene, FA flexors with FA extensors and SCM showing increase or decrease.
	Muscle dysfunction is generalized and affecting activities of daily living at home, leisure hobbies and sports, and distant muscles secondary to compensation.

Continued

Table 9-2
MSD Stages as They Relate to Physiologic Risk Factors—cont'd

Neural-Kinetic Fault Stages	As They Correspond with MSD Symptoms
C. Fatigue Characteristics	Profound delay (1-2 days) in recovery from fatigue; spectral cluster analysis fails to show any recovery with neural activity present, activation of slow twitch fibers altered, increasing inhibition's duration and extent. Fatigue occurs quickly as no compensation has evolved.
D. Functional and System Complaints	Profound functional limitation in all daily activities; inability to do simple activities of daily living at home; poor prognosis for returning full time to work that requires static load or repetitive task performance. Return to static or repetitive work requires daily maintenance work to sustain performance with progression of pathology and symptoms. Symptom tolerance is essential. Client reports increasing symptoms during week, with weekend needed for recovery. Leisure life suffers.
Stage 5: Task-Specific Inhibition with Compensation	Compensation assists where inhibition has occurred. Pain from compensation becomes the cause or perpetuating factor in unresolved pain. Strain is placed on multiple soft tissues that can develop into new pathology.
A. Trigger Points	New trigger points are added by compensation patterns as they evolve. The trigger points become "centers" from which secondary trigger points spread. All early trigger points have autonomic dysfunction and are more resistant to treatment.
B. Muscle Dysfunction	The extensive compensation now requires that whole new patterns of movement be developed with new motor control strategies. Postural stress syndromes may exceed the extremity or original area of injury. Compensation patterns are showing inhibition and failure.
C. Fatigue Characteristics	Fatigue is occurring now by first trying a compensation pattern of close by synergists, which are lost to pure inhibition. Now more distal sites add to duration of movement but at a large cost to soft tissues. Compensation also occurs by using fast-twitch fibers of prime muscles or compensatory muscles.
Stage 6: Fatigue without Recovery	Fatigue failure shows pattern of inability of supporting systems to provide physiologic recovery at one or multiple sites of fatigue. Therefore, pattern has many profiles and appearances, but inhibition may persist for hours to days. Sympathetic effects on neural system enhance the response to pain.
A. Trigger Points	All of above with anterior deltoid, triceps, and other trigger points depending on the direction the MSD symptoms took.
B. Muscle Dysfunction	Muscle dysfunction is global, influenced by central drive and MAS. Inhibition dominates primary and compensatory muscles.
C. Fatigue Characteristics	Recovery from fatigue failure does not appear within a time frame compatible with job demands. Static and repetitive work attempts only lead to refailure and increase in severity of symptoms.
D. Functional and System Complaints	The neural parameters governing activation of muscles are in failure with inability to recover if performing any typical ADL. Avoids tasks so well that they state they *don't* do them, not that they *can't*. Kinesthetic awareness is compromised; sensory discrimination is greatly diminished. These clients often have persistent compartment syndromes, MAS, inhibition that reaches adaptive failure with loss of adequate compensation systems. Homeostasis cannot be established, even with prolonged rest.

Table 9-2
MSD Stages as They Relate to Physiologic Risk Factors—cont'd

Neural-Kinetic Fault Stages	As They Correspond with MSD Symptoms
Stage 7: Global (Central Drive) Inhibition	Muscle or muscles are inhibited in all types of movements, static and loaded tasks, while still having normal innervation.
A. Trigger Points	Do not seem to exhibit in the profoundly inhibited muscles found at this stage. The muscles do begin to show the pain of these trigger points if the muscle can be reactivated. Sympathetic effects on neural system enhance the response to pain.
B. Muscle Dysfunction	Muscle dysfunction is profound, found in multiple areas not near the original injury, and the negative results of so many tests are negative. Health care providers have, in the past, looked for psychologic reason for these symptoms.
C. Fatigue Characteristics	Recovery or progression is very slow. The recovery of these muscles after 3-6 repetitions has been shown to require three days of rest (obvious that a job cannot be performed with recovery). Long periods of time off from work are needed with a model of therapy that progresses the therapy as changes show that the muscles or neural system can tolerate it. The program is very slow in progress, but return to work and repetitive work can be achieved at this stage if the right program is followed.
D. Functional and Symptom Complaints	Client may have already learned how to fail and has become a "victim." Objectification of the problems often helps with compliance. If injuries across the lifespan are involved, or other vulnerable areas are strong, full adaptive failure can be reached.
Stage 8: Adaptive Failure	Inhibition without recovery. Multiple complex perpetuating faults. Severe neural distress and starting recovery at the most basic levels of muscle and neural reactivation.
A. Trigger Points	With autonomic involvement trigger points can be painful, although they can seldom be palpated due to prolonged inhibition, extreme fatigue, and compensation. The pain they experience is from the strains of the soft tissues and joints from the soft tissue action on them.
B. Muscle Dysfunction	Muscle dysfunction is widespread, the involved extremity is very highly guarded as pain is its primary complaint. Other pathology may have evolved. Recovery from global inhibition may show some initial changes, and some activities may be recovered, but return to full static or repetitive work requires a return to homeostasis and that is unlikely.
C. Fatigue Characteristics	The needs of recovery are profound, very slow, and if helplessness or failure has been learned by clients, they may not succeed because of the slowness of recovery. All the fatigue characteristics are not known or explained. The author has not personally seen a client return to repetitive work from this level.
D. Functional and Symptom Complaints	Autonomic dysregulation is predominant and complex with multiple systems involved. The cost of long-term compensation has been too great, and the recovery from endurance-based fatigue does not seem to happen. Many clients become withdrawn, "give up," or expect less from life. A few can return to work if NO repetitive or static work is performed, breaks and changes of position can be frequent, and some time off given in the middle of the week to decrease the "week-long fatigue." This is progressive over the course of a week (all shown physiologically) and then some rest occurs over the days off, with the cycle beginning all over again when they return to work.

starting level, and a system to monitor response to treatment choices. With these determined by doing a FAME evaluation, the client is placed at a precise point on the "map to recovery," a map that can be followed, measuring the result of any treatment intervention. The results of these protocols demonstrate a significant difference between the clients and asymptomatic controls when scored by software without subjective interference (Headley, 1996c). The failure of muscles to recover within a reasonable time frame has also been reported as statistically significant in an examination of 55 clients with upper-quadrant MSD as compared with control subjects (Headley, 1996a). Observation using physiologic movement measures shows that the client moves faster to neural recovery following the standardized parameters. With MSD, knowing the muscles' physical tolerances prevents overloading—that is, placing the client in rehabilitation that is over his or her limits—which slows recovery.

The six stages of MSDs are presented in Table 9-2 as they relate to PRF and the stages of MSD. The muscles cited relate to individuals performing upper-quadrant static and repetitive tasks at very low loading (i.e., requiring muscle recruitment levels of less than 8% of their maximal voluntary contraction [MVC]). The more global deficit stages of myofascial pain syndrome, appropriate for all soft-tissue dysfunction, include other forms of MSD in both upper and lower quarters, and the spine. They also show the correlation among MSDs developing anywhere the body is being stressed and low-level, long-duration, or repetitive demands that affect muscle, neural drive, central drive, fatigue development, and its failure to recover.

Stage 1

Awkward posture is an accepted component in the development of MSDs, placing strain on soft tissues that are not capable of handling the load for long periods. Muscles working at improper lengths, without rest breaks or proper motor control strategies, develop Postural Stress Syndromes (PSSs) that can lead to the spread of symptoms by the postural perpetuating factors. Myofascial trigger points (MTrPs) develop from the primary muscle overworked to secondary ones, almost like a spider builds an ever-larger web. With this comes more symptoms and fatigue of additional muscles. It is the ever-expanding fatigue of muscle that results in the progression of the MSD and its functional impairments.

Posture-related pain, often referred to as PSS, was identified by Janda et al. (Janda, 1968; Janda, 1988; Janda, 1992; Lewit, 1985). It is one of the most common factors in the early stages of MSD. The Upper and Lower Cross Syndromes, defined by Janda and outlined by Chaitow (1996), show that some patterns of dysfunction do exist in PSS. Patterns of MAS can be useful in establishing standardization of workstations to correct known postural set patterns but should be recognized as being short of universal. A chain reaction of muscle length and tension is common but is influenced by MCS that evolves from previous injuries or habituated MCS in many individuals.

The computer mouse was introduced with the idea that the interruption of typing creates minibreaks (gaps) during which muscle activity drops to near zero for a fraction of a second and decreases fatigue, much like the carriage returns on typewriters. Jensen, Finsen, Hansen, and Christensen (1999) found that the number of gaps on the mouse side was significantly lower than the values for the upper trapezius muscle (UTR) on the non-mouse side, indicating that more continuous activity was present in the UTR muscle on the mouse side. The frequency of gaps was about tenfold on the side operating the mouse than on the other side, and the total gap time was sixfold shorter on the mouse side as compared to the other side.

Headley's findings (reported in 1996b), however, contradicted this previous study. Headley studied mouse activity for software being developed for a company that wanted to decrease MSD injuries. Headley was asked to use sEMG to prove the mouse was beneficial in symptom reduction. The data, however, supported the opposite, with excessive activity on the mouse side in the UTR and forearm muscles. In addition, data related to the lower trapezius muscle (LTR) suggested that loss of scapular stabilization often preceded hyperactivity of the UTR. In symptomatic clients this LTR inhibition is almost universal and progressive, as shown in Figure 9-4. Symptoms in the LTR appeared first and have progressed through the Neural-Kinetic Model Stage 6, whereas at this time the forearm muscles are still in a much earlier stage. Findings may differ because of the nature of a novel test in the study by the author, since the employees had not used the mouse at that point. Early stages of fatigue were the primary finding at this level, with loss of muscle skill and efficiency its primary characteristics. It is beyond the scope of this chapter to expand on each of the perpetuating faults of the Neural-Kinetic Model that serves as an "umbrella" for the stages of MSD, but the parallels are unmistakable, and fatigue of low-frequency (slow twitch) fibers is the key.

To determine the influences of various factors on fatigue development, the individual muscles in the shoulder were examined in MSD disorders. The chain of muscle failure is particularly important, as can be seen when the UTR fatigues more quickly than the fingers using the mouse, when the intent was to vary the job demands and facilitate job rotation and load sharing of MUs. Examination of two different manual tasks, however, has reinforced the difficulty of removing the static load of the more proximal muscles. A study of scrubbing and mopping demonstrated minimal change to the load placed on shoulder MUs despite distal differences (Sogaard, Laursen, Jensen, & Sjogaard, 2001).

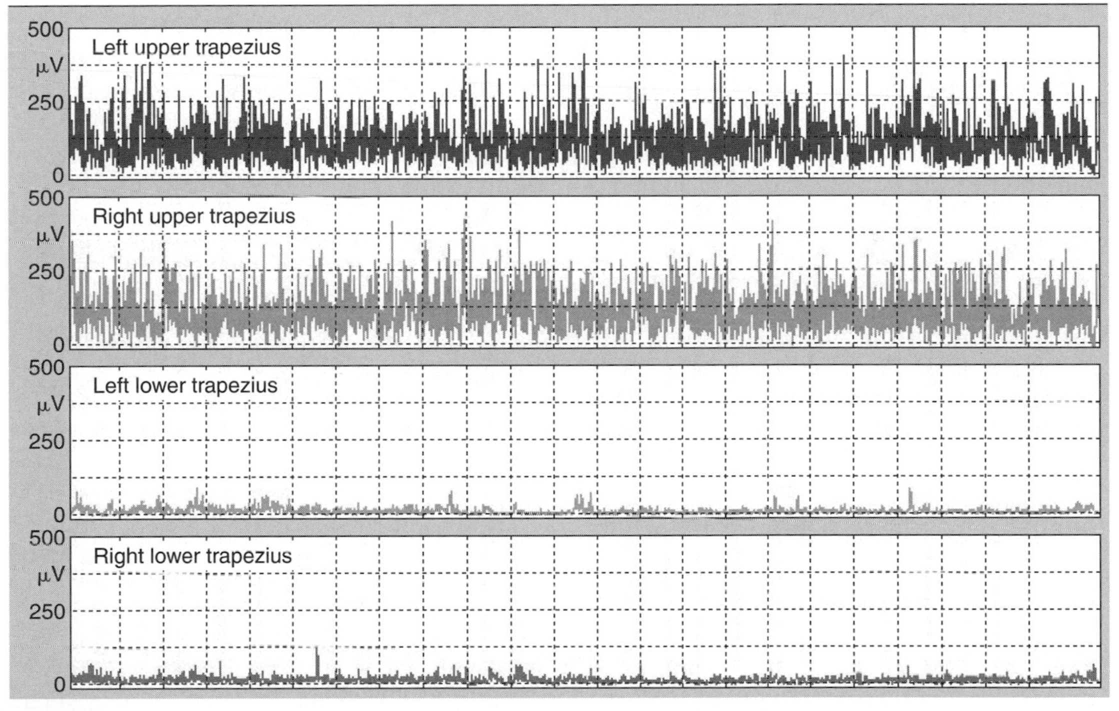

Figure 9-4 The first stage of MSD is often the loss of scapular stabilization by fatigue-related inhibition of the LTR following activation of an MTrP. As fatigue progresses through the six stages of cumulative trauma, the LTR inhibition becomes more global and UTR hyperresponsivity evolves as the first stage of MSD in the second muscle involved. From here it moves to the neck muscles, the forearm muscles, and the thenar muscles. Loss of the agonist-antagonist relationship of the UTR and LTR leaves the scapulohumeral rhythm to fail, followed by malpositioning of the shoulder joint and loss of efficient use of the arm.

Muscle compensation was eloquently described by Price, Clare, and Ewerhardt in 1948. When few knew of MTrPs, Price et al. described the changing pattern of symptoms, with high and low amplitude levels in the same muscle groups over time. Inhibition was common but not consistent over time to any one muscle group. Changing muscle activation also alters MAS as it applies to compensation and MTrPs. Changes in symptoms, and changes in level of function commonly occur. Compensation may produce hyperresponsive activation resulting from the lack of a defined motor control strategy, with efficient use of MUs still undefined as well as the use of too many muscles in order to establish a way to perform the task. Overflow may also be present, in which the contralateral side, in spite of being at complete rest, shows high amplitude as bilateral effort is put into the task by central drive mechanisms trying to accomplish the task. Overflow can fatigue the contralateral muscle while it is in its rest cycle and increase the rate of fatigue development. The rest cycle of a muscle is just as critical to homeostasis and health as the work cycle (Hansson et al., 2000). This stage, if identified as early MSD, can be treated quickly and easily, with changes made to the workstation, and training, if necessary, to enhance muscle skill and efficiency. The physiologic markers provide proof of positive change as well as the use of multiple parameters to maximize the effect of a multiparametric approach. The symptoms are often so minor, however, that few pay attention to them, and the employee moves into later stages of Neural-Kinetic deficit.

The influence of pain on muscle activation must have a threshold at which point the pain interferes with normal muscle function. Birch, Christensen, Arendt-Nielsen, Graven-Neilsen, and Sogaard (2000) found that when wrist muscular demands were performed at 10% MVC for 60 seconds, muscular fatigue set in. Muscle pain was introduced into one group by the addition of hypertonic saline to evoke muscle pain. They found the number of MUs recruited was almost identical for baseline and MUs with pain, and no effect of experimental muscle pain was found on the properties of the MUs (amplitude, area) or their firing characteristics (mean firing rate, firing variability) during low-force ramp contraction. During the sustained 10% MVC, no effect of pain was found for concentric or sEMG of the forearm muscles. At low-force levels no pain-induced modulations were found in MU activity, when the mechanical condition was similar to that of a control situation (Birch et al., 2000).

Stage 2

Yaksh (1996) and Mense et al. (2001) have made major contributions to identifying how peripheral muscle overloading leading to MTrPs is just one example of how neural afferent activity becomes altered at the peripheral and then central-processing level. Chronicity of MTrPs has been shown to have several neural distress characteristics in the innervation of the involved muscle. These include generation of spontaneous afferent activity, peripheral changes in terminal sensitivity and others, and sprouting. With peripheral nerve injury, low-threshold afferent input is encoded as a noxious event. The number of low-threshold afferents increases by spreading into other areas of the dorsal horn. These new afferents (sprouting) show spontaneous activity with significant mechanochemo sensitivity. Although blocking afferent activity temporarily shuts down the afferent hypersensitivity, reestablishment of transmission can lead to powerful allodynia, plus the afferent changes alter muscle activation response to stimuli. These changes can lead to severe pain behavior in spite of moderate triggering stimulus.

Changes in the patterns of neural drive may have a variety of influences on the force-generating capacity of muscle (Bigland-Ritchie & Woods, 1984). Neural involvement may include the autonomic nervous system, which can lead to such symptoms as hypersensitivity to touch and distortion of temperature. Treatment of these aberrant neural activity patterns often results in reduction of the need to treat the MTrP, except in acute flare-ups, suggesting that aberrant neural activity may be a major perpetuating factor in some MTrPs. Work can generally continue without maintenance on MTrPs every night if the treatment is focused on the fatigue and neural issues as well as awareness by the employee of when fatigue begins to set in and what he or she can do to relieve it.

The effect of MTrPs on muscle activity may be one of hyperirritability or inhibition, both local or referred. Both have been reported (Headley, 1990c; Simons, 1993). Studying muscle activation and the neural drivers of such behavior focuses on characteristics of MU activity and how it affects the loading of muscles. These reflex neural effects of trigger points may prove to be an important factor in the development of muscle dysfunction in clients with MPS and occupationally related pain complaints (Yaksh, 1996). Ivanichev (1990) has also reported disturbance of coordination in a muscle with active trigger points that has been observed by this author as well (Simons, 1993). An example is provided in Figure 9-5.

On a task level, as with practicing to develop skill on a balance beam, compensatory patterns can evolve into habituated and efficient but inappropriate MCS with practice to reduce overuse of MUs. In this case, the use of compensatory patterns is not desirable because of added stress to soft tissue and joints. The length, level arm, tension, and architecture of the compensatory muscles may compromise joint and soft tissue to stress, placing demands that cannot be met for any length of time. Compensatory movement has an eventual negative effect on afferent activity and the peripheral effects in Stage 1 evolution (Headley, 1990a).

Rather than changing to compensatory patterns, an employee benefits from having several MCSs to perform a task. A MCS is what allows us to brush our teeth easily with one hand and very clumsily with the other. Multiple healthy MCSs allow rotation of proper muscles without stress to soft tissue. Individuals with healthy MCSs can work longer without symptoms and pathologic problems. Staying healthy for years with good MCSs can often explain why one individual base is healthy at a workstation while another employee with poor MCSs can rapidly become symptomatic. Learning a job without pressure of speed often provides the critical opportunity for prevention of MSD.

This load sharing reduces the opportunity for MSDs to develop. McLean, Tingley, Scott, and Rickards (2000) found a cyclical nature to the mean frequency trend, and it was present whether or not the subjects took breaks. This cyclical

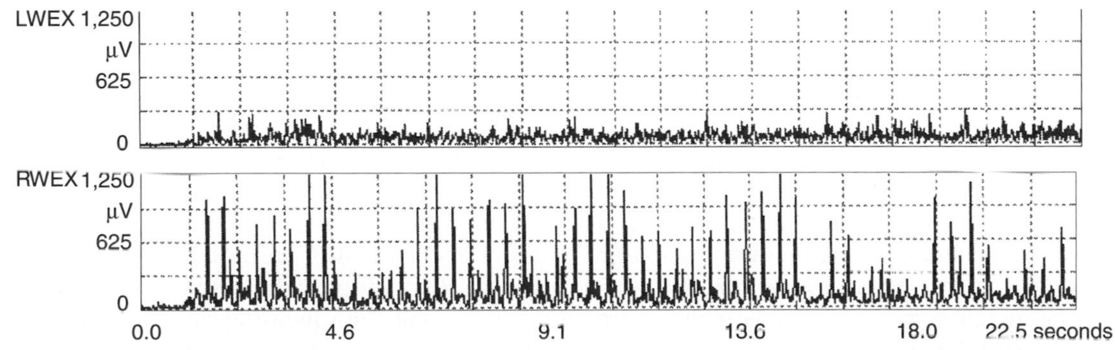

Figure 9-5 In a client identified as having tennis elbow in the left arm, the forearm extensor muscle group was monitored bilaterally during rapid pronation and supination. Right wrist extensor muscle group *(RWEX)* recruitment is hyperactive and erratic. A trigger point was present in the right extensor carpi radialis longus. Tracing is 22 seconds in duration; peak amplitude is 1250 μV. *LWEX,* Left wrist extensor muscle group.

trend suggests itself as such a strong indicator of cyclical recruitment of motor units during sustained postural contractions that it can be used as a mathematical algorithm to determine the extent and severity of the dysfunction, could help target severity and the stage of neural-kinetic deficits, and provide prognostic indicators. Jensen showed in a study of two different job tasks in manual handling workers that those who developed symptoms did so in part because of consistent use of the same muscle fiber bundles throughout the work cycle. Those who did not develop symptoms, on the other hand, were found to have several motor plans available to use that were efficient and that activated different, but similar, fiber bundles. The rest of the fiber bundles allowed the task to be performed while recovery of the MUs was also possible, and symptoms did not evolve with adequate recovery from fatigue (Jensen et al., 1999).

The research of Byl et al. (1996, 1997) supports these findings by changes in the sensory field of the brain when MCSs were used to facilitate recovery compared to using one MCS, which leads to MSD symptoms in animals. Dissection of the sensory cortex shows spread of the localization of areas within the brain in those who had no changes in MCS to obtain food compared to the monkeys who found several MCSs to perform the task to obtain food. One must be cautious to not confuse the hyper-responsivity seen with overflow or with lack of force production matching amplitude production with muscle spasm. The difference is that in the case of muscle spasm, constant, involuntary muscle activity is occurring whether the muscle is in a rest or work cycle. In inhibition no energy is required to maintain the shortened position of the muscle, maintained by a shutdown of energy use. Travell and Simons (1992) first described this phenomenon as a physiologic contracture, whereas Headley (1990b) referred to it as a functional contracture. It is imperative that when developing a stretching program that the taut band be released concurrently. Stretching of a muscle with a taut band may not change the length of the taut band, but it may force additional sarcomeres to develop at the MTJ in response to the passive stretching. This often results in a hyper-lengthened muscle with MTrPs untreated within the taut band.

As upper-quadrant muscle fatigue progresses, influenced by both LMF and fatigue of central origin, compensatory muscle patterns change as synergistic or accessory muscles fatigue and cervical muscles are involved secondarily. Muscle dysfunction with accompanying soft-tissue changes continues to progress in one of several patterns. Muscle dysfunction causes headaches in some individuals, whereas others experience mostly shoulder problems. For those who may eventually develop CTS, the compensatory muscle patterns and trigger points proceed distally into the arm, forearm, and hand. The combination of trigger points and muscle dysfunction seen in muscle-related MSD suggests a causative relationship in proximal to distal MSD between active trigger point development, muscle compensation, and fatigue.

Fatigue of muscle fibers at this stage is limited to the low-level, low-frequency fibers that perform the static or repetitive holding. The MUs selected for the low-level, low-frequency activity persist in performing in spite of high fatigue. These activities were designed to eliminate any rotational forces as this has not yet been discussed in research literature.

Therefore, long-term, low-force, continuous activation of the low-threshold MU could have mechanical as well as metabolic implications for these muscle fibers (Olsen, Christensen, & Sogaard, 2001). The entire muscle is not involved because fast twitch fibers are not yet called on in the compensation system. When this system of MUs fails, other MUs must be activated to support the task, or the performance will fail. With multiple sites of fatigue, and peripheral, central influences at work, there are many system failures required before task failure occurs, often from the extreme hypersensitivity to altered pain mechanism (Yaksh, 1996).

Employees without good rotation of MCS and/or job rotation, including proximal stabilizers, will see a spread of symptoms earlier. The ability of the muscle to rest is limited, taking more time and therefore eliminating many of the minigaps previously so helpful in providing brief periods of relaxation. Since the work does not seem "hard," the employees generally persist in working through the discomfort, although they may go home and find that activity levels are starting to change and they unconsciously begin to avoid tasks that burden the same fiber bundles as those used at work. With increased fatigue of the scapular stabilizers, more postural stress is added to more compensation of other MCSs. The spider web is not involving more than just the original muscles yet, and treatment at this stage is still uncommon because the employee can do a lot of work at home and has a poor understanding of the problem.

sEMG offers clarity here, since the level of muscle activity (spasm or inhibition) can be seen by the level of sEMG activity in functional tasks. Headley (1995) examined 40 low-back clients within three hours of injury and found no clients to be in muscle spasm. However, over 95% of the subjects exhibited inhibition. Further examination found that an acute active trigger point showing very high bursts of activity was found in the location of the surrounding inhibition (Hubbard & Berkoff, 1993). Mense et al. (2001) reiterated that the old concept of a pain-spasm-pain cycle does not stand up to experimental verification from either a physiologic or clinical point of view (Basmajian, 1978; Johnson, 1989; Price, Clare, & Ewerhardt, 1948). Referred spasm by MTrPs is a hallmark of identification, but the spasm is on a much lower level than that of an entire muscle in spasm. In the presence of trigger points, inhibition or referred spasm may originate in the same afferent fibers and cause the referred pain. In Figure 9-6, the trigger point located in the long head of the triceps not only referred pain to the UTR but created a localized spasm until the trigger point in the long head of the triceps was released.

sEMG also offers a unique means of examining the neural changes that occur in MSD with fatigue and how they alter muscle recruitment choice. Current research by the author is supportive of Yaksh's (1996) clinical findings of his predictive research model. A healthy response to sustained, low-level job demands is to begin load sharing, influenced by physiologic and environmental demands. Healthy changes in MCS use load sharing when fatigue begins. Failure to do so may increase the risk of work-related symptoms (Jensen et al., 2000). This means that as each repetition is evaluated for sEMG-PS parameters in multiple combinations, the activation by very different combinations of muscles, fiber bundles, and power spectrum contributions can be seen. Although these physiologic characteristics of MUs reveal neural distress, the hyperresponsivity may be the result of improper choices in MUs secondary to neural distress. One example is that when static load demands increase, the MU firing rate increases among those being used. During dynamic contractions, when the demand increases, additional MUs are activated (Sogaard et al., 1998). Hyper-

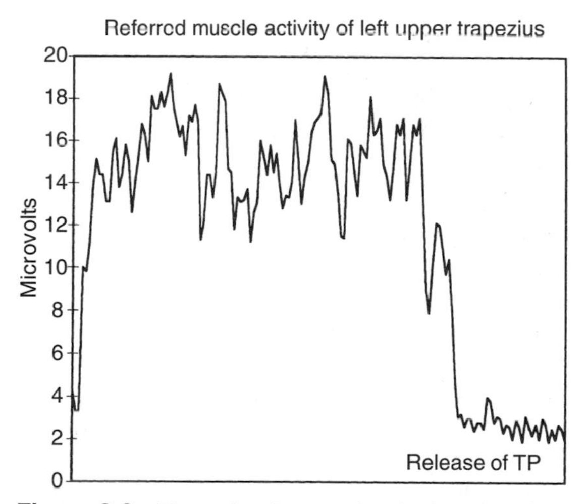

Figure 9-6 The patient is seated and relaxed, and an electrode is in place on the left upper trapezius muscle. The MTrP in the left long head of the triceps is stimulated with pressure for 20 seconds, and referred muscle activity in the left upper trapezius is recorded. Referred muscle activity drops quickly when the TP stimulation is stopped.

responsivity can often include a high ratio of fast twitch fibers that, for a brief time, can increase amplitude output. Without proper sensory feedback and changes of MCS, with each repetition the differences in activation patterns across just three repetitions can be dramatic (proprioceptive wandering). The author, examining each repetition's use of muscle sites with sEMG, found that the first repetition can include almost exclusive use of prime movers, whereas the second repetition would likely show a mixture of prime movers and compensatory muscles. In the third repetition the prime movers are no longer firing, and entire amplitude production is the result of compensatory muscles. Inhibition may or may not be visible unless sEMG-PS analysis is used.

Because of the need to describe different feedback modes, Sjogaard et al. (2000) studied the influence of different feedback modes, including proprioception, on muscle fatigue and perceived exertion. Proprioceptive feedback was the major mode when a weight was held in a static position. Visual feedback slowed fatigue onset. However, greater amplitude was achieved during proprioceptive feedback than during visual. He concluded that the feedback mode had a significant influence on fatigue. This may help explain the author's preliminary findings that radiofrequency denervation to reduce pain by burning a specific nerve, reducing sensory feedback as well as the desired motor output, leads frequently to the proprioceptive wandering described previously. Treatment specific to target these different influences on performance can enhance outcomes and recovery. Proprioceptive wandering may increase under Yaksh's model where any blockade of afferent fibers is withdrawn, or peripheral changes may proceed to central as with dorsal rami neuropathy, entrapment, neural tension, fascial restrictions, or sprouting (Butler, 1991; Pratt, 1986; Sihvonen, 1992; Yaksh, 1996).

Stage 3

Fatigue may now have progressed to the entire muscle, with fast twitch fibers giving out quickly. Symptoms may persist when the employee stops working. This is often the stage in which the employee may get through the day at work (commonly with medication to assist) and then go home and do little, worrying about getting through the rest of the week in increasing fatigue-related pain. When no diagnostic tests show the cause of the pain, doubts start to creep in about the validity of the problem, and, in some companies, the employee's credibility may be questioned. With the expansion of muscle dysfunction the opportunity for compensation patterns to endure the full task of stepping in for the prime movers begins to be compromised.

More and more muscles may develop MTrPs that contribute to muscle fatigue, and selective fatigue is generalizing so that amplitude begins to drop. This has been studied in relationship to specific tasks involved in static and repetitive loads. The activation involves the attempt to use the same small fraction of the motor neuron pool, but selective fatigue is giving way to a more generalized fatigue of the muscle as fast twitch fibers are also used in compensatory patterns. Sogaard, Sjogaard, Finsen, Olsen, and Christensen (2001) showed this to be true when wrist extension was absent. Headley (1990b) has seen multiple examples in which squeezing after typing has created dysfunction, with the loss of wrist extensor or finger flexion and in some chronic cases and later stages, both extrinsic groups, leaving only the intrinsic muscles to meet the functional needs. An example of using the intrinsic thenar muscles and the concurrent omission of extrinsic flexors show this pattern clearly in Figure 9-7. With neck muscle involvement, symptoms may spread to headaches, eye pain, and cervical pain, making it harder to hold the head without letting it drop into forward flexion. Postural compromises become greater. Involvement of the sternocleidomastoids (SCM) creates much of the headache symptoms, and dizziness may be added to the symptom list as the spider web grows increasingly larger. Muscles rest even less, recover more slowly, and central drive controlling activation is less specific, adding

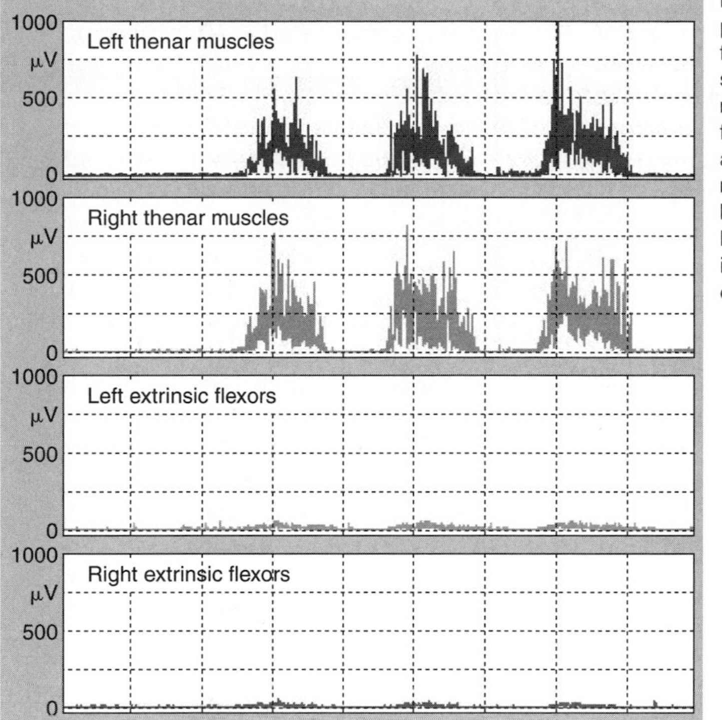

Figure 9-7 As the muscle dysfunction progresses distally and becomes global, the forearm flexors may no longer participate in squeezing a ball, whereas the thenar muscles remain active. The long finger flexors also show inhibition while typing with activation of the thenar muscles, the only muscles able to continue performing the keying function. Significant changes to the lever arm and stress to the soft tissue often increase the likelihood of carpal tunnel developing under this type of dysfunction.

additional muscles to the activation of muscles to the MCS.

Veiersted and Westgaard (1993) report similar findings on examining the development of trapezius myalgia in workers performing light manual work. New employees were examined every tenth week for 1 year. The development of symptoms to warrant classification of client status was high (17 of 30 employees). The development of complaints throughout the week showed a slight but significant increase during the first five days of the week, decreasing on weekends and holidays. The authors concluded that many new cases of nonchronic trapezius myalgia occur during the first year of employment, especially during the first six months, in a job with low static load. These findings suggest a delayed recovery during the week as compared to increased recovery from fatigue when the light static workload is not performed for two or more consecutive days (Veiersted & Westgaard, 1993).

With a number of different analyses available for the examination of physiologic risk factors, using sEMG suggests that many methods are available for the examination of muscle rest and recovery factors. Examination of the raw data of symptomatic clients currently in treatment and controls (asymptomatic) performed by Headley (1996b) suggests that any one physiologic parameter might not be discriminatory in identifying clients versus controls. The multivariate approach was used in a pilot study for seven different parameters to identify clusters of risk factors that might be more consistently predictive of impending muscle-related MSD (Headley & Nicholson, 1998). Such an approach has been used by Headley on MSD and motor vehicle clients to separate FAME evaluations of controls versus symptomatic clients using a blinded evaluator of the FAME auto-generated reports into appropriate groups. The studies were done with 100% accuracy (Headley & Centeno, 2001). sEMG then becomes a valuable marker for identifying employees' complaints and making decisions about work, workstations, and time at work. A balance must be struck between keeping the employee active and letting the muscles involved get needed rest. Job rotations must be examined carefully because many do not change the load to proximal stabilizers (Sogaard et al., 2001).

Stage 4

This stage represents a level of muscle failure at which symptoms are taken more seriously, they increase with afferent hypersensitivity, and employees are generally unable to "push through the pain." Employees may now find their way into the workers' compensation system, reduce work time, and seek health care provider resources. Home life is more affected, role changes have a negative impact on self-esteem, and stress is a constant aspect of life on both the employees and their support system as impairment increases and pain interferes with the most basic activities. Although earlier stages could be ignored, inhibition with failure in compensation systems reflects the progressive severity of the problem. Intervention is necessary. Employees ignoring help at this stage usually are fearful of losing their jobs, have multiple family systems to support, or fear never getting another job with benefits. Such external factors are powerful and can prohibit advancement to treatment at a time when reversing the symptoms can still be done, although longer time and effort will be required than in previous stages.

All fibers now show involvement in fatigue, and the muscles involved in the dysfunction show a greater decline than increase in amplitude, indicated by a more chronic fatigue involving all fiber types. A study by Fugl-Meyer, Gerdle, and Langstrom (1985) concluded that the relative pauses (gaps) between repetitive concentric contractions make it possible for slow twitch fibers to continue maximal contractions for a long time without decreased output. Inability to relax between concentric contractions, more closely resembling a static work load, results in poorer performance in the long run. Such continuous activity during all phases of work will overtax the low-threshold MUs. In a study in which subjects were asked to sustain a contraction of the knee extensor muscles at a constant force (5% torque), the force was maintained, although four different parts of the quadriceps femoris muscle were used during the 1-hour task (Sjogaard, Kiens, Jorgensen, & Saltin, 1986). An increase in central drive may be seen when a synergistic or contralateral muscle is activated as the prime-mover fatigues. Central factors may be contributing to the "overload" phenomenon seen in monitoring the UTR bilaterally. The graph in Figure 9-8 demonstrates that the right trapezius went through stages of hyper-responsivity, some initial response to stretching, and then total inhibition for the last 50 minutes.

Muscle dysfunction now moves from task-specific fatigue with inhibition to a more global response, reflecting both peripheral and central changes in activation patterns. The information on MSD emerging with sEMG indicates that muscles may test "within normal limits" during standardized manual muscle testing but not recruit appropriately during numerous functional tasks. The muscle does not show total inhibition but rather movement-specific functional inhibition. MCS changes may explain such inconsistencies. If these changes in motor planning could be identified as causative in generating discrepancies in movement patterns, it would challenge the tendency to label such inconsistencies as evidence of malingering, symptom magnification, or psychosocial in nature. In fact, motor control theory stresses that such dysfunction in the recruitment of muscle must be related to central drive.

In a study by Elert and Gerdle (1989), the shoulder stabilizers of 20 healthy subjects were studied using sEMG and isokinetic testing. MVC data were collected at four velocities and 150 repetitions of maximal shoulder flexion. Measures of perceived fatigue were also collected. The authors found a marked drop in force and a corresponding reduction in mean power

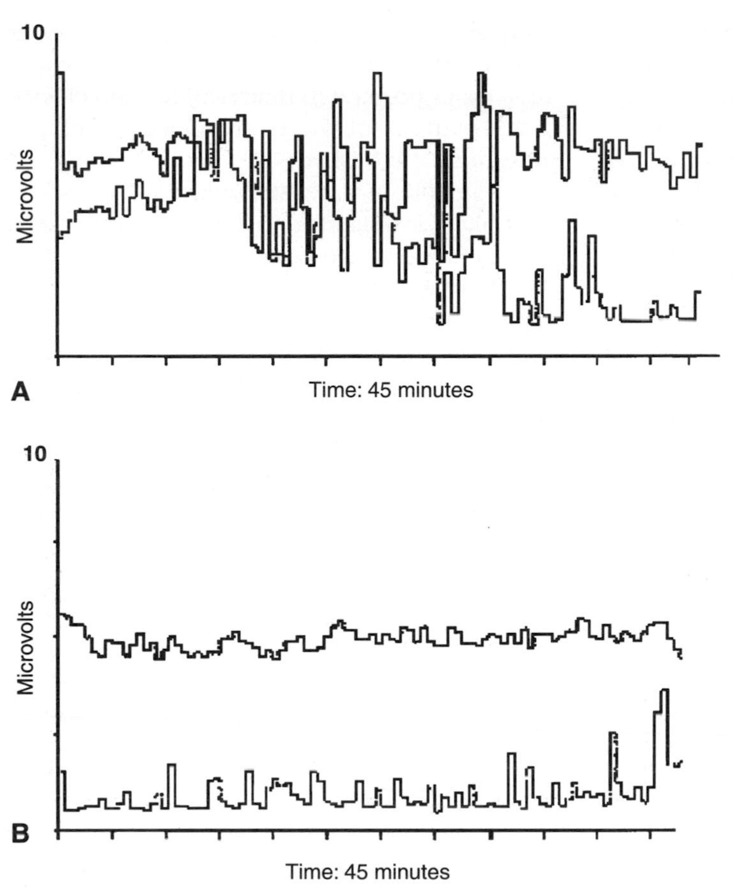

Figure 9-8 The upper trapezius muscles are monitored with a data logger while the person performs a bilateral, symmetric task at work. Each data-log collection period is 45 minutes in duration. **A,** The right upper trapezius, the symptomatic side, is working appropriately for the first 30 minutes but then begins to show some evidence of overload, dropping in amplitude. **B,** The right upper trapezius, 2 hours later, is inhibited in spite of stretching breaks every 15 minutes.

frequency of all four muscle groups monitored with sEMG. Another finding related to the repeated contractions was the differences in individual ability to relax between contractions. In examining the capacity of the muscle to rest during the passive extension phase, the presence of high sEMG levels in some individuals was associated with reduced force output. The concept of delayed latency refers to the time it takes a muscle to reduce muscle activity amplitudes fully after the command for relaxation has been given by the CNS. This lack of relaxation with a long latency may eliminate relaxation between work tasks, when the muscle is assumed to be unloaded and relaxed. The contraction level nonetheless serves as a static load and contributes to muscle fatigue (Elert & Gerdle, 1989).

Complex fatigue patterns at multiple sites are present at this stage, and the type of fatigue must be known in order to address its correction of perpetuating faults. The examination of muscle fatigue requires an understanding of the multiple sites of fatigue, of the impact of central and peripheral phenomenon, and of differences imposed by a variety of exercise formats. The complexity and variety of human movement suggest an interactive sequence of events, any one of which may produce fatigue under certain circumstances. Bigland-Ritchie and Woods (1984) suggested that muscle failure can occur from fatigue in three possible areas. First, sites of fatigue may lie within the central nervous system (CNS). Second, fatigue may occur at neural transmission sites linking the CNS to muscle.

Third, sites within individual muscle fibers may be responsible. As activity continues, functional changes may occur in any or all potential sites. Although the measurement of force reduction (or decreased work capacity) has been used as a method of quantifying muscle fatigue, fatigue is also accompanied by many other measurable changes, such as a shift in the sEMG-PS; slowing of muscle conduction velocity and contractile speed; and the accumulation of H^+, lactate, and other metabolites. It is important to determine which of these events determine performance and which are simply incidental by-products.

It would be unwise to consider muscle fatigue as a singular phenomenon with a single treatment target. Exercise type, muscle selection, and the nature of a task must be considered, since sites of muscle fatigue may be dependent on these and other factors. New research findings are shedding light on the order in which fatigue occurs at various sites, the influence on muscle activity, and how normalization of muscle can be restored by the choice of various interventions at appropriate times (Jensen et al., 2000; Laursen, Jensen, & Sjogaard, 1998; Sjogaard et al., 2000).

LMF, initiated in Stage 1 and contributing to early compensation MCS, is a self-protective mechanism against damage to the contractile elements that progress until significant inhibition is present in Stage 4. This means that the muscle will choose inhibition as a choice to protect itself against further trauma once it is injured. During muscle fatigue, the force-frequency ratio shifts toward the lower frequency range with the slowing of muscle contraction. This action allows all MUs to remain fully activated despite a substantial reduction in motoneuron discharge rate. This reduction probably guards against failure of neuromuscular transmission (Nyland, 1993). Headley's research has substantiated the neural faults found and the reversal of each stage coinciding with increases in functional gains and reduction of symptoms. Aberrations found also include autonomic dysregulation, high sympathetic tone, segmental dysfunction (both facilitated and inhibited), task-specific versus global inhibition, fast twitch activity characteristics in postural muscle samples, and chaotic firing patterns of the motor units (Headley & Hocking, Unpublished).

Invaluable in understanding the later stages of MSD with significant impairment, Sjogaard (1986) found that in healthy human subjects the MVC had fallen to 88% of the initial level after holding a 5% MVC for 1 hour. The data indicate that fast twitch fibers are not recruited during low-level contractions. Fast twitch fiber activity has been found clinically after sustained low-level contraction, suggesting slow twitch fibers have reached exhaustion and fast twitch fibers may represent different fiber bundles in the same or compensatory muscles.

These data suggest that although micropauses (gaps) recommended for the prevention of muscle fatigue at this stage may delay the time to fatigue, these brief pauses result in only partial metabolic recovery. Different metabolic components recover at varying rates; therefore, time needed for full recovery may in fact be increased by the micropauses.

With multiple factors—physiologic, environmental, mental, muscular, and neural—all contributing to the development of inhibition and fatigue failure, it is important to understand that the complexity of human movement increases in dysfunction. This has consequences that are very broad in scope and can lead to pathologic conditions far from the initial injury. As industries look to reduce the effects of MSDs, the internal parameters cannot be ignored. They can far outweigh the external circumstances that may seem to be the obvious culprit. The nature of the internal changes must be known to make effective changes.

When fatigue is present with slow twitch fibers no longer able to fire and no compensatory muscles working, or when compensatory muscles have taken over for the prime movers, it is unlikely that the individual will have a core stabilization mechanism that is working effectively, even if symptoms are limited to the upper extremities (Headley, 2001). Exploring the deep stabilizers has become a prominent factor in rehabilitation and must be just as important to the MSD clients.

The determination of activation of deep muscle stabilizers also provides insight into why and how fatigue develops. Findings in a study of four male subjects by Seidel, Beyer, and Brauer (1987) suggest that the "scope of recruitment" (i.e., the number of MUs recruited) varies within equal ranges of force, with less variation occurring at higher forces. They propose the possibility of "selective fatigue" following sustained isometric constant-force contractions (Olsen et al., 2001). This concept refers to the selection of a certain pool of MUs that is subject to fatigue when recruited according to force needs. Sustained contractions of only approximately 20% MVC quickly induced a functional insufficiency of muscles, thus requiring compensatory recruitment patterns. This concurs with the results found by Headley (2002) but represents one deficit stage of six. The body will continue to seek the means to provide the contraction asked and exhaust all methods before total inhibition results.

Several studies have examined the relationship of sustained, low-level contractions to muscle fatigue (Jorgensen, Fallentin, Krogh-Lund, & Jensen, 1988). It has been shown that the endurance capability for sustained contractions is approximately 1 hour for 10% MVC. "Indefinite" endurance at contractions below 15% to 20% of the MVC and cannot be maintained. A 12% reduction in maximal force was seen with significant decreases in the MU firing rate after a 1-hour contraction sustained at only 5% MVC. These changes vary with muscle type. Firing rate reduction, along with a marked reduction in MU rotation, increases the load on the MUs activated. The initial response is to increase the output of these MUs with the MUAP increasing by 38% initially, but if some means of compensation cannot support the ongoing demand, inhibition of the active MUs is likely (Jensen et al., 2000).

To understand the evolution of the stages of MSD, it is critical to know how selection of MUs is made for recruitment to perform a specific task. It is important to recognize that overload fatigue may occur only in task-specific MUs that may not be reached in a traditional rehabilitation program. Task-specific fatigue characterizes the early stages of MSD. Caldwell, Jamison, and Lee (1993) have described how muscles develop very task-specific fatigue of motor unit bundles in muscles around the elbow. In later stages, when central fatigue fails to sustain muscle activation and inhibition occurs in a task-specific pattern, an entire muscle may be removed selectively from one movement pattern (i.e., shoulder flexion) but continue to recruit normally in other

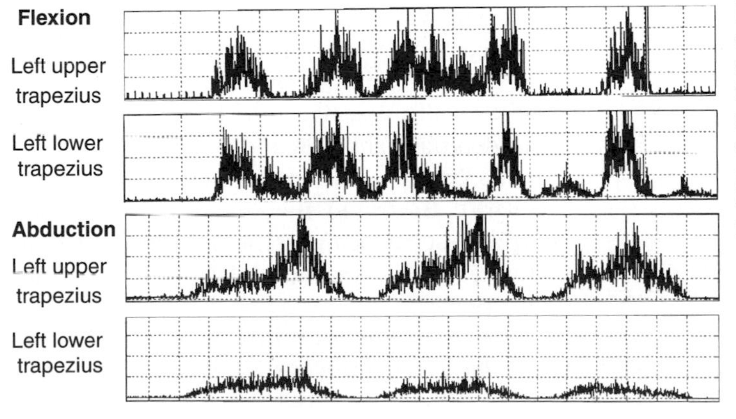

Figure 9-9 Monitored with four bilateral electrode sites, a client with distal forearm complaints was asked to perform shoulder flexion and abduction through full range of motion. The upper and lower trapezius sites are shown, and a good recruitment pattern is present in flexion by the left LTR, but significant inhibition of the left LTR is present in abduction. (Scale, 1-100)

movements. An example of such movement-specific fatigue in muscle recruitment is demonstrated in Figure 9-9. The LTR is recruited as expected in flexion but shows significant inhibition in abduction. If the fatigue persists, the inhibition may become more global, and any motor plan that generally includes the fatigued muscle may be altered to exclude it from recruiting. This may result in a clinical picture of apparent weakness in that muscle. The use of strengthening programs that emphasize power will often contribute to failure in rehabilitation and return-to-work attempts when central inhibition is contributing to the alteration of motor plans.

Jonsson (1988) describes a static load as a constant level of muscle contraction that exists because the muscle does not come to a full resting level despite changes in the dynamic workload. Task specificity programming with increasing fatigue creates an elevation of the static load until inhibition occurs. As shown in Figure 9-10, constant use of low-frequency MUs becomes critical in the development of proximal scapular muscle fatigue. In studies by Christensen (1986) and Jonsson (1988), symptomatic subjects were judged to have static levels that exceeded recommended levels. Bigland-Ritchie, Johansson, Lippold, and Woods (1983) found that fatigued muscle actually contracted and relaxed more slowly, with the time to peak tension and half-relaxation time dramatically increasing. Such a change would allow the muscle to generate higher forces at lower frequencies to maintain a consistent force output. CNS modulation through a feedback mechanism may sense the muscle speed and drive it with the appropriate stimulation frequency. Presumably, such regulation would require some sensory feedback from the individual muscles innervated (Bigland-Ritchie & Woods, 1984). Although these authors acknowledged MU activity changes are a contributory factor in static load, the work of Yaksh (1996) and Mense et al. (2001) may represent the model by which such MU activity increases and remains elevated.

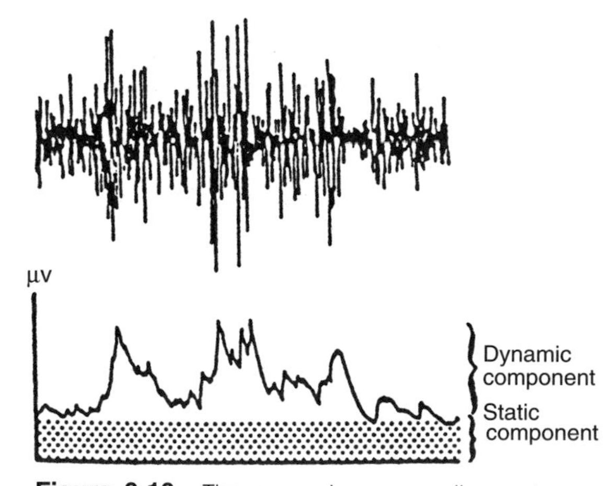

Figure 9-10 The raw and corresponding root mean square electromyographic signal for approximately 6 seconds of activity are shown. The muscular load may be subdivided into a static and a dynamic component. (Reprinted with permission from Jonsson, B. [1988]. The static load component in muscle work. *European Journal of Applied Physiology, 57*[3], 305.)

Jonsson (1988) designed a mathematical model using sEMG for the static workload because without high-peak values being achieved by employees performing low-load static tasks, there are few criteria to represent adequately the load assumed by the musculoskeletal system when prolonged low loading occurs (Hagberg, 1981; Jonsson, 1988). For this reason, sEMG-PS is seen as an important tool for detection of muscle loads in vocational situations and in evaluation for the severity or stage MSD has reached. The map created by FAMEs sEMG-PS analysis can determine where the system has been vulnerable to a high static load, what type and severity of inhibition is present, and the prognosis for reversing the negative effects. Jonsson (1988) recorded the right UTR and used the amplitude probability model to demonstrate recruitment similarity. He found that job rotation for the purpose of reducing static muscular load in some cases may be of limited value in light work situations.

"Down-training" of a high amplitude level is generally a straightforward procedure, but when it is controlled by central drive, it requires highly specific intervention strategies. In an example, the UTR and LTR muscles were being monitored during a data-entry task in which the mouse was also used. The static load on the right UTR is obvious by the lack of descent to the baseline, probably because the use of the mouse produces a high resting level representing this new typist's anticipatory response that keeps the muscle active. Figure 9-11 demonstrates an elevation of static load level resulting from the knowledge that the mouse is going to be used again. It is the anticipatory nature of the mouse activity that may give rise to the higher static load, as the employee continues to move back and forth from the mouse to the keyboard but loses the low level previously associated with use of the keyboard. Support for Headley's theories has been reported by Sogaard et al. (2001). But the neural facilitation described by Yaksh (1996) cannot be ignored. Once the MUs were turned on, they tended to remain active as long as a specific condition of awareness is maintained.

Stage 5

This stage is referred to as "adaptive failure" and represents a global failure of systems with the inability to recover the capability to perform the job. Employees who reach this level without proper treatment do not return to static or repetitive work, although new research is providing hope that this stage, like all the others, can be amenable to successful rehabilitation and return to work. Proper treatment does require a prolonged period off work at this stage as multiple system failure requires moving the failed systems through correction of all the perpetuating faults of previous stages. The failure of muscle to recover from fatigue, as seen in MSD, may increase the risk factor for other injuries as the time to return the muscle to a

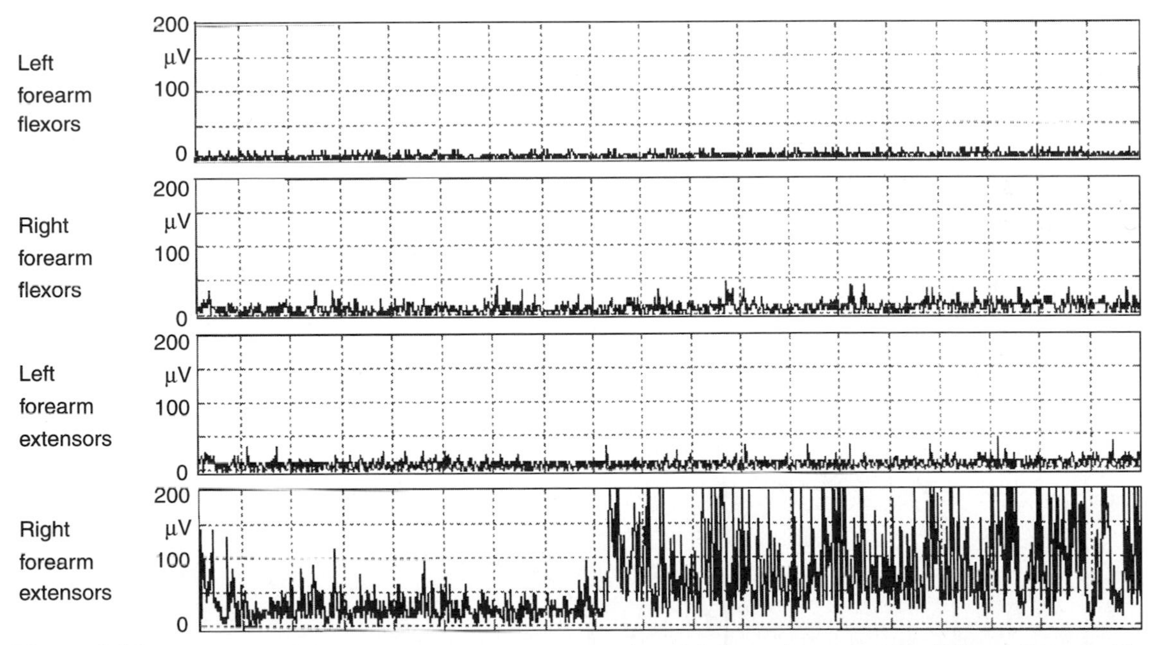

Figure 9-11 The forearm flexor and extensor groups are monitored during a data-entry task. Although the use of the mouse with the right hand is intermittent, the right extensor muscle group increases its activity level and does not decrease it when the hand returns to the keyboard. Overall, the static load on the right extensor group is significantly higher than that on the contralateral muscle group.

metabolically rested state is increased (Noonan & Garrett, 1992).

Studies of the flexor muscles (Jorgensen et al., 1988; Krogh-Lund & Jorgensen, 1992) demonstrate a basic recovery pattern that can be seen in several other studies. The flexor muscles of the elbow were studied at 30% MVC in both isolated and repetitive testing to examine changes in median frequency (MF), conduction velocity, and amplitude. Changes in the sEMG-PS with recovery are shown in Figure 9-12. In both the biceps and the brachioradialis muscles, the MF value dropped by 50% of its original value by the time of exhaustion. After 1 minute of rest, there was an 85% increase in the MF value, with full recovery occurring within 5 minutes. When multiple system adaptive failure (postexhaustion) has been reached, such recovery would not occur for days, demonstrating a lower starting point, faster drop into inhibition, and prolonged, slow recovery to the original low level. Aberrant neural activity can be seen in using multivariate analysis rather than just MF, providing information on use of fast twitch fibers, total site activation levels, and the faults contributing to adaptive failure with profound inhibition.

As shown in Figure 9-13, Headley (1996a) examined 55 clients with muscle-related MSD in a prospective study. Muscle fatigue and recovery were examined using sEMG-PS analysis. Bilateral LTR electrode sites were monitored pre- and postexercise and after a 7-minute rest period. There was a statistically significant difference ($p < 0.05$) between the pre- and postexercise values, indicating that muscle fatigue did occur. When the preexercise MF value was compared with the recovery values, again a statistically significant difference ($p < 0.05$) was demonstrated, indicating that recovery did not occur. An example of adaptive failure to recover is shown in Figure 9-14, in which the data of one of these clients has been plotted compared to a control. Clients were no better after 7 minutes of

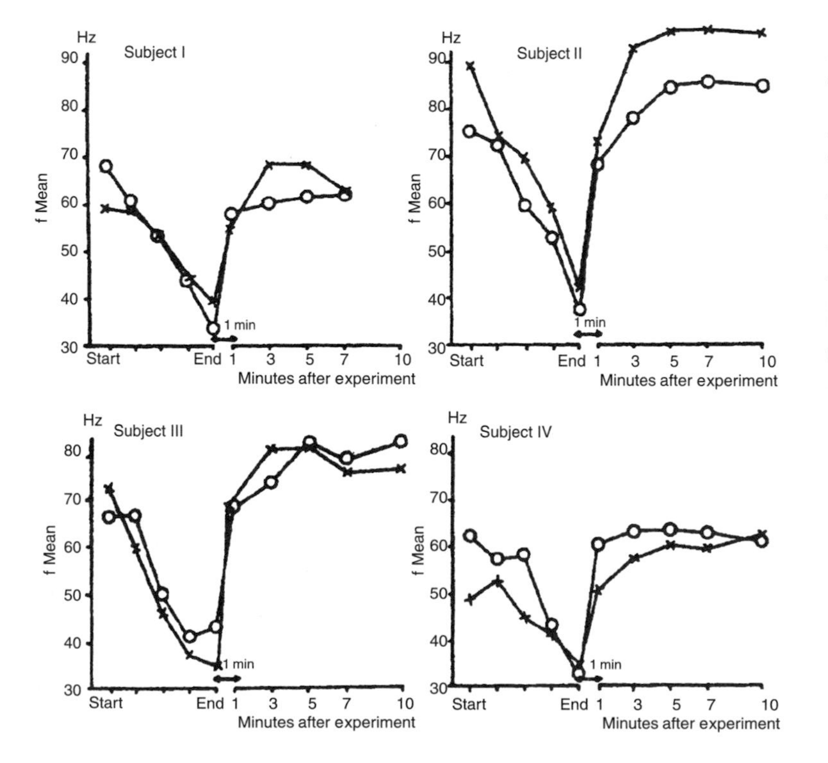

Figure 9-12 Median frequency data from the biceps muscles of four subjects is represented showing preexercise, postexercise, and rest values at 1, 3, 5, 7, and 10 minutes. The contractions were done at 60% and 50% (rest values) of maximum voluntary contraction. Two trials for each subject, collected one week apart, are plotted. (Reprinted with permission from Kuorinka, I. (1988). Restitution of EMG spectrum after muscular fatigue. *European Journal of Applied Physiology*, *57*(3), 313.)

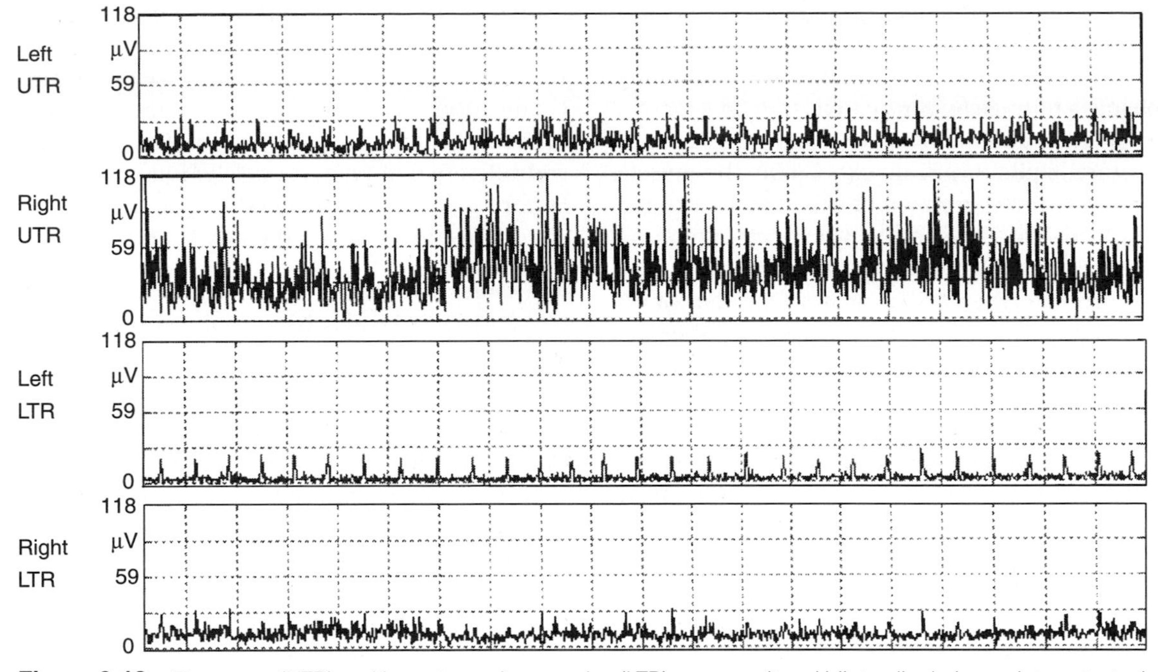

Figure 9-13 The upper (UTR) and lower trapezius muscles (LTR) were monitored bilaterally during a data-entry task. The UTR demonstrates a higher static level of activity with no return to the baseline throughout the task (8 minutes), even though the mouse was used only intermittently.

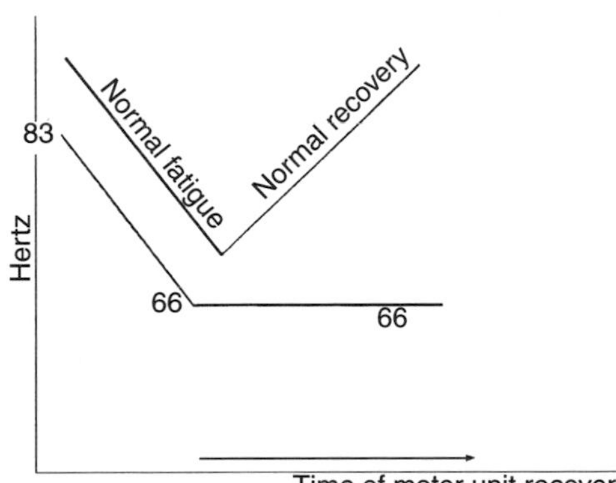

Figure 9-14 Subject's left lower trapezius muscle had an acceptable median frequency value initially. With exercise, the value dropped to 66 Hz, as one would expect with fatigue. However, after 7 minutes of rest, the muscle shows no recovery, a characteristic of this client population with a cumulative trauma disorder.

rest than immediately after the fatigue test. These findings differ from normal muscle recovery expectations, when 70% to 90% of MF fatigue recovery is shown to occur within the first minute of rest (Krogh-Lund & Jorgensen 1992, 1993; Solomonow et al., 1990). Some clients have been monitored by the author for up to 3 hours after a 5- to 7-minute low-frequency task demand with no signs of recovery. Other clients were tested the next day as part of the FAME-PAC functional capacity test and found to have no recovery, demonstrating the profound loss of function at the adaptive failure stage. Knowing recovery time is essential in established work capabilities.

Another characteristic of this stage is a profound loss of kinesthetic awareness, which frequently begins in earlier stages. Flor, Schugens, and Birbaumer (1992) examined groups of individuals with pain and found that poor muscle tension discrimination also extends to areas not involved in the pain complaints. New research on the neural influences on muscle recruitment has identified recovery from neural correction as a prerequisite to making any long-lasting changes to muscle. A research study in progress by Headley has demonstrated that muscular and postural faults return quickly if only the muscle is treated, but correction of neural activity to the involved muscle can provide long-lasting recovery (Headley & Hocking, Unpublished).

Fortunately, sEMG-PS analysis in the FAME program allows for such analysis of aberrant neural activity with identification of location. Examining amplitude is of little use at this stage unless data are collected for a long duration. Otherwise, amplitude caused by compensation or neural hypersensitivity can be misidentified as normal recruitment. Studying bilateral tasks, the difference in work demands between the two sides must be known and accounted for, as well as skill of dominant hand, static loads, and other factors that affect amplitude. Data loggers have been used to track muscle activity over an entire workday or during particular job rotations with these factors taken into account (Headley, 2001). In such cases, this capability provides an additional type of quantitative assessment of muscle activity in industry.

By the adaptive failure stage, compensatory recruitment patterns are also failing; exhaustion of compensation patterns used by the employee may find thc simplest of job demands difficult. The plasticity of the human brain will seek to find an adaptive response, but the energy demands lead to rapid exhaustion. If treatment is successful in reactivating the primary or compensatory muscles, MCSs may continue to exclude the prime movers, and the long-used compensatory MCS may prevail. It is important to restore neuromuscular efficiency if any gain in function is to be maintained.

Adaptive failure of central origin relates to loss of one or several mechanisms to maintain muscle activation (Enoka, 1995). In the CNS, there may be a modulation factor that facilitates recruitment in fatigued muscle by altering the rate of muscle fiber recruitment. Observations (Enoka, 1995) suggest that the generation of a sufficient central command is not a trivial matter and that if a subject (or employee) is not motivated, this lack of motivation will cause premature termination of a fatiguing task. Other factors, such as discomfort, a negative work environment, and tolerance of pain, cannot be ignored. These factors may be influenced by a change in conditions under which the task is performed.

INTERVENTION: MSD RECOVERY MODEL

The common denominator of MSDs is proximal loss of stability in one or more muscle groups. Carpal tunnel symptoms may be seen in some clients as the end product of proximal to distal muscle dysfunction and fatigue failure. In the population that initially experiences proximal symptoms, symptoms similar to carpal tunnel may arise first from proximal trigger points and only in the chronic stage represent true carpal tunnel syndrome. Surgery to address the compression of the median nerve in the carpal tunnel space in this population subgroup will be seen as only partially successful, and clients will then turn their attention to early proximal symptoms that were not addressed because of their progression to profound inhibition. Only when the muscle begins to fire again will initial discomfort be felt and proximal problems recognized.

Training at a task can do much to circumvent the faults that create the earliest stages of deficit progression. Learning a movement pattern for low-frequency task demands occurs more easily at lower speeds. This might not only suggest that training for repetitive tasks should be done to allow for the building of efficient MCS but that for highly repetitive work the training should take place at a slower pace initially. The slower pace will improve the ability of the muscle to take advantage of short pauses that actually can exist during task performance. Progression in speed would have to be accomplished with respect to motor strategy training to ensure continued use of the proper motor plan as performance reaches expected levels for the job.

It has been assumed that increases in overall strength provide some protection against the development of MSD. Exploration of this assumption is critical to our use of strengthening in both prevention and rehabilitation. The relationship of task specificity and its implications in MSD may be examined in work done by Kilbom (1988). Two groups of employees were studied; the first group performed a variety of postures and exertions related to lifting and assembling automotive parts, and the second group worked on the assembly of circuit boards, working only in a seated position and exposed mainly to postural static loads. This study examined the assumption that individuals with high muscle strength have a lower risk of anaerobic intramuscular compromise and fatigue than do those with low muscle strength. One-year longitudinal studies were done on these two employee populations with pre- and posttest measurements of MVC and static endurance. The static strength test was in the range of 20% to 50% MVC. The results showed that low muscle strength was a risk factor for development of shoulder-neck-arm disorders in those employees working in the automotive industry. However, no such relationship could be demonstrated in the assembly employees. Although both groups reported a high incidence of symptoms, the mechanisms of injury are likely to be different, given the differences in job tasks, measured predictors, and outcome findings.

The most critical factor in understanding a rehabilitation strategy for recovery is system interaction. Replacing the pain-tension-spasm cycle is a new cycle of neural distress-altered muscle spindle feedback-postural and movement adaptation-inhibition. Historically, an attempt to summarize this was presented by Liebenson (1990).

Once joint movement is free, hypertonic muscles relaxed, and connective tissue lengthened, a muscle strengthening and movement coordination program can begin. It is important not to commence strengthening too soon because tight, overactive muscles (from aberrant neural activity) reflexively inhibit their antagonists, thereby altering basic movement patterns. It is inappropriate to initiate muscle strengthening programs while movement performance is disturbed, since the patient will achieve strength gains by use of "trick" movements.

The importance of not strengthening muscles before neural distress has allowed restoration of muscle length, tension, and tone, releasing muscles from inhibition and allowing activation is clear. Compensatory patterns could be strengthened with increased likelihood of symptoms and pathologic problems spreading to other anatomic locations. Clients treated for 200 or more sessions in the current, traditional model of physical therapy were found to score more faults until the paradigm of a neural-kinetic model made rapid positive changes in the same client by refocusing treatment (Headley, 2002). The traditional model emphasizes compensation as necessary. But to perform sustained activity, the stress and strain of compensation must be removed and movement normalized. Otherwise fatigue, neural, and muscular dysfunction will produce a reduction in function and increase in symptoms over time.

CASE STUDY

A 47-year-old female presented with complaints of forearm pain and swelling, describing her forearms has "hard and swollen." Swelling could not be demonstrated, but a fullness could be palpated in the proximal forearm areas of both the flexor and extensor muscle groups. This was identified as a compartment syndrome, with fatigue-induced inhibition of the long flexor and extensor muscle groups. Although not currently symptomatic, the client was found to have inhibition of the LTR muscles bilaterally, hyperresponsivity of the UTR muscle sites bilaterally, and task-specific inhibition of the cervical paraspinal and scalene muscles of the cervical area.

She was able to perform some but not all of her chores at home and found that as the week progressed she had to ask the family to do more and more for her. Over the weekend she would begin to feel better, but on Monday her symptoms would quickly return. She was dropping objects with her right hand, as well as having some trouble identifying objects in her right hand when she could not see them. She experienced some numbness and tingling bilaterally in her fingers. She reported she had trouble keeping her "head on straight," feeling that she knew it was drifting forward but she could do nothing to stop it. Her arms felt increasingly "heavy," and she had concerns she was developing carpal tunnel.

Examination revealed she did have a forward head and forward, rounded shoulders, and with her protracted scapula, she had difficulty keeping her posture within normal limits. She also felt her right hand was much cooler than her left hand, although measurement showed that her left hand was actually 2° cooler than her right.

Questions

1. What was her stage of dysfunction?
2. What muscle dysfunction most likely came first?
3. How might treatment be started on the most severely inhibited muscles to not increase the use of the MCS that included inhibition?
4. What chores is she most likely able to do at home and not have symptoms?

Answers

1. Overload, or Stage 3 of MSD
2. The loss of LTR activation and subsequent inhibition.
3. Use a novel exercise, limit the repetitions, and stop when any sign of fatigue is present.
4. Chores involving use of power (fast twitch) fibers rather than slow twitch that are used for long-duration typing.

REFERENCES

Basmajian, J. V. (1978). Cyclobenzaprine hydrochloride effect on skeletal muscle spasm in the lumbar region and neck: Two double-blind controlled clinical and laboratory studies. *Archives of Physical Medicine and Rehabilitation, 59*(2), 58–63.

Basmajian, J. V., & DeLuca C. J. (1985). *Muscles alive. Their functions revealed by electromyography* (5th ed.). Baltimore: Williams & Wilkins.

Bigland-Ritchie, B., Johansson, R., Lippold, O., & Woods, J. (1983). Contractile speed and EMG changes during fatigue of sustained maximal voluntary contractions. *Journal of Neurophysiology, 50*(1), 313–324.

Bigland-Ritchie, B., & Woods, J. (1984). Changes in muscle contractile properties and neural control during human muscular fatigue. *Muscle & Nerve, 7*(9), 691–699.

Birch, L., Christensen, H., Arendt-Nielsen, L., Graven-Neilsen T., & Sogaard K. (2000). The influence of experimental muscle pain on motor unit activity during low-level contraction. *European Journal of Applied Physiology, 83*(2–3), 200–206.

Butler, D. S. (1991). *Mobilisation of the nervous system*. New York: Churchill Livingstone.

Byl, N., Merzenich, M. M., Cheung, S., Bedenbaugh, P., Nagarajan, S. S., & Jenkins W. M. (1997). A primate model for studying focal dystonia and repetitive strain injury: Effects on the primary somatosensory cortex. *Physical Therapy, 77*(3), 269–284.

Byl, N., Wilson, F., Merzenich, M., Melnick, M., Scott, P., Oakes, A. et al. (1996). Sensory dysfunction associated with repetitive strain injuries of tendinitis and focal hand dystonia: A comparative study. *Journal of Orthopaedic and Sports Physical Therapy, 4,* 234–244.

Caldwell, G., Jamison, J., & Lee, S. (1993). Amplitude and frequency measures of surface electromyography during dual task elbow torque production. *European Journal of Applied Physiology, 66*(4), 349–356.

Chaitow, L. (1996). *Muscle energy techniques.* New York: Churchill Livingstone.

Christensen, H. (1986). Muscle activity and fatigue in the shoulder muscles of assembly-plant employees. *Scandinavian Journal of Work, Environment and Health, 12*(6), 582–587.

Christova, P., & Kossev, A. (2001). Human motor unit recruitment and derecruitment during long lasting intermittent contractions. *Journal of Electromyography and Kinesiology, 11*(3), 189–196.

Elert, J., & Gerdle, B. (1989). The relationship between contraction and relaxation during fatiguing isokinetic shoulder flexions. An electromyographic study. *European Journal of Applied Physiology, 59*(4), 303–309.

Enoka, R. M. (1995). Mechanisms of muscle fatigue: Central factors and task dependency. *Journal of Electromyography and Kinesiology,* 141–149.

Flor, H., Schugens, M. M., & Birbaumer, N. (1992). Discrimination of muscle tension in chronic pain patients and healthy controls. *Biofeedback and Self-Regulation, 17*(3), 165–177.

Fugl-Meyer, A., Gerdle, B., & Langstrom, M. (1985). Characteristics of repeated isokinetic plantar flexions in middle-aged and elderly subjects with special regard to muscular work. *Acta Physiologia Scandinavica, 124*(2), 213–222.

Hagberg, M. (1981). Electromyographic signs of shoulder muscular fatigue in two elevated arm positions. *American Journal of Physical Medicine, 60*(3), 111-121.

Hagberg, M., & Kvarnstrom, S. (1984). Muscular endurance and electromyographic fatigue in myofascial shoulder pain. *Archives of Physical Medicine and Rehabilitation, 65*(9), 522-525.

Hansson, G., Nordander, C., Asterland, P., Ohlsson, K., Stromberg, U., Skerfving, S. et al. (2000). Sensitivity of trapezius electromyography to differences between work tasks-influence of gap definition and normalization methods. *Journal of Electromyography and Kinesiology, 10*(2), 103-115.

Headley, B. (2002). Neural-kinetic model of dysfunction. Unpublished Vol.

Headley, B. J. (1990a). EMG and postural dysfunction. *Clinical Management, 10,* 14-17.

Headley, B. J. (1990b). Evaluation and treatment of myofascial pain syndrome utilizing biofeedback. In J. R. Cram & J. V. Basmajian (Eds.), *Clinical EMG for surface recordings*. Nevada City: Clinical Resources.

Headley, B. J. (1990c). EMG and myofascial pain. *Clinical Management, 10,* 43-46.

Headley, B. J. (2001). Chronic pain. In S. B. O'Sullivan & T. J. Schmitz (Eds.), *Physical rehabilitation: Assessment and treatment* (4th ed.). Philadelphia: FA Davis Company.

Headley, B. J. (1995). *Towards a new understanding of movement dysfunction: Acute and chronic patient populations*. Jackson, MS: Mississippi Fall APTA Conference.

Headley, B. J. (1996a). *The failure of muscles to recover as a factor in upper quarter CTD*. Presented at the American Physical Therapy Association-Combined Sections, Atlanta.

Headley, B. J. (1996b). *Multivariate analysis of physiological risk factors related to CTD using surface EMG*. Presented at the American Physical Therapy Association-Combined Sections, Atlanta.

Headley, B. J. (1996c). *Muscle dysfunction: a comparison of symptomatic patients and controls*. Presented at the American Physical Therapy Association-Combined Sections, Atlanta.

Headley, B. J. (1997). *FAME: Functional assessment of movement with electromyography*. Fond du Lac, WI: St Agnes Sports & Spine.

Headley, B. J. (2001). *Trunk core stabilization as a factor in the reduction of recurrent low back pain*. San Antonio, TX: Combined Sections Meeting of American Physical Therapy Association.

Headley, B. J., & Centeno, C. J. (2001). *A surface electromyography assessment of motor vehicle patients and controls to establish presence of soft-tissue injury: A pilot study*. San Antonio, TX: Combined Sections Meeting of the American Physical Therapy Association.

Headley, B. J., & Nicholson, E. R. (1998). *Multivariate analysis of physiological risk factors to identify cumulative trauma disorders (CTD) using surface EMG: A pilot study*. Phoenix: SOTAC.

Headley, B. J., & Hocking, B. (Unpublished). *Examination of muscle-related changes pre & post treatment with electro therapeutic point stimulation (ETPS) neuro-mechanical acupuncture treatment of low back pain*.

Hubbard, D. R., & Berkoff, G. M. (1993). Myofascial trigger points show spontaneous needle EMG activity. *Spine, 18*(13), 1803-1807.

Ivanichev, G. (1990). *Painful muscle hypertonus* [Russian]. Kazan: Kazan University Press.

Janda, V. (1968). *Postural and phasic muscles in the pathogenesis of low back pain*. XIth Congress, Dublin.

Janda, V. (1988). Muscles and cervicogenic pain syndromes. In R. Grant (Ed.), *Physical therapy of the cervical and thoracic spine*. New York: Churchill Livingstone.

Janda, V. (1992). Treatment of chronic back pain. *Journal of Manual Medicine,* 166-168.

Jensen, B., Laursen, B., & Sjogaard, G. (2000). Aspects of shoulder function in relation to exposure demands and fatigue—a mini review. *Clinical Biomechanics, 15* (Suppl 1), S17-S20.

Jensen, B., Pilegaard, M., & Sjogaard, G. (2000). Motor unit recruitment and rate coding in response to fatiguing shoulder abductions and subsequent recovery. *European Journal of Applied Physiology, 83*(2-3), 190-199.

Jensen, C., Finsen, L., Hansen, K., & Christensen, H. (1999). Upper trapezius muscle activity patterns during repetitive manual material handling and work with a computer mouse. *Journal of Electromyography and Kinesiology, 9*(5), 317-325.

Johnson, E. W. (1989). The myth of skeletal muscle spasm. *American Journal of Physical Medicine, 68*(1), 1.

Jonsson, B. (1988). The static load component in muscle work. *European Journal of Applied Physiology, 57*(3), 305-310.

Jorgensen, K., Fallentin, N., Krogh-Lund C., & Jensen, B. (1988). Electromyography and fatigue during prolonged, low-level static contractions. *European Journal of Applied Physiology, 57*(3), 316-321.

Kilbom, A. (1988). Isometric strength and occupational muscle disorders. *European Journal of Applied Physiology, 57*(3), 322-326.

Kilbom, S., Armstrong, T., Buckle, P., Fine, L., Hagbert, M., Haring-Sweeney, M. et al. (1996). Musculoskeletal disorders: Work-related risk factors and prevention. *International Journal of Occupational and Environmental Health, 2*(3), 239-246.

Krogh-Lund, C., & Jorgensen, K. (1992). Modification of myo-electric power spectrum in fatigue from 15% maximal voluntary contraction of human elbow flexor muscles, to limit of endurance: Reflection of conduction velocity variation and/or centrally mediated mechanisms? *European Journal of Applied Physiology, 64*(4), 359-370.

Krogh-Lund, C., & Jorgensen, K. (1993). Myo-electric fatigue manifestations revisited: Power spectrum, conduction velocity, and amplitude of human elbow flexor muscles during isolated and repetitive endurance contractions at 30% maximal voluntary contraction. *European Journal of Applied Physiology, 66*(2), 161-173.

Laursen, B., Jensen, B., & Sjogaard, G. (1998). Effect of speed and precision demands on human shoulder muscle electromyography during a repetitive task. *European Journal of Applied Physiology and Occupational Physiology, 78*(6), 544-548.

Lewit, K. (1985). Muscular and articular factors in movement restriction. *Manual Medicine,* 83-85.

Liebenson, C. (1990). Active muscular relaxation techniques (part 2): Clinical application. *Journal of Manipulative and Physiological Therapeutics, 13*(1), 2-6.

McLean, L., Tingley, M., Scott, R., & Rickards, J. (2000). Myoelectric signal measurement during prolonged computer terminal work. *Journal of Electromyography and Kinesiology, 10*(1), 33-45.

Mense, S., Simons, D., & Russell, I. J. (2001). *Muscle pain. Understanding its nature, diagnosis, and treatment.* Philadelphia: Lippincott Williams & Wilkins.

Middaugh, S., & Kee, W. (1987). Advances in electromyographic monitoring and biofeedback in treatment of chronic cervical and low back pain. In M. Eisenberg (Ed.), *Advances in clinical rehabilitation*. New York: Springer Publishing Co.

Middaugh, S. J., Kee, W. G., & Nicholson, J. A. (1994). Muscle overuse and posture as factors in the development and maintenance of chronic musculoskeletal pain. In R. C. Grzesiak & D. S. Ciccone (Eds.), *Psychological vulnerability to pain*. New York: Springer Publishing.

Noonan, T. J., & Garrett, W. E. (1992). Injuries at the myotendinous junction. *Clinics in Sports Medicine, 11*(4), 783-806.

Nyland, J. (1993). Relation between local muscular fatigue and the electromyographic signal with emphasis on power spectrum changes. *Isokinetics and Exercise Science*, 171-180.

Olsen, H., Christensen, H., & Sogaard, K. (2001). An analysis of motor unit firing pattern during sustained low force contraction in fatigued muscle. *Acta Physiologica et Pharmacologica Bulgacia, 26*(1-2), 73-78.

Pratt, N. E. (1986). Neurovascular entrapment in the regions of the shoulder and posterior triangle of the neck. *Physical Therapy, 66*(12), 1894-1900.

Price, J. P., Clare, M. H., & Ewerhardt, R. H. (1948). Studies in low backache with persistent muscle spasm. *Archives of Physical Medicine and Rehabilitation,* 703-709.

Seidel, H., Beyer, H., & Brauer, D. (1987). Electromyographic evaluation of back muscle fatigue with repeated sustained contractions of different strengths. *European Journal of Applied Physiology, 56*(5), 592-602.

Sihvonen, T. (1992). The segmental dorsal ramus neuropathy as a common cause of chronic and recurrent low back pain. *Electromyography and Clinical Neurophysiology, 32*(10-11), 507-510.

Simons, D. G. (Ed.). (1993). *Referred phenomena of myofascial trigger points. New trends in referred pain and hyperalgesia*. Amsterdam: Elsevier Science.

Sjogaard, G. (1986). Water and electrolyte fluxes during exercise and their relation to muscle fatigue. *Acta Physiologica Scandinavica, 556,* 129-136.

Sjogaard, G., Jorgensen, L., Ekner, D., & Sogaard, K. (2000). Muscle involvement during intermittent contraction patterns with different target force feedback modes. *Clinical Biomechanics, 15*(Suppl 1), S25-S29.

Sjogaard, G., Kiens, B., Jorgensen, K., & Saltin, B. (1986). Intramuscular pressure, EMG and blood flow during low-level prolonged static contractions in man. *Acta Physiologica Scandinavica, 128*(3), 475-484.

Sogaard, K., Christensen, H., Fallentin, N., Mizuno, M., Quistorff, B., & Sjogaard G., (1998). Motor unit activation patterns during concentric wrist flexion in humans with different muscle fibre composition. *European Journal of Applied Physiology and Occupational Physiology, 78*(5), 411-416.

Sogaard, K., Laursen, B., Jensen, B., & Sjogaard, G. (2001). Dynamic loads on the upper extremities during two different floor cleaning methods. *Clinical Biomechanics, 16*(10), 866-879.

Sogaard, K., Sjogaard, G., Finsen, L., Olsen, H. B., & Christensen, H. (2001). Motor unit activity during stereotyped finger tasks and computer mouse work. *Journal of Electromyography and Kinesiology, 11*(3), 197-206.

Solomonow, M., Baten, C., Smit, J., Baratta, R., Hermens, H., D'Ambrosia, R. et al. (1990). Electromyogram power spectra frequencies associated with motor unit recruitment strategies. *Journal of Applied Physiology, 68*(3), 1177-1185.

Travell, J., & Simons, D. (1992). *Myofascial pain and dysfunction. The trigger point manual*. Baltimore: Williams & Wilkins.

Veiersted, K. B., & Westgaard, R. H. (1993). Development of trapezius myalgia among female workers performing light manual work. *Scandinavian Journal of Work, Environment and Health, 19*(4) 277-283.

Westgaard, R. H. (1988). Measurement and evaluation of postural load in occupational work situations. *European Journal of Applied Physiology, 57*(3), 291-304.

Wolf, S L., Basmajian, J. V., Russe, T. C., & Kutner, M. (1979). Normative data on low back mobility and activity levels. *American Journal of Physical Medicine, 58*(5), 217-229.

Yaksh, T. L. (1996). Pharmacology of facilitated nociceptive processing. *Journal of Musculoskeletal Pain,* (1-2), 201-221.

CHAPTER 10

Biomechanical Risk Factors

Nick Warren
Martha J. Sanders

As early as 1717, health care practitioners speculated on factors within the work environment that contribute to musculoskeletal disorders (MSDs). Ramazzini (1717) first identified "violent and irregular motions," "bent posture," and "tonic strain on the muscles" as contributing factors. Centuries later, researchers agree that force and awkward or static postures contribute in some way to MSDs (Armstrong, 1986; Bernard, 1997; Bullock, 1990; Putz-Anderson, 1988). However, our ability to quantify and determine the relative weight of each factor in the overall scheme of MSD natural history still remains limited. The following case exemplifies the multiple factors involved in MSD etiology and the difficulty in determining a single, precipitating event.

Carl, a 64-year-old man who had been employed as a heavy equipment operator for 20 years, described a work history of jackhammering on road crews, welding, and wiring commercial buildings. Over a period of 2 years, Carl noticed that he could no longer sense the amount of pressure he was exerting on the controls and that he was dumping loads of gravel too quickly and "jerking" the heavy machinery dangerously. He stated that his fingers were numb by the end of the day and that his hands felt weak. In fact, Carl had increasing difficulty pulling himself into the cab. (He weighed 370 lb) Once in his cab, he sat all day except during coffee breaks. Although he was close to retirement, he loved his job and planned on working as long as he was able.

Carl appeared to be developing signs and symptoms of carpal tunnel syndrome (CTS). However, determining the most important CTS risk factor is not a straightforward exercise. Was the repetitive grasping and manipulating of controls the source of the problem, or did the operation of the controls require high hand forces? Was Carl's sitting in a slumped posture all day the cause, or was Carl's history of jackhammering and electrical work to blame? How did Carl's weight affect his risk for CTS? Most likely, all factors played a role, although we cannot be certain which factor or factors played the primary role in Carl's situation.

Much current research in biomechanics as related to MSDs attempts to identify the relevant risk factors, delineate the relative weight of each risk factor, and identify safe limits for workers. By definition, a *risk factor* is an attribute of a situation that increases the probability of an exposed worker developing a certain disease or disorder. This chapter deals solely with *extrinsic* biomechanical risk factors—physical characteristics of the work environment—rather than *intrinsic* risk factors (characteristics of the individual that either predispose toward or protect against disease development). Although the relationships are probably not linear, the greater the magnitude or duration of exposure to a risk factor, the greater the risk for developing a disorder. Exposure to several factors may substantially increase the risk of MSD development (e.g., Punnett, 1998), although research is often unable to determine how multiple risk factors interact. In Carl's case, his history of working with vibrating tools combined with his present job probably increased his risk for developing CTS, as compared to someone whose work involves more varied tasks with lower levels of stressors.

This example highlights several sources of uncertainty in occupational ergonomic research (presented in more detail in Chapter 8), including the following.

- Some research suggests that the combined effect of exposure to two or more risk factors may be multiplicative (i.e., a true interaction) rather than additive (Armstrong & Ulin, 1995; Silverstein, Fine, & Armstrong, 1986, 1987).
- The relative contribution of psychosocial, organizational, and the more commonly assessed biomechanical risk factors to MSD development is often difficult to determine.
- It is challenging to identify and measure the contribution of nonoccupational exposures, although most workers do not encounter these with the same intensity or duration as experienced over the workday.
- Uncertainty remains about the mechanisms through which personal characteristics (e.g., gender, age, individual physiology, anatomy, psychology, skill level, work technique, and recovery processes, etc.) modify or influence the effect of exposure to extrinsic risk factors (American National Standards Institute, 1998; Faucett & Werner, 1998; Harber et al., 1993; Radwin & Lavender, 1998).

Because research is inconclusive about which risk factor or combination of factors places a particular person at most risk for developing MSDs, our best means of assessing the risk of injury is to measure as many exposures as possible, including psychosocial risk factors and characteristics of the work organization and the company (Warren, Dillon, Morse, Hall, & Warren, 2000) (discussed in Chapter 12). With this information, we can monitor individual workers as well as compile information from jobs that can help set levels of exposure that are safe for most workers (Armstrong & Ulin, 1995; Joseph & Bloswick, 1991; Putz-Anderson, 1988).

In this chapter, the biomechanical risk factors and modifiers are reviewed, using as a framework the taxonomy presented in the Preamble to the short-lived Ergonomic Program Standard. The seven risk factors recognized by the Occupational Safety and Health Administration (OSHA), National Institute for Occupational Safety and Health (NIOSH), American Conference of Governmental Industrial Hygienists (ACGIH), and most researchers are the following.

1. Repetition
2. Force
3. Awkward postures
4. Static postures
5. Dynamic factors
6. Mechanical compression
7. Vibration

Full biomechanical analysis of a job requires identification of which risk factors are present, as well as characterization of the following four important modifying factors.

1. *Intensity or magnitude*: the strength of the exposure—for example, how many pounds of force, how deviated from neutral the joint angle, how large the acceleration of vibration, and so on.
2. *Duration*: the length of exposure. Depending on analysis goals, duration can be assessed over the work cycle or workday, as well as cumulative exposure over a year, a career, or working life.
3. *Temporal profile*: the pattern in which the exposure is distributed over the work cycle, workday, workweek, and longer time cycles. The same cumulative exposure could, for example, be concentrated into a few intense periods in the workday or distributed evenly, at lower concentrations, over the workday. These patterns have different implications for disease development.
4. *Cold temperatures*: cold is a well-established exacerbating factor for vibration exposure (NIOSH, 1989) that may exacerbate the effects of other biomechanical risk factors primarily through vascular effects.

The biomechanical risk factors and modifiers discussed in this chapter are characteristics of the work environment. Their effects on an individual worker are, of course, strongly influenced by personal factors (workstyle, anatomy, physiology, etc.). See Chapter 8 for a more detailed discussion of personal risk factors.

This chapter relates each risk factor to the development of MSDs and will identify the means to measure each risk factor. This information will enable the health care practitioner to understand and critically analyze the interaction of risk factors. A broad discussion of methods to measure risk factors will apply to all further discussions on risk factor measurement.

MEASURING AND REPORTING OUTCOMES FOR BIOMECHANICAL RISK FACTOR EXPOSURES

A wide range of tools exists that can help identify the biomechanical risks that may be present in a workplace. Measurement tools generally include self-reports, simple checklists, direct measurements, observational methods, and standardized tests representing increasing levels of validity in identifying exposures.

Checklists and self-report survey instruments are quick and inexpensive to administer, making them ideal for large studies and a preliminary identification of potential risk factors. Checklists can be used as a screen to determine whether a particular risk is present or absent and which tasks should be analyzed in greater detail. Checklists alone may not be sufficient to effectively guide preventive actions unless the exposures of interest are obvious in their presence and intensity. However, they may be the first step in identifying workplace risks. Self-reports have been used to provide estimations of exposures, perceived exertions, and indications of bodily discomfort. Controversy exists as to the validity of self-reports due to subjective bias, lack of reproducibility, and lack of precision in most self-reported questionnaires. They are often used in conjunction with other methods (Speilholz, Silverstein, Morgan, Checkowy, & Kaufman, 2001).

The other analysis methods are more time intensive but can provide much more precise risk factor identification. Observational methods include both field-based and video-based approaches. They can be especially useful for postural analysis and work sampling studies particularly when analyzed by an ergonomics team. Video methods allow repeated analysis in slow motion to characterize rapid, complex jobs. Limitations to video-based recording include the potential for occluded views of the worker (Keyserling, Armstrong, & Punnett, 1991). Standardized tests such as the Strain Index and Rapid Upper Limb Assessment (RULA) use both checklists and observational methods to indicate the levels of risk for the tasks being evaluated and to predict the potential for developing an MSD. At this point, most tests do not have strong predictive validity or reliability studies completed.

Direct measurement such as measuring loads with a spring scale or hand dynamometer can provide specific detailed information. However, the more portable, lower-tech equipment does not always measure the true risk factor exposure (e.g., a spring scale measures load, not muscle forces). (Please see the "Force" section in this chapter for a complete discussion.) More sophisticated measures such as electromyography (EMG), electrogoniometry, or digital motion capture recording of joint motion, force- or pressure-sensitive transducers provide detailed information but generally involve costly equipment.

The strength of association between exposures and outcomes (e.g., the strength of the association between high levels of wrist bending and the development of carpal tunnel syndrome) is often expressed as an odds ratio (OR). An odds ratio quantifies the increased risk of developing a negative outcome (e.g., carpal tunnel syndrome) in a group of workers exposed to the risk factor of interest, compared to a group that is unexposed or exposed at a much lower level (the control or reference group). An OR of 1.00 means that there is no difference between the exposed group and the control or reference group. An OR above 1.00 means that the exposed group does have a higher prevalence or incidence of disease, relative to the control or reference group; the higher the number, the greater the risk. An OR less than 1.00 means that the exposed group has a lower prevalence or incidence of disease. ORs presented in this book are a standard measure of association between exposure and outcome (disease or symptom). Because estimation is always subject to error, in scientific literature ORs are presented as a single estimated number with an accompanying range, called the 95% confidence interval (CI). This is the range within which we have 95% statistical confidence that the effect was actually due to the difference in exposure level rather than due to chance. For simplicity, in this chapter we do not present the 95% CI but instead present ORs that are statistically significant. (This means that the lower limit of the 95% CI is greater than 1.00—the level at which there is no difference between exposed and control groups. A result significant at this level would be expected to appear by chance only 5% of the time, or less).

REPETITION

Repetition refers to the performance of the same motions over and over within a given time period. Repetitive work became the hallmark of the industrial revolution as management attempted to increase manufacturing efficiency by eliminating and simplifying motions. Today, the information age continues this propensity toward repetition through computer use, instrument control panels, and service occupations. However, the musculoskeletal problems associated with repetitive work have become a concern to certain occupational groups such as supermarket checkers (Margolis & Kraus, 1987), dental hygienists (Akesson, Johnson, Rylander, Moritz, & Skirfving, 1999), workers in fish processing (Chiang et al., 1993), and telecommunications workers (Putz-Anderson, Doyle, & Hales, 1992).

Repetition is reported as a risk factor in itself (Kourinka & Forcier, 1995) or as an exposure intensifier (Radwin & Lavender, 1998). Acting as a modifier, repetition can exacerbate the basic risk factors of force and posture. But acting as a basic risk factor, high repetition also may have its own tissue effects (combined with the dynamic factors described below). For example, increased friction-induced irritation of finger flexor and extensor tendons in their sheaths can result in tendinitis and lead to increased pressure in the carpal canal.

Although other risk factors may demonstrate a roughly linear exposure-response relationship, repetition is unique in demonstrating a U-shaped exposure/response curve. Very low levels of repetition approximate the effects of static postures (following), whereas high levels can overload tissues. A moderate level of repetition may be seen as protective, since it can increase muscle strength and flexibility (this is the concept behind exercise). It can also assist blood flow through muscles, thus relieving the stressful nature of static muscle contractions. Ideal work cycles keep overall repetition rates in a middle zone between the injurious extremes of static contraction and excessive repetition, as demonstrated in Figure 10-1.

The physiologic problems that arise from repetitive work or overuse of certain muscles, tendons, and soft-tissue structures have been addressed in terms of muscle fatigue (Sjogaard,

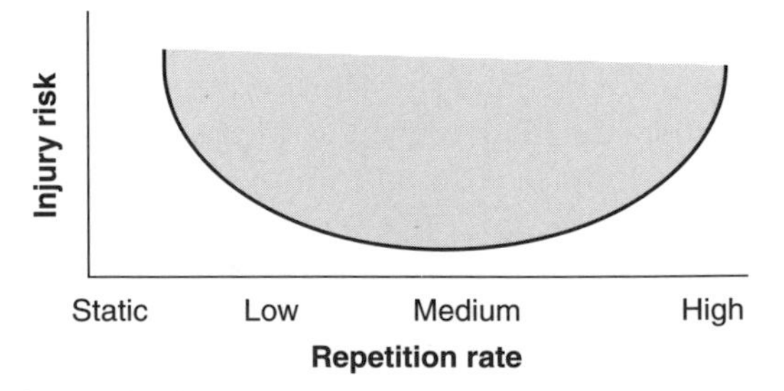

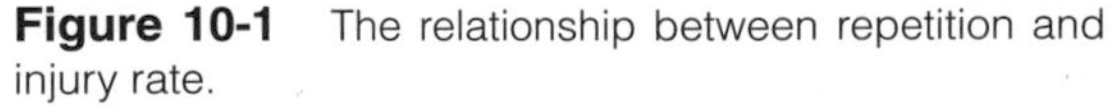

Figure 10-1 The relationship between repetition and injury rate.

Savard, & Juel, 1988; see Chapter 9 in this book), tissue density changes (Armstrong, Castelli, Evans, & Diaz-Perez, 1984), and tissue strain (Goldstein, Armstrong, Chaffin, & Matthews, 1987; Rodgers, 1987), among others. Tissue strain theory will be discussed and related to MSDs. The reader is referred to Armstrong et al. (1984) for a discussion of histologic changes in tissue density that result from repetitive work.

Tissue Strain and Repetition

Tissue strain concept incorporates the combination of two risk factors: repetition and force. The stress-strain curve provides a means of explaining the natural process that occurs in tendons after repetitive exposures (LeVeau, 1992) (Figure 10-2). According to the stress-strain curve, external loads applied to tendons during repetitive work will elongate the tendon and create microtears in the tissue. Initially, these viscoelastic tendons recover, repair, and return to their original length (elastic range). This mechanism allows the worker to function with no apparent problem at a moderate pace with time for rest. However, if external loads are applied too often or too quickly, leaving inadequate time for complete recovery, a residual strain develops in the tendons. Over time, tendons accumulate strain that may weaken, deform, or create a chronic inflammatory response in the tendon (Chaffin & Andersson, 1984; Kumar, 2001). The worker may begin to feel pain while performing the usual tasks and compensate by using inefficient muscle patterns or motor control strategies to accomplish the job. (See Chapter 9 for a complete discussion.)

At a certain point (such as during overtime or excessive work for several weeks), the accumulation of strain and the magnitude of the load supersede the ability of the tissues to repair. The worker is unable to keep up the work pace. The tissue becomes permanently deformed (plastic range) and thereafter needs less force or load to break or rupture. This model may explain why workers seem to report one particularly stressful event prior to seeking medical help, although the client may have performed repetitive work for years. It may also explain why workers seem to have a lower tolerance to repetition when returning to work after an MSD than when they originally started the job.

To more fully understand the relationship of accumulated tissue strain (referred to as *creep*) to repetitive work, Goldstein et al. (1987) studied

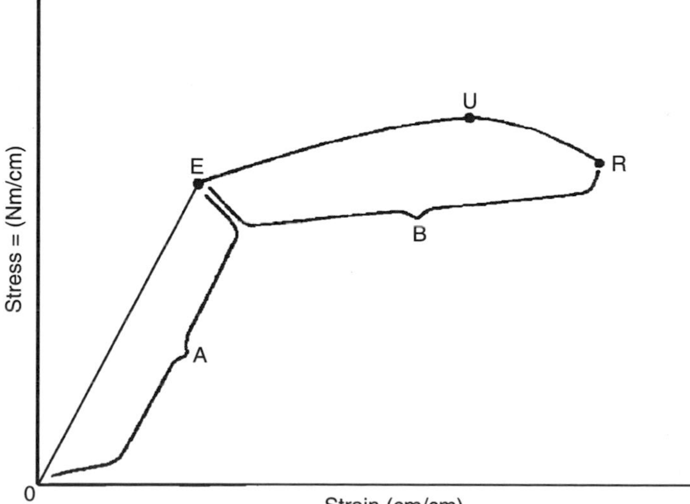

Figure 10-2 Stress-strain curve. *A*, elastic range; *E*, elastic limit; *B*, plastic range; *U*, ultimate strength; *R*, rupture or breaking point. (Redrawn with permission from B. F. Leveau, [1992]. *William's & Lissner's biomechanics of human motion* [3rd ed]. Philadelphia: Saunders.)

the strain in tendons during repetitive pinching activities at submaximal loads. Researchers subjected the finger flexor tendons of cadavers to various workloads and frequency cycles and then measured the strain accumulated within the tendons. Results indicated that the frequency cycles (or work-rest cycles) were correlated significantly with tendon strain. In a 2-second work cycle followed by a 9-second recovery period, no significant change in tendon strain was noted after 500 cycles. However, when work time was increased to 8 seconds and recovery time decreased to 2 seconds, the accumulated strain in the tendon was equivalent to an 80% increase in load after 500 cycles. Goldstein et al. (1987) contend that the recovery time between successive loads is the greatest indicator of tendon strain in repetitive work.

Fatigue Model

Recovery cycles are clearly important in the planning of work tasks. The concept of work and recovery cycles was introduced by Romhert (1973) and developed by Rodgers (1987, 1988) in relation to MSDs in industry. Rodgers (1987) noted that industry standards for repetitive tasks were based solely on the amount of time necessary to complete a motion, without regard for the amount of effort involved or recovery time needed. When workers were required to perform heavy tasks at the same rate as light tasks, they clearly fatigued much more quickly. Rodgers proposed that work cycles in industry (the total time required to perform a task and recover from the task before repeating it again) incorporate muscular effort as well as effort duration, allowing for longer recovery times for heavy, repetitive work.

Rodgers (1987, 1988) proposed the fatigue model (Figure 10-3), which identifies the interaction between the effort duration (x-axis), the effort intensity (graphed curves), and the total cycle time necessary to perform the task (y-axis). In this model, the effort duration or holding time refers to static work, demonstrating the close relationship between all work-related factors. The effort intensity corresponds to the percentage of a person's maximum voluntary capacity (MVC) in that working posture or aerobic work capacity. Effort intensity can be measured as a function of perceived exertion (Rodgers, 1987, 1988) such as light (30%), moderate (50%), and heavy (80%), because direct measurements are not always possible.

Recovery time is calculated in Figure 10-3 by subtracting the effort duration or continuous holding time from the total cycle time. For example, a light-effort task that requires a

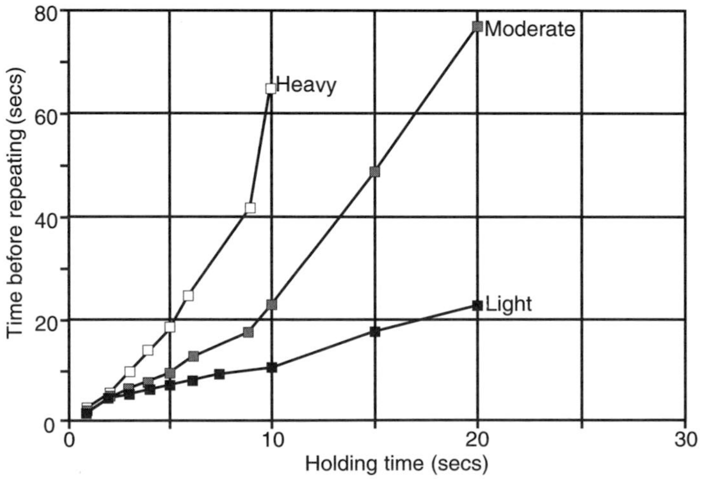

Figure 10-3 Work-recovery times for static work. The total cycle time (time before repeating, y-axis) is a function of the effort duration (or holding time, x-axis) and the effort intensity (graphed curves). (Reprinted with permission from Rodgers, S. [1987]. Recovery time needs for repetitive work. *Semin Occup Med, 2*[1], 19–24.)

10-second continuous holding time will require a 12-second repetition cycle, which allows 2 seconds for recovery. However, if the task requires heavy effort, a 10-second holding time will necessitate a cycle time of 70 seconds to allow for a 60-second muscle recovery period. The fatigue model can assist the health care practitioner in determining cycle times or the extent of effort required to sustain the predetermined cycle time.

Research on Repetition and Musculoskeletal Disorders

As noted previously, it is extremely difficult to isolate risk factors because several risk factors usually occur together in work environments. In a seminal piece of work, Silverstein et al. (1986, 1987) attempted to document repetition and force and then to identify the risk of developing a work-related MSD on the basis of exposure to these factors. In a cross-sectional study, researchers examined the prevalence of CTS among 652 workers in 39 different jobs, as related to force and repetitive hand use on the job. All workers were observed, videotaped, and classified into four groups on the basis of their exposure to force and repetition in the workplace. The four groups were low force-low repetition, high force-low repetition, low force-high repetition, and high force-high repetition. A sample of workers from each job underwent a structured interview and physical examination in order to determine the presence of symptoms associated with CTS.

Results indicated that the prevalence of CTS was 5.6% in the high force-high repetition group and 0.6% in the low force-low repetition group (Silverstein et al., 1987). Odds ratios (ORs) indicated that the risk of developing CTS was 15.5 times greater in the high force-high repetition group than in the low force-low repetition group. The low force-high repetition jobs presented a slightly higher risk than the high force-low repetition jobs; therefore, repetition was considered to be a greater risk factor in the analysis than was force. Deviations in posture and use of vibrating tools were not controlled in the study.

As further evidence for the contribution of repetition to hand-wrist problems, a cross-sectional study of female assembly-line packers, compared with department store shop assistants (Luopajärvi, Kourinka, Virolainen, & Holmberg, 1979), found a prevalence of hand-wrist tendinitis 7.1 times greater in the packer group. (In this study, exposure was a combination of awkward postures, static postures, and repetitive motions, demonstrating the difficulty of studying one risk factor in isolation.) Kourinka and Forcier (1995) also reported several studies demonstrating a strong association between CTS and repetition.

Strong associations have also been found between repetition and neck and shoulder disorders. The NIOSH summary, *Musculoskeletal Disorders and Workplace Factors* (Bernard, 1997) found a significant relationship between repetition and neck disorders in 20 of the 26 rigorously selected studies for the NIOSH summary. Ohlsson et al. (1995) compared 82 female industrial workers exposed to short-cycle tasks (less than 30 seconds) to 64 referents with no exposure to repetitive work. Exposed workers had an OR of 3.6 to 5 times the likelihood of developing a variety of neck and shoulder symptoms. In a further review of the epidemiologic evidence for three neck-related MSDs, Kourinka and Forcier (1995) reported weak-to-moderate but consistent associations between exposures to repetitive work and outcomes of tension neck syndrome and thoracic outlet syndrome (TOS). Overall, Hansson et al. (2000) found elevated prevalences of neck, shoulder, and wrist-hand disorders (OR 2 to 7.5) in women who performed repetitive work in the laminate industry as compared to a referent group.

Although most research has focused on tendinous structures, articular structures are not impervious to repetition-induced injury. Bard, Sylvestre, and Dussault (1984) describe osteoarthritis of the distal interphalangeal and metacarpophalangeal joints that occurs in pianists. Williams et al. (1987) describe a metacarpophalangeal arthropathy associated with manual labor. Dillon, Petersen, and Tanaka (2002), on compiling data from the National Health Interview Survey, found an OR of 1.43 for developing hand-wrist arthritis in work that requires repetitive hand flexing and twisting. Occupations with the greatest prevalence of hand-wrist arthritis were technicians, machine operators, assemblers, and farmers. (See Chapter 7 for extensive review of joint-related MSDs as related to repetitive work.)

Measurement of Repetition

Repetition has been measured in a number of ways. Health professionals tend to focus on the number of similar movements in a given time period, whereas engineers focus on the work quantity (expressed as the amount of time to complete a task) (Armstrong, 1986). It would appear that as work quantity increases, so does the repetition. However, the repetition increases only if all the motions in the task involve similar muscle groups. Hence, one must carefully examine the actual repetitive nature of the job in order to determine whether repetition indeed increases.

Silverstein et al. (1987) developed a method by which to categorize jobs into low- or high-repetition groups on the basis of the estimated cycle time for a job task and the percentage of time performing the same fundamental cycle. *Cycle time* refers to the amount of time necessary to complete a task. Within a cycle, there may be a series of steps or movements that are repeated. These movements are referred to as the *fundamental cycle* (Silverstein et al., 1987). According to the method of Silverstein et al. (1987), jobs are classified as *low repetitive* if the cycle time is more than 30 seconds and if less than 50% of the cycle time involves performing the same kind of fundamental cycle. (In other words, similar movements are repeated less than 50% of the time.) A job is considered to be *high repetitive* if the cycle time is less than 30 seconds or more than 50% of the cycle time involves performing the same kind of fundamental cycle. This classification has been used widely in research studies (Silverstein et al., 1987; Chiang et al., 1993).

Other approaches measure the repetition *rate*, the average number of motions performed within a unit of time, such as motions per shift (Putz-Anderson, 1988). Hammer (1934) measured repetition in terms of the number of manipulations per hour and concluded that more than 2000 manipulations per hour, or 30 to 40 manipulations per minute, were considered to be repetitive.

Although cycles and repetition rates attempt to quantify job repetitiveness, these systems consider only the speed at which the worker performs the movements rather than the quality of movements. Armstrong and Ulin (1995) introduced a qualitative scale that rates the degree of repetition as related to the worker's ability to keep up with the work. In rough form, this scale was later incorporated into the Hand Activity Level standard (following). Work is rated as follows.

- *Very high:* The worker's body parts are in rapid, steady motion; the worker has difficulty keeping up with the pace.
- *High:* The worker's body parts are in steady motion; any difficulty causes the worker to fall behind.
- *Medium:* The worker's body parts are in steady motion, but he or she is able to keep up, with time for brief pauses or rest.
- *Low:* The worker has no difficulty keeping up; there are frequent pauses during work to wait for another job or machinery cycle.
- *Very low:* The worker is inactive most of the time but occasionally uses his or her hands.

Armstrong and Ulin note that this scale can compare jobs with vastly different productivity standards. For a complete discussion of this scale, the reader should see Armstrong & Ulin (1995).

Measurement as a Basis for a Standard: the ACGIH HAL (Hand Activity Level) Voluntary Standard (ACGIH 2001)

The difficulty of establishing a Threshold Limit Value (TLV) for any biomechanical exposure because of the interaction among risk factors was noted in Chapter 8. Using the concept of multiple exposures, the ACGIH has created a standard for hand exposure to combinations of force and repetition in so-called monotasks (tasks involving only one job operation). (See Chapter 4 for further discussion.) The observer rates both average hand activity and peak force using a 1-10 visual analog scale (VAS). In a rating procedure similar to that just described (Armstrong & Ulin, 1995), hand repetition is rated on a scale with anchor points as identified in Figure 4-6.

The originators of the scale, Dr. Tom Armstrong and Dr. Wendi Latko, at the University of Michigan (ACGIH, 2001), have found that with basic training, reliability of estimates among observers is quite high. Worker or observer rating of peak hand force uses a well-validated Borg scale. Ideally, the worker performing the task performs force ratings, with the following verbal anchors (or force is assessed by direct measurement). If this is not practical, the observer rates peak force from visual cues. Finally, taking cycle time and task length into account, the observer uses the combination of hand repetition and peak hand force to determine whether the job is acceptable or in need of intervention.

FORCE

Nearly all activities require some degree of force. *Force* is the mechanical effort required to carry out a movement or to prevent movement. Force may be exerted against a work piece or tool, or against gravity, to stabilize body segments. Force does not necessarily imply motion. The dynamic act of lifting a work piece and the static act of holding that piece in position both require force, generated by muscles, transmitted through tendons, and exerted by body segments on the work piece.

Ashton-Miller (1998), summarizing a large body of laboratory evidence assessing the effects of loading on body tissues, concludes that muscle, tendon, and ligamentous tissues can fail when subjected to sufficient force under certain conditions. Excessive force can cause muscle fiber damage, either by disruption of the contractile proteins or of the boundary (Z-lines) between the contractile units in the muscle fibril. Muscles are particularly likely to be injured through exertion of excessive force in eccentric contractions as the muscle lengthens. This may occur when stopping the motion of the body or an external object (Brooks, Zerba, & Faulkner, 1995).

Forceful muscle contractions also raise intramuscular pressure (IMP), which may compress nerves and blood vessels within the active muscle. Palermud, Forsman, Sporrong, Herberts, and Kadefors (2000) studied the IMP of shoulder musculature at different static arm positions and hand loads. The intramuscular pressure of the infraspinatus and supraspinatus muscles was found to increase gradually as flexion of the shoulder increased from 0 degrees to 90 degrees. Even positions of moderate shoulder flexion (greater than 30 degrees) caused reduced recovery from local muscle fatigue and blood flow impairment. Researchers found that an additional 1-kg hand load increased the IMP 132% in the infraspinatus muscle and 65% in the supraspinatus muscle.

Studies using both human cadavers (Cobb, Cooney, & An, 1996) and healthy volunteers (Kier, Bach, & Rempel, 1998; Rempel, Keir, Smutz, & Hargans, 1997) demonstrate that forceful loading of fingertips results in elevated carpal tunnel pressures likely to cause damage to neurons. Abundant human and animal studies (Rempel, Dahlin, & Lundborg, 1998) demonstrate that many of these changes can occur over relatively short exposure times and in the presence of relatively low-pressure elevations.

External and Internal Force Considerations

It is useful to consider external and internal force requirements separately in order to determine the risk posed by force requirements of the task. *External forces* (also called *output forces)* are the loads exerted on or by the surface of the body during work-related activities such as lifting, pushing, or grasping objects. *Internal forces* refer to the tension generated within the muscles, tendons, and ligaments that resist or move external loads. External loads are more readily measured and tend to be the reference point for industry. In industry, force is commonly expressed as the amount of effort required by a worker to overcome external loads through pushing, pulling, grasping, or handling objects. However, estimating internal forces from external characteristics of the task can be complicated.

First, many external job characteristics can affect muscle force requirements, and some of these characteristics may not be recognized in a job analysis. For example, Kourinka and Forcier (1995) note several factors that affect muscle force required for a grip including the presence of other risk factors (such as awkward postures required by grip type and handle size), the coefficient of friction between the work piece surface and the hand, whether gloves are required, and individual variations in technique. Haselgrave (1991) found that the maximal force that workers generated for a job varied with the workers' positions—standing, kneeling, or lying on their backs. Haselgrave suggested that the variability in force was due to changes in the workers' abilities to use their body weight, to brace their feet or shoulders against a surface (thus providing joint stability), and to use stronger muscle groups to accomplish the job.

Second, the lever arm (the distance from point of force application to the fulcrum—the joint center) for most muscles is generally much smaller than that of the external load (Radwin & Lavender, 1998). This means that internal forces are usually several times greater than the external load. Accurate modeling requires precise estimation or modeling of actual lever arm lengths.

Third, fatigue affects muscle fiber recruitment patterns within a single muscle, as well as recruitment (substitution) patterns of alternative muscles (Parnianpour, Nordin, Kahanovitz, & Frankel, 1988). When secondary muscles are recruited to assist a fatigued primary muscle, the recruited secondary muscles may be more vulnerable to injury because of less advantageous lever arm length, smaller size, or less-than-optimal fiber length in the work posture. (See Chapter 9 for further discussion.)

As stated, posture is an important variable that affects the generation of muscle force. Deviations from a so-called "neutral posture" can dramatically reduce the amount of muscle force translated into output force. The "lost" force is generally seen in inefficient coupling of the contractile proteins in muscle fibers, in lateral force exerted by muscles and tendons against adjacent anatomic structures where force transmission changes direction, or in stabilizing a joint during joint movement (LeVeau, 1992). Table 10-1 demonstrates this concept relating handgrip strength to hand posture. In a neutral position, one's grip strength is 100%. However, when the wrist flexes to 45 degrees, for example, the grip strength is only 60% of its entire strength. That figure drops to 45% when the wrist flexes to 65 degrees (Rodgers, 1987). In this position, the individual must work more than twice as hard to accomplish the same task. Three to four more times the force is required to exert the same force level in a pinch versus a power grip (Armstrong, 1986; Tichauer, 1978).

In addition, most holding and moving tasks involve input from several muscles, often working in opposition. Skilled, small-motor

Table 10-1

Effects of Wrist Angle on Power Grip Strength

Wrist Angle (Degrees)	Percentage of Power Grip
Neutral	100
Flexion 45	60
Flexion 65	45
Extension 45	75
Extension 60	63
Ulnar deviation 45	75
Radial deviation 25	80

Adapted from Rodgers, S. (1987). Recovery time needs for repetitive work. *Seminars in Occupational Medicine, 2*(1), 19–24.

activities involve cocontraction of antagonist muscles to generate precisely graded movements, joint stabilization, or holding forces. Thus, substantial muscle activity can be associated with very little net output or external force. In addition, these cocontractile forces act additively on the joint components (ligaments, cartilage, and bone). For the researcher, this has important implications. For example, measurements of the weight of a work piece or the finger forces necessary to move a computer mouse may substantially underestimate the potential damage to the muscles, tendons, joints, and other soft tissues involved. Guidelines for manual materials handling (Snook & Ciriello, 1991; NIOSH, 1981, 1994) clearly note that the weight of the load, in isolation, is not a sufficient measure of musculoskeletal stress.

Research on Force and MSDs

Force has been implicated as a risk factor in MSD etiology, especially when combined with other risk factors. Investigators suggest that the risk of MSDs increases with an increase in force (Armstrong & Chaffin, 1979; Armstrong et al., 1984; Silverstein et al., 1987). However, as discussed previously, parameters for acceptable forces in industry have not been established.

The Silverstein et al. (1987) study noted previously found a prevalence of CTS 15.5 times greater in high force-high repetition jobs, compared to jobs with low levels of both. The interaction of force and repetition was important in this study. In separate models, force alone had a nonsignificant association with CTS; only when combined with high repetition did its association become significant in this study. The NIOSH summary (Bernard, 1997) of upper-extremity MSDs found evidence of a causal relationship between exposure to force and disorders of the neck and elbow, as well as CTS and hand-wrist tendinitis.

Other epidemiologic studies point to an association between force requirements and work-related MSDs. Ekberg et al. (1994) investigated the relationship between neck and shoulder pain in workers and the physical, organizational, and psychosocial aspects of the job. The researchers found that workers who performed light lifting were 13.6 times more likely to develop neck and shoulder symptoms than were those who performed no lifting. Interestingly, those who reported ambiguity in the work role were 16.5 times more likely to develop neck and shoulder pain. This report is thus also evidence for the relationship between physical and psychosocial variables in MSD etiology.

Vingärd, Alfredsson, Goldie, and Hogstedt (1991), in a registry-based cohort study of people hospitalized for osteoarthritis within a 3-year period, compared men and women with high exposure to dynamic and static forces at the knee to those with low exposure. Occupations with significantly elevated relative risk of developing osteoarthritis were firefighters, farmers, and construction workers for men, and cleaners for women.

Finally, Armstrong and Chaffin (1979) studied the effects of hand size and work methods on the presence of CTS in two groups of female production sewers: one group with a history of CTS and the other group with no such history. These researchers found no correlation between hand size and CTS. However, individuals with a history of CTS were found to use higher hand forces and more frequent pinch grips during work than individuals with no history of CTS. Although we cannot be certain whether the use of higher forces and pinch grips is the cause or effect of CTS, it appears that force may play a role in MSDs in this group of workers.

The body's ability to generate and sustain muscle forces varies with body posture and body orientation and with grip determinants, such as the frictional characteristics of materials, and the wearing of gloves.

Frictional Forces

Frictional forces develop when one surface slides over another surface. Frictional forces that develop between two surfaces can play an additional role in the total force needed to move an object. The amount of force needed to produce motion of one surface relative to the other depends on how tightly the surfaces are pressed together and the texture and composition of each surface (LeVeau, 1992).

The *coefficient of friction* refers to the slipperiness between two objects or the effect of the texture of the materials on the overall force needed to move an object. Surfaces with a low coefficient of friction glide easily over each other, such as greased metal on metal and joint surfaces bathed by synovial fluid. Surfaces with a high coefficient of friction resist movement yet provide greater stability between the two objects. Examples of surfaces with a high coefficient of friction include rubber crutch tips on a wooden floor and sandpaper on skin (Buchholz, Frederick, & Armstrong, 1988a; LeVeau, 1992).

Friction is an important factor in determining the ability to grip and manipulate objects. When the coefficient of friction between an object and the hand is low, the object tends to slide out of the hand and thus requires higher grip forces to grasp and hold. For example, it is more difficult to open a jar with wet hands than with dry hands because the hands slip on the jar top. When a higher coefficient of friction exists between an object and the hands, lower hand forces are required to move or hold the surfaces. Therefore, use of a rubber pad to open a jar will make the task easier. Comaish and Bottoms (1971) suggest that individuals sense frictional forces between objects and adjust grip forces accordingly.

Knowledge of the coefficient of friction is relevant to the design of tool handles, controls, and assembly jobs. Each condition must be examined carefully, since the moistness of the hands will differentially interact with the properties of the materials to increase or decrease the overall coefficient of friction and related grasp. Buchholz et al. (1988a) and O'Meara and Smith (2001) studied coefficient of friction properties between common materials and human skin. Buchholz et al. (1988a) found that pinch forces decrease when moist hands rather than dry hands grasp *porous materials* such as suede, adhesive tape, and paper because the coefficient of friction between moist hands and these materials is relatively high. Table 10-2 outlines the coefficient of friction for human skin against common materials.

O'Meara and Smith (2001) examined the coefficient of friction between human skin and five grab rail materials (chrome, stainless steel, powder-coated steel, textured aluminum, and knurled steel) under conditions of dry, wet, and soapy hands. As expected, the grip force required to grasp the grab rails when the hands were soapy was significantly higher than when the hands were dry. When researchers examined the best grab rail materials for soapy hands, the two textured materials—textured aluminum and knurled steel—displayed superior frictional properties.

Researchers recommend that adhesive tape, suede, or texturing be added to surfaces for handling materials in industrial environments with high moisture or heat indices (Buchholz et al., 1988a; O'Meara & Smith, 2001) (see Chapter 11 for further discussion on tool handles).

Gloves

Most research suggests that gloves increase grip force requirements for several reasons. First, the addition of glove material between hand and

Table 10-2

Coefficients of Friction for Common Materials Against Human Skin

Material	Dry (n = 42)	Moist (n = 42)	Combined (n = 84)
Sandpaper (no. 320)	—	—	0.61 + 0.10
Smooth vinyl	—	—	0.53 + 0.18
Textured vinyl	—	—	0.50 + 0.11
Adhesive tape	0.41 + 0.10	0.66 + 0.14	—
Suede	0.39 + 0.06	0.66 + .011	—
Aluminum	—	—	0.38 + 0.13
Paper	0.27 + 0.09	0.42 + 0.07	—

tool handle increases the effective diameter of the handle, often outside the diameter range allowing maximal output grip force for a given muscle force (Buchholz, Wells, & Armstrong, 1988b). Thus, to maintain the required output force, greater internal muscle forces are required. In fact, Hertzberg's (1955) study of airline pilots found that pilots exerted 25% to 30% more force to overcome the bulkiness of the gloves. More broadly, Tichauer (1978) explains that the use of bulky gloves may lead to inadequate control of the hands when operating tools or dials and difficulty sustaining objects in the hand. In addition, gloves may interfere with the tactile feedback necessary to determine the appropriate grip force; therefore, individuals tend to grip harder than is necessary to accomplish a task. Finally, Buchholz et al. (1988a) suggest that gloves often reduce the coefficient of friction between the hand and the surface and thus require higher grip forces.

Armstrong and Ulin (1995) suggest that the use of gloves be reviewed to ensure the proper use and design. For example, when only palm protection is required, the fingers to the gloves may be removed. Likewise, if only finger protection is required, tape may be applied to the fingers for sufficient protection. Testing should be performed prior to use for the optimum performance.

Measurement of Force

Force can be measured or estimated in a number of ways. Most job analyses estimate the external forces needed to accomplish a given task by identifying the weight of an object, the location of an object, the distance carried, and the duration of the action. Portable equipment for measuring force includes scales, torque wrenches, and force gauges (Keyserling et al., 1991). Spring scales measure the weight of objects being lifted or held. Torque wrenches identify the torque required to loosen or tighten a threaded fastener. Handheld digital force gauges measure the push or pull forces in a worksite. Hoozemans, van der Beek, Frings-Dresen, and van der Molen (2001) report that the use of a handheld force gauge yields valid results for workplace job analyses when firmly applied to the object being pushed. This approach identifies the workplace demands or external force that a worker must generate to complete a task. However, this method does not indicate the exertion perceived by the individual worker. The preceding discussion outlines the pitfalls in translating external force measurement into an estimate of internal forces, the true measure of tissue risk.

Another method of analyzing external force involves placing a pressure-sensitive gauge at the point of contact of the force. To measure hand or finger forces, small force-sensitive resistors (FSRs) are attached to the hands or gloves while the individual performs a task. This allows for direct measurement of the forces on the hands or fingers (Joseph & Bloswick, 1991).

The internal forces (or the actual muscle requirements of the job) can be estimated using surface electromyography (sEMG). (See Chapter 9 for a discussion of sEMG.) Surface electrodes are placed over the muscles involved, and these record the sum of all motor unit potentials reaching the electrode (Chaffin & Andersson, 1984). For a more precise estimation of motor units or deep muscle activity, fine-wire EMG measurements can be obtained by inserting thin electrodes into the actual tissue of interest, rather than relying on the surface measurement of electrical activity.

Psychophysical Methods to Estimate Force

Studies often associate lifting tasks with scales of perceived exertion to rate the degree of discomfort or force that workers associate with the task. Psychophysical methods have been used to identify workers' perceptions of acceptable lifting load limits (Ciriello, Snook, Blick, & Wilkinson, 1990), to determine the extent of bodily discomfort associated with their tasks (Dimov et al., 2000), and to predict overexertion injury at work (Herrin, Jaraiedi, & Anderson,

1986). The Borg Rating of Perceived Exertion (RPE) and the Borg CR-10 scales are the most widely used in industry. The RPE scale is a 15-unit scale (ratings from 6 to 20) designed to rate exercise intensity, perception of physical strain, and fatigue (Figure 10-4) (Borg, 1990; Borg, 1982). The more recent Borg CR-10 scale (Category-Ratio) is a 10-level scale developed to meet demands of ratio scaling with estimations of intensity levels (Figure 10-5). The CR-10 scale equates verbal descriptors with positions on the scale according to a quantitative meaning. Both scales have shown strong correlations between the amount of weight a person lifts and the level of discomfort experienced. Ulin, Armstrong, Snook, and Franzblau (1993) suggest that workers' perceived exertion ratings be used similarly to develop the optimal work position and tool shape combination.

Borg's RPE Scale

6	No exertion at all
7	Extremely light
8	
9	Very light
10	
11	Light
12	
13	Somewhat hard
14	
15	Hard
16	
17	Very hard
18	
19	Extremely hard
20	Maximal exertion

Figure 10-4 Borg Rating of Perceived Exertion (RPE) Scale. A 15-level scale.

POSTURE

Posture is one of the most frequently cited risk factors for MSDs (Armstrong, 1986; Pheasant, 1991). Although the protective influence of neutral posture on employee health and productivity is recognized widely in ergonomic and manufacturing circles, a clear definition of what constitutes neutral posture remains elusive.

Norkin and Levangie (1992) discuss static and dynamic posture in biomechanical terms, noting that very little effort is required to sustain an upright, static posture. The motor control necessary to maintain dynamic posture, however, is very complex, dependent on tactile, articular, and proprioceptive feedback mechanisms. Optimal posture, in biomechanical terms, is that in which body segments are aligned vertically and the center of gravity passes through all joint axes. The compression forces of body segments in optimal posture are distributed evenly over weight-bearing surfaces, with no excessive

Borg's CR-10 Scale

0	Nothing at all	
.5	Extremely weak (just noticeable)	
1	Very weak	
2	Weak	(light)
3	Moderate	
4		
5	Strong	(heavy)
6		
7	Very strong	
8		
9		
10	Extremely strong (almost maximal)	
•	Maximal	

Figure 10-5 Borg CR-10 Scale. A category scale with ratio properties.

tension exerted on the ligaments and muscles. Although this definition is imprecise, it provides a basis for examining posture in any part of the body.

Corlett (1981) addresses posture in functional terms relative to the task being performed. Among the principles Corlett offers for workplace design that promotes good posture during work are upright head and neck positions for visual tasks, sitting or standing options, equal distribution of weight while standing, use of joints in midrange, work performed "below the level of the heart," and the ability of the worker to assume several safe and varied postures throughout the day.

Kroemer and Grandjean (2001) and Chaffin and Andersson (1984) present recommendations for specific body positions during work. These researchers more specifically suggest that the head and neck should be positioned at 10 to 15 degrees of neck flexion during visual work, shoulders flexed or abducted to no more than 30 degrees, elbows flexed to no more than 90 degrees, and other joints should be positioned in neutral for execution of tasks. The positions listed in Table 10-3 should be avoided if they will have to be maintained for long periods. Unfortunately, much of what has been touted as good posture in industry is derived from laboratory experiments that rarely simulate actual work settings.

Table 10-3

Work Postures to Avoid for Long Durations

Body Part	Posture to Avoid
Neck	Forward flexion ≥20 degrees
Shoulder	Flexion or abduction ≥30 degrees
	Extension and internal rotation
Elbow	Extreme elbow flexion
	Extreme supination and pronation with grasp
Wrist	Extreme flexion
	Extreme extension
	Ulnar or radial deviation with grasp
Fingers	Pinching or pressing with the fingertips
	Thumb extension

Haselgrave (1994) sought to bring functional and biomechanical aspects of posture together in a model influenced by Corlett (1981). This model proposes that individuals adopt a posture during work tasks according to the functional demands of the tasks and the individuals' anthropometric capabilities. This posture is modified by the physical and spatial constraints within the working environment. Haselgrave (1994) explains that workers first position themselves according to the primary demands of the task. For example, sewing machine operators must view the material closely and therefore work in extremes of neck and trunk flexion and shoulder abduction. Because visual demands are the greatest priority, neck and trunk flexion postures take precedence over other body postures.

The primary demands of the task are also the primary points of interaction between the worker and the workplace. When the task demands (e.g., high precision and high speed) are in conflict, the worker assumes a position of compromise between the least body discomfort and the quickest manner in which to perform the task, which may also be the most hazardous. Haselgrave (1994) summarizes that "posture therefore arises from the functional demands of vision, reach, manipulation, strength, and endurance, and is constrained by the geometric relationship between the person's own anthropometry and the layout of the workplace." (See Haselgrave [1994] for a complete discussion of this model.)

Two technical aspects of posture are related to MSDs. Static postures involve maintaining the same position for relatively long periods of time; awkward postures involve working in a position that is deviated from neutral. Both concepts are discussed next.

Awkward Postures

Concepts Related to "Neutral Posture"

Although most ergonomic textbooks advise the practitioner to design work that limits time spent in nonneutral joint angles, the term *nonneutral posture* should be seen only as a first approximation of a stressful, awkward posture for several reasons. First, neutral posture is generally defined in terms of muscle length, although joint angles have implications for other tissues. What is considered optimal for one tissue may not be the optimal joint angle for another. For example, a roughly 90 degrees elbow angle satisfies both of the preceding criteria (best biomechanical geometry and physiologic muscle length) for optimal biceps activity. But that posture may stretch the ulnar nerve against the elbow, suggesting that a more open elbow angle is necessary for optimal nerve function and safety. Similarly, a position of 90 degrees of abduction and external rotation of the shoulder may put some shoulder muscles (e.g., the deltoids) in a relatively "neutral" posture but can expose the brachioplexus to compressive forces from other muscles and anatomic structures. This posture can also entrap the tendon of the supraspinatus muscle between the acromion and the head of the humerus (Hagberg, 1981). To fully characterize the degree to which a posture is awkward, it is necessary to take an integrated overview of the tissues involved, defining which muscles and other tissues are involved in the position and what the implications are for tissue damage.

Second, most body exertions involve more than one muscle, each of which may be in optimal biomechanical and length relationship at a different joint angle. Third, the body can adopt postures that are not necessarily the optimal biomechanical or length-tension relationships for muscles but that result in the lowest sum of muscle activation to stabilize body parts against gravity.

With these concerns in mind, Kourinka and Forcier (1995) separate awkward postures into the following three concepts, which may characterize a particular posture in combination or alone.

- *Extreme postures*. The NIOSH review of epidemiologic evidence (Bernard, 1997) uses this term to describe joint positions close to the ends of the range of motion. They require more support, either by passive tissues (e.g., ligaments and passive elements of the muscles) or increased muscle force. These positions may also exert compressive forces on either blood vessels or nerves or both. Note, however, that some joints, such as the knee, are designed to be used close to the range-of-motion extremes.
- *Nonextreme postures that expose the joint to loading from gravitational forces, requiring increased forces from muscles or load on other tissues*. For instance, holding the arm at 90 degrees to the body does not represent an extreme posture in terms of muscle length. But the position allows gravitational forces to exert a pull requiring roughly 10% of maximal strength from the associated muscles (Takala & Viikari-Juntura, 1991).
- *Nonextreme postures that change musculoskeletal geometry, increasing loading on tissues or reducing the tolerance of these tissues*. This third factor includes the reduction in available lever arm for muscles, described previously. An example of increased loading is provided by research (Smith, Sonstegard, & Anderson, 1977), demonstrating that even nonextreme wrist flexion can press the finger flexor tendons against the median nerve.

In addition, extreme postures can require elevated muscle activity simply to overcome the resistance of passive tissues. Zipp, Haider, Halpern, and Fohmert (1983) found that adopting an extremely pronated forearm position (such as that required by computer keyboard operation) requires high muscle activity, even without any external loading. Even nonextreme postures can trap tissues in injurious positions, as demonstrated again by the compression of the median nerve by finger flexor tendons when the wrist is in nonextreme flexion (Smith et al., 1977). Histologic changes (edema, thickening, fibrosis) occur in nerves at the site of compression injury and possibly at sites of bending around bony structures (e.g., the ulnar nerve at the elbow)

(Armstrong et al., 1984). Buchholz et al. (1988b) detail a sophisticated modeling approach that explains the measured increased muscle force demands associated with nonoptimal grip diameters (putting the fingers into awkward biomechanical relationships).

Work in awkward postures can be harmful when movements extend tissues beyond the normal range of motion, causing a tear or strain. Work is especially harmful when awkward movements are combined with force. The implications of nonneutral joint angles and muscle strength are discussed from two perspectives: physiologic and biomechanical.

Biomechanical and Physiologic Perspectives on Awkward Posture

Physiologic and biomechanical mechanisms affect the relationship between various postures the body assumes and its ability to generate forces. From a physiologic perspective, the *length-tension relationship* describes the ability of a muscle to generate tension and exert force on a bony lever. Norkin and Levangie (1992) explain that there is a direct relationship between the tension developed within the muscle and the length of the muscle at the time of contraction. A muscle contraction occurs when the smallest components of a muscle fiber—actin and myosin protein filaments—bind together to form a *cross-bridge*. The cross-bridge is considered the basic unit of active muscle tension. When the muscle is at its resting length (usually in midrange or neutral), actin and myosin filaments form the maximum number of cross-bridges and thus develop the maximal amount of muscle tension. When a muscle is lengthened, there is less overlap of the filaments and fewer cross-bridges form. Thus, only moderate tension develops within the muscle in its lengthened position. When the muscle is shortened, the cross-bridges have already been formed, so the muscle develops less tension. Therefore, as stated, use of a muscle in a lengthened or shortened position will require greater internal muscle forces than would be required to use a muscle in neutral (Chaffin & Andersson, 1984; Kroemer & Grandjean, 2001; LeVeau, 1992; Norkin & Levangie 1992). Figure 10-6 demonstrates that the maximal flexion forces at the elbow are generated closest to 90 degrees when the biceps muscle is at midrange (Kroemer & Grandjean, 2001). Ashton-Miller (1998) cites a number of studies demonstrating that a change of force direction as tendons pass around a pulley or over bony or ligamentous structures creates not only an increase in required muscle force but also shear forces and frictional forces experienced by tendons and tendon sheaths (Uchiyama, Coert, Berglund, Amadio, & An, 1995).

Biomechanical concepts related to lever systems and torque throughout the body also affect posture and the ability to develop muscle force. Torque *(T)*, or rotational force about a joint, is a function of the internal muscle force *(F)* multiplied by distance *(D)*, the shortest distance or length between the action line of

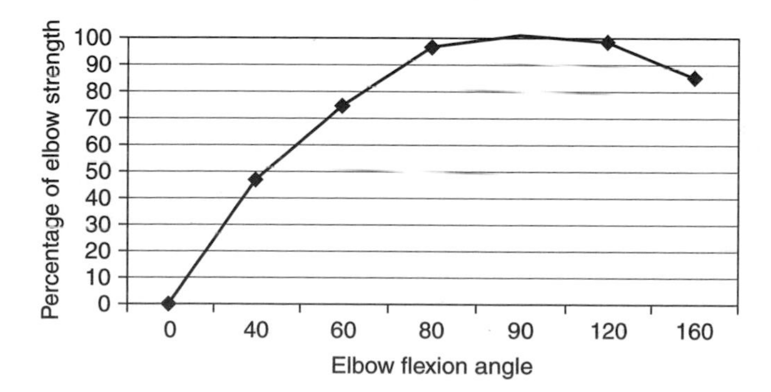

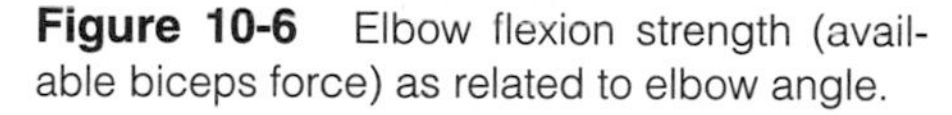
Figure 10-6 Elbow flexion strength (available biceps force) as related to elbow angle.

the muscle and the joint axis. This distance is also known as the *moment arm*. The moment arm is found by measuring the length of a line drawn from the joint axis perpendicular to the force vector of the muscle (Norkin & Levangie, 1992). When two bony segments are aligned at 90 degrees to each other, as in a neutral elbow posture, the moment arm is longest, and therefore the muscle produces the most torque. Figure 10-7 demonstrates that as two bony segments rotate from neutral into full flexion or extension, the moment arms become smaller. Thus, at a given muscle force, less torque is developed and less rotational force is executed on the segment (Chaffin & Andersson, 1984; LeVeau, 1992; Norkin & Levangie, 1992).

The following discussion addresses research relating to awkward and static postures of the neck and shoulder combined, shoulder, elbow, and wrist-hand.

Neck and Shoulders

Individuals unconsciously develop awkward neck and shoulder postures as a result of poor workplace ergonomics and personal work style (Barry, Woodhall, & Mahan, 1992). Typical neck and shoulder postures are forward flexion of the neck and protraction and internal rotation of the shoulders. These postures may cause localized pain as well as symptoms in the distal extremity, as evidenced in the NIOSH summary of upper-extremity MSDs (Bernard, 1997). The summary found evidence of a causal relationship between exposure to static or extreme postures and disorders of the neck and shoulder. Of the 15 studies that addressed postures, many with significant results were carried out on VDT workers (Bernard, Sauter, Petersen, Fine, & Hales, 1993; Kukkonen, Luopajärvi, & Riihimäki, 1983). The research on one of the largest study populations (Linton, 1990) examined 22,180 Swedish employees undergoing screening examinations at their occupational health care service. Combined exposures to uncomfortable posture and poor psychosocial work environment showed a risk for neck pain 3.5 times higher than employees in low-exposure jobs.

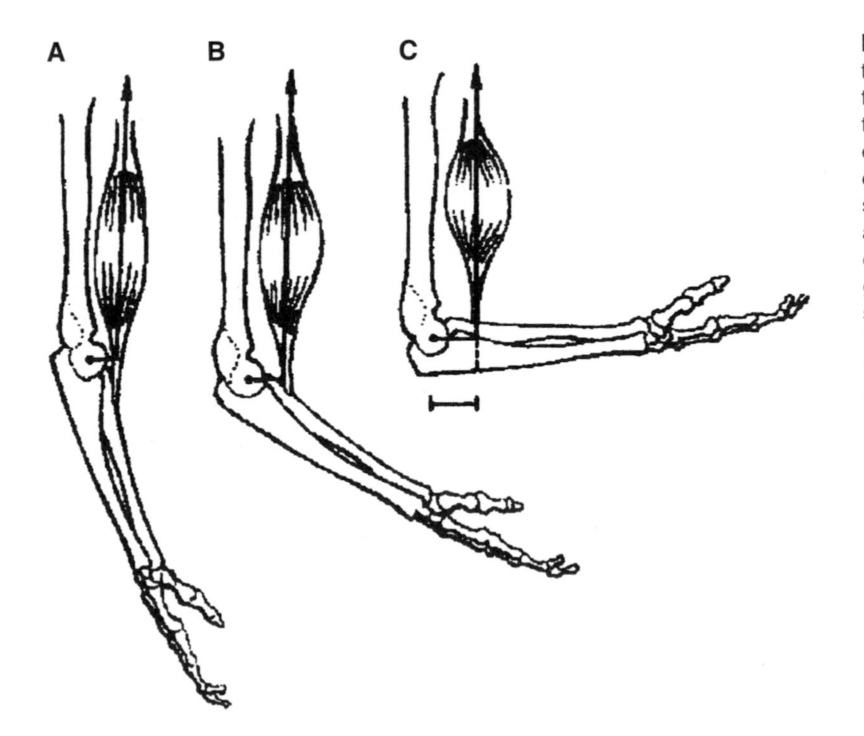

Figure 10-7 Moment arm of the biceps (the distance from the action line of muscle force to the joint axis) changes with elbow position. **A,** The elbow is extended and moment arm is small. **B,** At 45 degrees, moment arm becomes greater. **C,** At 90 degrees, the moment arm is greatest. (Redrawn with permission from LeVeau, B. F. [1992]. *Williams & Lissner's biomechanics of human motion* [3rd ed.]. Philadelphia: Saunders.)

Maeda, Hunting, and Grandjean (1980) examined the relationship between upper-extremity postures and musculoskeletal symptoms of 179 female keyboard operators and salespeople. The keyboard operators worked in a seated position with their necks flexed and rotated to the left for visual and inputting tasks. The salespeople spent each workday walking, standing, and bending down. Results of a survey indicated that the keyboard operators complained of stiffness and pain in the lumbar area and left side of the neck, as well as arm and hand pain (more so on the dominant side). Salespeople complained predominantly of torso and low-back pain. This study noted the effect of neck posture and static sitting on musculoskeletal complaints.

Dental hygienists also report a high prevalence of neck and shoulder pain during clinical work. In fact, up to 68% of all dental hygienists report painful neck and shoulder conditions that emanate from static, flexed postures throughout the day (Oberg & Oberg, 1993; Osborn, Newell, & Rudney, 1990). When Oberg (1993) performed a case analysis of the biomechanical factors that influenced one dental hygienist's pain, he found that a work position of 45 degrees neck flexion and 30 degrees lateral flexion to the right was associated with neck and shoulder pain. Biomechanical computation revealed that twice the muscle force is needed to support the head in forward flexion (50 N) than in a neutral, upright position (26.7 N). The total muscle force at the shoulder needed to support a position of 90 degrees shoulder abduction with 60 degrees elbow flexion during work is 186.7 N (Oberg, 1993). (See Chapter 22 for a complete discussion of dental hygiene.)

Shoulder

Workers use their shoulders in awkward positions when the work task involves overhead reaching, unsupported use of the hands away from the body, or performing a seated task in a chair that is too low, to name a few. The repetitive or prolonged use of shoulder flexion or abduction has been associated with localized fatigue and tendinitis in the biceps and supraspinatus muscles, as well as with decreased productivity (Hagberg, 1981; Putz-Anderson, 1988; Tichauer, 1978).

Hagberg (1981) demonstrated that workers who work with their shoulders in greater than 90 degrees of abduction rapidly develop fatigue in the upper trapezius muscle along with compensatory muscle patterns. Chaffin (1973) examined the relationship between muscle fatigue and arm abduction angle in healthy men and found that subjects fatigued in 15 minutes when using the arms at 90 degrees of abduction and in 30 minutes when using the arms at 60 degrees but did not fatigue after an hour when the arms were abducted to only 30 degrees.

When Tichauer (1978) examined the relationship between chair height and shoulder abduction angle, similar problems of fatigue and decreased efficiency were noted. Chair height that was 3 inches too low for the worker produced an arm abduction angle of 45 degrees and excessive shoulder movements in an effort to place the hand. Several hours of work in this position reduced workplace efficiency by as much as 50%.

Other epidemiologic studies demonstrate an association between awkward or extreme shoulder postures and work-related MSDs. Bjelle, Hagberg, and Michaelsson (1979) found a strong relationship between industrial work with hands at or above shoulder level and outcomes of shoulder tendinitis (OR: 11 times the risk of unexposed controls). Similar findings appeared in studies by Herberts, Kadefors, Andersson, and Petersen (1981) on shipyard welders (13 times increased risk) and shipyard plate workers (11 times increased risk). The referent group in these studies consisted of office workers. Results of these studies suggest that workers should maintain a position of less than 30 degrees of shoulder flexion or abduction during work activities.

Elbow

Although fewer studies have been performed on elbow postures than on the other parts of the body, results are notable. Tichauer (1978) studied the effect of various elbow positions on the elbow soreness of 38 workers who performed constant screwdriving. Sixty percent (23) of the workers who used their elbows in at least 130 degrees of elbow extension reported complaints of elbow pain, whereas no workers who used the elbow in 85 degrees or less of elbow flexion reported pain. Tichauer explained that the elbow-extended position incites excessive compressive forces within the joint that ultimately cause the pain. Tichauer notes that during rotational tasks, such as clockwise screwdriving, the biceps act to supinate the forearm. To maximize the ability of the biceps to exert this rotational force, the elbow should be positioned in 90 degrees of flexion.

Wrist

Work that incorporates extremes of wrist flexion and extension and radial and ulnar deviation may cause problems over time, especially when combined with grasp. During extremes of wrist flexion and extension, the nerves and structures within the carpal canal are displaced against the carpal bones and the flexor retinaculum. The human cadaver studies (Cobb et al., 1996) and healthy volunteer studies (Kier et al., 1998; Rempel et al., 1997) cited previously also demonstrate that nonneutral hand postures, combined with forceful loading of fingertips, result in elevated carpal tunnel pressures well within the range demonstrated to cause damage to animal neurons. Rempel et al. (1998) cite eight human studies measuring pressure in the carpal tunnel when the wrist is in a flexed or extended posture relative to a neutral posture. Most of these studies show elevation of carpal pressure, again into the range that causes damage in the animal studies.

Constant stretching and compression of the nerves against adjacent tissues may contribute to CTS. De Krom, Kester, Knipschild, and Spaans (1990) found this to be the case in a study identifying the risk factors for CTS. These researchers found CTS to be associated with exposure to activities with flexed or extended wrists. The risk ratio increased 4 to 5 times for those subjects engaged in such activities for more than 20 hours per week.

The effects of wrist deviation on hand force and symptom development have been widely studied. Tichauer (1978) studied the outbreak of de Quervain's disease in wiring operators at a Western Electric plant and found the outbreak to be associated with the use of needle-nosed pliers. When Tichauer redesigned the pliers to include a bent handle, the prevalence of tenosynovitis dropped considerably. Only 10% of the new workers who used the bent-handled tool developed tenosynovitis after 12 weeks of work, whereas 60% of those workers who used the traditional pliers developed tenosynovitis after 12 weeks.

Similarly, Armstrong, Foulke, Joseph, and Goldstein (1982) found that poultry workers were developing CTS-like symptoms at an alarming incidence rate of 17.4 cases per 200,000 hours (the plant average was 12.8). A worksite evaluation revealed that workers were using a straight-handled knife to cut poultry thighs vertically, which demanded extremes of wrist flexion and ulnar deviation. Further, high forces were used to hold and cut the thighs. Researchers recommended a pistol-grip knife design with a wraparound handle to neutralize the wrist posture and allow the hand to relax between exertions. The Luopajärvi et al. (1979) study cited in the Repetition section assessed a combined exposure of awkward postures, static postures, and repetitive motions. This cross-sectional study of female assembly-line packers, compared with department store shop assistants, found a 7.1 times increased risk for hand-wrist tendinitis. Results of these studies indicate that the wrist should be used in neutral position whenever possible

In summary, the preceding studies also support the conclusion that a combination of risk factors carries increased risk for the development of a MSD. In particular, the studies reviewed provide strong evidence for the causal relationship of combined risk factors (especially force, postural stressors, and repetition) with disorders of the elbow, CTS, and hand-wrist tendinitis.

Static Postures

The impact of static muscle loads on musculoskeletal pain has come to the forefront, particularly in precise or sedentary work that requires proximal low-level muscle tension or constrained work postures over long periods. Static postures are those postures held over a period of time that resist the force of gravity or stabilize a work piece or body part. Static postures require isometric muscle force (exertion without accompanying movement). Examples of static work include performing fine manipulations away from the body, holding objects in the arms, placing body weight on one leg while operating a pedal with the other, maintaining an extended or flexed position of the head for long periods of time, and standing in one place for long periods (Kroemer & Grandjean, 2001). Both static and dynamic muscle components are inherent in precision work as the body must be stabilized proximally for distal control. Research cited in the preceding section highlights the fact that awkward and static postures often occur together in the occupational setting, together with repetitive work (Luopajärvi, 1990; Milerad & Erickson, 1994). Many of the mechanisms relevant to awkward postures apply, but the duration of muscle exertion is increased, blood flow is more drastically reduced, and the temporal profile of exposure is usually made worse by the reduction in rest breaks and opportunity for recovery time.

Although static work would appear less fatiguing than dynamic work, the opposite is actually true. Dynamic work involves a rhythmic contraction and relaxation of the muscle that enables an exchange of blood flow, nutrients, and muscle wastes (Kroemer & Grandjean, 2001). Static work can be particularly stressful to the musculoskeletal system. Static work involves a prolonged state of contraction during which no movement is being performed. During static contractions, the internal pressure of muscle tissue compresses blood vessels and reduces blood flow to that muscle so that the oxygen and energy supply to the muscle is decreased. The waste products from the muscle accumulate, causing muscle fatigue and, eventually, pain. The blood flow is constricted in proportion to the exertion and duration of forces (Kroemer & Grandjean, 2001; Luopajärvi, 1990).

Laboratory studies provide plausible hypotheses for the mechanism that may explain the mechanism through which chronic reduction of blood flow from static contractions may lead to MSDs. Several studies have found that the small, slow motor units in clients with chronic muscle pain show changes consistent with reduced local oxygen concentrations (Dennett & Fry, 1988; Larsson, Bengtsson, Bodegard, Hendriksson, & Larsson, 1988). Reduced blood flow and disruption of the transportation of nutrients and oxygen can produce intramuscular edema (Sjogaard et al., 1988). The effect can be compounded in situations in which recovery time between static contractions is insufficient. Eventually, a number of changes can result: muscle membrane damage, abnormal calcium homeostasis, an increase in free radicals, a rise in other inflammatory mediators, and degenerative changes (Sjogaard et al., 1988).

Further, the increased intramuscular pressure exerted on neural tissue may result in chronic decrement in nerve function. Lundborg, Gelberman, Minteer-Convery, Lee, and Hargens (1982) showed that a constant hydrostatic pressure (i.e., during a static muscle contraction) of between 30 and 60 mm Hg reduces microcirculation of the nerve and compromises nerve conduction. This suggests the possibility of chronic blood vessel and nerve compression during static tasks.

Maximal Holding Time

Researchers use the term *maximal holding time* to refer to the duration that a static posture can be maintained continuously before fatigue sets in (Rodgers, 1987, 1988). The maximal holding time of a muscle as related to percent MVC has been the subject of many research studies with great variation in terms of recommendations. The maximal holding time varies with the muscle effort required of the most highly loaded muscle groups. Some investigators (Rohmert, 1973; Byström & Kilböm, 1990) find that muscle contractions can be maintained for prolonged periods if kept below 20% of MVC. However, Kroemer and Grandjean (2001) and Armstrong and Chaffin (1979) contend that muscles cannot sustain static contractions of 15% to 20% MVC for more than a few minutes before interruptions of blood flow and muscle fatigue ensue. Other investigators (Westgaard & Aarås, 1984) find chronic deleterious effects of contractions even when lower than 5% of MVC. Luopajärvi (1990) suggests that no more than 5% to 6% of the MVC should be sustained for work lasting more than 1 hour. This latter finding is supported by the observation that low-level static loading (such as shoulder loading in keyboard tasks) is associated with shoulder MSDs (Aarås, Horgen, Bjorset, Ro, & Thoresen, 1998).

Sjogaard et al. (1988) studied the effect of static work on blood flow, blood pressure, and intramuscular pressure in exercising muscles performed at contractions of 5% to 50% of the subjects' MVC. Blood flow was sufficient to maintain the muscle at low-level contractions (10% MVC). However, intramuscular changes (such as changes in water content or potassium depletion) caused muscle fatigue at prolonged low levels of exertion. Impaired blood flow appeared to be the cause of fatigue at sustained high levels of effort (>30% MVC).

Related Research on Static Posture and MSDs

Since the NIOSH summary (Bernard, 1997) did not distinguish between awkward and static postures, the summary cited previously applies here as well. In addition to the NIOSH summary, other epidemiologic studies demonstrate an association between static contractions or prolonged static load and work-related MSDs. In a review of the epidemiologic evidence for three neck-related MSDs, the contributors to Kourinka and Forcier (1995) report consistent associations between exposures to static head and arm postures and outcomes of tension neck syndrome. Grieco, Molteni, De Vito, and Sias (1998) also report associations between static work and tension neck syndrome in several different occupations. Looking at the neck region more generally, Hales and Bernard (1996) report several studies showing consistent association between neck disorders and work involving static or constrained postures. A review of neck studies by Hidalgo, Genaidy, Huston, and Arantes (1992) proposes that prolonged static contraction of neck muscles be limited to force levels at or below 1% of MVC, since the evidence indicates that MSDs can occur even at that level of static contraction. In an intervention study, Aarås et al. (1998) found that introduction of a workstation arrangement that allowed forearm support (thus lowering static load on the shoulders) reduced trapezius muscle activity from 1.5% to 0.3% of MVC and was associated with a reduction in neck pain.

Posture Assessment

The primary means of assessing posture are observation and recording of workers through observation or through the use of video camera equipment. Once postures are observed, various schemes have been developed to record and describe workers' postures for clinical and research purposes. In most schemes, joint angles, duration times, and frequency of efforts are measured. Rodgers (1988) suggests that several workers, including highly skilled and less skilled workers, should be videotaped when one is assessing the physical components of a job to determine variability in work methods.

Posture Targeting

Posture targeting is an assessment method developed by Corlett, Madeley, and Manenica (1979) and used in numerous studies in Scandinavia (Oberg & Oberg, 1993). As demonstrated in Figure 10-8, this method uses a body diagram with 10 prearranged concentric circles or targets placed alongside the body parts. The individual is observed, and the posture for each body part is recorded as 45 degrees, 90 degrees, or 135 degrees from the target center. The postures are estimated from the standard, anatomic position provided by the body diagram. Movements in the sagittal plane (forward or backward) require a mark along the vertical axis; movements to the side of the body are marked along the horizontal axis. Changes in the postures of specific body parts can be documented throughout the duration of a shift. The reader is referred to Corlett (1990; Corlett et al., 1979) for complete discussions of this approach.

Postural Analysis Tools

More recently, tools have been developed to analyze workers' postures with the goal of easily identifying those postures (with minimal equipment) that most place a worker at risk for developing an MSD. The Ovaco Steelworks in Finland developed a simple postural analysis tool to be used by ergonomics teams in identifying risks called the Ovaco Working Posture Analysis System (OWAS) (Karhu, Kansi, & Kuorinka, 1977). This method provides the analyst with a graphic presentation of body silhouettes, allowing rating of upper extremity, trunk, and leg postures. This method is particularly applicable to large muscle, whole body positions. Building on this method, researchers at the University of Massachusetts, Lowell, developed the PATH (Posture, Activity, Tool &

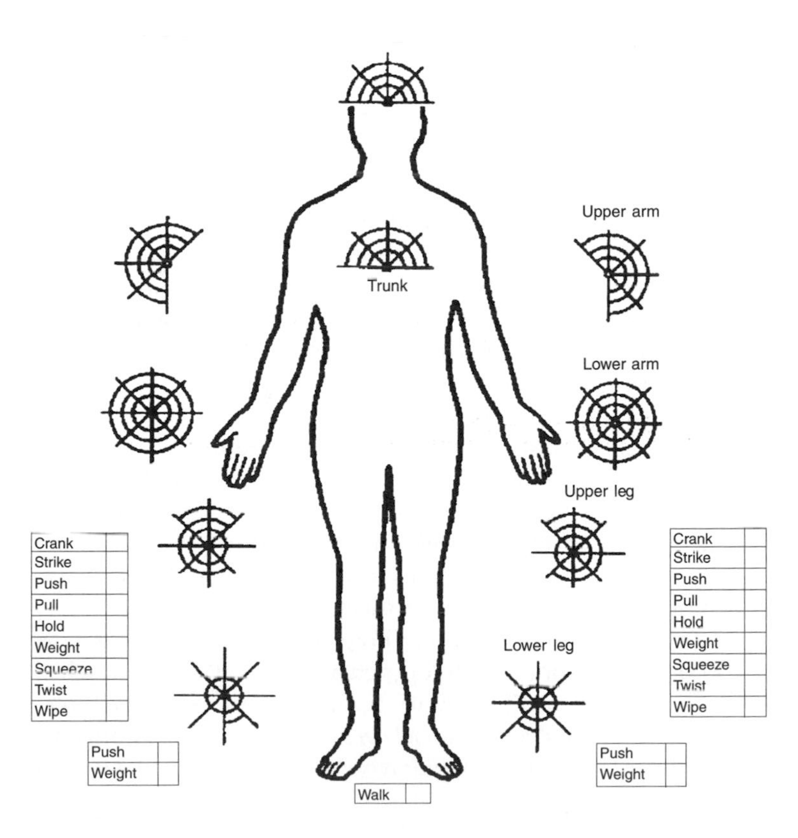

Figure 10-8 Posture-targeting diagram. Targets adjacent to each body part are used to record deviations from the standard position. (Reprinted with permission from Corlett, E. N., Madeley, S. J., & Manenica, I. [1979]. Posture targeting: A technique for recording working postures. *Ergonomics, 22,* 357–366.)

Hand) assessment tool, combining a simple checklist with a work sampling procedure (analyzing mental snapshots at fixed intervals) to provide more detailed posture and activity assessment for nonrepetitive jobs (Buchholz, Pacquet, Punnett, Lee, & Moir, 1996).

The proposed 1999 OSHA Ergonomic Rule suggested the use of six existing posture analysis tools, outlined in Table 10-4, as being appropriate for use by the recommended joint labor-management ergonomic teams. Several of these posture analysis tools are as follows.

- Rapid Upper Limb Assessment (RULA) was developed as a quick assessment of the postures of the neck, trunk, and upper extremities incorporating muscle function and loads placed on the body. Postures are identified from diagrams and coded according to ranges of motion (McAtamney & Corlett, 1993).
- Rapid Entire Body Assessment (REBA) divides the body into six parts to be coded with body diagrams that depict gross measures of movement. It is designed to be used in a variety of tasks that involve static, dynamic, and rapidly changing postures such as health care (Hignett & McAtamney, 2000).
- Revised NIOSH Lifting Equation is a comprehensive lifting equation that estimates a safe weight limit for a worker to lift, given six specific features of a given job task: horizontal distance of the load from the worker's ankles, vertical distance from the floor (at lift origin or destination, whichever is more stressful), distance lifted, frequency of lifting, angle of body rotation, and quality of the grip (Waters, Putz-Anderson, & Garg, 1994).
- Strain Index (SI) is a semiquantitative tool that assesses the risk of developing a distal upper-extremity MSD for a given job. The tool assesses six task variables, assigns a rating for each variable, and then determines an overall Strain Index score (Moore & Garg, 1995).

  Other assessments include the following.
- Concise Exposure Index (OCRA) calculates the exposure to repetitive movements of the upper extremity and groups together various combinations of exposure to risks that may contribute to MSDs (Occipinti, 1998). OCRA has shown predictive qualities in its assessment of performance risk for MSDs (Grieco, 1998).

Self-Analysis Checklist

Luopajärvi (1990) notes that workers themselves need to be more involved with the identification and correction of postures in the workplace. Self-analysis checklists have been developed for typists, data operators, and cashiers as part of an informational booklet that describes the optimal work environment, ergonomic recommendations, and advice on how to improve the existing work situation. The purpose of the booklet is to encourage both the worker and the supervisor to collaborate in making improvements in the workplace. Numerous self-report instruments have been developed for use in large epidemiologic studies. There is an ongoing discussion about the limits of their accuracy and validity; they appear to be useful in generating at least broad-brush profiles of exposure. Punnett & van der Beek (2000) found that the sum of self-reported exposures was strongly associated with subsequent incidence of MSDs. In addition, self-report instruments use the individual's ability to create a summary measure of risk, integrating many sources of risk simultaneously, some of which might be missed by an external observer.

Film- and Video-Based Systems

Awkward and static postures can be documented through the use of Polaroid film with a grid background to identify asymmetries in worker postures. The Healthcam offers a reliable method for measuring posture at specific joints, using a grid as a point of reference. Several more sophisticated programs are avail-able that allow practitioners to capture frames from videotapes and automatically generate joint angles from lines the observer draws on the image by clicking the

Table 10-4
Job Hazard Analysis Tools

Job Hazard Analysis Tools	Source*	Risk Factors Evaluated	Areas of Body Addressed	Examples of Jobs to which Tool Applies
Job Strain Index	"The Strain Index: A Proposed Method to Analyze Jobs for Risk of Distal Upper Extremity Disorders." Moore, J. S., & Garg, A., (1995). *AIHA Journal, 56*(5), 443–458. You may obtain a copy from: American Industrial Hygienists Association, 2700 Prosperity Ave., Suite 250, Fairfax, VA 22031. Phone: (703) 849-8888. http://www.aiha.org/ See also: http://sg-www.satx.disa.mil/hscoemo/tools/strain.htm and http://hsu.usf.edu/~tbernard/HollowHills/StrainIndexM12.pdf	Repetition Force Awkward postures	Hands Wrists	Small parts assembly Inspecting Meatpacking Data processing Sewing Packaging Keyboarding Jobs involving highly repetitive hand motions Dental hygiene
Revised NIOSH Lifting Equation	"Applications Manual for the Revised NIOSH Lifting Equation." Waters, T. R., Putz-Anderson, V., & Garg, A. (1994). National Institute for Occupational Safety and Health, January (DHHS, NIOSH Publication No. 94-110). Obtain a copy from: U.S. Department of Commerce, Technology Administration National Technical Information, 5285 Port Royal Road, Springfield, VA 22161. (NTIS Pub. No. PB01 176030) Phone: (703) 487-4650. www.cdc.gov/niosh/ See also: http://industrialhygiene.com/calc/lift.htm for a web-based version of this tool.	Repetition Force Awkward postures	Lower back	Package sorting, handling Package delivery Beverage delivery Assembly work Manual handling Lifting weights >10 lbs. Production jobs Laundry work Stationary lifting
Rapid Entire Body Assessment (REBA)	"Rapid Entire Body Assessment (REBA)," Hignett, S., & McAtamney, L. (2000). *Applied Ergonomics, 31,* 201–205. You may obtain a copy from: Elsevier Science, Regional Sales Office, Customer Support Department, P.O. Box 945, New York, NY 10159. Phone: (212) 633-3730. Web site: http://www.elsevier.com/	Repetition Force Awkward postures	Wrists Forearms Elbows Shoulders Neck Trunk Back Legs Knees	Patient lifting, transfer Nurses Nurses aides Orderlies Janitors Housekeeping Grocery warehouse Grocery cashier Telephone operator Ultrasound technicians Dentists Dental hygienists Veterinarians

Continued

Table 10-4
Job Hazard Analysis Tools—cont'd

Job Hazard Analysis Tools	Source*	Risk Factors Evaluated	Areas of Body Addressed	Examples of Jobs to which Tool Applies
Rapid Upper Limb Assessment (RULA)	"RULA: A Survey Method for the Investigation of Work-Related Upper Limb Disorders," McAtamney, L., & Corlett, E. N. (1993). *Applied Ergonomics, 24*(2), 91–99. You may obtain a copy from: Elsevier Science, Regional Sales Office, Customer Support Department, P.O. Box 945, New York, NY 10159. Phone: (212) 633-3730. Web site: http://www.elsevier.com/	Repetition Force Awkward postures	Wrists Forearms Elbows Shoulders Neck Trunk	Assembly work Production work Sewing Janitorial Maintenance Meatpacking Grocery cashier Telephone operator Dentists Dental hygienists
ACGIH Hand/ Arm Vibration TLV	1998 Threshold Limit Values for Physical Agents in the Work Environment, 1998 *TL Vs® and BEIs® Threshold Limit Values for Chemical Substances and Physical Agents Biological Exposure Indices,* pp. 109–131, American Conference of Governmental Industrial Hygienists. You may obtain a copy from: American Conference of Governmental Industrial Hygienists, Inc., 1330 Kemper Meadow Dr., Suite 600, Cincinnati, OH 45240. Phone: (513) 742-2020. Web site: http://www.acgih.org/	Vibration	Hands Arms Shoulders	Grinding Sanding Chipping Drilling Sawing Jigsawing Hand tools Chainsawing Production work using vibrating or power hand tools Regular use of vibrating hand tools
Washington State Appendix B	WAC 296-62-05174, "Appendix B: Criteria for Analyzing and Reducing WMSD Hazards for Employers Who Choose the Specific Performance Approach," Washington State Department of Labor and Industries, May 2000. You may obtain a copy from: Washington Department of Labor and Industries, P.O. Box 44001, Olympia, Washington 98504. Phone: (360) 902-4200 Web site: http://www.lni.wa.gov/wisha/	Repetition Force Awkward postures Contact stress Vibration	Hands Wrists Forearms Elbows Shoulders Neck Trunk Back Legs Knees	Assembly work Production work Sewing Meatpacking Keyboarding data Small parts assembly Maintenance Patient lifting Package delivery Packaging Garbage collection Food service Regular use of vibrating hand tools

*This table originally appeared as Appendix D-1 in the Ergonomic Standard, §1910.900 that was rescinded in 2001. These documents may be inspected at the Occupational Safety and Health Administration, Technical Data Center, Room N2625, 200 Constitution Ave., N.W., Washington, DC 20210, or at the Office of the Federal Register, 800 North Capitol Street, N.W., Suite 700, Washington, DC. Some URLs have been updated.

mouse on joint centers or markers. Investigators at the University of Wisconsin have developed a computerized system to analyze motion and postures in real time from running videotape (Ergonomics Analysis and Design Research Consortium, 1998). This system has the obvious advantage over still-frame systems of allowing characterization of repetition rates, speed of motion, and relative percentage of time spent in dynamic and static postures.

Computerized Motion Analysis Systems

Recent biomechanical analyses routinely use systems developed originally for gait analysis. These digital image capture systems rely on tracking markers placed on joint centers with several cameras, thus producing a real-time, 3-D computer model of the worker. These systems thus allow extremely detailed analysis of joint positions, as well as velocity and acceleration of body segments. Some systems use active markers that produce their own light. Others use reflective markers to capture reflected infrared light emitted by sources in the cameras. Electrogoniometry and accelerometer, methods that rely on small transducers taped to joints or body segments to measure joint motion, also allow precise measurement of motion parameters. Marras and Granata (1995), Marras et al. (1995), and Marras and Schoenmarklin (1993) have adapted electrogoniometry to back motion analysis, using a triaxial goniometric device resembling a spine strapped to the subject. This level of detail is expensive and not cost-effective for most job analyses or epidemiologic studies, but the instrumentation is ideal for laboratory research on human biodynamics and applied research characterizing risk profiles of, for example, tools and consumer products.

DYNAMIC FACTORS

It is only recently that research has added characteristics of motion, itself, to the list of biomechanical risk factors. Motion of body segments consists of both linear motion and rotational motion around a joint. Present research addresses the effects of kinematic posture measures: both angular and linear velocity (speed of motion) and acceleration (rate at which velocity increases or decreases). It is possible that, to a degree, measured acceleration and velocity are surrogates for increased force and postural risk factors. For example, Marras and Granata (1995, 1997) find that increased velocity and acceleration in trunk lateral bending and twisting result in measurable increases in both compressive and shear forces experienced by the intervertebral disks. But dynamic factors themselves may result in increased tendon travel and irritation. Viscoelastic soft tissues, such as tendons, spinal discs, and ligaments, have a fixed, intrinsic capacity to regain resting dimensions after stretching. Brief movement cycles may involve peak accelerations that can exceed tissue elasticity limits during an otherwise moderate task. The biodynamic literature suggests that, even in tasks performed for a short time, the acceleration and velocity of movements may pose risks that would not be predicted by the muscle forces or joint angles alone.

Most research on dynamic factors has been carried out on low-back injury. Sudden maximal lifting effort and unguarded movements appear to be risks for developing work-related low-back pain (Magora & Schwartz, 1976). Marras and Schoenmarklin (1993) also implicate dynamic factors in wrist MSDs. Using a job-based analytic design, they found that angular velocity of wrist extension and angular acceleration of wrist flexion could distinguish between jobs having high and low prevalence of CTS. Szabo and Chidgey (1989) found that repetitive, passive wrist flexion and extension resulted in higher pressures in the carpal tunnel. These elevated pressures took longer to return to normal in their CTS clients than in normal subjects. These investigators also found evidence that, if the wrist and finger motions are active (in other words, if the subject rather than the investigator moves the wrist), the effect may be larger.

MECHANICAL COMPRESSION

Earlier discussions have indicated the role in MSD etiology played by internal compressive forces, caused by intramuscular pressure and compression of tissues against adjacent anatomical structures. Internal pressure that results from injury-related swelling can also cause or exacerbate other MSDs.

External pressure placed on human tissue (from tool edges, tool handles, equipment, and workstation components) can also contribute to tendon, nerve and other soft-tissue injuries (Armstrong et al., 1982; Tichauer, 1966). During tool use, grip forces are transmitted to the soft-tissue structures underlying the tool. If a tool grip is even moderately sharp, the forces will be concentrated and transmitted to a small surface area, thus hastening pain and tissue damage to that area. These changes may themselves result in disease or predispose tissues to damage from other stressors. (See Chapter 11 for a complete discussion of tool design and recommendations.)

Common conditions that result from direct pressure on tissues are tenosynovitis and trigger finger. Tools such as short-handled pliers place pressure on the thenar eminence and may compress median nerve branches. Tools with inappropriately short handles, such as pliers and paint scrapers, can also apply substantial compressive forces to the blood vessels and in the palmar area, resulting in occlusion of the ulnar artery and possible ulnar neuropathy (Tichauer, 1966; Tichauer & Gage, 1977). Tools with ridged handles place pressure on the finger pulley system at the metacarpophalangeal and distal phalangeal joints. This pressure may cause irritation as the finger tendons move beneath the compressed pulleys.

Finger loops on tools such as scissors or tin cutters place direct pressure on the digital nerves lateral to the fingers. Prolonged pressure may cause localized paresthesias and tenderness. Gloves with elasticized wrists and expandable wristwatch bands place direct pressure on the median nerve at the carpal tunnel. Finally, leaning one's wrists or elbows on a table edge can also cause direct pressure to superficial structures.

Research Related to Mechanical Compression

A few epidemiologic studies have assessed the role of compression as a risk factor. Hypothenar hammer syndrome, characterized by signs of blood deprivation in the fingers, is caused by thrombosis or aneurysm in the ulnar artery or the superficial palmar arterial arch. This condition has been linked to the practice of using the palm as a hammer, exposing the palm to repetitive, forceful compression. Comparing vehicle maintenance workers who used their hands as a hammer to those who did not, Little and Ferguson (1972) calculated an increased risk for objectively verified (by a Doppler flow detector) ulnar artery block of 16.3. Nilsson, Hagberg, and Burström (1990) found a smaller effect (2.8 increased risk), comparing 890 plate workers to 61 office workers in the same plant. This study also found a dose-response relationship with increasing years on the job. However, inappropriate palm use and vibration exposure occurred together in this population.

Finelli (1975) describes the compression of an ulnar nerve branch in the palm by both occupational (tool handles) and nonoccupational (bicycle handle grips) exposures. Several investigators describe compression of the ulnar nerve at the elbow, caused by leaning the ulnar side of the elbow on a hard surface (Aguayo, 1975). In the shoulder, Nevasier (1980) found examples of tendinitis in individuals who habitually carried heavy loads (such as lumber) on their shoulders.

VIBRATION

Prolonged exposure to vibration from vibrating hand tools or surfaces has been known to affect workers' overall health and to contribute to hand-arm vibration syndrome (HAVS) in an average of 50% of all workers who use vibrating tools (NIOSH, 1989). In this section, we review the basic physical concepts of vibration, discuss the effects of vibration on the human body, and provide recommendations to decrease workers' exposure to vibration.

Physical Concepts of Vibration

Vibration is described as an oscillating motion of a body about its resting position. Vibration can be understood as a series of waves that oscillate at regular or irregular intervals in distinct patterns specific to the body or vibration source (Chaffin & Andersson, 1984; Kroemer & Grandjean, 2001). Vibration, when applied to the human body, causes oscillations in the body tissues and produces a bodily response. The response depends on a number of factors including the frequency, direction, intensity, acceleration, and point of application of the vibration and the posture of the body at the point of vibration contact.

Frequency and acceleration are commonly used to measure and define the vibrational waveform in meters per seconds squared. Acceleration is equated with the vibrational load or vibrational energy in a body; frequency and acceleration combine to produce a level of discomfort in the human body (Chaffin & Andersson, 1984; Kroemer & Grandjean, 2001; NIOSH, 1989).

Vibration sources can be broadly classified into two categories: free and forced vibration. *Free vibration* refers to the internal, natural oscillations of any body with elastic properties, such as human tissue. *Forced vibration* refers to the external, vibrating forces that are introduced to a body through sources such as vibrating tools or seats in trucks and heavy equipment. If an external vibrating force is applied to a body at or near its own natural frequency, the body will *resonate*, or vibrate at a higher amplitude than the original vibrating force applied. If vibration is applied to the body at other frequencies, the body will absorb or reduce the intensity of the vibration. This occurrence is called *damping* or *attenuation* (Chaffin & Andersson, 1984). Clearly, the frequencies of forced vibrations, such as those imposed by hand tools, that fall into the range of the natural resonant frequencies of the human body are of special concern to health care practitioners and safety specialists.

Classifications for human exposure to vibration are divided into two major categories, segmental and whole-body vibration. *Segmental vibration* is vibration transmitted through the hands. Segmental vibration appears to damage both the small, unmyelinated nerve fibers and the small blood vessels in the fingers, resulting in two specific diseases: vibration-induced white finger (VWF) and vibratory neuropathy. Together, these are called the hand-arm vibration syndrome (HAVS, see following). Segmental vibration is usually associated with use of high-frequency (= 50-Hz) power tools such as pneumatic drills, grinders, nut-runners, or chain saws.

Whole-body vibration is vibration transmitted through the lower extremities, buttocks, back, or the entire body, depending on whether the person is sitting or standing. Whole-body vibration is implicated in low-back disorders and a host of less well-understood symptoms. Whole-body vibration damage is associated with very low-frequency (= 4-Hz) oscillations, as are found in trucks, buses, or cars (Eastman Kodak Company, 1983; Kroemer & Grandjean, 2001).

Recent research suggests that vibration should be further subdivided into the following types, with different levels of association with HAVS.

- Harmonic or oscillatory vibration (caused by a constant driving source, such as a grinding wheel)
- Impact vibration (from a single impact)
- Percussive vibration (bursts of separable impacts, such as those produced by a pneumatic riveting tool)

It is possible that the thresholds for health effects of these three types of vibration are quite different, with impact and percussive vibration having physiologic effects at much lower measured exposure times (Cherniack & Mohr, 1994).

Effects of Vibration on the Body

As mentioned, human body parts oscillate at different natural frequencies and therefore react differently to various external, forced vibrations. Certain low-level, whole-body vibrations simulate the natural frequency of the neck and trunk and therefore resonate to other parts of the body. For example, frequencies from 4 to 8 Hz cause resonance in the head and trunk and amplify vibrational load to other body parts by more than 200%. Vibrations at higher frequencies are dampened by local body tissues, causing the vibrational energy to stay localized. Kroemer and Grandjean (2001) summarize the reaction of body parts to the following vertical, whole-body vibrations.

- 3 to 4 Hz: Resonance in the cervical vertebrae
- 4 Hz: Resonance in the lumbar vertebrae
- 5 Hz: Resonance in the shoulder girdle
- 5 to 30 Hz: Resonance between the head
- >30 Hz: Resonance in the arms, hands, and fingers
- 20 to 70 Hz: Resonance in the eyeballs
- 100 to 200 Hz: Resonance in the lower jaw

When vibration is applied to a specific muscle belly or tendon, a reflex contraction of the muscle occurs, called the *tonic vibration reflex* (TVR). The TVR reaches a plateau and is maintained after approximately 30 seconds of the application of vibration. Thereafter, the muscle contracts as long as the muscle is in contact with the vibrating source. Radwin, Armstrong, and Chaffin (1987) suggest that workers may use higher grip forces to accomplish a job because of the influence of the TVR and decreased tactile sensation in the fingers as a result of prolonged exposure.

Physiologic Effect

Whole-Body Vibration

Although each person reacts differently, somatic complaints from vibration seem to be frequency specific and related to the resonance produced in specific body parts. Whole-body vibration at very low frequencies (= 1 Hz) tends to produce feelings of seasickness. Frequencies between 1 and 4 Hz may cause difficulty breathing, whereas frequencies between 4 and 12 Hz may cause chest pain, back pain, and severe discomfort. Between 10 and 30 Hz, impairment in the visual field is most pronounced, causing blurred vision, headaches, and poor visual acuity. This may be especially worrisome to tractor, truck, and construction equipment drivers (Kroemer & Grandjean, 2001).

Laboratory research has demonstrated short-term and long-term vibration-related changes to human neural tissue. These effects include intraneural edema, structural changes in nonmyelinated fibers, demyelination, fibrosis, and even loss of axons (Stromberg, Dahlin, Brun, & Lundborg, 1997; Takeuchi, Takaya, & Imanishi, 1988).

Segmental Vibration

Three classes of effect caused by segmental vibration are indicated by the research literature.

- *Vascular effects.* Damage leading to premature vasoconstriction and insufficient circulation in the fingers gives rise to the original name for occupationally induced (sometimes called secondary) Raynaud's syndrome: vibration-induced white finger (VWF). In 1987, a consensus panel, meeting in Stockholm, coined the term hand-arm vibration syndrome (HAVS) to give equal weighting to neurologic symptoms (Gemne, Pyykko, Taylor, & Palmear, 1987).
- *Neurologic effects.* These effects involve damage to both the median nerve and to the small, unmyelinated nerve fibers in the fingers.
- *Musculoskeletal effects.* Kourinka and Forcier (1995) list a number of possible effects in this category, including impaired muscle strength and osteoarthrosis of some upper-extremity joints.

CTS and tendinitis are of great concern to workers using vibrating hand tools. Vibrational forces cause peripheral vascular and neural changes in the tissues affected by the vibration that may or may not return to normal, depending on the duration and intensity of the exposure. Reduced tactile sensitivity and the tonic vibration reflex combine to contribute to the use of high grip forces during repetitive manual tasks, which further increases the risk of chronic tendon and nerve disorders (Radwin et al., 1987).

HAVS (sometimes called secondary Raynaud's phenomenon or vibration white finger syndrome [VWF] is the term for chronic disorders most specifically associated with segmental vibration exposure. Raynaud's phenomena is a symptom of a vasospastic disorder characterized by cyanotic coloring or blanching of the skin in response to cold temperatures or stress with a gradual return of color with warming. HAVS involves peripheral neurovascular changes in response to long-term or intense vibration exposure. The vibration causes damage to the blood vessels in the affected area. The damage becomes particularly apparent during cold temperatures, when blood vessels have difficulty reopening after constricting. This chronic constriction of blood flow causes numbness and tingling in the fingers, blanching of the fingers on exposure to cold, pain following the eventual return of circulation, and reduced grip strength and finger dexterity.

These symptoms disappear initially when the hands are warmed and vibration exposure is reduced. However, finger pain, loss of sensitivity, and progressive loss of function remain potential threats if the condition is left untreated (Armstrong, Fine, Radwin, & Silverstein, 1987; NIOSH, 1989). Symptoms of HAVS, primary Raynaud's disease, and CTS can be difficult to differentiate because of the similarities of loss of tactile sensitivity and peripheral changes in all three conditions. If a worker has only conditions associated with vasospasm such as Raynaud's phenomena, then the worker has Raynaud's disease. Whereas primary Raynaud's disease is symmetric (NIOSH, 1989), the distribution of HAVS is usually asymmetric. The occurrence of HAVS may be affected by numerous variables, including the level of acceleration (vibrational load), frequency, and duration of tool use per day and cumulatively per month and year, and the ergonomics of tool use itself (NIOSH, 1989).

Research

Epidemiologic research has demonstrated a strong relationship between the use of vibrating tools and the occurrence of MSDs, including HAVS. A NIOSH summary (Bernard, 1997) finds strong evidence for a causal relationship between segmental vibration and HAVS. The best-designed study in this summary (Bovenzi et al., 1995) compared forestry workers with more than 400 hours of sawing to shipyard workers with no vibration exposure. These authors found increasing effect sizes, depending on the intensity of vibration exposure. Forestry workers using antivibration saws and those using no antivibration measures had an increased risk of 6.2 and 32.3, respectively. This study also found a dose-response relationship to number of years exposed. Nilsson et al. (1990), comparing platers with current vibration exposure to office workers in the same workplace, calculated an 85 times increased risk. Although these numbers have a wide range of variation, large effect sizes are characteristic of many vibration studies.

Studies of select populations using vibrating tools find high concentrations of vascular and neurologic symptoms compared to these in other working populations. Examples include shipyard workers (Cherniack, Letz, Gerr, Brammer, & Pace, 1990), surgeons (Cherniack & Mohr, 1994), and dental technicians (Hjortsburg, Rosen, Orbaek, Lundborg, & Valogh, 1989).

The NIOSH summary also found evidence for a causal link between segmental vibration and CTS. Chatterjee, Barwidk, and Petrie (1982), comparing 16 rock drillers to 15 controls unexposed to vibration, found a 10.9 times elevated risk for CTS, identified by nerve conduction. Weislander, Norbäck, Göthe, and Juhlin (1989), comparing 32 male CTS clients to population referents, found an increased risk for vibrating tool use of 6.1. Several other studies have also found an association between CTS and vibration exposure in jobs involving the use of vibrating tools, such as grinders and chipping hammers (Hagberg, Morgenstern, & Kelsh, 1992; Nathan, Meadows, & Doyle, 1988; Nilsson et al., 1990). In this literature, however, it is extremely difficult to separate the association of CTS and vibration from the association of CTS and the other biomechanical stressors that often are associated with these tools: awkward and static postures, repetition, and high force requirements.

Radwin et al. (1987) examined the relationship among tool vibration, tool weight, and grip force. In 14 subjects, these researchers investigated the effect of hand-tool vibration and tool weight on grip force and the effect of hand-tool vibration on the contraction of hand flexor muscles and extensor muscles during grip force. Results indicated that average grip increased from 25.3 N without vibration to 32.1 N at 40 Hz (27% increase) and to 27.1 N (7% increase) at 160 Hz. The TVR was found to be associated with activation of forearm muscles at specific grip forces.

Dimberg et al. (1989) studied the relationship between neck and upper-extremity symptoms and work-related factors in 2814 industrial workers. These investigators found that neck and upper-extremity symptoms were twice as prevalent in workers who used vibrating hand tools. Researchers suggested that the use of vibrating tools might also be associated with awkward hand positions, edema from the vibration, and reduced sensation, all of which necessitate increased grip force to hold the tool. (See NIOSH (1989) for a complete summary of research to that date.)

Finally, some literature has addressed the consequences of whole-body vibration exposure to other body parts. Jensen, Tuchsen, and Orhede (1996), studying a cohort of more than 89,000 drivers hospitalized for prolapsed cervical disks over 10 years, found a Standardized Hospitalization Ratio (SHR, similar in concept to an OR) of 142 compared to other male workers. The drivers' self-reported vibration exposure was 7.1 times that of the other workers.

Measurement

Assessment of vibration exposure is difficult because of the differences in hand-tool vibration frequencies, varied techniques among operators, and the problems of measuring vibration duration. Radwin et al. (1987) assert that vibration exposure must include not only the vibrational load from the tool itself but also the duration of the exposure and the worker's posture assumed while operating the tool. One must distinguish further between impact and nonimpact tools and include measurements of the vibration quantities along the three orthogonal axes.

Piezoelectric accelerometers are commonly used to measure vibration associated with hand-held tools (Bruel & Kjaer Instruments, 1993; NIOSH, 1989; Radwin & Armstrong, 1985). The vibrational measurement is taken at the point of contact with the body by placing sensors on the body part. The vibration oscillations impinge on the piezoelectric accelerometer and move a small mass against a crystal element. This crystal element produces an electrical current, the voltage of which is proportional to the acceleration of vibration. An amplifier may be used to overcome signal loss problems (NIOSH, 1989).

Once the vibration acceleration is determined, researchers can determine the daily exposure dose and the length of time after which a certain percentage of workers will demonstrate symptoms of HAVS. Recommendations for safe exposure limits calculate the duration of the exposure and the dose (acceleration in meters per second squared) energy equivalents as a logarithmic function. Charts that display acceleration limits as a function of frequency and exposure are found in the references provided.

NIOSH (1989) has not issued specific exposure limits but recommends strict medical monitoring to prevent the occurrence of HAVS or MSDs. NIOSH suggests that vibrational measurements should be based on a time-corrected, 4-hour equivalent to facilitate comparison of data between studies.

Recommendations to Decrease Vibration Exposures

Recommendations for decreasing vibration exposure involve engineering controls, workplace practices, protective clothing, and worker training (NIOSH, 1989). The following suggestions have been gleaned from Bonney (1981), NIOSH (1989), Brown (1990), and Hampel (1992).

Engineering Controls

- Keep machines well maintained. Imbalanced tools or loose fittings may increase vibration.
- Reduce tool vibrational load to the lowest level possible for efficient operation of the task.
- Provide counterbalances to reduce the forces needed to hold and manipulate the tool.

Protective Equipment

- Use damping materials in floor mats, seats, and handgrips to reduce the transmission of vibration to the body. Closed-cell foam most effectively isolates vibration; silicone and elastomers are also used for damping.
- Wear gloves with damping materials incorporated into the palms and fingers.
- Wear proper clothing to maintain body temperature and prevent vasoconstriction of the fingers induced by cold temperatures.
- Ensure that gloves fit properly.

Workplace Practices

- Alternate work tasks to reduce vibration exposure.
- Reduce the number of hours per day and days per week that a worker uses vibrating tools.
- Reduce grip force necessary to operate the tool.

Worker Training

- Train workers about the sources of vibration exposure and means of transmission to the body.
- Train workers to recognize the early signs of HAVS, CTS, or Raynaud's phenomenon and to understand the long-term effects.
- Review use of protective clothing, tool maintenance, and proper tool use.
- Reinforce the need to warm the hands before starting a job and to keep the body warm thereafter.

COOL TEMPERATURES

Temperature has a modifying role in the relationship between other biomechanical risk factors and MSD outcomes. Temperature is a clear modifying factor in vibration-related MSDs. All of the effects attributed to vibration exposure are exacerbated by simultaneous exposure to cold temperatures. The primary problems associated with industrial work in cool temperatures are local discomfort in the hands and feet and decreased manual dexterity after several hours of exposure (Eastman Kodak Company, 1983; Parsons, 1981). More severe problems such as frostbite, reduced circulation, and decreased tactile sensitivity may occur after prolonged exposure to very cold temperatures (Armstrong, 1986; Fox, 1967; Parsons, 1981).

Workers' exposures to cold temperatures commonly occur in the following working conditions: work in refrigerated or cold-storage units; construction work in poorly heated buildings; outdoor maintenance, service, or construction work in cold climates; and cleaning with cold water (Eastman Kodak Company, 1983). Additionally, fingers and distal extremities may be cooled as a result of manipulating cold materials (such as meat), using tools with cold handles, working in a cool environment (such as a cool office), or being exposed to cool-air exhaust from air-powered tools.

Cool temperatures have been demonstrated to affect tactile sensitivity, manual dexterity, reaction time, and the ability to perform complex tasks (Eastman Kodak Company, 1983; Fox, 1967). Studies indicate a strong relationship among ambient temperature, finger numbness, and tactile discrimination (Grandjean, 1988). Researchers found that after several hours of exposure to cold at 15.5° C, workers' hands began to lose flexibility and dexterity; after exposure to cold at 7° C (45° F) workers lost up to 20% dexterity in manual tasks (Eastman Kodak Company, 1983). Fox (1967) discusses a critical hand-skin temperature (HST) above which performance is relatively unaffected and below which there is a severe decline in performance. For tactile sensitivity, the critical HST is near 8° C; for manual dexterity, the critical HST is higher, between 12° and 16° C.

Clinically, individuals report subjectively increasing their muscle tension and contracting muscles in the cold. This behavior may increase the forces involved in task performance. Investigators further note the psychologic stress that cold exposure produces, which might distract individuals during task performance. Fox (1967) discusses that the effects of both temperature and wind velocity (known as wind-chill) must be taken into account when addressing the hand surface temperatures. Wind velocity may be a more important factor than air temperature in decreasing the tactile sensitivity of outside workers.

In general, hand temperatures of less than 10° to 15° C are usually uncomfortable, although they do not produce injury. To date, there are no standards for temperatures in work environments; however, it is recommended that temperatures be maintained above 25° C to promote workers' comfort and good performance (Armstrong, 1986).

Recommendations for minimizing the effects of cold temperatures include the following (Armstrong, 1986; Eastman Kodak Company, 1983; Parsons, 1981):

- Wear well-fitting gloves.
- Use tool handles with low thermal conductivity.
- Work in an area not directly affected by exhaust air.
- Maintain a warm core body temperature; wear sufficiently layered clothing.
- Work in an area free from local drafts.
- Use windproof gloves or clothing if wind velocity is high.
- Maintain dry gloves and clothing; change garments as needed. Moisture from sweating will reduce the effects of insulated gloves or clothing.
- Warm hands and feet on an ongoing basis; do not wait until numbness sets in.

REFERENCES

Aarås, A., Horgen, G., Bjorset, H. H., Ro, O., & Thoresen, M. (1998). Musculoskeletal, visual and psychosocial stress in VDU operators before and after multidisciplinary ergonomic interventions. *Applied Ergonomics, 29*(5), 335-354.

Aguayo, A. J. (1975). Neuropathy due to compression and entrapment. In P. J. Dyck, P. K. Thomas, & E. H. Lambert (Eds.), *Peripheral neuropathy*. Philadelphia: W.B. Saunders Co.

Akesson, I., Johnson, B., Rylander, L., Moritz, U., & Skirfving S. (1999). Musculoskeletal disorders among female dental personnel—clinical examination and a 5-year follow-up study of symptoms. *International Archives Occupational Environmental Health, 72*(6), 395-403.

American Conference of Governmental Industrial Hygienists (ACGIH) (2001). Hand Activity Level-Draft.

American National Standards Institute (1998). Control of work-related cumulative trauma disorders: I. Upper extremities. ANSI Z-365. Working draft.

Armstrong, T. J. (1986). Ergonomics and cumulative trauma disorders. *Hand Clinics, 2*(3), 553-565.

Armstrong, T. J., Castelli, W. A., Evans, G., & Diaz-Perez, R. (1984). Some histological changes in carpal tunnel contents and their biomechanical implications. *Journal of Occupational Medicine, 26*(3), 197-201.

Armstrong, T. J. & Chaffin, D. B. (1979). Carpal tunnel syndrome and selected personal attributes. *Journal of Occupational Medicine, 21*(7), 481-486.

Armstrong, T. J., Fine, L. J., Radwin, R. G., & Silverstein, B. S. (1987). Ergonomics and the effects of vibration in hand-intensive work. *Scandinavian Journal of Work, Environment and Health, 13*(4), 286-289.

Armstrong, T. J., Foulke, J. A., Joseph, B. S., & Goldstein, S. A. (1982). Investigation of cumulative trauma disorders in a poultry processing plant. *American Industrial Hygiene Association Journal, 43*(2), 103-115.

Armstrong, T. J. & Ulin, S. S. (1995). Analysis and design of jobs for control of work-related upper limb disorders. In J. M. Hunter, E. J. Mackin, & A. D. Callahan (Eds.), *Rehabilitation of the hand: Surgery and therapy* (4th ed.). St. Louis: Mosby.

Ashton-Miller, J. A. (1998). Response of muscle and tendon to injury and overuse. In National Academy of Sciences. *Work-Related musculoskeletal disorders: The research base*. Washington, DC: National Academy Press.

Bard, C. C., Sylvestre, J. J., & Dussault, R. G. (1984). Hand osteoarthropathy in pianists. *Journal of the Canadian Association of Radiology, 35*(2), 154-158.

Barry, R. M., Woodhall, W. R., & Mahan, M. (1992). Postural changes in dental hygienists: Four-year longitudinal study. *Journal of Dental Hygiene, 66*(3), 147-150.

Bernard, B. (Ed.). (1997). *Musculoskeletal disorders and workplace factors*. U.S. Department of Health and Human Services, Public Health Service, Centers for Disease

Control, National Institute for Occupational Safety and Health. DHHS (NIOSH) Publication # 97-141.

Bernard, B., Sauter, S., Petersen, M., Fine, L., & Hales, T. (1993). *Health hazard evaluation report. Los Angeles Times, Los Angeles, California*. U.S. Department of Health and Human Services, Public Health Service, Centers for Disease Control, National Institute for Occupational Safety and Health. HETA Publication #90-013-2277.

Bjelle, A., Hagberg, M., & Michaelsson, G. (1979). Clinical and ergonomic factors in prolonged shoulder pain among industrial workers. *Scandinavian Journal of Work, Environment and Health, 5*, 205–210.

Bonney, R.A. (1981). Human responses to vibration: Principles and methods. In E. N. Corlett & J. Richardson (Eds.), *Stress, work design and productivity*. New York: Wiley.

Borg, G.A.V. (1982). Psychophysical bases of perceived exertion. *Medicine and Science in Sports and Exercise, 14*(5), 377–381.

Borg, G.A.V. (1990). Psychophysical scaling with applications in physical work and the perception of exertion. *Scandinavian Journal of Work, Environment and Health, 16*(Suppl 1), 55–58.

Bovenzi, M., Franzinelli, A., Mancini, R., Cannava, M. G., Maiorano, M., & Ceccarelli, F. (1995). Dose-response relation for vascular disorders induced by vibration in the fingers of forestry workers. *Occupational and Environmental Medicine, 52*(11), 722–730.

Brooks, S.V., Zerba, E., & Faulkner, J.A. (1995). Injury to fibers after single stretches of passive and maximally stimulated muscles in mice. *Journal of Physiology, 488*(Pt 2), 459–469.

Brown, A. P. (1990). The effects of anti-vibration gloves on vibration-induced disorders: A case study. *Journal of Hand Therapy*, *3*(2), 94–100.

Bruel & Kjaer Instruments (1993). *Good vibrations? Instrumentation for human vibration measurements*. Naerum, Denmark: Bruel & Kjaer.

Buchholz, B., Frederick, L. J., & Armstrong, T. J. (1988a). An investigation of human palmar skin friction and the effects of materials, pinch force, and moisture. *Ergonomics*, *31*, 317–325.

Buchholz, B., Wells, R. P., & Armstrong, T. J. (1988b). The influence of object size on grasp strength: Results of a computer simulation of cylindrical Grasp. In M. Hubbard, (Ed.), *Proceedings of the 12th Annual Meeting of the American Society for Biomechanics*. Held in Urbana, Illinois, September 28–30. Oxford: Pergamon.

Buchholz, B., Pacquet, V., Punnett, L., Lee, D. & Moir, S, (1996). PATH: A work sampling based approach to ergonomic job analysis for construction and other non-repetitive work. *Applied Ergonomics*, *27*, 177–187.

Bullock, M. I. (Ed.). (1990). *Ergonomics: The physiotherapist in the workplace*. New York: Churchill Livingstone.

Byström, S., & Kilböm, A. (1990). Physiological response in the forearm during and after isometric intermittent handgrip. *European Journal of Applied Physiology, 60*(6), 457–466.

Chaffin, D. B. (1973). Localized muscle fatigue—definition and measurement. *Journal of Occupational Medicine, 15*, 346–354.

Chaffin, D. B., & Andersson, G. (1984). *Occupational biomechanics*. New York: Wiley.

Chatterjee, D. S., Barwidk, D. D., & Petrie, A. (1982). Exploratory electromyography in the study of vibration-induced white finger in rock drillers. *British Journal of Industrial Medicine, 39*(1), 89–97.

Cherniack, M. G., Letz, R., Gerr, F., Brammer, A., & Pace, P. (1990). Detailed clinical assessment of neurological function in symptomatic shipyard workers. *British Journal of Industrial Medicine, 47*(8), 566–572.

Cherniack, M., & Mohr, S. (1994). Raynaud's phenomenon associated with the use of pneumatically powered surgical instruments. *Journal of Hand Surgery, 19A*, 1008–1015.

Chiang, H., Ko, Y., Chen, C., Yu, H., Wu, T., & Chang, P. (1993). Prevalence of shoulder and upper-limb disorders among workers in the fish-processing industry. *Scandinavian Journal of Work, Environment and Health, 19*(2), 126–131.

Ciriello, V. M., Snook, S. H., Blick, A. C., & Wilkinson, P. L. (1990). The effects of task duration on psychophysically determined maximum acceptable weights and forces. *Ergonomics, 33*(2), 187–200.

Cobb, T. K., Cooney, W. P., & An, K-N. (1996). Aetiology of work-related carpal tunnel syndrome: the role of lumbrical muscles and tool size on carpal tunnel pressure. *Ergonomics, 39*, 103–107.

Comaish, S., & Bottoms, E. (1971). The skin and friction: Deviation from Amonton's laws and the effects of hydration and lubrication. *British Journal of Dermatology, 84*, 37–43.

Corlett, E. N. (1981). Pain, posture and performance. In E. N. Corlett & J. Richardson (Eds.), *Stress, work design and productivity*. New York: Wiley.

Corlett, E. N. (1990). Static muscle loading and the evaluation of posture. In J. Richardson & E. N. Corlett (Eds.), *Evaluation of human work: A practical ergonomics methodology*. London: Taylor & Francis.

Corlett, E. N., Madeley, S. J., & Manenica, I. (1979). Posture targeting: A technique for recording working postures. *Ergonomics, 22*, 357–366.

de Krom, M. C., Kester, A. D., Knipschild, P. G., & Spaans, F. (1990). Risk factors for carpal tunnel syndrome. *American Journal of Epidemiology, 132*(6), 1102–1110.

Dennet, X., Fry, H. J. H. (1988). Overuse syndrome: a muscle biopsy study. *Lancet*, 1(8581):905–908.

Dillon, C., Petersen, M., & Tanaka, S. (2002). Self-reported hand and wrist arthritis and occupation: Data from the U.S. National Health Interview Survey-Occupational Health Supplement. *American Journal of Industrial Medicine, 42,* 318-327.

Dimberg, L., Glafsson, A., Stephansson, E., Aagard, H., Odén, A., Andersson, G. B. J. et al. (1989). The correlation between work environment and the occurrence of cervicobrachial symptoms. *Journal of Occupational Medicine, 31*(5), 447-453.

Dimov, M., Bhattacharya, A., Lematers, G., Atterbury, M., Greathouse, L., Ollila-Glenn, N. (2000). Exertion and body discomfort perceived symptoms associated with carpentry tasks: An onsite evaluation. *American Industrial Hygiene Association Journal, 61*(5), 685-691.

Eastman Kodak Company (1983). *Ergonomic design for people at work,* Vol 1. New York: Van Nostrand Reinhold.

Ekberg, K., Bjorkqvist, B., Malm, P., Bjerre-Kiely, B., Karlsson, M., & Axelsdon, O. (1994). Case-control study of risk factors for disease in the neck and shoulder area. *Occupational and Environental Medicine, 51*(4), 262-266.

Ergonomics Analysis and Design Research Consortium (1998). User's Manual for Multimedia Video Task Analysis (MVTA), University of Wisconsin-Madison, Madison.

Faucett, J., & Werner, R. A. (1998). Non-biomechanical factors potentially affecting musculoskeletal disorders. In National Academy of Sciences, *Work-related musculoskeletal disorders: The research base*. Washington, DC: National Academy Press.

Finelli, P. F. (1975). Mononeuropathy of the deep palmar branch of the ulnar nerve. *Archives of Neurology, 32,* 564-565.

Fox W. F. (1967). Human performance in the cold. *Human Factors, 9*(3), 203-220.

Gemne, G., Pyykko, I., Taylor, W., & Palmear, P. (1987). The Stockholm Workshop scale for the classification of cold-induced Raynaud's phenomenon in the hand-arm vibration syndrome (revision of the Taylor-Palmear scale). *Scandinavian Journal of Work, Environment and Health, 13,* 275-278.

Goldstein S. A., Armstrong T. J., Chaffin D. B., & Matthews L. S. (1987). Analysis of cumulative strain in tendon and tendon sheaths. *Journal of Biomechanics, 20*(1), 1-6.

Grandjean, E. (1988). *Fitting the task to the man* (4th ed.). London: Taylor & Francis.

Grieco, A. (1998). Application of the concise exposure index (OCRA) to tasks involving repetitive movement of the upper limbs in a variety of manufacturing industries; preliminary validations, *Ergonomics, 41,* 1347-1356.

Grieco, A., Molteni, G., De Vito, G., & Sias, N. (1998). Epidemiology of musculoskeletal disorders due to biomechanical overload. *Ergonomics, 41*(9), 1253-1260.

Hagberg, M. (1981). Workload and fatigue in repetitive arm elevations. *Ergonomics, 24,* 543-555.

Hagberg, M., Morgenstern, J., & Kelsh, M. (1992). Impact of occupations and job tasks on the prevalence of carpal tunnel syndrome: A review. *Scandinavian Journal of Work, Environment and Health, 18*(6), 337-345.

Hales, T. R., & Bernard, B. P. (1996). Epidemiology of work-related musculoskeletal disorders. *Orthopedic Clinics of North America, 27*(4), 679-709.

Hammer, A. (1934). Tenosynovitis. *Medical Record, 140,* 353-355.

Hampel, G. A. (1992). Hand-arm vibration isolation materials: A range of performance evaluation. *Applied Occupational and Environmental Hygiene, 7,* 441-452.

Harber, P., Bloswick, D., Beck, J., Pena L., Baker, D., & Lee, J. (1993). Supermarket checker motions and cumulative trauma risk. *Journal of Occupational Medicine, 35*(8), 805-811.

Hansson, G-A., Balough, I., Ohlsson, K., Palsson, B., Rylander, L. & Skerfving, S. (2000). Impact of physical exposure on neck and upper limb disorders in female workers, *Applied Ergonomics, 31*(3), 301-310.

Haselgrave, C. M. (1991). Consequences of variability in posture adopted for handling tasks. In M. Kumashiro & E. D. Megaw (Eds.), *Towards human work*. London: Taylor & Francis.

Haselgrave, C. M. (1994). What do we mean by working posture? *Ergonomics, 37,* 781-799.

Herberts, P., Kadefors, R., Andersson, G., & Petersen, I. (1981). Shoulder pain in industry: An epidemiological study on welders. *Acta Orthopaedica Scandinavica, 52*(3), 299-306.

Hertzberg, H. T. E. (1955). Some contributions of applied physical anthropology to human engineering. *Annals of the New York Academy of Science, 63,* 616-629.

Herrin, G. D., Jaraiedi, M., & Anderson, C. K. (1986). Prediction of overexertion injuries using biomechanical and psychophysical models. *American Industrial Hygiene Association Journal, 47*(6), 322-330.

Hidalgo, J. A., Genaidy, A. M., Huston, R., & Arantes, J. (1992). Occupational biomechanics of the neck: A review and recommendations. *Journal of Human Ergology, 21*(2), 165-181.

Hignett, S., & McAtamney, L. (2000). Rapid entire body assessment (REBA). *Applied Ergonomics, 31*(2), 201-205.

Hjortsberg, U., Rosen, I., Orbaek, P., Lundborg, G., & Valogh, I. (1989). Finger receptor dysfunction in dental technicians exposed to high-frequency vibration. *Scandinavian Journal of Work, Environment and Health, 15*(5), 339-344.

Hoozemans, M. J. M., van der Beek, A. J., Frings-Dresen, M. H. W., & van der Molen, H. F. (2001). Evaluation of methods to assess push-pull forces in a construction task, *Applied Ergonomics, 32*(5), 509-516.

Jensen, M.V., Tuchsen, F., & Orhede, E. (1996). Prolapsed cervical intervertebral disc in male professional drivers in Denmark, 1981-1990. A longitudinal study of hospitalizations. *Spine, 21*(20), 2352-2355.

Joseph, B. S., & Bloswick, D. S. (1991). Ergonomic considerations and job design. In M. Kasdan (Ed.), *Occupational hand and upper extremity injuries and diseases.* Philadelphia: Hanley & Belfus.

Keyserling, W. M., Armstrong, T. A. & Punnett, L. (1991). Ergonomic job analysis: A structured approach for identifying risk factors associated with overexertion injuries and disorders. *Applied Occupational and Environmental Hygiene, 6*(5), 353-363.

Karhu, O., Kansi, P., & Kuorinka, I. (1977). Correcting working postures in industry, a practical method for analysis. *Applied Ergonomics, 8,* 199-201.

Kier, P., Bach, J., & Rempel, D. M. (1998). Fingertip loading and carpal tunnel pressure: Differences between a pinching and a pressing task. *Journal of Orthopaedic Research, 16*(1), 112-115.

Kourinka, I., & Forcier, L. (Eds.). (1995). *Work-related musculoskeletal disorders (WMSDs): A reference book for prevention.* London: Taylor & Francis.

Kroemer, K. H. E., & Grandjean, E. (2001). *Fitting the task to the human.* London: Taylor & Francis.

Kukkonen, R., Luopajärvi, T., & Riihimäki, V. (1983). Prevention of fatigue amongst data entry operators. In T. O. Kvalseth (Ed.), *Ergonomics of workstation design.* London: Butterworth-Heinemann.

Kumar, S. (Ed.). (2001). *Biomechanics in ergonomics,* London: Taylor & Francis.

Larsson, S. E., Bengtsson, A., Bodegard, L., Hendriksson, K. G., & Larsson, J. (1988). Muscle changes in work-related chronic myalgia. *Acta Orthopaedica Scandinavica, 59*(5), 552-556.

LeVeau, B. F. (1992). *Williams's and Lissner's biomechanics of human motion* (3rd ed.). Philadelphia: Saunders.

Linton, S. J. (1990). Risk factors for neck and back pain in a working population in Sweden. *Work and Stress, 4*(1), 41-49.

Little, J. M., & Ferguson, K. A. (1972). The incidence of the hypothenar hammer syndrome. *Archives of Surgery, 105*(5), 684-685.

Lundborg, G., Gelberman, R. H., Minteer-Convery, M., Lee, Y. F., & Hargens, A. R. (1982). Median nerve compression in the carpal tunnel: Functional response to experimentally induced controlled pressure. *Journal of Hand Surgery, 7*(3), 252-259.

Luopajärvi, T. (1990). Ergonomic analysis of workplace and postural load. In M. Bullock (Ed.), *Ergonomics: The physiotherapist in the workplace.* New York: Churchill Livingstone.

Luopajärvi, T., Kourinka, I., Virolainen, M., & Holmberg, M. (1979). Prevalence of teno-synovitis and other injuries of the upper extremities in repetitive work. *Scandinavian Journal of Work, Environment and Health, 5*(Suppl 3), 58-55

Maeda, K., Hunting, W., & Grandjean, E. (1980). Localized fatigue in accounting-machine operators. *Journal of Occupational Medicine, 22*(12), 811-816.

Magora, A., & Schwartz, A. (1976). Relation between the low-back pain syndrome and x-ray findings: Degenerative osteoarthritis. *Scandinavian Journal of Rehabilitation Medicine, 8,* 115-125.

Margolis, W., & Kraus, J. F. (1987). The prevalence of carpal tunnel syndrome symptoms in female supermarket checkers. *Journal of Occupational Medicine, 29*(12), 953-956.

Marras, W. S., & Granata, K. P. (1995). A biomechanical assessment and model of axial twisting in the thoracolumbar spine. *Spine, 20*(13), 1440-1451.

Marras, W. S., & Granata, K. P. (1997). Spine loading during trunk lateral bending motions. *Journal of Biomechanics, 30*(7), 697-703.

Marras, W. S., Lavender, S. A., Leurgans, S. E., Fathallah, F. A., Ferguson, S. A., Allread, W. G. et al. (1995). Biomechanical risk factors for occupationally related low back disorders. *Ergonomics, 38*(2), 377-410.

Marras, W. S., & Schoenmarklin, R. W. (1993). Wrist motions in industry. *Ergonomics, 36*(4), 341-351.

McAtamney, L., & Corlett, E. N. (1993). RULA: A survey method for the investigation of work-related upper limb disorders. *Applied Ergonomics, 24*(2), 91-99.

Milerad, E., & Erickson, M. O. (1994). Effects of precision and force demands, grip diameter, and arm support during manual work: An electromyographic study. *Ergonomics, 37,* 255-264.

Moore, J., & Garg, A. (1995). The strain index: A proposed method to analyze jobs for risk of distal upper extremity disorders. *American Industrial Hygiene Association Journal, 56*(5), 443-463.

Nathan, P. A., Meadows, K. D., & Doyle, L. S. (1988). Occupation as a risk factor for impaired sensory conduction of the median nerve at the carpal tunnel. *Journal of Hand Surgery, 13B*(2), 167-170.

National Institute of Occupational Safety and Health (NIOSH). (1981). *Work practices guide for manual lifting.* Cincinnati, OH: U.S. Department of Health and Human Services, Public Health Service, Centers for Disease Control, National Institute for Occupational Safety and Health. DHHS (NIOSH) Publication #81-122.

National Institute of Occupational Safety and Health (NIOSH). (1989). *Occupational exposure to hand-arm vibration* [DHHS pub no. 89-106]. Cincinnati: U.S. Department of Health and Human Services.

National Institute of Occupational Safety and Health (NIOSH). (1994). *Revised NIOSH lifting equation.*

Cincinnati, OH: U.S. Department of Health and Human Services, Public Health Service, Centers for Disease Control, National Institute for Occupational Safety and Health. DHHS (NIOSH) Publication #94-110.

Nevasier, J. S. (1980). Adhesive capsulitis and the stiff and painful shoulder. *Orthopedic Clinics of North America, 11*(2), 327-331

Nilsson, T., Hagberg, M., & Burström, L. (1990). Prevalence and odds ratios of numbness and carpal tunnel syndrome in different exposure categories of platers. In A. Okada & W.T. H. Dupuis (Eds.), *Hand-arm vibration*. Kanazawa, Japan: Kyoei Press Co.

Norkin, C. C., & Levangie, P. K. (1992). *Joint structure and function: A comprehensive analysis.* Philadelphia: F. A. Davis.

Oberg, T. (1993). Ergonomic evaluation and construction of a reference workplace in dental hygiene. *Journal of Dental Hygiene, 67*(5), 262-267.

Oberg, T., & Oberg, U. (1993). Musculoskeletal complaints in dental hygiene: A survey study from a Swedish country. *Journal of Dental Hygiene, 67*(5), 257-261.

Occipinti, E. (1998). OCRA: A concise index for the assessment of exposure to repetitive movement of the upper limbs, *Ergonomics, 41*(9), 1290-1311.

Ohlsson, K., Attewell, R., Paisson, B., Karsllon, B, Balogh, I., Johnsson, B., et al. (1995). Repetitive industrial work and neck and upper limb disorders in females. *American Journal of Industrial Medicine, 27*(5), 731-747.

O'Meara, D. M., & Smith, R. M. (2001). Static friction properties between human palmar skin and five grabrail materials. *Ergonomics, 44*(11), 973-988.

Osborn, J. B., Newell, K. J., & Rudney J. D. (1990). Musculoskeletal pain among Minnesota dental hygienists. *Journal of Dental Hygiene, 64*(3), 132-138.

OSHA. (1999). Health Effects Section of Proposed Ergonomic Rule. Federal Register Tuesday, Nov. 23. Dept. of Labor. OSHA. 29CFR Part 1910.

Palermud, G., Forsman, M., Sporrong, H., Herberts, P. & Kadefors, R. (2000). Intramuscular pressure of the infra- and supraspinatus muscles in relation to hand load and arm posture. *European Journal of Applied Physiology, 83,* 223-230.

Parnianpour, M., Nordin, M., Kahanovitz, N., & Frankel, V. (1988). The triaxial coupling of torque generation of trunk muscles during isometric exertions and the effect of fatiguing isoinertial movements ion the motor output and movement patterns. *Spine, 13,* 982-992.

Parsons, K. (1981). Human responses to thermal environments: Principles and methods. In E. N. Corlett & J. Richardson (Eds.), *Stress, work design and productivity*. New York: Wiley.

Pheasant, S. (1991). *Ergonomics, work, and health.* Gaithersburg, MD: Aspen.

Punnett, L. (1998). Ergonomic stressors and upper extremity disorders in vehicle manufacturing: cross sectional exposure-response trends. *Occupational and Environmental Medicine, 55*(6), 414-420.

Punnett, L., & van der Beek, A. J. (2000) A comparison of approaches to modeling the relationship between ergonomic exposures and upper extremity disorders. *American Journal of Industrial Medicine, 37*(6), 645-655

Putz-Anderson, V. (Ed.). (1988). *Cumulative trauma disorders: A manual for musculoskeletal diseases of the upper limbs.* Philadelphia: Taylor & Francis.

Putz-Anderson, V., Doyle, G. T., & Hales, T. R. (1992). Ergonomic analysis to characterize task constraint and repetitiveness as risk factors for musculoskeletal disorders in telecommunication office work. *Scandinavian Journal of Work, Environment and Health, 18*(Suppl 2), 123-126.

Radwin, R. G., & Armstrong, T. J. (1985). Assessment of hand vibration exposure on an assembly line. *American Industrial Hygiene Association Journal, 46*(4), 211-219.

Radwin, R. G., Armstrong, T. J., & Chaffin, D. B. (1987). Power hand tool vibration effects on grip exertions. *Ergonomics, 30,* 833-855.

Radwin, R. G., & Lavender, S. A. (1998). Work factors, personal factors, and internal loads: Biomechanics of work stressors. In National Academy of Sciences, *Work-related musculoskeletal disorders: The research base*. Washington, DC: National Academy Press.

Ramazzini, B. (1717). De morbis artificum diatriba. In W. Wright (Trans, 1940), *The diseases of workers.* Chicago: University of Chicago Press.

Rempel, D., Keir, P. J., Smutz, W. P., & Hargans, A. R. (1997). Effects of static fingertip loading on carpal tunnel pressure. *Journal of Orthopaedic Research, 15*(3), 422-426.

Rempel, E., Dahlin, L., & Lundborg G. (1998). Biological response of peripheral nerves to loading: Pathophysiology of nerve compression syndromes and vibration induced neuropathy. In National Academy of Sciences, *Work-related musculoskeletal disorders: The research base*. Washington, DC.: National Academy Press.

Rodgers, S. (1987). Recovery time needs for repetitive work. *Seminars in Occupational Medicine, 2*(1), 19-24.

Rodgers, S. (1988). Job evaluation in worker fitness determination. *Occupational Medicine, 3*(2), 219-239.

Rohmert, W. (1973). Problems in determining rest allowances: I. Use of modern methods to evaluate stress and strain in static muscular work. *Applied Ergonomics, 4,* 91-95.

Silverstein, B. A., Fine, L. J., & Armstrong, T. J. (1986). Hand wrist cumulative trauma disorders in industry. *British Journal of Environmental Medicine, 43*(11), 779-784.

Silverstein, B. A., Fine, L. J., & Armstrong, T. J. (1987). Occupational factors and carpal tunnel syndrome. *American Journal of Industrial Medicine, 11*(3), 343-358.

Sjogaard, G., Savard, G., & Juel, C. (1988). Muscle blood flow during isometric activity and its relations to muscle fatigue. *European Journal of Applied Physiology, 57,* 327-335.

Smith, E. M., Sonstegard, D., & Anderson, W. (1977). Carpal tunnel syndrome: Contribution of the flexor tendons. *Archives of Physical and Medical Rehabilitation, 58*(9), 379-385.

Snook, S. H., & Ciriello, V. M. (1991). The design of manual handling tasks: Revised tables of maximum acceptable weights and forces. *Ergonomics, 34*(9), 1197-1213.

Spielholz, P., Silverstein, B., Morgan, M., Checkowy, H. & Kaufman, J. (2001). Comparison of self-report, video observation and direct measurement methods for upper extremity musculoskeletal disorder physical risk factors, *Ergonomics, 44*(6), 588-613.

Stromberg, T., Dahlin, L. B., Brun, A., & Lundborg, G. (1997). Structural nerve changes at wrist level in workers exposed to vibration. *Occupational and Environmental Medicine, 54*(5), 307-311.

Szabo, R. M., & Chidgey, L. K. (1989). Stress carpal tunnel pressures in patients with carpal tunnel syndrome and normal patients, *Journal of Hand Surgery, 14A*(4), 624-627.

Takala, E. P., & Viikari-Juntura, E. (1991). Muscle force, endurance and neck-shoulder symptoms of sedentary workers: An experimental study on bank cashiers with and without symptoms. *International Journal of Industrial Ergonomics, 7,* 123-132.

Takeuchi, T., Takaya, M., & Imanishi, H. (1988). Ultrastructural changes in peripheral nerves of the fingers of three vibration-exposed persons with Raynaud's phenomenon. *Scandinavian Journal of Work, Environment and Health, 14,* 31-35.

Tichauer, E. (1966). Some aspects of stress on forearm and hand in industry. *Journal of Occupational Medicine, 8*(2), 630-671.

Tichauer, E. R. (1978). *The biomechanical basis of ergonomics*. New York: Wiley.

Tichauer, E. R., & Gage, H. (1977). Ergonomic principles basic to hand tool design. *American Industrial Hygiene Association Journal, 38*(11), 622-634.

Uchiyama, S., Coert, J. H., Berglund, L., Amadio, P. C., & An, K-N. (1995). Method for measurement of friction between a tendon and its pulley. *Journal of Orthopaedic Research, 13*(1), 83-89.

Ulin, S., Armstrong, T. J., Snook, S., & Franzblau, A. (1993). Effect of tool shape and work location on perceived exertion for work on horizontal surfaces. *American Industrial Hygiene Association Journal, 54*(7), 383-392.

Vingärd, E., Alfredsson, L., Goldie, I., & Hogstedt, C. (1991). Occupation and osteoarthrosis of the hip and knee: A registry based cohort study. *International Journal of Epidemiology, 20*(4), 1025-1031.

Warren, N., Dillon, C., Morse, T., Hall, C., & Warren, A. (2000). Biomechanical, psychosocial and organizational risk factors for WRMSD; Population-based estimates from the Connecticut Upper Extremity Surveillance Project (CUSP). *Journal of Occupational Health Psychology, 5*(1), 164-181.

Waters, T. R., Putz-Anderson, V., & Garg, A. (1994). Applications Manual for the Revised NIOSH Lifting Equation. U.S. Dept. of Health and Human Services, Cincinnati. Publication # 94-110.

Westgaard, R. H., & Aarås, A. (1984). Postural muscle strain as a causal factor in the development of musculoskeletal illness. *Applied Ergonomics, 15*(3), 162-174.

Wieslander, G., Norbäck, D., Göthe, C. J., & Juhlin, L. (1989). Carpal tunnel syndrome (CTS) and exposure to vibration, repetitive wrist movements, and heavy manual work: A case-referent study. *British Journal of Industrial Medicine, 46*(1), 43-47.

Williams, W. V., Cope, R., Gaunt, W. D., Adelstein, E. H., Hoyt, T. S., Singh, A. et al. (1987). Metacarpophalangeal arthopathy associated with manual labor (Missouri metacarpal syndrome). Clinical, radiographic, and pathologic characteristics of an unusual degeneration process, *Arthritis and Rheumatism, 30,* 1362-1371.

Zipp, P., Haider, E., Halpern, N., & Fohmert, W. (1983). Keyboard design through physiological strain measurements. *Applied Ergonomics, 14*(2), 117-122.

CHAPTER 11

Job Design

Martha J. Sanders

Successful injury prevention programs involve both preparing the worker for the job and providing a safe, comfortable, work environment. Medical therapies, rehabilitation programs, job training, preemployment testing, and fitness-for-duty programs fit the worker to the job. In other words, these programs traditionally match or increase the capacities of a worker to meet the job demands.

The focus of ergonomics, on the other hand, is to fit the job to the worker. Ergonomics seeks to design work environments and work tasks that are also user-friendly, efficient, safe, comfortable, and cognitively engaging for every worker. Ergonomics encompasses the design of workstations and equipment, the identification and elimination of tasks that are potentially unsafe or dangerous, the control of environmental factors, the concern for organizational factors that influence the design of the job, and psychosocial factors within the job tasks that may affect the ability of the worker to perform the job (see Chapter 8 for a complete discussion).

As the workforce becomes increasingly diverse with larger numbers of older, female, and disabled workers entering the workforce, ergonomic programs are challenged to design a work environment for the user who does not fall within the "typical" size or capacity norms but who can perform the job functions (Pheasant, 1991). Thus, the need for properly sized and designed equipment is vital to work efficiency and productivity today (Morse & Hinds, 1993).

This chapter provides an overview of selected factors in the physical design of jobs that may contribute to musculoskeletal disorders (MSDs), including anthropometrics, workstation design, tools, lighting, and work hours.

ANTHROPOMETRICS

Anthropometrics refers to the study of human dimensions or body size. Human dimensions include height, limb length, and limb girth, as well as physical capacities such as lifting, carrying, and grasping (Pheasant, 1991; Pheasant, 2001). Anthropometrics is fundamental to ergonomics in that it applies workers' body dimensions to the design of jobs, workplaces, equipment, tools, and personal protective equipment. Health care practitioners should be familiar with the basics of anthropometrics to make recommendations that minimize worker fatigue and the overall risk for MSDs.

Initial steps in applying anthropometric data to ergonomic design include identifying both the user population and the criteria to effectively perform the desired task (Pheasant, 1991). For example, if a machine shop's management team decides to buy chairs for all the shop's machinists and assembly persons, the procurement specialist must identify who will be using the chairs (two distinct groups: machinists and assembly persons) and which criteria will constitute a good chair for each group. Among the criteria to be considered may be comfort, support, ability to get close to the machine, and general preference. It is important to remember that the criteria will not be the same for the two user groups. Finally, the degree to which the chair can be adjusted for the individual worker must be determined. One generic chair style will rarely fit the needs of all workers.

Originally, anthropometric data were derived from a sample of military personnel in the 1950s representing a select population of young, presumably fit, men. Recently, data have been gathered from females, individuals of various ages (including children and infants), ethnic backgrounds, and wheelchair user groups (Diffrient, Tilley, & Bradagjy, 1990; Pheasant, 2001). However, older individuals, those with disabilities, and persons of certain ethnic backgrounds may continue to be underrepresented in anthropometric charts (Morse & Hinds, 1993). Nevertheless, experts suggest that anthropometric norms can be applied to the industrial population by increasing the frequency and ranges of extreme body measurements (Eastman Kodak Company, 1983).

Anthropometric charts are used in the following manner to design the optimal workstation. First, anthropometric measurements are gathered from a large sample population and are analyzed statistically to identify a range and frequency distribution of workers' sizes or capacities. Anthropometric data are then communicated in percentiles for men and women according to age. From these data, designers determine the necessary clearance, reach, and optimal location of controls for the majority of the population. For example, in Figure 11-1, for the dimension of seated functional overhead reach (see line 16 in Figure 11-1), the 95th percentile indicates that 95% of the population will have a reach span of 54.8 inches or less; 5% will have a reach span of less than 43.6 inches.

Ideally, the workstation should be designed to fit each worker. However, with a changing workforce, manufacturers are more likely to design a workstation that will accommodate most workers, including the largest man (95th percentile) and the smallest woman (5th percentile) for reasons of cost-effectiveness. The chosen cutoff percentiles are called *design limits* (Pheasant, 1991).

Body measurements gathered for anthropometric charts include static and dynamic dimensions (Bullock, 1990). *Static* or structural dimensions are measurements of specific anatomic structures such as limb length, width, and circumference. These measurements are applied to the design and size specifications of workstations or tools. *Dynamic* or functional dimensions refer to measurements taken for daily activities such as lifting, grasping, or reaching objects that relate directly to the job. Dynamic dimensions are more difficult to document and measure because of the wide variety of individual movement patterns. These measurements are especially important for designing jobs, identifying the work flow, conducting employment screenings after a job has been offered, selecting the most appropriate tools for the job, or adapting workstations for a varied population.

The following four main categories of anthropometric criteria are used in ergonomic design.

- *Clearance*, referring to headroom, legroom, and elbowroom.
- *Reach*, referring to the location of controls, storage materials, and the need to reach over an object to perform a task.
- *Posture*, referring to body positions relative to the height of the work surface and controls.
- *Strength*, referring to grip strengths and muscle strength related to lifting or carrying weighted loads.

To accommodate the limited user, *clearances* should always be designed for the largest user (95th percentile), whereas *reaches* should always be designed for the smallest user (5th percentile) (Pheasant, 1991).

Figures 11-1 and 11-2 provide normative data for anthropometric information related to sitting, standing, and reaching. Figure 11-3 summarizes anthropometric information relative to handtool and equipment design. The referenced dimen-

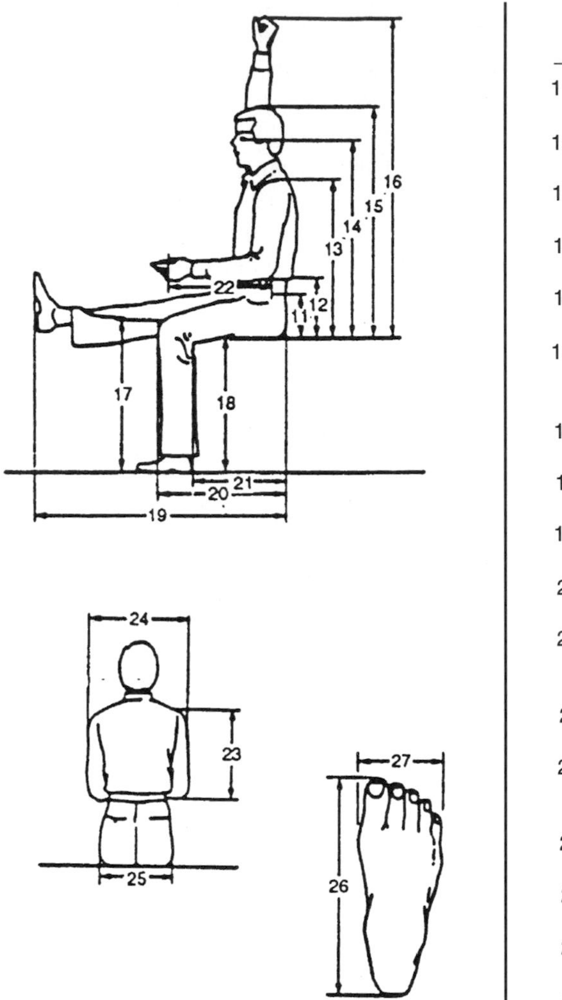

Measurement Number and Description	Percentile 5	50	95
11. Thigh clearance height	4.3	5.3	6.5
12. Elbow rest height	7.3	9.3	11.4
13. Mid-shoulder height	21.4	23.6	26.1
14. Eye height	27.4	29.9	32.8
15. Sitting height, normal	32.0	34.6	37.4
16. Functional overhead reach	43.6	48.7	54.8
17. Knee height	18.7	20.7	22.7
18. Popliteal height	15.1	16.6	18.4
19. Leg length	37.3	40.5	43.9
20. Upper-leg length	21.1	23.0	24.9
21. Buttocks-to-popliteal length	17.2	19.1	20.9
22. Elbow-to-fist length	12.6 (11.4)	14.5 (13.8)	16.2 (16.2)
23. Upper-arm length	12.9 (12.1)	13.8 (13.8)	15.5 (16.0)
24. Shoulder breadth	14.3	16.7	18.8
25. Hip breadth	12.8	14.5	16.3
26. Foot length	8.9	10.0	11.2
27. Foot breadth	3.2	3.7	4.2

Figure 11-1 Anthropometric data (in inches) for men and women seated. Statistics in parentheses represent an industrial population. (Reprinted with permission from Falkenburg, S. A., & Shultz, D. J. [1993]. Ergonomics for the upper extremity. *Hand Clinics, 9*[2], 268.)

sions include data from both men and women combined, for the 5th, 50th, and 95th percentiles. Pheasant (2001) provides expanded anthropometric data gathered from various ages and countries.

WORKSTATION DESIGN

The efficient design of a workstation (or workspace) is critical to workers' productivity and energy level throughout the day. The workstation influences a worker's postures, work patterns, and sequence of actions for the job. The workstation design includes the work surface, sitting or standing area, objects manipulated, layout or arrangement of these objects, and the visual display area. A well-designed workstation should minimize the worker's static work patterns, provide several ergonomically correct positions that the worker may assume throughout the day, and provide a logical flow for the work process (Pheasant, 2001; Putz-Anderson, 1988).

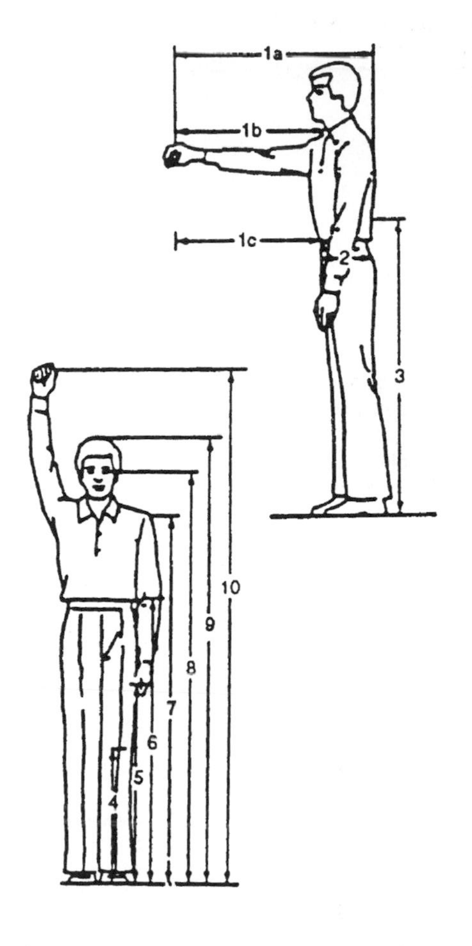

Measurement Number and Description	Percentile 5	50	95
1. Forward functional reach	27.2	30.7	35.0
a. back to functional pinch	(25.7)	(29.5)	(34.1)
b. shoulder to functional pinch	22.6	25.6	29.3
c. abdomen to function pinch	(19.1)	(24.1)	(29.3)
2. Abdominal depth	7.1	8.7	10.2
3. Waist height	37.4 (35.8)	40.9 (39.9)	44.7 (44.5)
4. Knee height	15.3	17.2	19.4
5. Knuckle height	25.9	28.8	31.9
6. Elbow height	38.0 (39.5)	42.0 (43.6)	45.8 (48.6)
7. Shoulder height	48.4 (49.8)	54.5 (55.3)	59.7 (61.6)
8. Eye height	56.8	62.1	67.8
9. Stature	60.8 (61.1)	66.2 (67.1)	72.0 (74.3)
10. Functional overhead reach	74.0	80.5	86.9

Figure 11-2 Anthropometric data (in inches) for men and women standing. Statistics in parentheses represent an industrial population. (Reprinted with permission from Falkenburg, S. A., & Shultz, D. J. [1993]. Ergonomics for the upper extremity. *Hand Clinics, 9*[2], 267.)

Many workers will modify their workstations independently with makeshift arrangements such as pillows or cardboard boxes. Ergonomic consultants should therefore carefully examine each worker's modifications to gain insight into the worker's perceived discomfort and his or her solutions to the problem.

The following general guidelines apply to all workstations.

- The area should be large enough to permit the full range of movements required for the task.
- The workstation should promote typical use of the extremities in a neutral position.
- The workstation should provide proximal support for the seated worker, a prop for rest for the standing worker, and padded or rounded edges for the work surface.
- The workstation design should be specific to the task being performed.
- The equipment must be easily adjustable to accommodate all workers.
- Mechanical aids and equipment should be available (Kroemer & Grandjean, 2001; Pheasant, 1991, 2001; Putz-Anderson 1988).

It is important that workplace design strives to decrease static loading on proximal muscles

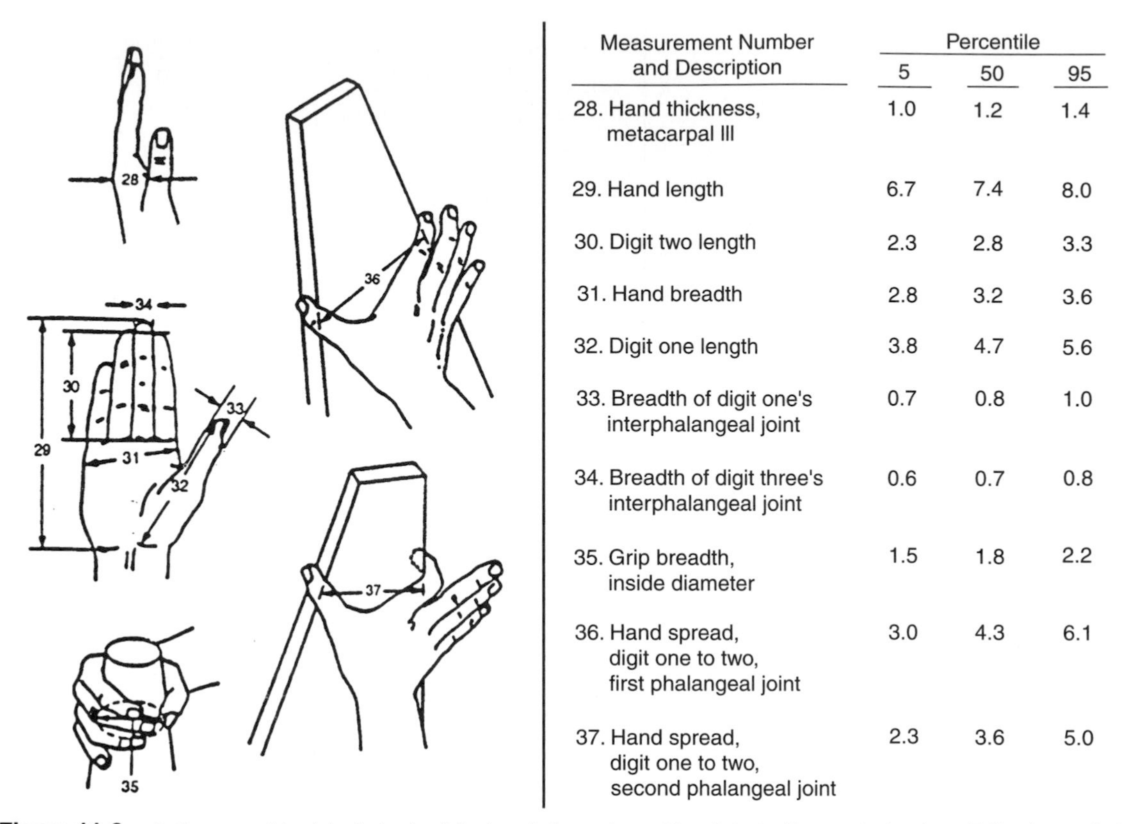

Measurement Number and Description	Percentile 5	50	95
28. Hand thickness, metacarpal III	1.0	1.2	1.4
29. Hand length	6.7	7.4	8.0
30. Digit two length	2.3	2.8	3.3
31. Hand breadth	2.8	3.2	3.6
32. Digit one length	3.8	4.7	5.6
33. Breadth of digit one's interphalangeal joint	0.7	0.8	1.0
34. Breadth of digit three's interphalangeal joint	0.6	0.7	0.8
35. Grip breadth, inside diameter	1.5	1.8	2.2
36. Hand spread, digit one to two, first phalangeal joint	3.0	4.3	6.1
37. Hand spread, digit one to two, second phalangeal joint	2.3	3.6	5.0

Figure 11-3 Anthropometric data (in inches) for hand dimensions. (Reprinted with permission from Falkenburg, S. A., & Shultz, D. J. [1993]. Ergonomics for the upper extremity. *Hand Clinics, 9*[2], 269.)

whenever possible (through support or proper posture) since such loading contributes to pain and muscle fatigue. Loading on the muscles of the neck and shoulder is the most obvious concern. Kroemer & Grandjean (2001) suggest that static effort should be reduced to not more than 15% of an individual's maximum voluntary capacity for short durations and to 8% for tasks of longer duration. Other researchers concur that even at 10% maximum voluntary capacity, the muscle will fatigue over time (Sjogaard, Savard, & Juel, 1988; see Chapter 9).

Workplace Layout

Well-designed workplaces are efficient because there is no wasted effort on the part of the workers. Workers are able to establish a working rhythm that follows the natural movement of extremities and a logical sequence for the task. Although most workplaccs are laid out well initially, over time the job might expand and the work area might become personalized (with pictures, pen holders, flowers, etc.) such that a logical workflow is interrupted. Experience has shown that most workers will acknowledge workplace clutter but do not realize the impact clutter has on their job tasks or postures.

Workstation layout or "what to put where" strives to place each work object in its optimum location to serve the designated purpose. Unfortunately, not all objects can exist in the same ideal space, therefore basic principles can help guide the process of prioritizing what goes where. The following principles address both the general location of the work objects as well as the specific arrangement of the objects within that general location (Pheasant, 2001; Sanders & McCormick, 1993). Decisions must be made relative to which objects or components are most vital or important to completion of the entire process, such as the following.

- Importance principle: Place the most important items in the most accessible locations.
- Frequency-of-use principle: Place the most frequently used items in convenient locations.
- Function principle: Place items with similar functions together.
- Sequence-of-use principle: Lay out items in the same sequence that they are used.

Workstation Height

The height of the work surface is critically important. A work surface that is too high may cause increased shoulder fatigue, whereas a work surface that is too low may cause low-back problems. The proper work height is determined by both the worker's height and the task requirements of the job. *Precise work* requires a higher work surface to provide proximal stabilization. *Heavier work* requires a lower work surface to increase the muscle forces available. These principles apply to work done while seated or standing.

Ideally, the workstation should combine both sitting and standing positions. In the early twentieth century, the majority of workers stood while they were working and moved about frequently on the job. Today, an estimated three-fourths of all workers are sedentary and remain seated for prolonged periods. Although sitting requires decreased physiologic effort and provides greater stability for the worker, sitting also increases spinal compression forces and the potential for static loading on the neck and shoulders (Kroemer & Grandjean, 2001; Pheasant 1991). The following discussion highlights general guidelines for seated and standing workstations.

Seated Workstations

A most important aspect of a seated workstation is the chair design and fit. A good chair design can minimize long-term neck, back, and even leg problems when adjusted properly. Kroemer & Grandjean (2001) point out that chairs have historically been a status symbol, with the chief occupying the ceremonial stool or throne. Although an elegant chair sends a message of authority and prominence even today, the importance of chair design on everyday productivity and comfort is often overlooked. A good ergonomic chair can cost as little as $300 and as much as $1500 or even more.

Researchers emphasize that sitting is not a static activity (Pheasant, 1991). If one observes seated workers for an extended period of time, one will note that individuals shift regularly from side to side, lean forward and backward, and stretch their legs throughout the day. The dynamic nature of sitting therefore requires a chair design that offers options for adjustment. The following are guidelines for designing a seated workstation (compiled from Eastman Kodak Company, 1983; Kroemer & Grandjean, 2001; Pheasant, 1991). (See Chapter 24 for further discussion on seating relative to office environments.)

- *Adjustable chair height:* Chair seat height should be equal to or slightly lower than knee height to allow for adequate leg clearance and to allow the feet to be flat on the floor. For light tasks, the work surface should be slightly below the elbow (2 to 4 inches; Figure 11-4).
- *Seat pan:* The seat pan depth should measure from the buttocks to the knee and be wide enough to provide thigh support. A seat pan that is too deep causes the user to sit forward and lose contact with the backrest. A seat pan that is too short causes increased pressure under the knee or thighs. The edges should be rounded and the seat upholstered.
- *Seat angle:* A seat angle of 100 to 110 degrees is a good compromise between minimizing disc pressures and allowing for use of the hands. The seat angle should be adjustable forward and backward by 5 degrees and have a locking device.

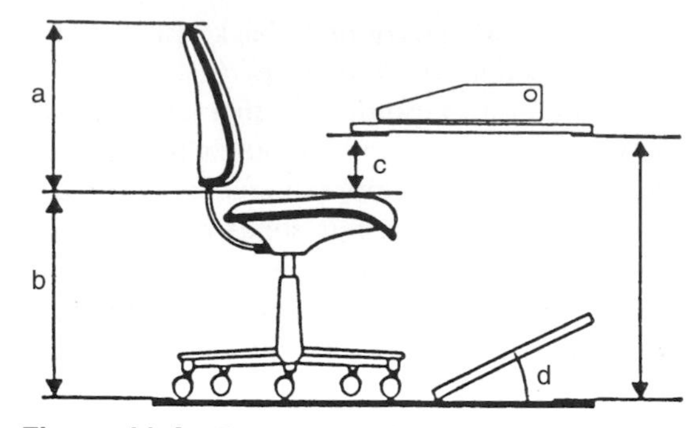

Figure 11-4 Recommended guidelines for a seated workstation. *a,* backrest: 18 to 20 in (48 to 50 cm); *b,* seat height: 15 to 22 in (38 to 54 cm); *c,* leg clearance: min 7 in (17 cm); *d,* footrest angle: 10 to 25 degrees. (Reprinted with permission from Kroemer, E., & Grandjean, E. [2001]. *Fitting the task to the person* [5th ed.]. London: Taylor & Francis.)

- *Backrest:* A backrest should support the lumbar and midthoracic spine for the greatest postural support. For office workers, the chair should have a high backrest with a lumbar pad. For industrial workers who work upright, the chair should have at least a lumbar support, with adequate space for the buttocks between the backrest and the seat pan.
- *Footrest:* Footrests are necessary to relieve pressure on the thigh and low back, particularly if the feet are not flat on the floor. Rings on high work chairs may or may not accommodate a short person if the rings do not adjust. Inexpensive footrests can be purchased or made from wooden platforms.
- *Armrest:* Armrests are recommended when the arms are held in the same position, particularly *away* from the body, for much of the task. Armrests can be part of the chair or clamped to the front edge of the desk. Armrests should swivel and tilt as needed to relieve the static loading of the neck and shoulders and provide the proper work position. Edges should be padded and round. Care should be taken to ensure that armrests do not prevent the user from getting close enough to the desk or keyboard.
- *Upholstery:* A contoured seat pan and good padding will help to distribute the pressure of the ischial tuberosities. Seat material should be porous, stain-resistant, and compressible to approximately 1 to 2 inches. The material should reduce static electricity and avoid heat transfer.
- *Base:* The chair base should have five points or casters for the greatest stability.

Standing Workstations

Standing is very efficient and places only low-level static forces on the lower extremity. However, standing still is not a static activity. Observations of standing workers indicate that workers sway slowly back and forth and from side to side, similar to seated workers. The body's center of gravity alternately shifts from over the ankles to slightly behind the hip joints (Pheasant, 1991). Many workers complain of leg pain after standing for long periods. Such complaints are related to increased venous pressure on the lower extremity while standing and the lack of venous return to the heart. The result is pooling of the blood in the legs, an actual increase in leg volume, and a feeling of discomfort or heaviness in the lower extremity (Pheasant, 1991).

Standing has also been associated with low-back and foot problems. Foot pain, particularly plantar fasciitis and heel spurs, have been associated with prolonged standing on a hard surface. A hard surface such as concrete does not promote the subtle muscular contractions in the feet and legs that pump blood to the heart. Further, the foot musculature becomes stressed by constant pounding on a hard surface. In terms of low-back pain, individuals tend to assume positions that increase the lumbar lordosis. However, there is no consensus regarding the relationship between lumbar lordosis while standing and low-back pain (Pheasant, 1991).

Despite these problems, standing workstations may be the best option for jobs that require higher forces, extended reaches, or frequent movement between several workstations (Eastman Kodak Company, 1983; Putz-Anderson, 1988). A small prop seat, leaning area, or stool must be provided for workers who continually work while standing.

Workers and health care practitioners must also pay attention to the visual and manipulative demands of a task. Invariably, the placement of visual displays and objects that must be manipulated determines the position of the head and neck. According to Kroemer and Grandjean (2001), visual display monitors should be angled approximately 0 to 15 degrees below eye level (see Chapter 24).

The following are guidelines for the design of standing workstations.

- *Proper work height* depends on the height of the person and the type of task performed. Unless specified, the elbow should be flexed to approximately 90 degrees, the shoulders abducted or flexed less than 20 to 25 degrees, and the neck slightly flexed (Figure 11-5).
- For *precise or delicate work*, the work surface should be approximately 2 to 4 inches (5 to 10 cm) above the elbow.
- For *light assembly work,* the work surface should be approximately 2 to 4 inches (5 to 10 cm) below the elbow.
- For *heavy work,* the work surface should be approximately 4 to 5 inches (10 to 15 cm) below the elbow.
- *Work surface edges* should be rounded or padded to avoid mechanical (or contact) stresses to underlying structures.
- *Hard floor surfaces* (such as concrete) should be cushioned with antifatigue mats or rubber matting to decrease the stress on the legs and low back. Specific floor mats are available for most industries.
- *Shoes* worn by the worker should have adequate instep support and a slip-resistant sole. A polyurethane or viscoelastic polymer insert will help cushion and absorb the forces from walking or standing on a hard surface.
- *Footrests* are necessary to relieve stress on the low back and to provide a change of position for the legs. Options include a foot rail, a low inclined stool, or footrests similar to those for seated work.

Frequently Used Equipment and Controls

Work equipment or controls that are used on a regular basis should be located within comfortable reach for the worker. Putz-Anderson (1988) advocates that frequently used supplies and equipment be kept within an area that can be easily reached by a "sweep of the forearm" when the upper arm is in neutral. Although an individual's reach can be extended by standing, moving forward, leaning, or flexing the trunk, a worker will fatigue if the reach is overextended for long periods of time.

Individual reach capabilities can be envisioned as a three-dimensional semicircular shell in front of the worker (Eastman Kodak Company, 1983). Figure 11-6 indicates that the reach distance in front of the body is approximately 17 to 18 inches, depending on the person's body

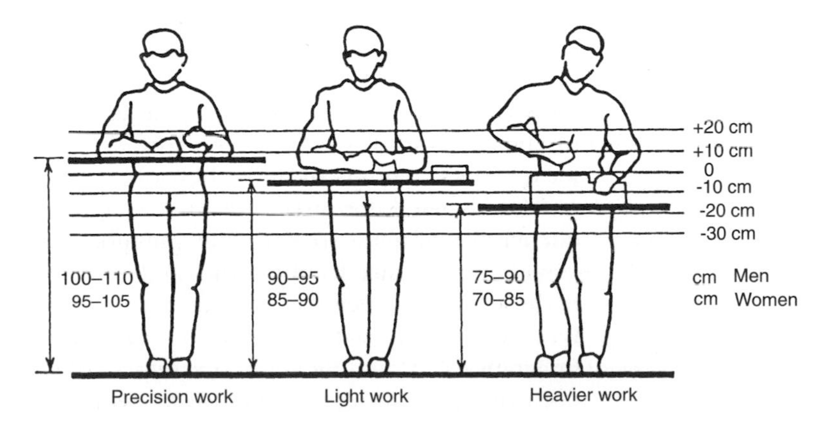

Figure 11-5 Recommended heights for standing workstations. Height varies with type of work performed. (Reprinted with permission from Kroemer, E., & Grandjean, E. [2001]. Fitting the task to the person [5th ed.]. London: Taylor & Francis.)

size and whether he or she is standing or sitting. The reach distances to the side will be slightly less than those for the front. Reach distances should be reduced by 2 inches (5 cm) for tasks that require hand grasp (Eastman Kodak Company, 1983).

A reach distance for repetitive use should be nearly half the maximum distance from the shoulder to the extended fingers. The worker should not reach above shoulder height or behind the back on a frequent basis.

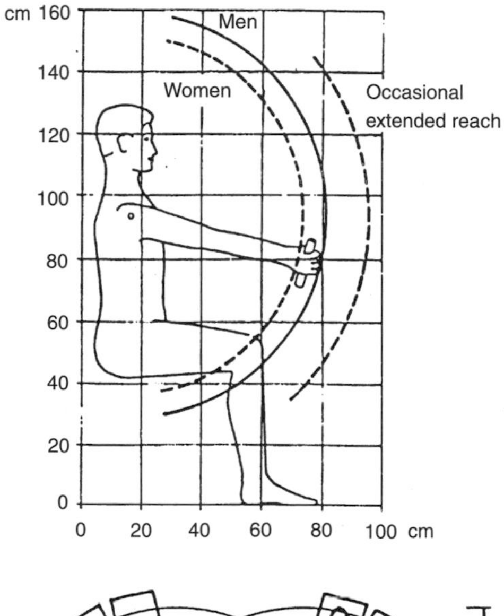

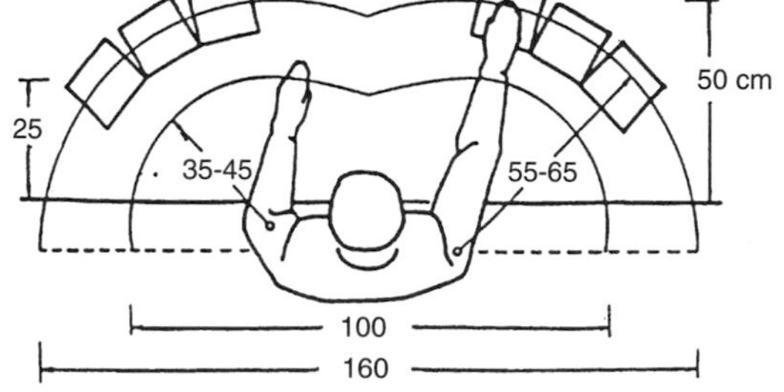

Figure 11-6 Recommended vertical (top) and horizontal (bottom) distances for reaching and grasping from a seated workstation (in cm). Reach distances are measured form the shoulder to hand; grasp distances are measured from the elbow to hand. Values include men and women from the 5th percentile. (Reprinted with permission from Kroemer, E., & Grandjean, E. [2001]. *Fitting the task to the person* [5th ed.]. London: Taylor & Francis.)

The following guidelines (compiled from Kroemer & Grandjean, 2001; Pheasant, 2001; Putz-Anderson, 1988) provide an additional checklist of workstation areas to consider for frequently used tasks or controls.

- Perform frequently repeated tasks within an arm's length in front of oneself and avoid reaching above shoulder height or behind the body.
- Perform manipulative work with the elbows flexed to 90 degrees and held close to the body.
- Keep motions symmetric or opposite during work tasks to reduce static loads on the trunk.
- Minimize work performed with the trunk flexed and the extremities in awkward positions.
- Avoid maintaining the arms outstretched for long periods. This posture will cause muscle fatigue rapidly and will reduce the accuracy of fine hand and arm movements.
- Alternate between sitting and standing workstations.
- Position work at a height that is optimal for the worker's visual acuity to prevent neck and eye strain.
- Create a natural rhythm for the work, using curvilinear rather than straight-line motions to accomplish tasks.

HAND AND POWERED TOOLS

Despite automation, workers continue to use tools on a daily basis for assembly and precision tasks that require careful monitoring or expertise (Cochran & Riley, 1986). Workers' use of tools has evolved from the use of varied tools throughout the day to reliance on specific tools for extended periods of time (Tichauer, 1966). As the demand for precision and high productivity continues, so does the potential for cumulative trauma to the hand and forearm because of improper tool design and use. The Bureau of Labor Statistics indicates that hand tool injuries account for approximately 5% of all occupational injuries. The industries with the highest incidence of hand tool injuries are construction, agriculture, mining, and manufacturing (BLS, 2002).

Fortunately, the ergonomic tool industry has stepped up research and design efforts to meet these strong consumer demands. However, consumers must be vigilant to truly separate the cosmetic styling from true ergonomic design. This discussion elucidates the basic issues of hand biomechanics and prehension relative to tool design. It offers the guidelines to identify the salient features of ergonomically sound tools.

Prehension Patterns

Basic to a discussion of tools is a common language or classification system for the grasps used to describe tool handling. Napier (1956) proposed a simple yet clear distinction between power and precision grasps that has been globally accepted. A *power* (or cylindric) grasp refers to clutching an object in the palm of the hand with the thumb wrapped around the object. Figure 11-7 demonstrates that to perform a power grasp, the wrist must assume a position of ulnar deviation and extension to align the index finger and thumb with the longitudinal axis of the forearm and tool (Fraser, 1989; Napier, 1956; Neumann, 2002).

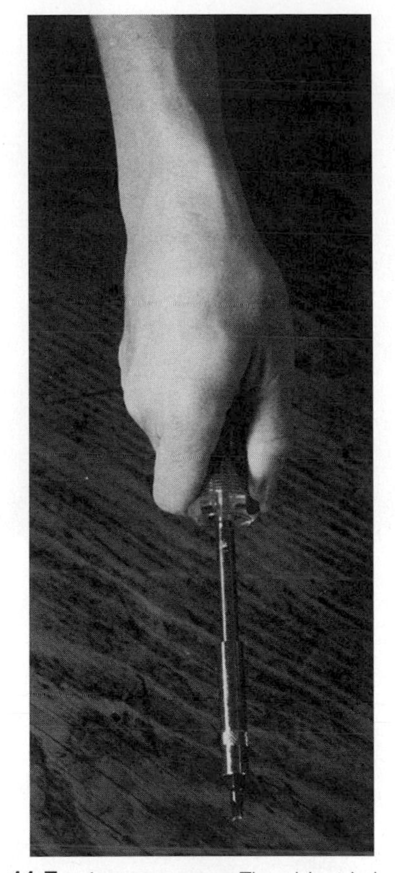

Figure 11-7 A power grasp. The object is held firmly in the palm of the hand. The wrist is ulnarly deviated to align the hand with the longitudinal axis of the tool.

A *precision* grasp refers to holding an object between the thumb and opposing fingers. This grasp allows for sensory input to the fingers and active manipulation of objects. To perform a precision grasp, the wrist is positioned in slight extension, and the thumb and fingers are partially flexed and opposed around the object (Figure 11-8). Types of precision grasps include *lateral* (Figure 11-9), *palmar* (also named a *three-jaw chuck* or *tripod*; see Figure 11-8), *pincer* (Figure 11-10), and *spherical grasps* (Figure 11-11). A hook grasp does not include the thumb. The lateral pinch grasp is the strongest of all precision grasps. When a precision grasp is needed, a modified palmar grasp is used 75% of the time.

Although this classification distinguishes between grasps, the power and precision grasps are rarely used independently of each other. In a combined grasp such as knitting, the ulnar fingers secure the object (in this case, needles) in the palm while the thumb and index fingers are free to manipulate (Napier, 1956) (Figure 11-12). (See Chapter 20 for a complete discussion of knitting.) While performing a given task, the operator may combine or switch grasps on a tool, depending on the purpose. For example, when using a screwdriver to hang a picture, an individual may initiate the project with a precision grasp to set the screw but will most likely switch to a power grasp to embed the screw in the surface. Similarly, when opening a bottle, one will use both power and precision grasps.

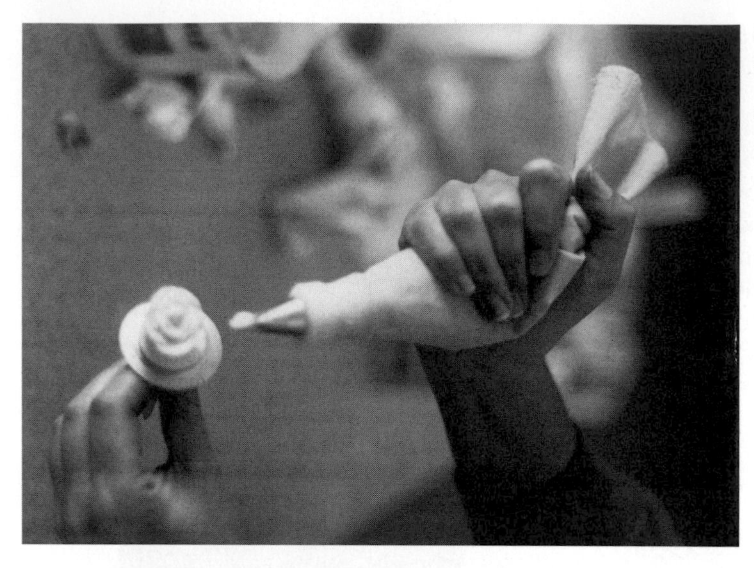

Figure 11-8 In a palmar pinch (left) the thumb opposes an object against the index and middle fingers. A power grasp is demonstrated in the right hand.

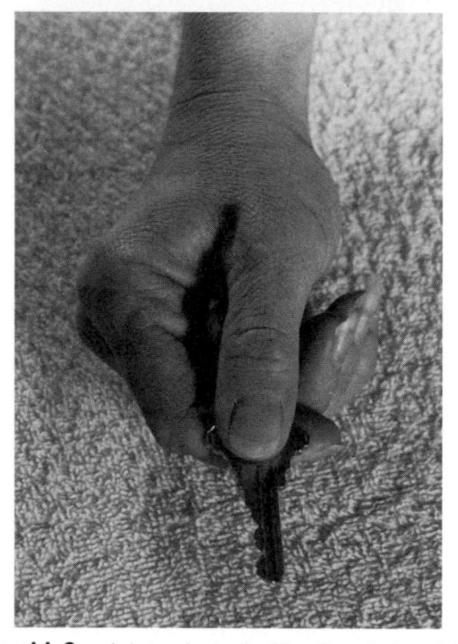

Figure 11-9 A lateral pinch. The thumb is adducted against the radial border of the index finger. The lateral pinch is the strongest of all pinches.

Grip and Prehension Forces

Individuals exhibit a wide range of power grip and prehension strengths. Knowledge of grip strength is clearly important for investigating tasks that involve tool activation, grasping and holding objects, opening and closing containers, and operating controls. The average power grip strength is approximately 100 to 115 pounds for men and 60 to 65 pounds for women. Average prehension grasp strengths are 17 to 24 pounds for men (pincer grasp is least strong and lateral grasp is strongest) and 11 to 16 pounds for women (Mital & Pennathur, 2001; Chaffin & Anderson, 1984). A wide range of "normal" exists depending on one's age, occupation, avocation, and personal stature.

Although most containers are designed to be opened with a minimal amount of force, Terrono, Nalebuff, and Phillips (1995) suggest that a grip strength of at least 20 pounds and a pinch strength of 5 to 7 pounds is required to perform most daily living tasks. However, this suggestion has not been systematically examined. Older individuals and those with disabilities are the user groups most affected by tasks requiring high prehension forces. When Robert Feaney Associates (2003) investigated the grasping forces needed to open paper and plastic packages in individuals over 50 years old, they found that the technique used to open the packages influenced the prehension forces generated. In packages with a larger area available for grasping, individuals could use a power grip, thereby

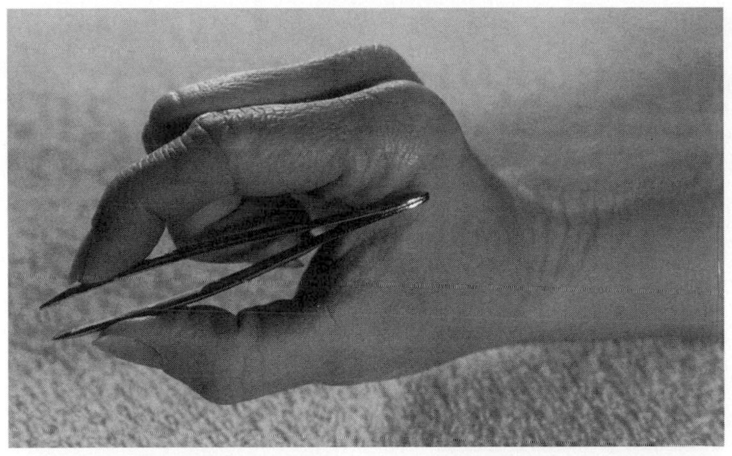

Figure 11-10 A pincer grasp. Opposition is performed using the tip of the thumb and index fingers.

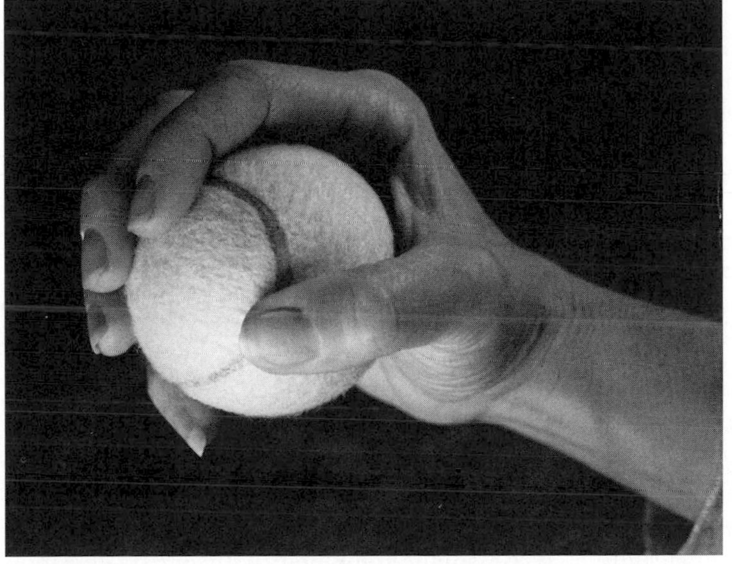

Figure 11-11 A spherical grasp. The object is held in the palm with fingers abducted securely around it.

applying more force to the package (please see reference for more details). These results have been applied to the packaging industry.

Further, Rahman, Thomas, and Rice (2002) found no clear relationship between the individual's maximum grip strength and the amount of force exerted on a container when opening the container. Interestingly, men used significantly more force than women to open containers and older individuals used less force than younger individuals to open the same containers. Authors suggest that clients modify techniques to use hands more gently and efficiently.

Principles for Hand and Tool Use

Clearly, the relationship between the type of grasp, the position of the hand, and hand anatomy is integral to proper tool use. The following principles (compiled from Hunter, Schneider, Mackin, & Callahan, 1990; Neumann, 2002; Pheasant, 2001; Rodgers, 1987; Spaulding, 1989;

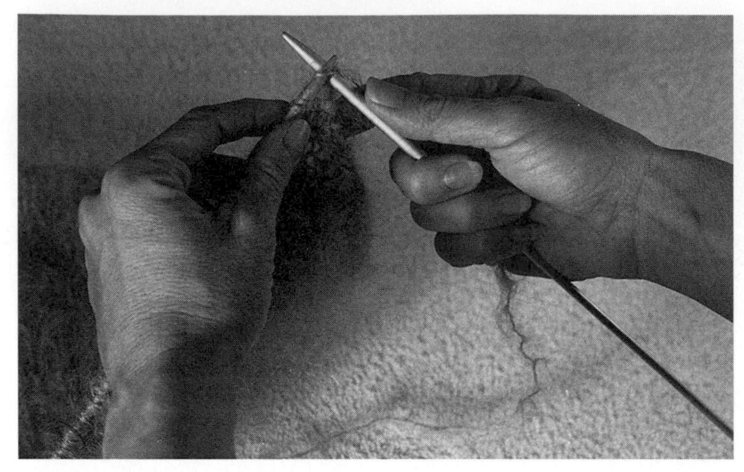

Figure 11-12 Both power and precision tasks are used simultaneously. Knitting requires use of a pincer grasp to manipulate the yarn and a power grasp to hold the needle in the palm of the hand.

Tichauer, 1966) for hand and tool use will assist managers, ergonomic consultants, and workers in understanding the implications for using and choosing tools.

Some *biomechanical considerations* are as follows.

- A power grasp is four times stronger than a precision grasp. Use a power grip whenever possible.
- Maximal grip strength is generated at 0 to 15 degrees of wrist extension.
- Wrist deviation reduces the grip force available. At 45 degrees of wrist extension, grip strength is 75% of maximal; at 45 degrees of wrist flexion, grip strength is reduced to 60% of maximal (see Table 10-1). With the wrist deviated, workers must generate significantly more force to accomplish the task.
- Grip strength is the weakest in flexion since the wrist and finger flexors are shortened, which diminishes the ability to generate tension.
- Elbow extension should be combined with pronation, and elbow flexion should be combined with supination for synergistic action and optimal force development in arm musculature.
- All hand grasping requires isometric contractions of the wrist extensor muscles to position the wrist. Stronger grasping requires stronger muscle contractions and thus greater strain to elbow extensor musculature.

The *neurovascular considerations* are as follows.

- The median nerve is superficial in the palm of the hand and at the base of the thumb.
- The radial digital nerves and arteries run lateral to each finger and are unprotected by fat pads.
- The ulnar nerve passes between the medial epicondyle and the olecranon at the elbow and just deep to the pisiform bone at the ulnar border of the wrist.

Some other *musculoskeletal considerations* are as follows:

- Grasping combined with wrist deviation places added stress on wrist musculature and the median nerve in the carpal canal.
- Lateral pinch combined with wrist deviation stresses the abductor pollicis longus and extensor pollicis brevis tendons.
- Digital creases are not protected by fat pads. Consequently, the finger pulley systems underlying digital creases are prone to direct or repetitive trauma.
- Intrinsic muscles provide optimum stability for grasping at midrange between full finger flexion and extension.

Tool Design

Today, industry consultants and managers must consider not only the most appropriate tool for the specific job but also the range of tool sizes necessary for a diverse workforce. Most obviously, tools that are balanced and sized for men with larger muscle mass will demand more force from female users with smaller hand mass. Conversely, the operation of precision tools that are balanced and designed for a smaller hand (such as dental hygiene instruments) will cause excessive strain for men with larger hand mass.

As Meagher (1987) explained, "One size does *not* fit all." Tools must be sized to fit the worker, and consideration must be given to the normal biomechanics of the hand. Further, workers should try out the tools before committing to their long-term use. Meagher (1987) suggests that the most important elements of tool design with regard to human usage are handle size, shape, and texture, ease of operation, shock absorption, and weight.

Handle Diameter and Span

The handle size refers to either the diameter of the tool handle, for cylindric tools (such as a hammer or pneumatic tools), or the span between handles, for crimping tools or tools with two handles (such as pliers, scissors, or clippers). The correct tool handle size allows the worker to generate optimal strength for the job without straining the flexor tendons or intrinsic muscles.

Cylindrical Tools

To generate the maximum grip strength, the flexor digitorum superficialis and flexor digitorum profundus provide flexion forces, and the intrinsic muscles stabilize the tool in the hand. When a power grasp is used on a tool with a cylindric handle, the proximal and distal interphalangeal joints should be in midflexion; the distal joint of the middle and ring fingers should overlap the distal joint (or part of phalange) of the thumb.

The optimal diameter for torque development in a cylindric tool varies slightly according to type of effort exerted. Axial thrust (turning a tool about its own axis, such as screwdriver) involves shear forces acting on the cylindrical surface and is best generated with a handle size of 1.5 inches (4 cm) with ranges from 1.25 to 2 inches (3 to 5 cm), depending on the individual's hand size (Cochran & Riley, 1986; Eastman Kodak Company, 1983; Pheasant, 2001). For tools that are gripped and turned about a perpendicular axis (T-wrench) or straight-on (hammer) (Figure 11-13), the optimal grip diameter may be larger (2 to 2.5 inches, or 5 to 6 cm) since the force generation is less dependent on the handle size and shape. Grip strength generally increases with diameter up to a certain point and then decreases (Mital & Pennathur, 2001). Gripping can be enhanced with a thumb stall to reduce slippage (Robinson & Lyon, 1994).

Two-Handled Tools

The span between handles for crimping tools or double-handled tools should be 2.5 to 3.5

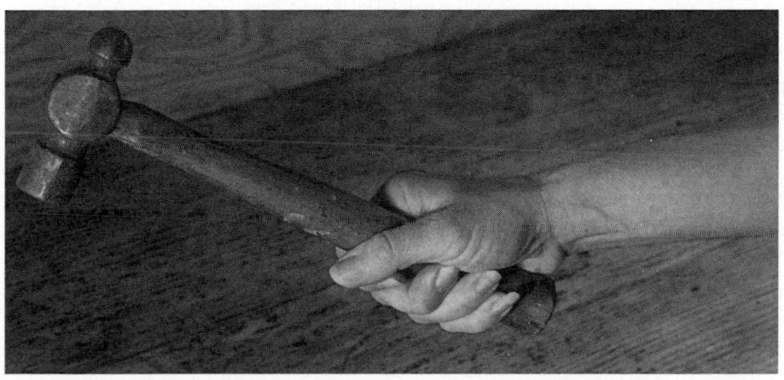

Figure 11-13 Handle size for a cylindrical tool. Both distal interphalangeal (DIP) and proximal interphalangeal (PIP) joints should be in midflexion.

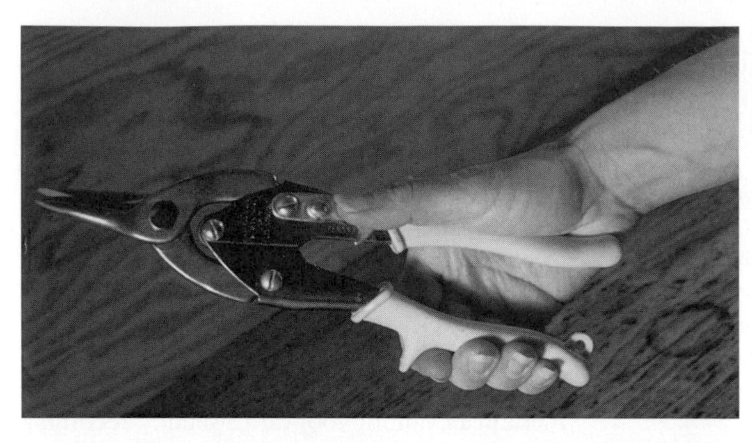

Figure 11-14 Handle size for a two-handled tool. Proximal interphalangeal (PIP) joints should be in midflexion at the application of force.

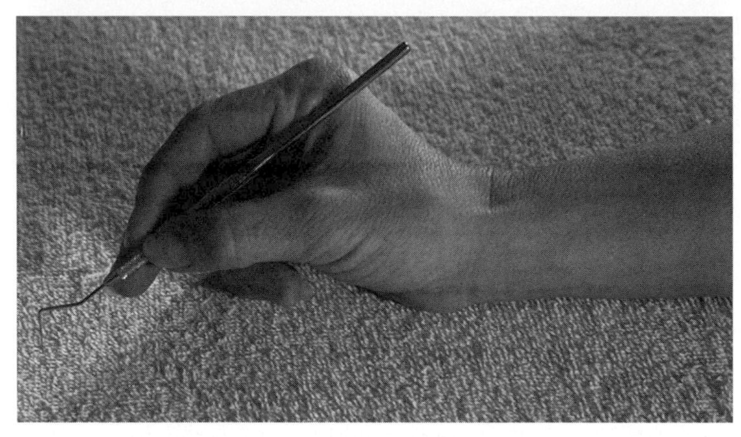

Figure 11-15 Handle size for precision tools. A modified palmar (or tripod) grasp is commonly used for precision work. Precision tools have a small diameter and smooth tip for accurate work.

inches (6.5 to 9.0 cm) at the application of force (Eastman Kodak Company, 1983). The maximal flexor force should be leveraged at the proximal interphalangeal joint to use the stronger flexor digitorum superficialis tendons for flexion. Crimping tools should have a spring opening so as not to injure the dorsal structures of the hand against the handle when opening the jaws of the tool. The spring should open the handles no more than 3.5 to 4.5 inches (9 to 11.5 cm) to prevent stretching the thumb collateral ligaments (Figure 11-14).

Precision Tools

Most precision tools require some type of a modified palmar or tripod grasp. To allow better control and manipulation, precision tools should have a small diameter and a smooth front end. The optimum diameter for precision tools is suggested to be 0.45 inches (12 mm), the acceptable range being from 0.3 to 0.6 inches (8 to 16 mm) (Figure 11-15) (Eastman Kodak Company, 1983; Robinson & Lyon, 1994). However, dental hygiene instruments are being manufactured at diameters up to ¾ inches in efforts to decrease strain on fingers during instrumentation (see Chapter 22).

Inappropriately Sized Tools

If a tool's handle diameter is not appropriately sized, the hand muscles and ligaments become strained and easily fatigued when using the tool. For example, if the tool diameter or span between handles is too large, the force is

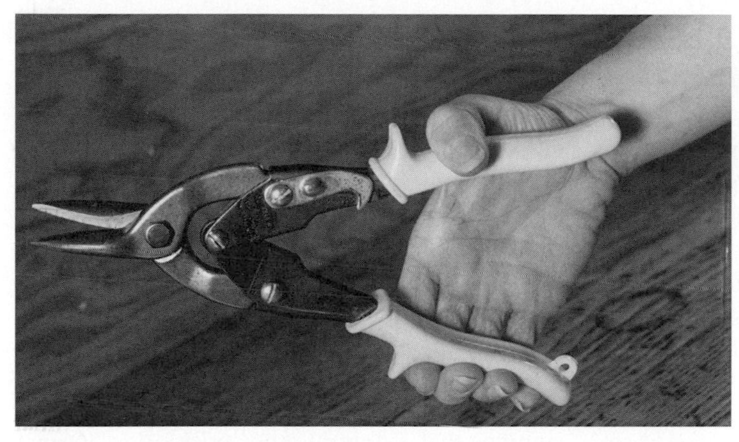

Figure 11-16 Overly wide handle openings. Excessive strain is placed on the collateral ligaments of the thumb carpometacarpal (CMC) and metacarpophalangeal (MCP) joints when handle openings are too wide. Force is applied at the DIP joints rather than the PIP joint in this photo.

applied at the distal phalanx. The weaker flexor muscle, the flexor digitorum profundus, becomes the primary flexor. When force is applied at the distal phalanx, the tendon force is two to three times greater than when forces are applied at the middle phalanx. Handle openings on crimping tools that are too wide also place excess stress on the collateral ligaments of the thumb carpometacarpal and metacarpophalangeal joints (Figure 11-16).

If the handle is too small, the finger flexors and intrinsics must generate more force because the muscles are already contracted maximally and thus are at a mechanical disadvantage. The intrinsics must generate added force to maintain the position (Johnson, 1990).

Handle Contour

The shape or contour of a tool's handle should follow the transverse arch of the hand to use the stronger ulnar musculature and to permit an even application of force between all fingers. The handle should rest on the thenar and hypothenar eminences to prohibit compression of the neurovascular bundles between the fingers (Meagher, 1987). Most tool handles are cylindric in shape, although a slightly curved or cone shape better facilitates gripping by following the transverse arch (Fraser, 1989).

Optimal Shape

Studies regarding the relationship between handle shape and muscle force suggest that the optimal shape for developing torque on a tool relates to the direction of the forces exerted and type of task performed. The area of the grip should be maximized in order to avoid localized pressure. Studies suggest the following (Cochran & Riley, 1986; Mital & Pennathur, 2001).

- Triangular handles or rectangular handles are superior for forward push-pull forces or for using the wrist in extremes of wrist flexion or extension (if absolutely necessary).
- T-shaped handles can increase torque generation for screwdrivers.
- Circular or rectangular handles or handles that are circular with two flat sides should be used for sideways or orthogonal forces such as are used for slicing meat.
- Circular or square handles are best for use in tasks that demand lower forces for longer periods of time.

Digital Separators

Digital separators or finger recesses present both biomechanical and neurovascular problems. Separators force the fingers into abduction, which strains the intrinsic musculature and flattens the hypothenar eminence. Further, the separators may apply pressure to neurovascular bundles (the digital arteries and nerves) lateral to each finger. Although the separators were originally designed to promote handle control, the separators actually limit a worker's options for moving or adjusting the tool in his or her hand (Eastman Kodak Company, 1983; Mital & Pennathur, 2001; Tichauer, 1966).

Finger Rings

Finger rings pose the same problem as do digital separators in terms of compressing the neurovascular bundles lateral to each finger. The finger loops (as in scissors or tin snips) place pressure on a small surface area and can injure dorsal or volar structures below the loops. Loop-design scissors allow for a more even distribution of pressure in the hand (Figure 11-17).

Handle Orientation

A tool handle that is not well oriented to the body causes the worker to assume awkward postures during work tasks and to use more force to accomplish the task. Workers often compensate for wrist deviation by elevating the elbows and abducting the shoulders, thus transferring stresses to another area of the body. Many tools, such as hammers or pliers, necessitate positioning the hand in ulnar deviation to accomplish a task (Robinson & Lyon, 1994).

Tichauer (1978) found a high incidence of tenosynovitis among workers performing wiring operations at an electronics manufacturing plant. When the traditional straight-handled pliers were replaced with bent-handle designs, the incidence of tenosynovitis decreased from 60% to 10% for those using the bent-handle design. The adage "Bend the tool, not the hand" signifies that a neutral wrist position is optimal for tool use. Handle curves are recommended for tools that require the hand to be positioned in ulnar deviation during use, such as hammers, pliers, and saws. For most tools, at least a 20-degree curve positions the hand in neutral and,

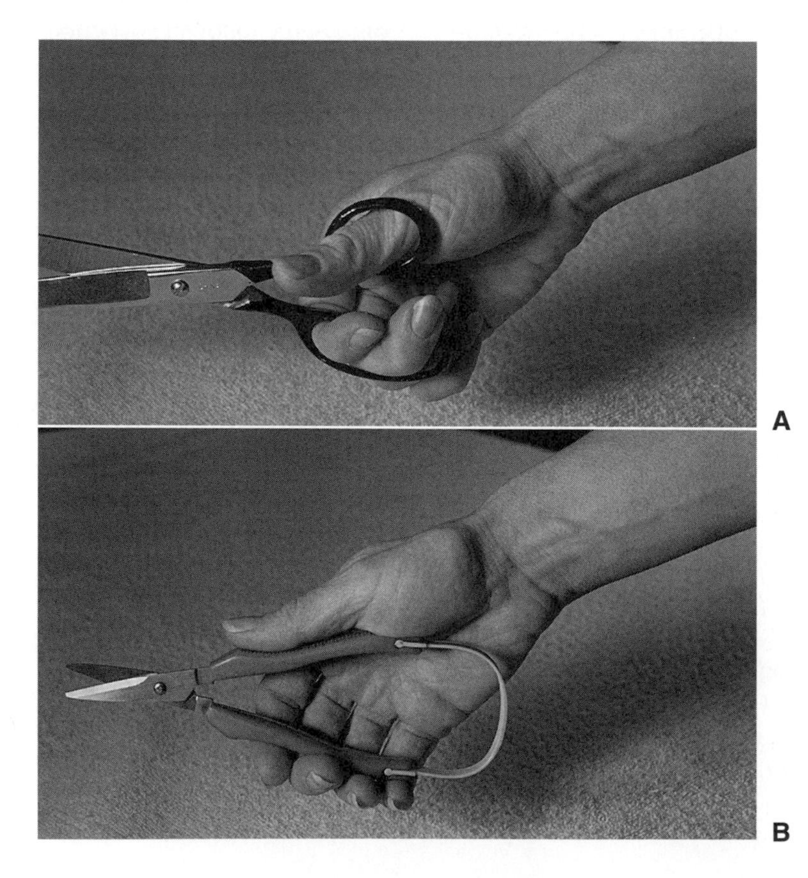

Figure 11-17 Handle contour. **A,** Finger loops on scissors may compress the digital neurovascular bundles lateral to the thumb and index fingers. **B,** Loop design scissors distribute pressure evenly across the thenar eminence and fingers.

thus, decreases ulnar deviation (Schoenmarklin & Marras, 1989; Tichauer, 1966). Novice workers seem to derive more benefit from handle curves than do experienced workers. Today, tools such as hammers, pliers, scissors, and knives with curved handles can be purchased.

Curved handles are most effective when all work is performed on the same plane. However, the proper handle orientation also depends on the work surface being used. In-line cylindric tools can be used for drill work being performed on a horizontal surface, such as a workbench, whereas a pistol grip is effective for work performed on a vertical surface. Figure 11-18 demonstrates the improved position for the wrist when using a pistol grip on a knife. For pistol grips, the angle of the handle in relation to the longitudinal axis should be 70 to 80 degrees (Mital & Pennathur, 2001; Robinson & Lyon, 1994). Tools such as paint rollers, paintbrushes, hoes, and garden equipment can be adapted with pistol grips (see Chapter 20) (Johnson, 1990).

Handle Length

Sufficient length of a tool is necessary to distribute the pressure of forces evenly across the hand and to prevent direct pressure on the median nerve in the palm of the hand or at the base of the thumb. A tool handle should be long enough to extend proximal to the thenar emi-

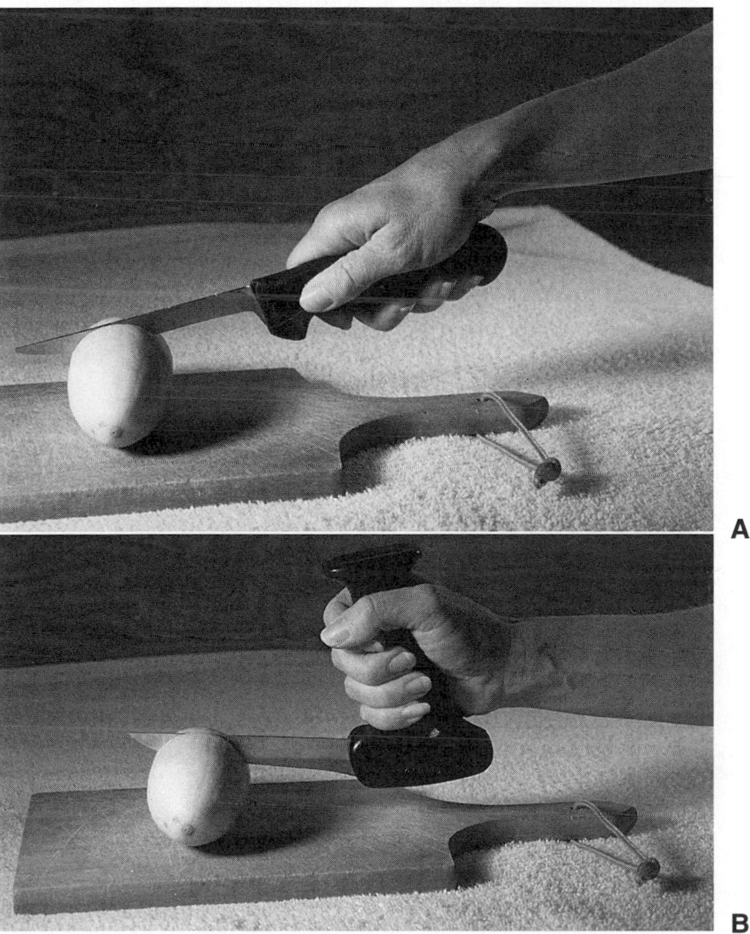

Figure 11-18 Handle orientation. **A,** A straight-handle design causes the wrist to deviate ulnarly once force is applied. **B,** A pistol-grip design promotes a neutral position of the wrist and the use of arm musculature to power the task.

nence and permit adequate freedom of movement on the handle (Putz-Anderson, 1988). A short tool handle (Figure 11-19, *A*) may injure not only the superficial median or ulnar nerves but also the tendon sheaths, causing trigger finger and digital neuritis. Figure 11-19, *B*, shows a more even distribution of forces on the thenar eminence structures.

Anthropometric data suggest that the range of palm width is 2.8 to 3.6 inches (Eastman Kodak Company, 1983). The minimum tool length recommended for most tasks is 4 inches (10 cm), although a length of 5 inches (13 cm) is preferred. When gloves are to be worn during tool use, an additional 0.5 inches (13 mm) should be added to the tool's length (Putz-Anderson, 1988).

Handle Surface, Texture, and Materials

The surface and texture of the tool handle directly affects the transfer of force from the worker to the tool. A tool handle must allow for insulation against heat, shock absorption, and pressure distribution, and it must provide some friction for ease of grasping the handle. The general recommendations suggest that a grip surface should be slightly compressible, nonconductive, and free from ridges (Mital & Pennathur, 2001). Compressible materials both dampen vibration and distribute pressure over a

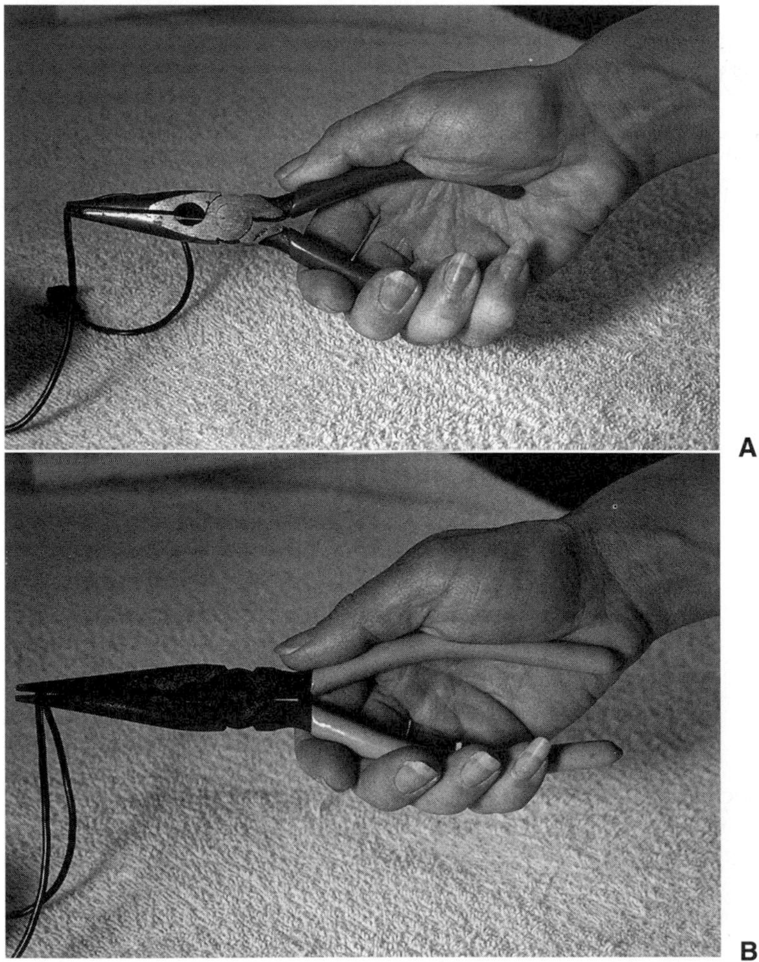

Figure 11-19 Handle length. **A,** A short handle may injure superficial structures in the thenar eminence, such as the median nerve. **B,** Handles should extend proximally through the thenar eminence to avoid contact forces and distribute the pressure through the palm.

larger surface. Wood has traditionally offered such advantages, but wood has low resistance in that it eventually cracks or separates from the metal component. New polystyrene and stain-resistant plastics have replaced wood. However, these materials should be covered with rubber, leather, or synthetic layers of material for comfort and ease of grasping the tool (Fraser, 1989; Mital & Pennathur, 2001). A tool handle with a lightly compressible, thin rubber coating provides good proprioceptive feedback, friction, and moisture for gripping.

Slipperiness

The *coefficient of friction* refers to the slipperiness of an object and has been calculated for many surfaces (see Chapter 10). A tool handle that is too slippery or too dry will require extra force to maintain the tool in the hand. Such has been the case in poultry workers who have developed MSDs in part because of the excessive force needed to grasp and cut slippery poultry carcasses.

Generally, a higher coefficient of friction will improve the ability to grip an object and thus lower the grip force requirements. Tool handles should have the ability to maintain frictional forces when moist, since many workers develop sweaty palms during the day. Buchholz, Frederick, and Armstrong (1988) studied the effects of material type and moisture on pinch forces. Buchholz's group identified that porous materials, such as cloth-based tapes and suede, had a higher coefficient of friction when wet and would therefore be good choices for tool handles in environments with much moisture. Rubber coating is a good all-around choice for wet or dry environments. Clearly, materials with a very high coefficient of friction, such as sandpaper, may cause abrasion and should be avoided.

Surface Pattern

Tool surfaces should not be perfectly smooth because the tool will rotate or slip in the hand during use. However, tool handles that are too coarse or knurled can lead to discomfort or skin irritation and therefore decrease work efficiency (Fraser, 1989). Handles should not have deep fluted edges or ridges that may injure underlying hand structures.

Fraser (1989) suggests a dull roughening or distinctive surface pattern to provide sensory input and to assist the user in maintaining grip. Greenberg and Chaffin (1977) suggest that patterns in the tool handle should be perpendicular to the force exerted to avoid slippage and improve surface friction. A study of instrumentation among dental hygienists revealed a preference for waffle-iron serrations on dental instruments; these were claimed to provide adequate friction without irritating the fingers (Atwood & Michalak, 1992).

Vibration Absorption

Chronic exposure to power tools or hand-held tools with low-frequency vibrating components may constrict blood flow or injure the digital arteries of the fingers and hand, causing such conditions as vibration white-finger syndrome, hand-arm vibration syndrome, Raynaud's disease, or carpal tunnel syndrome (refer to Chapter 10 for a complete discussion). Repetitive impact from a hammer also can cause blood vessel spasms, clots, or hypothenar hammer syndrome (National Institute of Occupational Safety and Health, 1989).

Research suggests that use of vibrating tools stimulates the tonic vibration reflex in hand and forearm muscles, which stimulates additional muscle contractions during tool use. Researchers also speculate that vibration decreases the worker's tactile sensitivity. Therefore, the worker must grip harder because of the lack of proprioceptive feedback (Armstrong, Fine, Radwin, & Silverstein, 1987; Radwin, Armstrong, & Chaffin, 1987). Finally, heavy tools that vibrate may cause the worker to grip the tool more tightly, and, consequently, the vibration will resonate to the elbow and shoulder.

To decrease the effects of vibration, tool handles should be padded or covered with rubber housing, vibration components dampened, and exposure monitored. Padded gloves may protect hands by absorbing vibration energy, provided the gloves fit properly (Brown, 1990). Most tool companies offer kits to decrease vibration effects and also offer specially dampened, custom-made tools. Certain vibration-dampening materials are more effective at certain frequencies. For example, closed-cell foam materials may provide better vibration-dampening qualities above 160 Hz (Hampel, 1992; Robinson & Lyon, 1994). Hickory wood is recommended as a good material for absorbing shock. Although parameters for vibration do not yet exist, the American National Standards Institute recommends that individuals operate tools for no more than 30 minutes at a time and, cumulatively, for only 4 hours per day (NIOSH, 1989).

Tool Weight and Balance

In general, tools should weigh as little as possible. Particularly for precision tasks, a lighter tool will require less force to support than will a heavy tool. In some cases, such as power tools, reducing the weight of a tool will require that more force be exerted to operate the tool, and this will increase shoulder tension. The decision regarding whether to increase or decrease the weight of a tool will depend on how that tool is used.

Guidelines suggest that tools weigh no more than 5 pounds (2.3 kg) if the tool must be supported by the hand and arm or if the tool is being operated away from the body. Tools used in precision work should weigh no more than 1 pound (0.4 kg). Tools that are heavier should be counterbalanced with an overhead sling that is positioned perpendicular to the task. Tools should be well balanced to reduce hand fatigue. The center of gravity of the tool should be located close to the hand grip (Armstrong, 1990; Eastman Kodak Company, 1983; Robinson & Lyon, 1994).

Tool Position

Operating a tool requires a combined effort of supporting and controlling the tool. Often, the body is forced into awkward positions during one of these two acts because of the position of the task or the tool. As stated previously, the body should be in neutral for the best biomechanical advantage. Shoulders should be positioned at less than 25 to 30 degrees of abduction, and the wrist should be in neutral. Through use of a vice, the worker can maintain neutral wrist and arm positions and leverage body weight. An assortment of vices, jigs, tilted surfaces, and overhead pulley systems and fixtures can aid the worker in improving the tool position and minimizing the weight needed to support the tool or task itself (Armstrong, 1990).

Tool Operation and Activation

A variety of trigger options are available for tool operation. Trigger designs should allow several fingers to activate the trigger and allow both joints of the fingers to depress the mechanism. The proximal joint should activate the trigger initially, thereby using the flexor digitorum superficialis for most of the work.

Many trigger designs require single-finger activation or activation by the distal interphalangeal joint only. With such designs, the potential exists for tenosynovitis or a nodule to develop on the flexor tendon from its repetitive and forceful use (Johnson, 1990). In contrast, a strip trigger is approximately 2 inches long and allows two or three fingers to activate the trigger (Robinson & Lyon, 1994).

Robinson and Lyon (1994) suggest that trigger forces be determined on the basis of the tool's application. Tools used for high-precision operations or those operated over an extended period of time should require light trigger-force activation, whereas tools used for heavier tasks, such as power tools, may require higher trigger forces.

Ergonomic Tool Selection

New Directions

Clearly, an ergonomically designed tool is more than the size and shape of the handle. The proper choice of tools depends on the task orientation and task demands, as well as the environmental conditions of air quality, humidity, and temperature. Tool manufactures have spent copious hours in observing workers and conducting focus groups to identify the specific user needs and hazards in both professional contractor and home tool user groups. To that end, manufacturers have built sound ergonomic design into high-end tools so that professional contractors now expect design features such as balance, light weight, and comfort as integral to the functionality of their tools (Spaulding, 2001).

Many tools are now powered, which decreases the amount of force and exertion needed to perform a task. Some of the newer features of powered tools include low levels of noise and vibration output, high power-to-weight ratios, pistol grips, automatic shut-off (which decreases the chance of overtightening for pneumatic screwdrivers), and the use of torque arms. Torque arms with torque-controlled tools shut off automatically, which decreases torque reactions or kickback of high forces to the hands. These high forces are particularly stressful because workers must forcefully grip the tool harder to maintain the tool in the hands (Atlas Copco, 2002; Carson, 1995). Powered screwdrivers with a pistol grip orientation keep the hand in a neutral position; the counterbalance decreases the forces necessary to hold and operate the tool.

An expanded user population has also driven the need to develop more ergonomic features for the home project tool user. Women and older workers have created a consumer market for power tools—that is, the application of power to traditional tools such as wrenches, saws, and even tape measures. Such populations are willing to pay more for increased ease and less discomfort. A variety of grip sizes and options are now offered. Smaller grip sizes and cushioned grips have been adapted for screwdrivers, pliers, and hammers.

The future of ergonomic tools is speculated to be "smart tools" with microchip controls to improve the power distribution and balance when the tool is in operation. Further developments will include lighter weight and more durable materials (Spaulding, 2001).

Ergonomic Tool Analysis and Guidelines

Although tool use is ubiquitous, few job analysis methods have been developed to examine work with hand tools. The Hand Tool Work Analysis Method (HTWAM) has been developed as part of the Eurohandtool Project to analyze hand-operated, nonpowered tools within a work system (Peterson, Wakula, Landau, 1999/2000). The goals are to provide recommendations for the ergonomic design of hand tools in specific industries and to provide users with information needed to perform jobs more safely.

Although in its early stages of statistical testing, the HTWAM has shown promising effectiveness in the viticulture industry identifying the most stressful exposures in hand tool use. For example, Wakula, Beckman, Hett, and Landau (1999/2000) were able to identify that cutting with a pneumatic tool was 30% more effective than using nonpowered tools to cut grapevines.

The following performance goals for the development and use of ergonomic tools can help determine the degree to which tools are truly ergonomic.

- Low torque reaction and impulse vibration
- Use of neutral hand and wrist positions
- Lowest possible muscle effort during use
- Even distribution of pressure forces with low peak pressures across the grip
- Operating temperature between 68° and 77° F for thermal comfort
- Trigger pressure less than 22 psi
- Correct tool balance for this application

Boxes 11-1 and 11-2 offer further guidelines or criteria for the selection and use of manual and hand-powered tools.

LIGHTING IN THE WORKPLACE

Proper lighting of the workplace is essential to visual comfort and good work performance. Discussion of poor lighting might call to mind an image of a weary watchmaker or jeweler hunched over a high bench with a single lightbulb hanging directly overhead. Such an image underscores the strong impact of lighting on

BOX 11-1
Guidelines for Selecting Manual Tools

1. Use of a power versus a pinch grip
2. Rounded edges and corners for all contact areas
3. Grip forces distributed over a wide area
4. Handles that extend beyond the palm
5. Ample finger room on the handle
6. No finger grooves
7. Handle material that is semisoft, nonslip, and compressible
8. A flange present when downward forces are used
9. Spring openings on two-handled tools
10. Well-balanced handle located close to tool's center of gravity
11. No potential of pinching hand between closing parts

BOX 11-2
Guidelines for Using Powered Tools

1. Minimize vibration exposures
2. Use flexible cords that do not interfere with the job
3. Suspend tools on an overhead balancer
4. Use torque-controlled settings
5. Select push-to-start mechanism to eliminate triggers
6. If push-to-start is not available, use thumb or long triggers

posture, eye strain, visual acuity, and overall safety in the work environment.

Most health care professionals are familiar with basic lighting principles from personal experience; most of us have had to deal with computer glare from backlighting or difficulty reading notes when sunlight is being reflected off a white desk. Health care professionals and ergonomic consultants also realize that the visual demand of the task often determines head and neck postures. However, many are not familiar with the illumination levels appropriate for certain jobs and with ergonomic approaches for good lighting. In the following sections, the basic concepts of workplace lighting are introduced.

Terminology

The terms used to describe and measure lighting are essential to this discussion. *Illumination* is the measure of the quantity of light falling on a surface from a source such as the sun, a lamp, a candle, or a flashlight. It is measured with a photometer that is set directly on the surface. Illumination is recorded in footcandles (fc) in the United States or lux (1 fc = 10 lux) in other countries. Quantities range from .05 fc (0.5 lux) on a moonlit night to 16,000 fc (160,000 lux) at noon in summer (Eastman Kodak Company, 1983). Table 11-1 identifies some common sources of illumination and the associated levels.

Luminance is the perception of brightness of a surface or the light energy that is reflected back from a surface. Luminance depends on various factors in the surrounding environment, such as color, material, and contrasting articles that reflect different amounts of light energy. Generally, brighter, contrasting colors and shiny surfaces reflect more light and therefore give more luminance to an area. Luminance can also be measured by a photometer that is placed at a distance from the surface and pointed toward that surface. A photometer is similar to a camera lightmeter except that it provides a direct readout in fc or lux and is color corrected. Luminance is expressed as candela per square meter (cd/m^2) and can be envisioned as a certain number of lighted candles illuminating 1 m^2 (Eastman Kodak Company, 1983). Table 11-2 identifies the reflective value of common materials in a room.

To draw a distinction between illumination and luminance, imagine that an office with dark

Table 11-1
Levels of Illumination from Common Sources

Illumination Source	Footcandles	Lux
Outdoors, noonday sun	16,000	160,000
Outdoors, clear day	5,000	50,000
Outdoors, overcast day	500	5,000
Brightly lit office	100	1,000
Well-lit office	50	500
Reading light	30	300
Living room	5	50
Street lighting	1	10
Moonlight	0.05	0.5

furniture and many windows is illuminated to 30 fc (300 lux). The luminance in this room will vary from 50 cd/m^2 near the dark-colored desk to 2500 cd/m^2 near the unshaded window. Although the illumination is the same, the luminance will vary according to the reflective value of the walls (e.g., bright white or mauve), surface of the desk (e.g., dark wood or white panel), paper on the desk, and availability of light (e.g., window blinds open or shaded) (Pheasant, 1991).

Contrast ratio is the difference in luminance between two adjacent surfaces (Helander, 1997). Contrast ratio is determined as Luminance A/Luminance B. For tasks such as reading at a desk, a high contrast between the background and figures (e.g., dark figures on a light background) is beneficial to enhance legibility and ease of reading. However, in the work environment, sharp contrasts in luminance between large surfaces reduces visual comfort and visibility and may cause discomfort glare. For example, stark white walls contrasted with dark floor coverings, dark furniture, and dark business machines should be avoided in an office. The contrast between a window and the adjacent wall may be as high as 1:100 and therefore workstations are usually not facing the window. It is commonly recommended that the ratio between the task and large items in the work environment be less than 10:1 (Helander, 1997). The recommended luminance or reflective values should be high for ceilings (80% to 90%) but much lower for business machines, furniture (less than 50%), and flooring (less than 40%) (Kroemer & Grandjean, 2001).

Table 11-2
Reflective Values of Common Materials

Material	Reflective Value (%)
Fresh white plaster	95
White paint or white paper	85
Light gray or cream paint	75
Newsprint, concrete	55
Plain light wood	45
Dark gray paint	30
Printer's ink	15
Matte black paper	5

Most recommended values for lighting are expressed in terms of illumination (Helander, 1997; Pheasant, 1991). However, an understanding of luminance is necessary if one is to determine the best means of decorating and arranging the work environment to provide proper lighting.

Recommended Levels for Workplace Lighting

Recommended levels for workplace lighting have steadily increased throughout history. Pheasant (1991) states that in the 1930s most offices were lit by incandescent lamps that provided illumination of 10 fc (100 lux). Today, because of more efficient lighting, a typical office is lit to 50 fc (500 lux). Clearly, more precise, detailed, and exacting work demands better lighting. The extent to which illumination affects performance varies with the accuracy demands of the task, frequency of the task's performance, and safety demands. For example, surgical work, which is characterized by very detailed, low contrast, and small object manipulation may require 1000 to 2000 fc for the optimal illumination.

The generally accepted rule for lighting has been "more is better," but this is not necessarily true. Pheasant (1991) argues that once a worker has enough light to perform the task optimally, more lighting will not necessarily improve the performance. In fact, Kroemer and Grandjean (2001) found that office workers preferred lower lighting levels 40 to 80 fc (400 to 850 lux) for office tasks. Further, a high prevalence of office workers complained of eye problems when working at illumination levels greater than 100 fc (1000 lux). Although one cannot directly associate bright lighting and eye problems, the reflective glare and contrasting shadows may cause eye strain or blurriness at illumination levels in excess of 100 fc (1000 lux).

Older workers may experience changes in sight from the loss of focusing power (accommodation) and to clouding of vision (Anshel, 1998; Helander, 1997). Loss of accommodation, apparent after age 40, may cause individuals to have more difficulty than previously reading materials close to their eyes or seeing distant objects. This may not be a problem for computer users, but it may affect the distance a worker must stand from a task and affect the posture while trying to view the task. Clouding of vision impairs clear vision, causing workers to be sensitive to glare sources or stray illumination. Anshel (1998) recommends increasing the illumination levels for older workers, and using task lighting to minimize glare and add further illumination as needed.

Recommendations for lighting vary greatly throughout the world. The U.S. standards are much higher than those in Europe. Regardless of the standards chosen, lighting must meet the minimum lighting level—that is, a level that is sufficient for workers to perform the most critical part of the task. In designing lighting for a workplace, one must remember to consider the size of the task and object to be viewed, the contrast ratios and reflective value of the surrounding materials, the need for speed or accuracy, the age of workers, the level of detail required, and the need for artificial lighting during the day. Table 11-3 offers a range of recommendations for lighting for varied work tasks and the associated visual demand.

Glare

Glare occurs when excessively bright objects interfere with the visual field. This brightness is seen as a reflection of a light source that is superimposed on the visual task. The brightness may interfere with the visual task or may cause discomfort only.

Direct glare occurs when a source of light in the visual field is much brighter than task materials at the workplace. Sources of direct glare for indoor offices or machine shops include light fixtures, bright sky showing through a window, or reflections from brass or polished materials.

Indirect glare is a term used for light that is reflected from materials at the work surface itself. Indirect glare reduces the contrast of materials at the workplace and may reduce task performance (Eastman Kodak Company, 1983; Pheasant, 1991).

Direct glare can be reduced by decreasing the illumination level of the light source with shades or by equalizing the luminance of materials near the workstation. The light source

Table 11-3

Recommended Illumination Levels According to Tasks and Visual Demands

Task	Visual Demand	Range of Illumination*
Orienting self in corridor	Orientation	5-10 fc = 50-100 lux
Waiting rooms, stairways	Visual tasks performed occasionally	10-20 fc = 100-200 lux
Machine work, video display terminal, reading	Visual tasks of high contrast or large size	20-50 fc = 200-500 lux
Office work, drafting, difficult inspection	Visual tasks of medium contrast or small size	50-100 fc = 500-1000 lux
Writing with hard pencil, very difficult inspection	Visual tasks of low contrast or small size	100-200 fc = 1000-2000 lux
Fine machine work, highly difficult inspection	Visual tasks of low contrast, very small size over a prolonged period	200-500 fc = 2000-5000 lux
Extra fine assembly work, most difficult inspection	Visual tasks that are prolonged and exacting	500-1000 fc = 5000-10,000 lux
Surgical procedures, sewing gowns	Very special tasks of low contrast and small size	1000-2000 fc = 10,000-20,000 lux

* Upper value for ages > 55 years.

should not be in the visual field of the worker. The angle formed between the horizontal surfaces and the light source should be greater than 30 degrees (Eastman Kodak Company, 1983; Kroemer & Grandjean, 2001).

Direct and Indirect Lighting

Direct and indirect lighting are two types of lighting arrangements. *Direct lighting* is usually from above and directs approximately 90% of light toward the visual surface. Direct light often produces strong contrasts and shadows and may produce glare. However, small lamps may be used for close reading and video-display-terminal work.

Indirect lighting is light that is reflected off the ceiling and walls and back to the room. Indirect light casts no shadows and thus produces no glare. Indirect lighting produces uniformity of lighting but is less efficient because some of the light energy is lost to reflection.

Designers widely recommend a combination of direct and indirect lighting. Such light sources have translucent shades that reflect approximately 40% to 50% of light to the ceilings and direct the rest downward. This combination of direct and indirect lighting minimizes shadows and permits even illumination. Other designers recommend generally lower levels of office illumination with small lamps directed at the task.

Artificial Light Sources

Daylight is always preferable to artificial light for its aesthetic qualities and for the change of scenery that a window to the outdoors affords. Unfortunately, daylight is not enough to illuminate deep rooms or offices, and thus artificial light is used. Two types of artificial lighting commonly used are electrical filament lamps and fluorescent tubes.

Electric filament lamps (lightbulbs, incandescent lamps) create a subdued, pleasant atmosphere with red and yellow rays. However, filaments are inefficient because they emit heat and usually last less than 1 year.

Fluorescent lighting is created by electricity passed through a gas or mercury vapor that is then converted to light energy. This type of lighting is very efficient; little energy is lost in the conversion from electricity to light. The advantages of fluorescent lighting are that the fluorescent tubes have a high output and long life, and the color of the lighting can be controlled by varying the chemical composition of the fluorescent substance lining the inside of the tube. The major disadvantage is a flicker that may not be noticeable in older or defective fluorescent tubes. Normally, fluorescent tubes produce a flicker from alternating current at a much higher frequency than is apparent to the human eye. However, a flicker that is visible can be extremely uncomfortable and annoying because of repetitive overexposure of the retina (Kroemer & Grandjean, 2001).

Guidelines for Proper Lighting in Workplaces

The following guidelines should assist in the proper design of workplaces. The light source should have the following.

- Direct lighting should be placed at right angles to the work task. Workstations should be at right angles to windows.
- A direct light source should not be in the visual field of the worker.
- For fine work the light source should be in front of the visual task.
- Fluctuating brightness of light sources or objects should be avoided especially when the worker must switch visual fields from one object to another.
- Use more lamps of low power than fewer lamps of high power for equal distribution of light and for diminished glare.
- Avoid glare whenever possible.

The work space design should have the following.

- Select colors of similar brightness for large surfaces.
- Choose matte finishes rather than glossy surfaces.

- Avoid reflective color on tabletops, control panels, and machines.

ORGANIZING WORK SCHEDULES: SHIFTWORK, WORKING HOURS, OVERTIME, AND WORK BREAKS

Shiftwork

Continuous production in the industrial arena has made shiftwork (working outside the normal daylight hours) a reality for about 14.5 million full-time wage and salary workers representing 14.5% of America's workforce. Specified by type of shift, 4.8% of the total work evening shifts, 3.3% work night shifts, 2.8% work employer-arranged irregular schedules, and 2.3% work rotating shifts (BLS, 2001).

Shiftwork has become increasingly common in industries requiring around-the-clock attention such as manufacturing, food service, health care, and maintenance. The prevalence of shift-work is greatest among workers in service-oriented occupations, such as protective services (49.0%), which includes police officers, firefighters, and guards; food service (40.4%); and those employed as operators, fabricators, and laborers (25.4%). Alternative shifts are least common among managers and professionals (6.7%); those in administrative support occupations (8.4%); and workers in farming, forestry, and fishing occupations (5.6%) (BLS, 2001).

Although companies argue that shiftwork is necessary for timely delivery of products and services, many companies fail to consider the effects of shiftwork on workers' quality of life and work. Shiftwork has the potential to affect many aspects of a worker's life, from health to social relationships. In fact, 20% to 30% of all shiftworkers are forced to leave shiftwork within the first 2 to 3 years because of medical problems (Scott & Ladou, 1990).

The effects of shiftwork on individuals result from a disturbance of a worker's own circadian rhythms and a mismatch between the normal activity of shiftworkers and that of society. *Circadian rhythms* are individuals' inherent biologic clocks that affect bodily functions, work readiness, and individuals' levels of general alertness over a 24-hour period. Shiftwork affects circadian rhythms in the following manner: During the day, a person is in the ergotropic (performance) phase, in which body temperature, heart rate, and mental and physical capacities are peaked; at night, a person is in the trophotropic (recuperation) phase, when bodily functions slow down. Within these cycles, circadian rhythms predispose individuals to be tired in the early morning (2 to 7 AM) and mid-afternoon (2 to 5 PM). Light-dark cycles are believed to be the major synchronizers of our circadian rhythms. Darkness stimulates the secretion of the hormone melatonin, which stimulates the onset of sleepiness (Colligan & Tepas, 1986; Kroemer & Grandjean, 2001; Pheasant 1991).

When individuals disrupt this rhythm by working at night, health and social relationships are affected. The term *shiftwork tolerance* was recently introduced to describe the relationship between circadian rhythms and subjective health effects of shiftwork, such as sleep-wake disturbances, digestion, irritability, and sleepiness (Harma, 1993).

The most obvious effect of shiftwork on individuals is the interruption of the quantity and quality of sleep. Individuals who work at night and sleep during the day generally do not get adequate deep, restorative sleep, because of daytime noise and general restlessness. Although the long-term effects of chronic sleep loss are not well documented, most researchers agree that the immune system of a shiftworker is compromised by a long-term sleep deficit. Researchers state that, on average, shiftworkers get 6 hours of sleep per night; informal reports reveal that many workers receive only 3 to 4 hours of sleep nightly (Colligan & Tepas, 1986; Smith, Colligan, & Tasto, 1982). Kroemer & Grandjean (2001) estimate that approximately two-thirds of all shiftworkers suffer from some type of health problem related to shiftwork because these employees are working out of synch with their natural body cycles.

General Health

Studies assert that shiftworkers are at an increased risk for developing sleep-wake disturbances, gastrointestinal disorders, and possibly cardiovascular disease because of a chronic disruption in circadian rhythms (Monk & Colligan, 1997; Moore-Ede & Richardson, 1985; Scott & Ladou, 1990). Sleep-wake disturbances occur because of chronic fatigue and the tendency for some workers to use stimulants or sleeping tablets. Gastrointestinal problems such as peptic ulcers, constipation, or diarrhea are common because the body's normal cycles of eating, digesting, and voiding are altered as the body normally suppresses appetite and renal functions at night. Inadequate food options for shiftworkers and poor food choices exacerbate the problem (Monk & Colligan, 1997; Westfall-Lake & McBride, 1998).

Women may be at greater risk for health problems than men. A recent study of the effects of shiftwork on nurses (Labyak, Lava, Turek, & Zee, 2002) indicates that shiftwork may also be associated with reproductive disturbances, menstrual irregularities, and risk of adverse pregnancy outcomes in women. In a study of 68 nurses working the night shift, 53% noted menstrual changes when working the night shift and reported difficulty falling asleep. Further studies are investigating the association between night shiftwork and the risk of breast cancer. Davis, Mirick, and Stevens (2001) found in a case control study of 1606 women that those working the night shift have a 60% greater risk of developing breast cancer than those not working at night. According to researchers, exposure to bright lights at night decreases the secretion of melatonin that may in turn increase the release of estrogen.

Colligan and Tepas (1986) also suggest that shiftwork may exacerbate certain health problems and interfere with the efficacy of prescribed medication. Shiftworkers who take medication at the wrong times during their circadian rhythms may not receive the proper effects of that medication, since the dose-response characteristics of medication cycles are based on a normal daily activity cycle.

Physical Performance

Most individuals accustomed to working during the day find it difficult to switch shifts and maintain the same quality of work. The effects of shiftwork have been studied on various occupational groups including truck drivers (Hamelin, 1987), food-processing workers (Smith et al., 1982), nurses (Minors & Waterhouse, 1985), and computer-monitoring operators (Rosa, Colligan, & Lewis, 1989).

Overall, shiftworkers have been shown to have a higher number of accidents; slower reaction times; and less proficient hand-eye coordination, math calculations, and visual search skills as compared to day workers (Kroemer & Grandjean, 2001; Monk, 1989; Rosa et al., 1989; Smith et al., 1982). In a study of shiftworkers who had recently switched to a night and rotating schedule, workers' alertness and performance skills decreased 10% over a 7-month period (Rosa et al., 1989).

Although night workers try to mentally override the body's tendency toward sleep, individuals become vulnerable to accidents or to falling asleep at the wheel at low times during their circadian rhythms (Pheasant, 1991). Pilots, security guards, and drivers have all reported difficulty staying awake on the job. In a series of confidential interviews reported by Moore-Ede and Richardson (1985), between one-third and two-thirds of all shiftworkers in an industrial plant indicated that they fell asleep at least once per week while on the job.

Decreased alertness would seem to have serious implications for individuals performing continuous monitoring jobs. However, Rosa et al. (1989) caution, "It is difficult to speculate on the magnitude of risk associated with the decrements in alertness, or the partial sleep deprivation we have observed." In other words, we cannot translate a certain percentage decrease in performance skills to an estimate of risk for health and safety issues.

Social Adjustment

Our society assumes a work-during-the-day and sleep-at-night 5-day workweek schedule. Workers who rotate shifts often become frustrated and exhausted in trying to coordinate work, family, and social life. Researchers report that shiftworkers feel dissatisfied with the amount of time spent with family and friends (Sanders, 1996; Tepas & Monk, 1987). In a survey of 1490 hourly workers, Tepas and Monk (1987) found a 50% increase in divorces and separations for those on the night shift as compared to those on the day shift. Shiftworkers report being chronically tired and apathetic about extracurricular activities.

Monk (1989) associates maladaptive coping with shiftwork with marital problems, working a second job, and excessive responsibilities at home. Research suggests that female shiftworkers are particularly susceptible to overwork and fatigue if they perform all the child-rearing and household responsibilities (Monk & Folkard, 1992) in addition to their jobs.

Although one would surmise that all shiftworkers would be dissatisfied with night work, studies on the satisfaction of shiftworkers yield varying results. Shiftworkers consistently report fatigue as a major problem. However, a minority of shiftworkers actually prefer shiftwork. The advantages cited are the slower pace of work, fewer hassles at night, and lack of management supervision at night. Shiftwork also provides individuals with an opportunity to care for children and to participate in hobbies or additional jobs during the day (Colligan & Tepas, 1986; Monk & Folkard, 1992). Interestingly, up to 33% of all shiftworkers hold second jobs, which would appear to further compromise sleep and social relationships.

Personality Types

Research suggests that individuals who adapt better to shiftwork are younger, flexible sleepers, with owl-like personalities—that is, individuals who enjoy staying up late in the evening and sleeping late in the morning. Monk and Folkard (1992) suggest that these individuals may have a longer free-running circadian clock of 25.5 hours that tends to extend the normal circadian cycles. Further, these "owls" may be less susceptible to physical or social cues that signal the time of day (see Zeitbergers, following). Older workers experience the most difficulty adapting to rotating schedules and night work in part because their normal circadian rhythms are becoming shorter and moving toward earlier bedtimes and wake times (Colligan & Tepas, 1986; Monk & Folkard, 1992).

Current Strategies for Adapting to Shiftwork

Workers' abilities to adapt to shiftwork are not as well understood as the effect of shiftwork on individuals. Studies suggest that it takes individuals anywhere from 1 week to 1 month to adapt to a new sleep and work schedule by reversing circadian rhythms. In most cases, a shiftworker's circadian rhythms are never reversed totally if the night worker returns to a normal nightly sleep routine on weekends (Monk, 1989; Smith et al., 1982). The most difficult schedule for worker adaptation is a rapidly rotating shift from night to day to evening. Workers rarely adjust to a certain shift and are therefore counseled to maintain a body schedule that simulates work during the day and sleep at night. Monk (1989) suggests that rotating shiftworkers should eat according to a day schedule and seek out light whenever possible.

Monk and Colligan (1997) propose that successful adjustment to shiftwork depends on a balance between the following three factors: sleep, circadian rhythms, and social and domestic life. Clearly, if workers are not receiving enough sleep, they are prone to absenteeism, irritability, and a poor attitude; if workers are preoccupied with domestic problems, they may be less productive and effective at work.

Sleep Strategies

Sleep must be recognized as a priority for

shiftworkers. Monk & Colligan (1997) stress that shiftworkers should try to sleep for one long period of time. A "snacking" approach to sleep—that is, napping whenever they can—should not be considered shiftworkers' main approach to sleep. Naps may be an emergency sleep supplement if needed. A shiftworker needs to establish a bedtime ritual similar to that at night: darken the room, change one's clothes, brush one's teeth, and so on. This ritual not only helps the worker's body prepare for sleep but also signals to the rest of the family that sleep is an important and respected entity.

Circadian Rhythms

There is no one solution to resetting one's biological rhythms to sleep during the day and stay awake at night. Although we cannot directly affect the circadian system itself, we can try to manipulate cues to the system to alter the body's biologic patterns using zeitbergers, daylight exposure, and light therapy.

Zeitbergers. *Zeitbergers* are time cues that allow one's circadian rhythms to distinguish between day and night. Shiftworkers on a fixed night shift may try to orient their circadian rhythms to night work by using zeitbergers to help set their biologic clocks. Whereas darkness or night sounds such as crickets may be zeitbergers for day workers, examples of zeitbergers for night workers may include a routine of warm milk and a shower in the morning to induce sleep or increased social interaction and lively music at night to increase alertness.

Daylight Exposure. Monk (1989) recommends that night shiftworkers avoid early-morning commitments after work and wear sunglasses on the way home from work. Those who are least exposed to sunlight before bedtime tend to fall asleep more quickly than those with exposure to daylight and a busy schedule after work.

Light Therapy. Light therapy is being investigated as a means of resetting biological clocks. Most offices use fluorescent lights illuminated at 50 fc. For night shiftworkers, this intensity does not simulate natural sunlight (5000 fc), causing workers to fatigue until the sun rises. To determine the relationship between light exposure and individuals' alerting mechanisms, investigators exposed shiftworkers to bright, full-spectrum light at night during work and asked that they maintain darkness during the day. Workers demonstrated increased levels of alertness and cognitive function during work hours and slept an average of 2 hours longer during the day (Czeisler et al., 1990). In the future, bright light may play a role in helping night shiftworkers adjust to working at night.

Social and Domestic Strategies

Cooperation from family is central to a shiftworker's positive adjustment to the work schedule. Practically, the family needs to guard a shiftworker's sleep times and help create a sleep environment for the shiftworker. Nonessential chores or appointments should not be delegated to the shiftworker during the day. Monk & Folkard (1992) suggest making a family calendar to mark the dates on which the shiftworker will be working days, evenings, or nights. Structured times should be set aside for activities with friends, children, and one's spouse. Communication is essential given that shiftwork can potentially create stressors for the entire family (Monk & Colligan, 1997).

Personal Strategies

Sanders (1996) found that most shiftworkers needed to devise their own personal strategies and routines to adapt effectively. For example, contrary to the suggested routine, many younger shiftworkers cautioned against trying to sleep immediately after work. Workers in this study usually performed simple chores, watched television, snacked, or exercised as calm-down time after work. Workers explained that a good social life depended on communicating with family members, delegating chores, planning weekend activities, and coordinating schedules.

Practical Suggestions for Adapting to Shiftwork

Health care practitioners can alert companies to the signs and symptoms of chronic fatigue in their workers in an effort to prevent the health and social problems associated with shiftwork. Symptoms of chronic fatigue include weariness even after sleep, depressive moods, and general loss of enthusiasm and motivation to work. Objective signs include loss of appetite, sleep disturbances, ulcers, and digestive problems (Kroemer & Grandjean, 2001).

The following suggestions facilitate shift-workers' physical and social adaptation to shift-work or rotating work hours (compiled from Colligan & Tepas, 1986; Monk & Colligan, 1997; Sanders, 1996; Westfall-Lake & McBride, 1998).

In order to get to sleep, try the following.

- Darken and quiet the sleep environment, perhaps using white noise (such as a fan), soundproof curtains, and thick carpets.
- Establish a ritual before sleeping, such as bathing, brushing teeth, and reading.
- Silence doorbells, telephones, and appliances.
- Exercise regularly.
- Sleep and rise at the same time every day.
- Avoid watching TV in bed.
- Avoid caffeine and alcohol at night (within 5 hours of sleep).

In order to eat healthfully, try the following.

- Eat low-fat, high-fiber meals.
- Eat a light meal halfway through the night shift.
- Eat small meals and frequent healthy snacks.
- Eat at the same time every day.
- Bring your own food to work, or encourage your employer to provide healthy eating resources.

In order to enjoy home and social life, take the following suggestions into account.

- Set aside quality time for family.
- Communicate your schedule to family and friends.
- Plan weekend activities.
- Delegate chores.
- Get extra sleep on weekends.

In order to improve work performance, try the following.

- Install bright lighting at work.
- Perform more monotonous tasks early in the shift and more interesting tasks later on.
- Schedule work breaks to avoid long periods of solitary work.
- Socialize with others during work.
- Rotate to other jobs.
- Walk around when possible.

Working Hours and Overtime

How many hours can a worker work and still be productive? The relationship between work hours and work output has been examined since the 1900s. Various schedules, including five 8-hour days, three 12-hour days, and four 10-hour days, have been examined from all perspectives. The 8-hour workday or 40-hour week consistently bears out as optimal for psychological health and fatigue recovery (Kroemer & Grandjean, 2001).

Kroemer and Grandjean (2001) suggest that workers reach and maintain a certain daily output for an 8-hour period. If the workday is shortened, hourly productivity appears to increase; if the workday is lengthened, the productivity appears to fall. Essentially, the length of the day affects workers' paces and their use of spontaneous rest breaks. In a longer workday, workers take more breaks toward the end of the day and slow the work pace.

The advantages and disadvantages of an extended workday (or compressed workweek) have been discussed by industrial planners and ergonomists. The potential advantages of an extended workday (or compressed workweek) for the company include decreased daily start-up time and decreased expenses; advantages for the worker include increased blocks of leisure time, an overall reduction in commuting time, fewer workdays, and less night work.

The potential disadvantages of an extended workweek seem to outweigh the advantages. Disadvantages for the company include overtime pay, potentially increased worker absenteeism because of illness, and decreased productivity; disadvantages to the worker include increased fatigue and related safety and health problems, increased exposure to toxic hazards, and difficulty scheduling child care and family functions. Further, a lengthened workday may cause workers to feel disconnected from others.

Providing an opportunity for a worker's balance of work, rest, and leisure is essential to planning workday hours (Colligan & Tepas, 1986).

Overtime presents a further dilemma from economic and medical perspectives. Although overtime pay may be necessary for some employees' financial survival, during periods of prolonged overtime, workers incur increased absences because of illness and risk the potential for poor health and overuse injury. When supervisors attempt to limit overtime hours for workers already injured or at risk for injury, the law suggests that a worker cannot be denied overtime because of an injury if the injury is job-related. Health care consultants agree that overtime increases the risk of overuse injuries to workers involved in repetitive or forceful work.

Work Breaks

Work breaks are an essential part of the worker's shift. Work breaks function to restore workers' energy, to alleviate the monotony of routine or vigilant tasks, and, importantly, to provide time for socialization. Pheasant (1991) suggests that 45 minutes to 1 hour is the maximum time span for human attention in a wide range of activities, although most people work well beyond this 1-hour span. Work breaks, when designed correctly, may increase overall productivity by deferring fatigue and monotony, which are associated with decreased work output.

Kroemer and Grandjean (2001) outline the following types of breaks that have been observed among workers throughout the workday.

- *Spontaneous pauses* are short pauses for rest that workers take on their own.
- *Disguised pauses* are breaks from a worker's routine to perform another, less taxing part of the job (such as emptying the wastepaper basket or consulting a fellow employee).
- *Work-related pauses* are short breaks inherent in the machine pace or work routine (such as waiting for a part or waiting in line).
- *Organizational pauses* are those breaks prescribed by management for certain times of the day.

Presently, there is no consensus as to the ideal number and duration of breaks during the day. The traditional standard for industry is a 15-minute break in the morning and afternoon and a 30-minute break for lunch. Ergonomists recommend a 3- to 5-minute pause or microbreak every hour, particularly for jobs that are static, repetitive, or paced, or for jobs that require intense alertness, such as assembly or computer work (Kroemer & Grandjean, 2001; Pheasant, 1991). Workers are sometimes reticent to take breaks, fearing that it will impact managers' perceptions of their efforts. McLean, Tingley, Scott, and Rickards (2001) recognized that both management and worker support would be necessary to advocate microbreaks. To that end, researchers performed a study to determine the effects of microbreaks on muscle activity, perceived discomfort, and productivity. Results indicated that microbreaks reduced discomfort in the cervical extensor, lumbar erector spinae, trapezius, and wrist and finger extensor musculature when breaks were taken at 20-minute intervals. Further, microbreaks did *not* negatively affect worker productivity. It has been suggested that longer breaks are needed for muscles to recover from work with high static forces. Further studies will help redefine the current break standard.

Although some organizations permit workers to leave early if no breaks are taken, workers should be encouraged to take regular breaks throughout the day to prevent accumulation of stress or fatigue. Observation indicates that the more organizational pauses that are integrated into a worker's schedule for stretches, the less time workers spend in spontaneous breaks (Kroemer & Grandjean, 2001).

Short breaks that involve gentle stretching appear to be more beneficial for increasing blood flow to muscle and increasing one's level of alertness than are breaks that involve only rest (Hansford, Blood, Kent, & Lutz, 1986; Pheasant, 1991). Breaks that included some neck motion were found to reduce fatigue and improve concentration among air traffic controllers

(Kroemer & Grandjean, 2001). Neck, shoulder, arm, and low-back stretches are recommended for computer workers (Pheasant, 1991). Neck, shoulder, and finger extension exercises are recommended for dental hygienists between each client (Atwood & Michalak, 1992) (see Chapter 22 for further information).

Machine Pacing and Worker Control

Machine-paced work is often a major stressor for assembly-line workers. *Machine pacing* refers to work in which the output, rate, and speed of the task is controlled by a machine. Most assembly-line jobs are machine-paced and have the additional problem of being monotonous. Machine pacing has been criticized as incompatible with human variability, since pacing sets a one-way standard against which the worker's performance is measured. The worker can either achieve or fail; there are no gradations. Machine pacing has been related to high stress levels in workers (Arndt, 1987; Karasek & Theorell, 1990), attributable to the short work cycle and the worker's lack of control over his or her work pace.

Whenever possible, a worker should control his or her own pace. This concept is especially true for overtime work and for critical work tasks (Eastman Kodak Company, 1983). Worker rotation to other stations, job enlargement, stretch breaks, and variety on the job (such as inventory, maintenance, or supervisory tasks) can help alleviate the monotony of and intense concentration demanded by machine-paced work.

The physical design of the workplace is crucial for worker comfort, productivity, safety, and morale. This chapter has provided practical ergonomic recommendations to apply to a wide variety of work settings in efforts of promoting optimal work environment and conditions.

REFERENCES

Anshel, J. (1998). *Visual ergonomics in the workplace.* London: Taylor & Francis.

Armstrong, T. J. (1990). Ergonomics and cumulative trauma disorders of the hand and wrist. In J. M. Hunter, L. H. Schneider, E. J. Mackin, & A. D. Callahan (Eds.), *Rehabilitation of the hand: Surgery and therapy.* St. Louis: Mosby.

Armstrong, T. J., Fine, L. J., Radwin, R. G., & Silverstein, B. S. (1987). Ergonomics and the effects of vibration in hand-intensive work. *Scandinavian Journal of Work, Environment, and Health, 13,* 286–289.

Arndt, R. (1987). Work pace, stress and cumulative trauma disorder. *Journal of Hand Surgery (Am), 12,* 866–869.

Atlas Copco (2002). Assembly tools. Retrieved on March 10, 2003 at: http://www.atlascopco.com/tools/products/AssemblyTools.nsf/va_Frames/Assembly+Tool.

Atwood, M., & Michalak, C. (1992). The occurrence of cumulative trauma disorders in dental hygienists. *Work, 2*(4), 1–31.

Brown, A. P. (1990). The effects of anti-vibration gloves on vibration-induced disorders: A case study. *Journal of Hand Therapy, 3*(2), 94–100.

Buchholz, B., Frederick, L. J., & Armstrong, T. J. (1988). An investigation of human palmar skin friction and effects of materials, pinch force and moisture. *Ergonomics, 31*(3), 317–325.

Bullock, M. I. (Ed.). (1990). *Ergonomics: The physiotherapist in the workplace*. New York: Churchill Livingstone.

Bureau of Labor Statistics (BLS). (2001). Workers on flexible and shift schedules in 2001 summary. Retrieved on March 11, 2003 at: http://www.bls.gov/news.release/flex.nr0.htm.

Carson, R. (1995, September). Ergonomically designed tools. *Occupational Hazards,* 49–54.

Cochran, D. J., & Riley, M. W. (1986). The effects of handle shape and size on exerted forces. *Human Factors, 28*(3), 251–265.

Colligan, M. J., & Tepas, D. I. (1986). The stress of hours of work. *American Industrial Hygiene Association Journal, 47*(11), 686–695.

Czcisler, C. A., Johnson, M. P., Duffy, J. F., Brown, E. N., Ronda, J. M., & Kronauer, R. E. (1990). Exposure to bright light and darkness to treat physiologic maladaptation to night work. *New England Journal of Medicine, 322*(18), 1253–1259.

Davis, S., Mirick, D. K., & Stevens, R. G. (2001). Night shiftwork, light at night, and risk of breast cancer. *Journal of the National Cancer Institute, 93*(20), 1557–1562.

Diffrient, N., Tilley, A. R., & Bradagjy, J. C. (1990). *Humanscale 1/2/3 Manual* (6th ed.) Cambridge, MA: The MIT Press.

Eastman Kodak Company. (1983). *Ergonomic design for people at work, vols. 1 and 2.* New York: Van Nostrand Reinhold.

Feaney, R. (2003). *Research into forces required to open paper and sheet plastic packaging-experiments, results and statistics in detail.* Robert Feaney Associates: Nottingham, UK. Retrieved on July 10, 2003 at http://www.virart.nott.ac.uk/pstg/peel%20pdfs/fullrep.pdf.

Fraser, T. M. (1989). *The worker at work: A textbook concerned with men and women in the workplace.* Philadelphia: Taylor & Francis.

Greenberg, L., & Chaffin, D. B. (1977). *Workers and their tools: A guide to the ergonomic design of hand tools and small presses.* Midland, MI: Pendell.

Hamelin, P. (1987). Lorry drivers' time habits in work and their involvement in traffic accidents. *Ergonomics, 30,* 1323–1333.

Hampel, G. A. (1992). Hand-arm vibration isolation materials: A range of performance evaluation. *Applied Occupational and Environmental Hygiene, 7,* 441–452.

Hansford, T., Blood, H., Kent, B., & Lutz, G. (1986). Blood flow changes at the wrist in manual workers after preventive interventions. *Journal of Hand Surgery (Am), 11*(4), 503–508.

Harma, M. (1993). Individual differences in tolerance to shiftwork: A review. *Ergonomics, 36,* 101–109.

Helander, M. (1997). *A guide to ergonomics of manufacturing.* London: Taylor & Francis.

Hunter, J. M., Schneider, L. H., Mackin, E. J., & Callahan, A. D. (Eds.). (1990). *Rehabilitation of the hand: Surgery and therapy.* St. Louis: Mosby.

Johnson, S. L. (1990). Ergonomic design of handheld tools to prevent trauma to the hand and upper extremity. *Journal of Hand Therapy, 3*(2), 86–93.

Karasek, R., & Theorell, T. (1990). *Healthy work: Stress, productivity and the reconstruction of working life.* New York: Basic Books.

Kroemer, E., & Grandjean, E. (2001). *Fitting the task to the person* (5th ed.). Philadelphia: Taylor & Francis.

Labyak, S., Lava, S., Turek, F., & Zee, P. (2002). Effects of shiftwork on sleep and menstrual function in nurses. *Health Care for Women International, 23*(6-7), 703–714.

McLean, L. Tingley, M., Scott, R. N., & Rickards, J. (2001). Computer terminal work and the benefit of microbreaks, *Applied Ergonomics, 32*(3), 225–237.

Meagher, S. W. (1987). Tool design for prevention of hand and wrist injuries. *Journal of Hand Surgery, 12*(5 Pt 2), 855–857.

Minors, D. S., & Waterhouse, J. M. (1985). Circadian rhythms in deep body temperature, urinary excretion and alertness in nurses on night work. *Ergonomics, 28,* 1523–1530.

Mital, A., & Pennathur, A. (2001). Hand tools. In S. Kumar (Ed.), *Biomechanics in ergonomics.* London: Taylor & Francis.

Monk, T. (1989). Human factors implications of shiftwork. *International Review of Ergonomics, 2,* 111–128.

Monk, T., & Colligan, M. J. (Eds.). (1997). *Plain language about shiftwork.* U.S. Department of Health and Human Services. DHHS (NIOSH) Pub No. 94-145. Retrieved on January 28, 2003 at: http://www.cdc.gov.niosh/pdfs/97-145pdf.

Monk, T., & Folkard, S. (1992). *Making shiftwork tolerable.* London: Taylor & Francis.

Moore-Ede, M. C., & Richardson, G. S. (1985). Medical implications of shift-work. *Annual Review of Medicine, 36,* 607–617.

Morse, L. H., & Hinds, L. J. (1993). Women and ergonomics. *Occupational Medicine, 8*(4), 721–731.

Napier, J. P. (1956). The prehensile movements of the human hand. *Journal of Bone and Joint Surgery (Br), 38,* 902–913.

National Institute of Occupational Safety and Health (NIOSH). (1989). Criteria for a recommended standard. Occupational exposure to hand-arm vibration [DHHS (NIOSH) pub no. 89-106]. Cincinnati: US Department of Health and Human Services.

Neumann, D. A. (2002). *Kinesiology of the musculoskeletal system.* Mosby: St. Louis.

Peterson, P., Wakula, J., & Landau, K. (1999/2000). Development of a hand tool work analysis method (HTWAM). *Occupational Ergonomics, 2*(3), 137–150.

Pheasant, S. (1991). *Ergonomics, work, and health.* Gaithersburg, MD: Aspen.

Pheasant, S. (2001). *Bodyspace: Anthropometry, ergonomics and the design of work* (2nd ed.). London: Taylor Francis.

Putz-Anderson, V. (Ed.). (1988). *Cumulative trauma disorders: A manual for musculoskeletal disease of the upper limbs.* London: Taylor & Francis.

Rahman, N., Thomas, J. J. & Rice, M. S. (2002). The relationship between hand strength and the forces used to access containers by well elderly persons. *American Journal of Occupational Therapy, 56,* 78-85.

Radwin, R. G., Armstrong, T. J., & Chaffin, D. B. (1987). Power hand tool vibration and tool vibration effects on grip exertion. *Ergonomics, 30,* 833–855.

Robinson, F. R., & Lyon, B. K. (1994). Ergonomic guidelines for hand-held tools. *Professional Safety,* August, 16–21.

Rodgers, S. H. (1987). Recovery time needs for repetitive work. *Seminars in Occupational Medicine, 2*(1), 19–24.

Rosa, R. R., Colligan, M. J., & Lewis, P. (1989). Extended workday: Effects of 8-hour and 12-hour rotating shift schedules on performance, subjective alertness, sleep patterns and psychosocial variables. *Work Stress, 3*(1), 21–32.

Sanders, M. (1996). Circadian rhythms: implications for shiftwork and occupational therapy. Presented at American Occupational Therapy Association National Convention. April 11, Chicago, IL.

Sanders, M. S., & McCormick, E. J. (1993). *Human factors in engineering and design* (7th ed.). New York: McGraw-Hill.

Schoenmarklin, R. W., & Marras, W. S. (1989). Effects of handle angle and work orientation on hammering: I. Wrist motion and hammering performance. *Human Factors, 31*(4), 397–411.

Scott, A. J., & Ladou, J. (1990). Shiftwork: Effects on sleep and health with recommendations for medical surveillance and screening. *Occupational Medicine, 5*(2), 273–299.

Sjogaard, G., Savard, G., & Juel, C. (1988). Muscle blood flow during isometric activity and its relation to muscle fatigue. *European Journal of Applied Physiology, 57*(3), 327–335.

Smith, M. J., Colligan, M. J., & Tasto, D. L. (1982). Health and safety consequences of shiftwork in the food processing industry. *Ergonomics, 25,* 133–144.

Spaulding, S. J. (1989). The biomechanics of prehension. *American Journal of Occupational Therapy, 43*(5), 302–307.

Spaulding, S. (2001, November). Contractor tool ergonomics. *Contractor,* 18–19.

Tepas, D., & Monk, T. H. (1987). Work schedules. In G. Salvendy (Ed.), *Handbook of human factors.* New York: Wiley.

Terrono, A. L., Nalebuff, E. A., & Philips, C. A. (1995). The rheumatoid thumb. In J. M. Hunter, E. M. J. Mackin, & A. D. Callahan (Eds.). *Rehabilitation of the hand: Surgery and therapy* (4th Ed.) Philadelphia: Mosby.

Tichauer, E. R. (1966). Some aspects of stress on forearm and hand in industry. *Journal of Occupational Medicine, 8*(2), 63–71.

Tichauer, E. R. (1978). *The biomechanical basis of ergonomics.* New York: Wiley-Interscience.

Wakula, J., Beckman, T., Hett, M., & Landau, K. (1999/2000). Ergonomic analysis of grapevine pruning and wine harvesting to define work and hand tools design requirement. *Occupational Ergonomics, 2*(3), 151–161.

Westfall-Lake, P., & McBride, G. (1998). *Shiftwork safety and performance: A manual for managers and trainers.* New York: Lewis Publishers.

CHAPTER 12

Psychosocial Factors

Dorothy Farrar Edwards

Musculoskeletal disorders (MSDs) are associated with persistent pain, loss of function, and increased work-related disabilities. In spite of comprehensive medical care and substantial attention to the biomechanical and ergonomic factors in the workplace, many persons with MSDs do not improve. Often, psychologic factors are implicated in the development of subacute and chronic musculoskeletal pain syndromes (Linton, 1995). In some cases, the psychologic risk factors in the workplace have been found to be more important than physical work factors as predictors of work related musculoskeletal disorders (Bigos et al., 1991; Bongers, Kremer, & ter Laak, 2002; Nachemson, 1992; National Research Council, 2001).

Interest in the interaction between psychosocial, musculoskeletal, and ergonomic mechanisms continues to grow (Feuerstein, 2002). Many studies addressing the contribution of psychosocial variables to work-related musculoskeletal disorders have been published since the first papers examining the association of psychologic factors to MSDs appeared in the 1970s. These studies continue to demonstrate the importance of job-related stress, social support, and the emotional climate of the workplace to MSDs.

The purpose of this chapter is to examine the effects of psychosocial factors on the etiology and management of work-related musculoskeletal disorders. An understanding of these factors is essential if one is to treat effectively or prevent the devastating consequences of MSDs (Faucett, 1994).

The relationship between psychosocial variables and musculoskeletal pain was first demonstrated in studies of individuals with low-back pain (Kelsey & Golden, 1988). Subsequent studies using similar research methods indicate that these processes generalize to the development of neck and shoulder pain as well as other upper-extremity disorders (Ariens, van Mechelen, Bongers, Bouter, & van der Wal, 2001; Haufler, Feuerstein, & Huang, 2000; Huang, Feuerstein, & Sauter, 2002). Generally, the psychosocial variables thought to be most highly associated with work-related MSDs are the psychologic aspects or emotional tone of the work environment, social support, perceptions of control, coping styles, cognitive responses to stress, and personality traits and states such as anxiety, defensiveness, and depression.

CONCEPTS AND DEFINITIONS

As more and more attention has been directed toward understanding the link between occupational stressors and MSDs, common concepts and definitions have been proposed. Adoption of consistent terminology facilitates comparisons across studies, stimulates the development of theoretical models, and enhances the translation of research findings into practical interventions.

Although terminology differences still occur, the following classifications and terminology are commonly used in the literature. It is also clear that some of the concepts are not mutually exclusive, and some are included in more than one category. The most common concepts used in the literature are work organization factors, psychosocial factors, and psychologic factors. (Also refer to Chapter 8.)

Work Organization

Work organization has been broadly described as the "the way processes are structured and managed" (NIOSH, 1996). Work organizational factors include both objective and subjective aspects of the workplace (Huang et al., 2002). Hagberg et al. (1995) describe work organization as the manner in which work is structured, organized, supervised, and carried out. This is evident in the taxonomy created for the National Occupational Research Agenda; proposed by NIOSH (1996), it includes five major components: scheduling, job design, career concerns, management style, and organizational characteristics. This classification is similar to models based on studies of the dynamics of work stress conducted in the 1970s (Cooper & Marshall, 1976).

Psychosocial Factors

The more subjective aspects of the work environment are often classified as psychosocial factors. Psychosocial stressors are conditions perceived as threatening, harmful, or bothersome, or that place demands on employees that provoke physiologic adaptation responses (Davis & Heaney, 2000). Specific types of stressors include quantitative work demands, availability of social support, job ambiguity, conflict, job control, job strain, job satisfaction, and job security. Although many studies address the contributions of psychosocial variables to work-related injuries and illness, the importance of these factors was identified through the demand-control model studies of Karasek and his colleagues (Karasek & Theorell, 1990).

Psychologic Factors

Many models and studies distinguish between psychosocial factors and psychologic factors. This distinction may seem artificial, since many of the psychosocial variables have an emotional or psychologic component. In these models, the psychosocial variables are associated with the individual's emotional response to worksite conditions or events, and the psychologic factors are intrinsic characteristics of the individual such as personality traits and types, mood, and cognitive and perceptual beliefs. Personality is a global concept that includes all of the characteristics that make a person unique. Traits are seen as relatively fixed features that strongly influence the way in which the individual perceives and interacts with his or her environment. The term *mood* refers to the feelings experienced by an individual; these feelings can range from positive emotional states like happiness to negative states like anxiety or depression. Cognitive factors include beliefs and values, coping styles, and problem-solving strategies (Linton, 2000).

STRESS AND WORK ENVIRONMENTS

Seyle's (1936) general adaptation syndrome describes three stages of stress: alarm, resistance, and exhaustion. The last stage, exhaustion, is induced by chronic stress. The term *strain* is used to describe this stage when the worker's psychosocial resources prove inadequate in the face of psychologic stressors such as time pressures or conflicts with superiors and coworkers.

The psychosocial characteristics of the work environment are defined as the employee's emotional response to workplace demands and stressors (Feuerstein, Callan-Harris, Dyer, Armbruster, & Carosella, 1993). Early studies of the industrial implications of stress defined stress as the state induced in an individual when his or her own needs, exertions, and aims are thwarted by the demands and expectations placed on him or her by a superior, work group, or organization. According to Bronner (1965), the employee finds him- or herself in a state of stress when he or she experiences a situation as threatening or frustrating and cannot adopt the behavior needed to reduce the frustration. Bronner associated worker stress in Swedish industrial workers with absenteeism, accidents, and increased emotional problems and psychosomatic disorders.

Interest in the contribution of work-related psychosocial factors to MSDs has increased as the prevalence of work-related musculoskeletal disorders continues to rise. Research evaluating ergonomic interventions designed to protect workers from job-related injury has shown that such interventions may not decrease work-related musculoskeletal disorders and absenteeism (Christmansson, Friden, & Sollerman, 1999). The evidence emerging from these studies suggests that a variety of psychologic, psychosocial, and organizational factors interact with physical and ergonomic demands, resulting in increased risk of work-related injury (Carayon, Smith, & Haims, 1999; MacDonald, Karasek, Punnett, & Scharf, 2001; Malchaire et al. 2001).

MODELS OF STRESS AND HEALTH

The work of Levi (1972, 1987) expands on the role of psychosocial factors in health and provides the foundation for most of the current theoretic and empiric models of workplace stress. According to Levi (1972), cognitive, behavioral, emotional, and physiologic reactions influence the development of pathogenic mechanisms that increase the risk of morbidity and decrease perceived health status. Levi (1987) further suggests that linear models of causality are not adequate. Complex, nonlinear systems models are required to account fully for the relationship of these elements to worker health. Levi's model, which was first presented in 1972, still is relevant today (Figure 12-1). The model illustrates the interactions among factors such as social systems, specific physical and psychosocial stimuli, and the individual's psychobiologic program.

Many elements of Levi's model have been incorporated into contemporary causal models of work-related stress and physical reactions such as cardiovascular disease or musculoskeletal pain. Since Levi's model was first presented, studies examining exposure to similar levels of ergonomic demands across different types of psychosocial environments have found differences in physiologic and psychologic markers of stress, as well as variability in muscular tension and neuromuscular pain (Bongers, Kremer, & ter Laak, 2002; Lundberg, 2002). Huang et al. (2002) described the critical features of explanatory models of job stress and musculoskeletal disorders. These critical features include the following.

- The models must be testable with clearly specified pathways and empirically defined variables.
- The models must include well-defined exposure and response constructs.
- The models must be multivariate and include feedback loops illustrating the interaction among the elements in the model.

There are many different models addressing the complex interaction among personal and work-related stressors. Huang et al. (2002) reviewed a selection of these models and evaluated the evidence supporting each model. Most of the models reviewed by Huang and his colleagues incorporate work organization, psychosocial, and psychologic factors. These models vary in the way the different factors interact to create musculoskeletal injuries. Three different models will be used to illustrate these complex relationships. It should be noted that although each of these models is based on information obtained from research on worksite stress, the evidence needed to fully support these models is still not available.

Model of Job Stress and Health

This transactional model proposed by Hurrell and McLaney (1988) is based on Levi's concepts

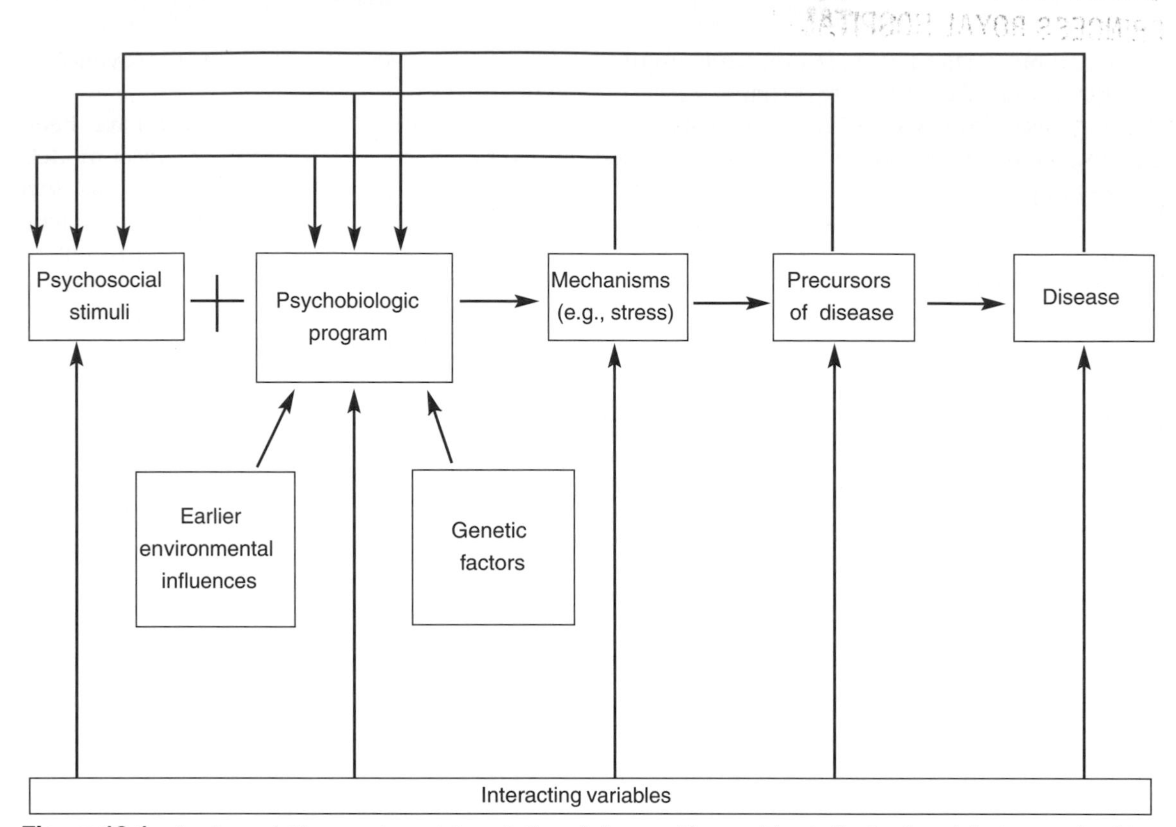

Figure 12-1 Levi's model for psychosocial mediation of disease. The combined effects of each factor may lead to a psychosocially influenced disease or condition such as musculoskeletal disorder. The model shows a system with continuous feedback among the factors. Psychosocial stimuli arise from the social and emotional environments of the person. These stimuli are interpreted based on personal, developmental, and genetic characteristics of the person, which, in turn, may create a stress response. In some cases, the stress response leads to the precursors of the disease or to the disease itself.

of job stress and health. Hurell and McLaney used evidence drawn from the occupational health literature to construct a framework that broadly integrates multiple sources of worksite stress with the additive effects of non-work-related problems and demands. This model suggests that these stressors interact to create acute strains or psychologic, physiologic, and behavioral reactions. Social support from friends, family, and coworkers can buffer the negative effects of job stressors. If the conditions causing the strain do not subside, the reactions can result in sustained work-related physical or psychologic disorders. Another strength of the model is the recognition of the additive effect of individual characteristics to work-related stressors in the development of disabling problems. The organization of this model emphasizes the primacy of worksite factors in the etiology of work-related musculoskeletal problems. It also supports the development of prevention programs addressing job-related stressors.

Epidemiologic Model of Musculoskeletal Disorders

This model proposed by Bongers et al. (1993, 2002) is based on a metaanalysis of a number of epidemiologic studies of musculoskeletal disorders. This model has several strengths relative to other multidimensional models. First, Bongers et al. incorporated constructs developed from psychologic studies of chronic pain. Second, many of the causal relationships presented in this model have been empirically validated. This model hypothesizes that work stress is the result of work-related psychosocial factors mediated by the individual's coping ability. This stress affects physiologic responses to the musculoskeletal job and task demands. Increased cortisol, epinephrine, and norepinephrine levels have been documented in persons with work-related musculoskeletal symptoms. These neuroendocrine reactions are known to occur in both psychologic and physiologic responses to stress. These responses create changes in muscle tone that may increase the severity of musculoskeletal symptoms.

Balance Theory of Job Design and Stress

The model proposed by Carayon et al. (1999) operationalizes the constructs of "balance theory" of worksite stress. This model is an elaboration of the concepts proposed by Levi in his studies of stress and health. Balance theory hypothesizes that stress is the result of loads generated by the imbalance between elements of the work system. These elements include characteristics of the individual and psychosocial and work organization factors. According to Carayon et al., individual psychologic and cognitive factors mediate both the short-term responses and long-term outcomes of work-related job stressors. When compared with other multidimensional models, the balance theory approach seems to place greater emphasis on individual factors in the development of long-term health and well-being outcomes of the worker.

These new conceptualizations of work-related stress and disability are also more holistic in that they consider the impact of stress from sources both internal and external to the individual. Chadwick (1980) suggested that investigators reject the "stress causes strain, which causes disease" formula in favor of the concept of person-environment fit. This concept incorporates the notion that optimal levels of performance and satisfaction are achieved when the worker skills and personal style are matched to the demands of the workplace (Csikszentmihalyi, 1993).

All of these models share many common elements. However, they differ in the directions of the interactions and the presence or absence of recursive (two-directional relationships) elements in the models. Although all address work-related upper-extremity problems, the level of detail and the evidence supporting the specific elements and organization of the models also varies from model to model.

OBJECTIVE AND SUBJECTIVE SOURCES OF OCCUPATIONAL STRESS

The investigation of occupational or work-related stress was advanced greatly by the passage of the Occupational Health and Safety Act of 1970 through the creation of the National Institute of Occupational Safety and Health (NIOSH) and the Occupational Safety and Health Administration (OSHA). Both these agencies were charged with the responsibility for conducting the research necessary to support industrial health and safety. NIOSH was directed to include the behavioral, social, and motivational factors associated with workplace safety and health.

The concept of occupational stress is often dismissed because of the difficulty of establishing operational definitions that are acceptable to all the parties involved in the research (Davis & Heaney, 2000; Smith, 1987). Smith, in his comprehensive review of occupational stress research, suggests that the chief source of confusion is whether to conceive of stress as a situational factor external to the worker or as a reaction experienced by the worker. Most of the work in the field of occupational stress has focused on the aspects of work that have, or threaten to have, negative consequences for the worker. He concluded that the prevalent research paradigm is that stress (independent variable) leads to undesirable consequences such as musculoskeletal pain (dependent variable) under certain conditions (mediating variables).

Traditionally, the studies examine either objectively or subjectively defined stress. Different types of stressors are believed to have a differential impact on health and well-being. Objectively defined stressors include the physical aspects of the work environment such as noise, temperature, and exposure to danger, as well as factors such as shiftwork that result in disturbed circadian rhythms and responses to machine-paced manufacturing. Subjectively defined stressors are those defined from the perspective of the worker. Variables such as role ambiguity, boredom, person-environment fit, uncertain job security, and supervisory style have been studied. Table 12-1 presents a list of the most frequently studied objective and subjective occupational stressors. The empiric benefits of separating stress into objective and subjective categories are unclear, since all responses are

Table 12-1

Subjective and Objective Sources of Job-Related Stress Associated with Musculoskeletal Disorders

Subjective Stressors	Role ambiguity
	Role conflict
	Boredom
	Person-environment fit
	Job insecurity
	Supervisory style
	Job and personal conflicts
	Demand and decision latitude
Objective Stressors	Noise
	Temperature
	Machine-paced tasks
	Electronic monitoring of performance
	Isolation
	Crowding
	Vibration
	Unsafe or hazardous working conditions
	Long hours, overtime

the result of the psychologic reactions of the worker to potentially stressful conditions. Individual differences in perception and response styles ultimately render all responses subjective, regardless of the source of the stressor.

A number of different physical and psychologic effects have been used in studies of subjective and objective occupational stressors. The physiologic and clinical aspects of cardiovascular disease in workers have been studied more often than any other stress-related medical condition. Other psychologic conditions studied include headaches, peptic ulcers, respiratory diseases, and arthritis. Interest in MSDs and other musculoskeletal disorders has stimulated many studies over the past 20 years. The published findings of studies of musculoskeletal disorders are generally consistent with similar investigations of other disease states and health problems. The majority of studies report associations between work-related organizational and psychosocial factors. However, the magnitude of these effects tend to be small, suggesting that the relationships are not very strong or that other causal factors have not been directly measured in the study.

METHODOLOGIC ISSUES IN WORKPLACE STRESS RESEARCH

Research on the relationship between subjective and objective stressors and health in the workplace is still complicated by controversies over design and analytic strategies. There are several major areas of concern. The first focuses on the continued use of simple and, at times, reductionist models to account for the complex interaction between stress and worker health. Although these studies generated important preliminary findings, there were many methodologic problems that limit the applicability of these findings. It is time to implement studies that more closely represent the actual working environments of individuals at risk of MSDs.

Second, many studies still use correlational analyses as compared to more sophisticated multidimensional statistical methods. Multidimensional designs require substantially larger sample sizes for valid data analysis. Simple correlational models can demonstrate only the associations among variables and should not be interpreted as causal. Because many studies include a number of highly correlated variables, the results can be confounded if the investigator does not use statistical techniques such as analysis of covariance to control for relationships that may mediate the association between stressors and health status. For example, it is generally believed that personality traits influence individual responses to stress. A simple design that does not measure these traits may conclude erroneously that worksite stress causes health problems, without considering the role that personality plays in influencing job choice, response to stress, or comfort in reporting health problems.

Another methodologic problem still present in research on worksite stress and personality factors in MSDs is the heavy reliance on cross-sectional rather than longitudinal designs. Cross-sectional studies do not allow the investigator to measure the temporal link between stressors and health problems, particularly when chronic problems such as musculoskeletal pain are the focus. Longitudinal surveillance of workers allows the study of changes in health status together with ongoing evaluation of the psychological environment of the workplace. Both types of studies are weakened by the tendency to use very small samples.

A recent review of the literature suggests that prospective longitudinal studies are beginning to make their way into the clinical literature. The benefits of such studies are clear. One such study conducted by Macfarlane, Hunt, and Silman (2000) examined the contributions of psychologic, work-related mechanical, and psychosocial factors to the onset of new forearm pain in 1953 workers in the United Kingdom over a 3-year period. They found that adverse psychosocial factors were independent predictors of forearm pain at follow-up. In other words, the relative risk of developing forearm pain over 3 years was 2.6 times greater for individuals who reported lack of support from supervisors and colleagues when compared with workers who reported adequate support.

In response to these methodologic criticisms, many investigators have moved beyond the generalized evaluations of occupational stressors to more complex models that examine occupational stress and health outcomes. Many of these studies of worker physical and mental health are based on the models of demand control and autonomy. This research on demand control and autonomy has had a dramatic impact on this field. Most of the multidimensional models discussed earlier in this chapter were influenced by the work of Karasek and Theorell and their studies of job demands, stress responses, and disabilities.

DEMAND CONTROL MODELS AND WORKER HEALTH AND MENTAL HEALTH

Karasek and Theorell (1990) have conducted a series of studies examining the impact of occupational stress on mental and physical health outcomes. This model, known as a *demand control model,* posits a relationship between the psychologic response to job demands and the worker's sense of control or autonomy. Such models have also been called *job strain models.* According to these models, stress-related illness is the product of the interactive effects of job demands and the worker's perceptions of control. Despite the emphasis on psychologic responses to job demands, this model calls for sociologic rather than a psychologic interventions. Interventions based on this model call for organizational and work environment changes rather than changes in individual worker behaviors (Soderfeldt et al., 1996).

Demand is defined as work-related feelings such as not having enough time to do one's work, being confronted with conflicting demands on the job, and having to work quickly (Marshall & Barnett, 1991). *Control* and *autonomy* are operationalized through two constructs: skill discretion and decision authority. Workers with high levels of skill have control over the specific skills they choose to exercise to accomplish a task. Karasek and Theorell (1990) suggest that the combination of these two constructs results in perceptions of control that influence worker health. The most adverse outcomes are seen in jobs that combine high levels of demand with low levels of control. High-strain jobs include machine-paced manufacturing, computer operations, and service jobs (Repetti, 1993). The same job tasks may be defined as low-strain if the worker is allowed to pace him- or herself, contribute information to management, or acquire new job skills. This model has been validated across a variety of work environments and in many different countries. The findings are remarkably consistent across job types and work settings (Evanoff & Rosenstock, 1994; MacDonald et al., 2001).

Musculoskeletal diseases have been studied with the demand control model. Most of the research has examined upper-extremity and neck and shoulder pain, although several studies have been directed toward low-back pain. Longitudinal and cross-sectional studies have found that monotonous work and work under time pressures are associated with neck and shoulder pain. In the most elaborate study of musculoskeletal pain using the demand control model (Bigos et al., 1991), jobs classified as having low decision latitude had odds ratios for hospitalization of 1.3 to 1.9 after adjusting for physical load. Other studies have combined the demand control model with measures of social support, but the findings are less clear (Nachemson, 1992; Peate, 1994). Social support appears to mediate the effects of high demands and low decision latitude, but the specific mechanisms are highly variable and very sensitive to individual differences. As previously stated, the demand control model has been used to study both mental and physical health outcomes. The combination of job demands and control has been shown to predict general symptoms of psychologic distress. A longitudinal study of male power-plant workers found that increased symptoms of psychologic distress were associated with the interaction between job demands and decision latitude (Bromet, Dew, Parkinson, & Schulberg, 1988). However, the same study found that decision latitude did not mediate the relationship between job demands and affective disorders. In other words, workers with high job demands and low decision latitude were not found to have higher rates of affective disorders than workers with high job demands and high decision latitude.

Marshall and Barnett (1991) suggest that it is also important to recognize the positive aspects of job challenge and decision authority. They conducted a series of factor-analytic studies and identified six work reward factors (helping others, decision authority, challenge, supervisor support, recognition, and satisfaction with salary) and five work concern factors (overload, dead-end job, hazard exposure, poor supervision, and discrimination). They then estimated separate regression models for well-being and psychologic distress as outcome (dependent) measures. This study found that not all work concerns or rewards are equally capable of producing or reducing job-related stress responses. The authors suggest that the narrowing of attention to only two workplace dimensions, such as demand and decision latitude, may be premature. Marshall and Barnett (1991) also found that men and women experience different aspects of work as problematic or rewarding. They concluded that models of workplace stressors and mediators of stress should be broadened to incorporate the growing evidence of gender differences in response.

IMMUNE RESPONSES TO WORKPLACE STRESS

Evidence from a number of studies points toward a link between neural activity and altered immune responses (Ader, Cohen, & Felten, 1987). Psychosocial factors such as bereavement, marital separation, depression, and examination stress in students are associated with altered measures of immune reactivity and altered health status. Both animal and human investigations show that the immune and nervous systems communicate through a dynamic process using a variety of hormones and neurotransmitters. This area of research is known as *psychoneuroimmunology* or biopsychology. Stress responses have been proposed as part of the etiology of fibromyalgia and low-back pain. Disturbed autonomic nervous system function has been clearly established in fibromyalgia (Simons, 1990). Simons cites several studies that demonstrate that abnormalities in the immune system produce alterations in serotonin pathways, accounting for many of the clinical manifestations. Although still speculative, the association between sleep disturbances, responses, and fibromyalgia may help explain the worksite findings of increased health problems (including musculoskeletal problems) in shiftworkers. Shiftwork is known to disrupt normal circadian rhythms and to change sleep-wake cycles (see Chapter 11 for further discussion).

One of the first models to emerge in psychoneuroimmunology uses new biomedical techniques to obtain ambulatory recordings of endocrine responses to conditions of daily life. This biopsychosocial model helps to identify stress-inducing environmental conditions and to analyze their influence on health, well-being, and efficiency (Frankenhaeuser, 1991; Frankenhaeuser & Johansson, 1986). Cognitive appraisal is a key element of this model. When an individual is confronted with an environmental challenge, he or she appraises the nature and strength of the challenge and weighs the importance and severity of the demands against his or her own coping abilities. A stimulus that is perceived as a threat or a situation that creates demands well beyond the perceived resources of the person evokes a complex series of physical and emotional reactions. Threatening stimuli generate the increased secretion of epinephrine and norepinephrine or stress hormones. The pituitary gland also secretes adrenocorticotropic hormone, which is an important element in the body's immune response. Lundberg (2002) was able to confirm these hypotheses. Lundberg linked lack of control and time pressure with reports of mental stress in workers. The mental stress associated with manual tasks was accompanied by elevated norepinephrine and cortisol and then followed by increases in muscle tension.

COPING, COGNITIVE APPRAISAL, AND MUSCULOSKELETAL DISORDERS

Many discussions of the psychosocial attributes of work-related MSDs emphasize the importance of coping styles in dealing with the day-to-day demands of the workplace (Ross, 1994). However, most of the research on cognitive appraisal and coping is more relevant to the treatment of MSDs than to understanding the development of musculoskeletal pain syndromes. A significant body of literature has examined the impact of cognitive appraisal and coping mechanisms in persons confronting the consequences of an injury or chronic illness. The findings of these studies are remarkably consistent.

Coping skills are called into action when a person experiences an injury or illness. According to Lazarus and Folkman (1984), coping allows a person to maintain a positive self-image, tolerate negative events, and maintain emotional equilibrium. Coping responses are described as coping styles. Two interrelated factors generally are considered in the investigation of coping styles. The first is appraisal, which involves a person's judgment about what is at stake in a stressful encounter, and the second is coping process, or the cognitive and behavioral efforts used to manage specific stressful episodes.

Lazarus and Folkman (1984) identified two stages in the appraisal process, *primary apprais-*

al, or the determination of the challenge, threat, or benefit of an event, and *secondary appraisal*, which reflects the individual's beliefs about the options available to deal with the situation. This appraisal process is believed to mediate an individual's reaction to an event. Measures of appraisal often include questions that tap a person's sense of control. For example, Peacock and Wong (1990) developed a measure—the Stress Appraisal Measure—that assesses both primary and secondary appraisal. They identified three aspects of secondary appraisal in their measure: controllable by self, controllable by others, and uncontrollable.

The type of coping style used depends on the personal characteristics of the individual, environmental factors such as availability of social support and presence of life stressors, and the individual's appraisal of the stressful situation (Parkes, 1986). Lazarus and Folkman (1984) identified two primary ways of coping: problem-focused and emotion-focused. Other investigators have reported similar classifications (Carver, Schier, & Weintraub, 1989; Endler & Parker, 1990; Feifel, Strack, & Nagy, 1987). *Problem-focused coping* is associated with efforts to manage the nature of the problem, whereas *emotion-focused coping* is directed at regulating the feelings that the problem or situation evokes. Coping styles are then classified further into approach strategies and avoidance strategies. *Approach strategies* include trying to identify and solve problems, seeking information, and seeking social and emotional support. *Avoidance strategies* include denial, resigned acceptance, hostility, and passivity.

Pellino and Oberst (1993) used a coping and cognitive appraisal model and found perceptions of situational control and appraisal of illness to be mediators of the outcome of treatment in a group of chronic low-back-pain clients. Those clients who considered the situation beyond their control were more likely to be depressed, reported more negative life events, and experienced more pain.

PERSONALITY AND ADJUSTMENT FACTORS

The previously described models all note the contributions of personality traits and emotional states to worker response to worksite stress and injury. It is important to remember the differences between personality traits and emotional states that arise in response to the consequences of an injury. The literature in this area often fails to distinguish clearly between the two.

Personality traits are defined as consistent characteristics of a person, including behavior patterns, emotional responses, and emotional predispositions. *Emotional* or *reactive states* are emotional reactions to a particular stimulus or situation. Both are thought to play a role in the etiology and response to treatment of musculoskeletal disorders; however, the empiric evidence in support of this belief is conflicting, despite more than 20 years of interest in the topic.

Personality Traits

Is there an MSD personality? Perhaps the investigations of type A personality and heart disease will shed some light on this problem. Studies of type A personality have identified individuals with high needs for control. This personality type was first investigated in persons with cardiovascular disease, although subsequent research has broadened the construct to include individuals with other diseases. Type A behaviors include competitiveness, aggressiveness, and hostility as coping responses elicited to perceived threats to control (Rhodewalt & Fairfield, 1990).

Of particular relevance to MSDs are the studies of type A-personality workers. There is substantial evidence that persons with type A personalities may choose high-pressure occupations. There also are substantial data that report type A workers as having unsupportive interactions with coworkers, enhanced feelings of time urgency, and decreased levels of perceived environmental control (Bedian,

Mossholder, & Touiliatos, 1990). Recent studies suggest that a subgroup of individuals with type A personality traits are particularly susceptible to musculoskeletal pain (Holmstrom, Lindell & Moritz, 1992). Floodmark and Aase (1992) reported that workers with type A behaviors such as anger, hostility, and extreme competitiveness had significantly more musculoskeletal symptoms than other workers with type A personalities but less pronounced behavioral characteristics. These findings are consistent with studies of the relationship between hostility and anger and cardiovascular disease in persons with type A personality.

Injury, illness, and treatment resulted in reactive, helpless behaviors and medical noncompliance in a group of injured type A recreational runners with foot injuries when compared to a type B group with similar injuries (Rhodewalt & Strube, 1985). The type A runners were more likely to express anger about the injury and to be dissatisfied with their rate of recovery. Smith and Rhodewalt (1986) suggest that type A behavior patterns are elicited by exposure to certain environmental stimuli based on concepts of person-environment fit. This proposition was supported by Hagihara, Tarumi, Miller, and Morimoto (1997). They studied the stressful aspects of work with a large group of Japanese office workers and found that type A and type B workers responded very differently to the characteristics and demands of the same work environment. Their findings suggest that certain personality types are at increased risk of work-related musculoskeletal disorders and that, once injured, these psychosocial states influence response to treatment, recovery, and return to work.

Few longitudinal studies have focused on personality traits and susceptibility to musculoskeletal disorders. In one of the most comprehensive studies, Vikari-Junitura, Vuori, Silverstein, Kalimo, and Videman (1991) followed a cohort of Finnish adolescents from 1955 to 1987. One hundred and fifty-four of the original group of 1084 persons completed a questionnaire about work characteristics and musculoskeletal symptoms and underwent a physical examination. Psychosocial measurements obtained in adolescence showed no consistent association with neck, back, or shoulder symptoms in adulthood. Vikari-Junitura et al. (1991) did find that weak "mental resources for promoting health," such as a poor sense of coherence, were associated consistently with neck and shoulder pain in adulthood.

Leino and Magni (1993) conducted a 10-year prospective study of working conditions, health habits, mental well-being, and physical health in a large cohort of metal workers in Finland. The study was designed to investigate whether distress and depression led to musculoskeletal disorders. They found that depressive and distress symptoms predicted musculoskeletal morbidity of the neck, shoulders, and low back, particularly in men. These investigators did not find the reverse temporal sequence for depression, although the onset of musculoskeletal symptoms was associated with increased distress. Poor adjustment has been associated with chronic musculoskeletal pain. Individuals who were anxious, angry, or depressed were found to be at significantly greater risk of a back injury than workers who were not in these states but who held similar jobs and had identical training (Hirschfeld & Behan, 1963).

Finally, more recently, Marras, Davis, Heaney, Maronitis, and Allread (2000) studied the influence of psychosocial stress, gender, and personality traits on measures of spine loading in a laboratory setting. Twenty-five participants who were asymptomatic for low back pain completed the Myers-Briggs Type Indicator (MBTI), a personality assessment, and the State-Trait Anxiety Inventory (STAI), a measure of anxiety, prior to performing a lifting task. The task was performed under stressful and nonstressful conditions relative to the experimenters' interactions with the participants. Results indicated that psychosocial stress increased spine loading in some individuals, males' and females' spinal kinematics reacted differently under stressful situations, and certain personality traits were associated with increases in spinal loads when psychosocial stress was introduced. Marras et al. suggest a potential pathway between psychosocial stress and spinal loading that may interact with certain personality traits.

Emotional States

A number of cross-sectional studies have compared self-reported measures of personality and adjustment among groups of clients experiencing different types of pain. Early studies classified the pain as either organic or functional. Functional pain was believed to be of psychogenic origin. Measurement of the psychiatric or psychologic problems was inconsistent, and the samples were often small. Not surprisingly, the results of these studies are conflicting. Joukamaa (1994) suggests that the use of standardized measures, such as the Minnesota Multiphasic Personality Inventory or the Millon Behavioral Health Inventory, coupled with large representative samples of musculoskeletal pain patients has increased our understanding of the complex relationship between psychologic states and chronic pain. Joukamaa concludes that all pain has psychologic consequences, that the relationship between psychopathology and pain is complex, and that depression and anxiety are the most common psychiatric disorders associated with low-back pain. He also proposes an atypical presentation of depression in some individuals with low-back pain, in whom the depression is masked by the absence of depressed mood.

Fernandez and Turk (1995) have proposed a similar model. However, they focus on the contribution of anger as opposed to depression as the most salient emotional correlate of pain. Many studies have identified hostility as a common feature of clients with low-back pain (Waddell, 1992). Fernandez and Turk believe that anger rather than hostility is the dominant emotion influencing the cognitive appraisals of chronic pain sufferers (Figure 12-2). Most clients inhibit their admission and expression of anger, perhaps because of the perceived social consequences of this emotion. This inhibited anger is believed to be a mediator of depression in persons with chronic pain. Angry, depressed, or hostile persons with painful musculoskeletal disorders are more likely to adopt maladaptive health habits and lifestyles that complicate treatment and prolong disability.

IMPACT OF MUSCULOSKELETAL DISORDERS ON QUALITY OF LIFE

MSDs have a major impact on occupational performance. *Occupation* is defined as "the day-to-day engagement in the activities, tasks, and roles that organize our lives, and meet our needs to maintain ourselves, to be productive, and to derive enjoyment and satisfaction within our environments" (Christianson, 1991). The primary focus of most health care professionals is on restoring a person's ability to work. However, it is also important to examine the emotional impact of MSDs as it relates to decreased independence in activities of daily living and leisure activities. The frustration and embarrassment resulting from one's inability to perform simple tasks independently (e.g., buttoning a shirt, tying a shoelace, combing ones hair, hooking a bra strap, opening a jar) are thought to increase the anger and depression experienced by most individuals. Anger and frustration take a toll on families and friends as well, decreasing the social networks essential for self-esteem and emotional support. As the number of pain-free activities diminishes, recreational and leisure activities are abandoned, giving rise to heightened social isolation. These factors increase the likelihood of sustained sick-role behaviors, particularly when activities of daily living provoke pain to some extent.

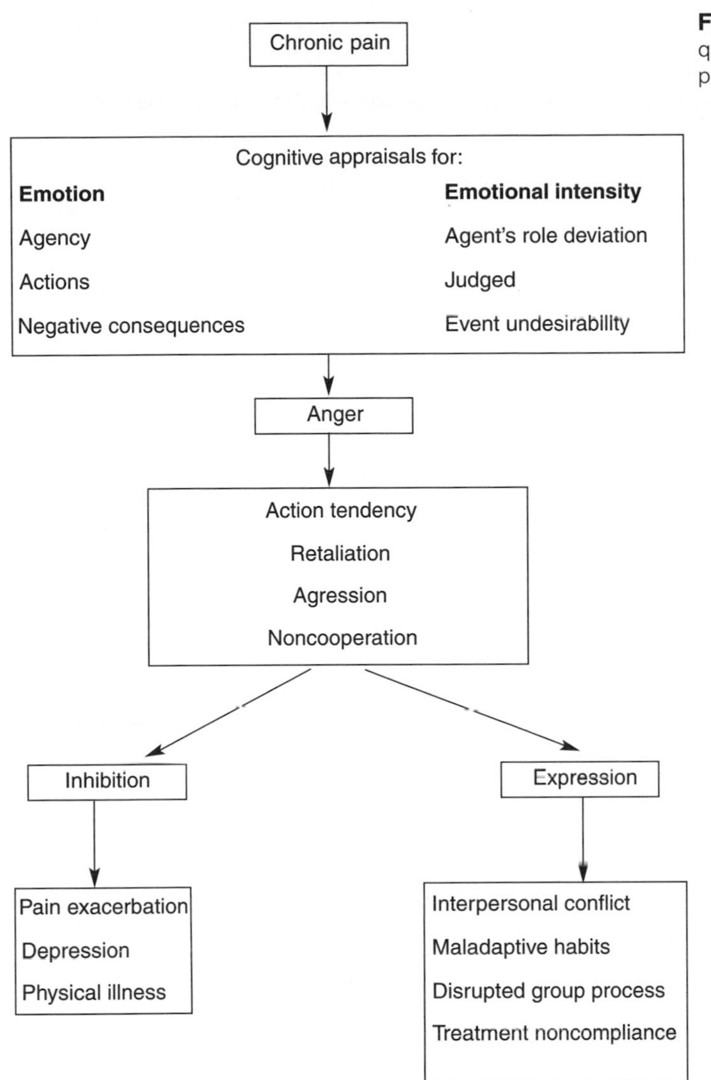

Figure 12-2 Antecedents and consequences of anger associated with chronic pain.

Unfortunately, the effect of MSDs on quality of life has still not been systematically explored. The growing emphasis on quality of life and functional outcomes as determinants of treatment efficacy will focus attention on the role of self-care, family and social group responsibilities, and leisure activity participation in the development of and recovery from upper-extremity MSDs.

REFERENCES

Ader, R., Cohen, N., & Felten, D. L. (1987). Brain, behavior and immunity. *Brain, Behavior, and Immunity, 1*(1), 1-6.

Ariens, G. A. M., van Mechelen, W., Bongers, P. M., Bouter, L. M., & van der Wal, G. (2001). Psychosocial risk factors for neck pain: A systematic review. *American Journal of Industrial Medicine, 39*(2), 180-193.

Bedian, A. G., Mossholder, K. W., & Touiliatos, J. (1990). Type A status and selected work experiences among male and female accountants. In M. J. Strube (Ed.), *Type A behavior.* Newbury Park, CA: Sage Publications.

Bigos, S. J., Battie, M. C., Spengler, D. M., Fisher, L. D., Fordyce, W. E., Hansson, T. et al. (1991). A prospective study of work perceptions and psychosocial factors affecting the report of back injury. *Spine, 16*(1), 1-6.

Bongers, P. M., de Winter, D. R., Kompier, M. A., & Hildebrandt, B. H. (1993). Psychosocial factors and work and musculoskeletal disease: A review of the literature. *Scandinavian Journal of Work, Environment, and Health, 19*(5), 297-312.

Bongers, P. M., Kremer, A. M., & ter Laak, J. (2002). Are psychological factors, risk factors for symptoms and signs of the shoulder, elbow or hand/wrist?: A review of the epidemiological literature. *American Journal of Industrial Medicine, 41*(5), 315-342.

Bromet, E. J., Dew, M. A., Parkinson, D. K., & Schulberg, H. C. (1988). Predictive effects of occupational and marital stress on the mental health of a male workforce. *Journal of Organizational Behavior, 9*, 1-13.

Bronner, K. (1965). Industrial implications of stress. In L. Levi (Ed.), *Emotional stress: Physiological and psychological reactions, medical, industrial and military implications.* New York: Elsevier.

Carayon, P., Smith, M. J., & Haims, M. C. (1999). Work organization, job stress, and work-related musculoskeletal disorders. *Human Factors, 41,* 644-663.

Carver, C. S., Schier, M. F., & Weintraub, J. K. (1989). Assessing coping strategies: A theoretically based approach. *Journal of Personality and Social Psychology, 56*(2), 267-283.

Chadwick, J. F. (1980). Psychological job stress and coronary heart disease: A current NIOSH project. In R. M. Schwartz (Ed.), *New developments in occupational stress.* Cincinnati: National Institute of Occupational Safety and Health.

Christianson, C. (1991). Occupational therapy: Intervention for life performance. In C. Christianson & C. Baum (Eds.), *Occupational therapy: Overcoming human performance deficits.* Thorofare, NJ: Slack.

Christmansson, M., Friden, J., & Sollerman, C. (1999). Task design, psycho-social work climate and upper extremity pain disorders-effects of an organisational redesign on manual repetitive assembly jobs. *Applied Ergonomics, 30*(5), 463-472.

Cooper, C. L., & Marshall, J. (1976). Occupational sources of stress: A review of the literature relating to coronary heart disease and mental ill health. *Journal of Occupational Psychology, 49*(1), 11-25.

Csikszentmihalyi, M. (1993). Activity and happiness: towards a science of occupation. *Journal of Occupational Science, 1,* 38-42.

Davis, K. G., & Heaney, C. A. (2000). The relationship between psychosocial work characteristics and low back pain: underlying methodological issues. *Clinical Biomechanics, 15,* 389-406

Endler, N. S., & Parker, J. D. (1990). A multidimensional assessment of coping: a critical evaluation. *Journal of Personality and Social Psychology, 58*(5), 844-854.

Evanoff, B., & Rosenstock, L. (1994). Psychophysiologic stressors and work organization. In L. Rosenstock & M. Cullen (Eds.), *Textbook of clinical occupational and environmental medicine.* Philadelphia: Saunders.

Faucett, J. A. (1994). Depression in painful clinical disorders: The role of pain and conflict about pain. *Journal of Pain and Symptom Management, 9,* 520-526.

Feifel, H., Strack, S., & Nagy, V. T. (1987). Coping strategies and associated features of medically ill patients. *Psychosomatic Medicine, 49*(6), 616-625.

Fernandez, E., & Turk, D. C. (1995). The scope and significance of anger in the experience of chronic pain. *Pain, 61*(2), 165-175.

Feuerstein, M. (2002). Biobehavioral mechanisms of work-related upper extremity disorders: A new agenda for research and practice. *American Journal of Industrial Medicine, 41*(5), 293-297.

Feuerstein, M., Callan-Harris, M. S., Dyer, D., Armbruster, W., & Carosella, A. M. (1993). Multidisciplinary rehabilitation of chronic work-related upper extremity disorders. *Journal of Occupational Medicine, 35*(4), 396-403.

Floodmark, B. T., & Aase, G. (1992). Musculoskeletal symptoms and Type A behavior in blue collar workers. *British Journal of Industrial Medicine, 49*, 683-687.

Frankenhaeuser, M., & Johansson, G. (1986). Stress at work: Psychobiological and psychosocial aspects. *International Review of Applied Psychology, 35*, 287-299.

Frankenhaeuser, M. (1991). The psychophysiology of sex differences as related to occupational stress. In M. Frankenhaeuser, U. Lundberg, & M. Chesney (Eds.), *Women, work, and health: Stress and opportunities.* New York: Plenum.

Hagberg, M., Silverstein, B., Wells, R., Smith, M. J., Hendrick, H. W., Carayon, P. et al. (1995). *Work-related musculoskeletal disorders (WMSDs): A reference book for prevention.* London: Taylor & Francis.

Hagihara, A., Tarumi, K., Miller, A., & Morimoto, K. (1997). Type A and type B behaviors, work stressors, and social support at work. *Preventive Medicine, 26,* 486-494.

Haufler, A. J., Feuerstein, M., & Huang, G. D. (2000). Job stress, upper extremity pain and functional limitations in symptomatic computer users. *American Journal of Industrial Medicine, 38*(5), 507-515.

Hirschfeld, A. H., & Behan, R. C. (1963). The accident process. *Journal of the American Medical Society, 186,* 1939-1945.

Holmstrom, E. B., Lindell, J., & Moritz, U. (1992) Low back and neck/shoulder pain in construction workers: Occupational workload and psychosocial risk factors. Part 2: Relationship to neck and shoulder pain. *Spine, 17*(6), 672-677.

Huang, G. D., Feuerstein, M., & Sauter, S. L. (2002). Occupational stress and work-related upper extremity disorders: Concepts and models. *American Journal of Industrial Medicine, 41*(5), 298-314.

Hurrell, J. J., & McLaney, M.A. (1988). Exposure to job stress—a new psychometric instrument. *Scandinavian Journal of Work, Environment, and Health, 14*(Suppl 1), 27-28.

Joukamaa, M. (1994). Depression and back pain. *Acta Psychiatry Scandinavica Supplementum, 377*, 83-86.

Karasek, R., & Theorell, T. (1990). *Healthy work: Stress, productivity and the reconstruction of working life*. New York: Basic Books.

Kelsey, J. L., & Golden, A. L. (1988). Occupational and workplace factors associated with low back pain. *Occupational Medicine, 3*(1), 7-16.

Lazarus, R., & Folkman, S. (1984). *Stress, appraisal, and coping*. New York: Springer.

Leino, P., & Magni, G. (1993). Depressive and distress symptoms as predictors of low back pain, neck-shoulder pain and other musculoskeletal morbidity: A 10-year follow-up of metal industry employees. *Pain, 53*(1), 89-94.

Levi, L. (1972). Stress and distress in response to psychosocial stimuli. *Acta Medica Scandinavica Supplementum, 191*, 528-538.

Levi, L. (1987). Definition and the conceptual aspects of health in relation to work. In R. Kalimo, M. A. El Batawi, & C. L. Cooper (Eds.), *Psychosocial factors at work*. Geneva: World Health Organization.

Linton, S. J. (1995). Overview of psychosocial and behavioral factors in neck and shoulder pain. *Scandinavian Journal of Rehabilitation Medicine Supplement, 32*, 67-77.

Linton, S. J. (2000). A review or psychological risk factors in back and neck pain. *Spine, 25*(9), 1148-1156.

Lundberg, U. (2002). Psychophysiology of work: Stress, gender, endocrine response, and work-related upper extremity disorders. *American Journal of Industrial Medicine, 41*, 383-392.

Marras, W. S., Davis, K. G., Heaney, C.A., Maronitis, A. B. & Allread, W. G. (2000). The influence of psychosocial stress, gender, and personality on mechanical loading of the lumbar spine. *Spine,* 25, 23, 3045-3054.

MacDonald, L. A., Karasek, R. A., Punnett, L., & Scharf, T. (2001). Covariation between workplace physical and psycholocial stressors: Evidence and implications for occupational health research and prevention. *Ergonomics, 44*, 696-718.

Macfarlane, G. J., Hunt, I. M., & Silman, A. J. (2000). Role of mechanical and psychosocial factors in the onset of forearm pain: prospective population based study. *British Medical Journal, 321*(7262), 676-680.

Malchaire, J. B., Roquelaure, Y., Cock, N., Piette, A., Vergracht, S., & Chiron, H. (2001). Musculoskeletal complaints, functional capacity, personality and psychosocial factors. *International Archives of Occupational and Environmental Health, 74*(8), 549-557.

Marshall, N., & Barnett, R. (1991). Race, class, and multiple role strains and gains among women employed in the service sector. *Women and Health, 17*, 1-19.

Nachemson, A. L. (1992). Newest knowledge of back pain: a critical look. *Clinical Orthopaedics and Related Research, 279*, 8-20.

National Institute for Occupational Safety and Health (NIOSH). (1996). National occupational research agenda (NORA). (NIOSH Publication No. 96-115). Cincinnati, OH: U.S. Department of Health and Human Services.

National Research Council (2001). *Musculoskeletal disorders and the workplace: Low back and upper extremities*. Washington, DC: National Academy Press.

Parkes, K. R. (1986). Coping in stressful episodes: The role of individual differences, environmental factors and situational characteristics. *Journal of Personality and Social Psychology, 51*(6), 1277-1292.

Peacock, E. J., & Wong, P.T., (1990). The Stress Appraisal Measure (SAM): A multidimensional approach to cognitive appraisal. *Stress Medicine, 6*, 227-327.

Peate, W. F. (1994). Occupational musculoskeletal disorders. *Primary Care, 21*(2), 313-327.

Pellino, T. A., & Oberst, M. T. (1993). Perception of control and appraisal of illness in low back pain. *Orthopaedic Nursing, 11*(1), 22-26.

Repetti, R. L. (1993). The effects of workload and the social environment at work on health. In L. Goldberger & S. Brenitz (Eds.), *Handbook of stress: Theoretical and clinical aspects*. New York: Free Press.

Rhodewalt, F., & Strube, M. (1985). A self attribution reactance model of recovery from injury in Type A individuals. *Journal of Applied Social Psycholog y, 15*, 330-344.

Rhodewalt, F., & Fairfield, M. (1990). An alternative approach to Type A behaviour and health: Psychological reactance and non-compliance. In M. Strube (Ed.), *Type A behavior*. Newbury Park, CA: Sage Publications.

Ross, P. (1994). Ergonomic hazards in the workplace, assessment and prevention. *American Association of Occupational Health Nurses Journal, 42*(4), 171-176.

Seyle, H. (1936). A syndrome produced by diverse noxious agents. *Nature, 138*, 2-4.

Simons, D. (1990). Muscular pain syndromes. *Advances in Pain Research and Therapy, 17*, 1-41.

Smith, M. (1987). Occupational stress. In M. Salvendy (Ed.), *Handbook of human factors*. New York: Wiley.

Smith, T. W., & Rhodewalt, F. (1986). On states, traits, and processes: A transactional alternative to the individual differences assumptions in Type A behavior and physiological reactivity. *Journal of Research in Personality, 20*, 229-251.

Soderfeldt, B., Soderfeldt, M., Muntaner, C., O'Campo, P., Warg, L., & Ohlson, C. (1996). Psychosocial work environment in human service organizations: A conceptual analysis and development of the demand-control model. *Social Science and Medicine, 42*(9), 1217-1226.

Vikari-Junitura, E., Vuori, J., Silverstein, B., Kalimo, R., & Videman, T. (1991). A lifelong prospective study on the role of psychosocial factors in neck-shoulder and low back pain. *Spine, 16,* 1056-1061.

Waddell, G. (1992). Biopsychosocial analysis of low back pain. *Bailliere's Clinical Rheumatology 6*(3), 523-557.

PART FOUR

Developing and Implementing Worksite Programs

CHAPTER 13

Job Analysis and Worksite Assessment

Melanie T. Ellexson

HISTORY

Work is a basis for skill acquisition; it is needed throughout all developmental stages for successful role function. Our occupations and the roles they support define who we are and what we consider to be our life's work.

People often describe themselves using their professional title or work activity. Rehabilitation programs, particularly occupational therapy programs, in the 1930s and early 1940s acknowledged the relationship between person and occupation by having hospital clients learn about work principles and perform work for very specific therapeutic reasons.

The division of services into prevocational and vocational programs marked the 1950s. Vocational programs used work samples and psychometric tests to determine work aptitudes, interests, and skills. Prevocational programs helped to prepare clients for the pressures and demands of vocational activity. These programs focused on developing work habits, tolerances, coordination, and acceptable production standards (Kirkland & Robertson, 1985).

In the late 1970s and early 1980s, U.S. industry began to recognize its responsibility for active management and prevention of injury in the workplace. Corporate owners acknowledged that a safer workplace could improve productivity and reduce costly claims. The primary activities for prevention and wellness are improving worker fitness; changing worker tolerances; educating management, supervisors, and workers; and modifying the workplace. These activities must have a basis in a functional analysis of the work activity and the worker's response to work and the work environment.

Government agencies and national law have provided industry with both demands and guidance for regulating workplace safety. In 1990, the Occupational Safety and Health Administration (OSHA) developed guidelines for control of cumulative trauma in the red meat industry. At the heart of these guidelines, which have now been applied to many different industries, is a thorough evaluation of work tasks.

In April 2002, OSHA released a protocol, "Developing Industry and Task Specific Ergonomic Guidelines," for the control of ergonomic problems in the workplace. OSHA places strong emphasis on the analysis and identification of work tasks. These guidelines are designed to develop industry-specific standards, with the goal of reducing injuries and illnesses in the workplace.

The American National Standards Institute (ANSI) has had a committee working on standards to reduce work-related musculoskeletal disorders (MSDs) in the workplace since 1990. Central to these draft standards is the analysis of the work, the worker, and the workplace.

The Americans with Disabilities Act (ADA), a civil rights law for individuals with handicaps, was signed into law in 1990. This act, with far-reaching implications for both employment and accessibility, identifies the functional job description as being a key document in determining compliance with the regulations set forth in the law. Knowing what tasks individuals are required to complete in the course of their work; what effects these tasks have on the human body and mind; and the role of tools, equipment, and the work environment has become good business (Kornblau & Ellexson, 1991).

WORK, WORKER, AND WORKPLACE

An accurate and complete functional job description must include analyses for three major components of work activity: the work, the worker, and the workplace. To make this assessment, one must analyze the task to be completed; the physical and mental requirements of the person doing the work; and the tools, equipment, and workspace of the specific company (Ellexson, 2000).

JOB ANALYSIS OVERVIEW

What follows is a discussion of the components of job analysis that are necessary for company compliance with laws and regulations and that serve as a basis for intervention and prevention programs. The chapter first outlines the steps for job analysis and then discusses the additional steps for assessment of work-related MSDs. The first step in analyzing a job is to determine the essential job functions.

Essential Job Functions

Essential functions or tasks are the basic job duties that an employee must be able to perform with or without reasonable accommodation. Each job must be carefully examined to determine which tasks are essential to job performance. The ADA provides the following examination guidelines for determining if a task is an essential function (Federal Register, 1991).

- Whether the reason the position exists is to perform that function
- The number of other employees available to perform the function or among whom the performance of the function can be distributed
- The degree of expertise or skill required to perform the function
- The work experience of present or past employees
- The time spent in performing a function
- The consequences of not requiring an employee to perform a function
- The terms of a collective bargaining agreement

The ADA states that it is the employer's right and responsibility to determine the essential functions of a job, but in fact, employers need help in identifying these essential job components. One successful approach is to arrange for a focus group facilitated by the therapist. The focus group should consist of at least two current employees, a working supervisor, and someone from the company who has decision-making authority. The group may include representatives from human resources, safety, labor, and management. The workers and the working supervisor should be asked to describe what they do during a normal workday. Tasks that occur only in the morning or afternoon, only on a particular day of the week, or only at certain times must be defined. It is also important to identify activities that are controlled by the environment and the time of year, such as snow removal for street and sanitation workers or planting flowers for park and recreation employees. This focus group discussion should require only about 1 hour, and it will provide the therapist with valuable information regarding when they need to be at the job site and how much time they need to spend looking at specific tasks. This extra step in developing the job analysis can reduce costly mistakes that occur when tasks are missed or jobs are not well defined (Ellexson, 1995).

Some examples of essential functions are a retail clerk ringing up sales and making change, an office receptionist answering the telephone, and a physical therapist working in orthopedics evaluating the spine.

Marginal Job Functions

Listing the marginal functions of the job is necessary to develop a clear picture of all tasks required of the worker. Marginal functions are those not essential to the specific job or those shared by different employees. The importance of identifying these functions becomes evident when the evaluator looks at the way employees spend time. These marginal functions may offer a certain amount of risk based on the infrequency with which they are performed and the activity itself. Marginal functions are identified by the focus group and listed separately from the essential functions. This is a particularly good idea because it helps identify the tasks that are truly essential and those that are not.

ACTIVITY DESCRIPTORS

When evaluating the workers in particular jobs, the therapist uses factors descriptive of activity. These factors include such terms as walking, standing, sitting, stooping, kneeling, crawling, climbing, lifting, reaching, handling, fingering, hearing, and seeing. These factors are correlated to each step of an essential function. In evaluating a job, one must look at the force necessary to move objects, tools, or equipment. The space assigned to various work tasks, clearances between equipment, aisle width, and distance from one work area to another must be measured. Accessibility to various work areas should be determined. Equipment evaluation may necessitate measuring the weight to be lifted, the reach, the height of the work surface, seating heights, widths, and depths, the height of sighting devices, and placement of controls.

Actual task performance should be measured, weighed, and evaluated for the force required in the operation. Vibration from tools or equipment or vibrations caused by moving over uneven surfaces must be considered. This measurement is difficult and sometimes expensive to make. The negative effect of any vibration on the worker must be determined. If there is no documented evidence of injury or cumulative trauma attributed to such vibration, one may choose to mention the vibration but not measure this exposure.

In an analysis of specific work tasks, the number of repetitions necessary in each essential function must be documented. For example, in evaluating a dockworker, it would be necessary to determine the average number of parcels to be loaded and unloaded from each truck. It would also be important to determine the number of trucks that a worker could expect to load and unload per shift.

One example of this is the toolmaker who is given a work order, sets up his or her machine, and cuts the order. How often the worker must reset the machine depends on the size of the order and could occur several times a day or several times a month. The frequency is important because this task is essential to the work to be done and because the physical requirements for setting up the machine may be of greater risk to the worker than processing the work itself. The analysis should include company production standards if they exist. Using the dockworker example, these might include how many trucks a worker is expected to load and unload per shift or the pay incentives based on the number of trucks serviced. Not all essential functions occur frequently.

It is necessary to gain an understanding of the work group and what assistance a worker may have available. The work group may include all employees with a particular job title or only a specified number of individuals assigned to work together. Frequently, workers from more than one job category may be able to perform tasks. Examples might be the journeyman carpenter, his or her apprentice, and the carpentry supervisor. Knowing who is available to carry out a particular task provides insight into why it is done in the manner observed at the job site. (See Chapter 2 for a discussion of work groups.)

The actual time spent in the performance of each essential function helps to complete the picture of the worker's daily activity. Some tasks must be assessed individually, and others need to have cumulative time documented. This is particularly important for tasks that are highly repetitive and for lifting tasks.

It is important to include information about license, certification, or registration requirements. These may vary from state to state and from municipality to municipality. Experience and/or educational requirements based on present and past practices or collective bargaining agreements should be noted. Knowing the education and experience of the workers will provide valuable insight into the reasons for particular practices in the workplace. It allows for future education and training to be developed at the appropriate level of understanding and learning.

The attitudes of workers can affect job performance. The effects of stress resulting from production standards, pay incentives, or precision requirements produce emotional arousal and trigger defensive behaviors. A worker with low job satisfaction may perceive his or her job as more difficult. High production standards may mean increased muscle fatigue and may lead to increased mental fatigue. Both types of fatigue lead to a decline in physical health and increased risk of injury. Individuals who are responsible for work completion or the activities of other workers may feel more stress because of this level of responsibility. Individuals are frequently promoted into positions of supervision without training or support. If they are not prepared for the added responsibility, there may be an increase in risk to themselves and those they supervise.

Although overall job satisfaction involves many aspects of the job including job content, skill match, and benefits structure (to name a few), the literature has found high correlations between a person's perception of his or her job difficulty and job satisfaction. Job satisfaction could therefore be assessed by using a simple scale from "very easy" to "very difficult" to rate each job task (Larson & Ellexson, 2000).

Physiologic considerations may include observations regarding respiratory compromise due to posture or position, static positioning that can influence blood pressure, bladder control problems secondary to urinary retention when breaks are only at scheduled times, and exposure to fumes or smells that irritate the nose and upper respiratory system. Noxious smells do not have to be toxic or dangerous. The process of cooking fruit or sugar can create odors that are irritating to the eyes and nose.

Temperature, exposure to weather conditions, lighting, noise, and air quality are all important factors in job analysis. Working indoors does not guarantee healthy temperatures. Many factories were built before modern heating and air conditioning systems and may be very cold or very hot. Lighting is frequently a problem in older factories and industrial structures and may dictate the way certain tasks are completed. Noise can certainly increase stress, create difficulty in communication, and ultimately cause hearing loss in certain frequencies. Audiometric testing may be appropriate if exposure is frequent or for prolonged periods.

Observations of the Worksite

The therapist will want to observe the general conditions of the worksite. These may include the following.

- Condition of the floor: Is the tile loose or broken?
- Condition of equipment: Is the equipment accessible? Are sighting devices at an appropriate level for the current workforce?
- Condition of materials: Are materials accessible? Are they easily placed?

Environmental conditions may also include psychosocial information regarding exposure or interface with other workers. Some production lines or assembly work may require very close physical contact with co-workers, whereas other jobs, such as overhead crane operator, may have little contact with others. Some individuals may thrive on close contact, others may like having co-workers nearby but not in their personal space, and still others may be content to have almost no contact with co-workers (Ellexson, 1995). This social aspect of the work environment is crucial to job satisfaction and worker health and safety. The degree of supervisor and peer support may exacerbate or buffer the perception of illness at work.

Personal protective equipment such as work boots, hard hats, aprons, gloves, and goggles are part of the worker's environment and must be recorded. Information about personal work equipment, such as tool belts, would be useful. Use of any chemicals and/or cleaning agents should be documented for further assessment as necessary (Ellexson, 1995, 1997).

Cognitive considerations include such items as the ability to follow directions, communicate verbally or in writing, count, make change, or read print material. The ability of the worker to solve problems, troubleshoot, or respond to an emergency may be important, depending on the particular work setting (Ellexson, 1995).

The Work

Analysis of the work activity is a systematic study of a specific job in terms of what is done with data, people, and objects. Such analysis requires breaking down each essential function into sequential steps that describe clearly what must be done to accomplish the function. The analysis should organize activity into meaningful units. The following example of this process details a packing position in a food manufacturing operation.

Job title: Packer

Essential function: Packing individual cobbler cups for shipping

Steps:

1. Select a box.
2. Place the box on the conveyor side rack.
3. Pick up one cobbler cup in each hand.
4. Place the cups into the packing box.
5. Repeat steps 3 and 4 until 36 cups are in the box.
6. Place the filled box on the sealing table.
7. Fold down the short flaps of the box top.
8. Fold down the longer flaps of the box top.
9. Tape down the long flaps of the box, using the manual taping machine.
10. Place the sealed box on the pallet.

In analysis of specific work tasks, the number of repetitions necessary in each core activity must be documented. The preceding example demonstrates that picking up the cobbler cups to fill each box is repeated 18 times with each hand. It would also be necessary to determine how many boxes must be filled in a given period and how many hours per day the packing actually takes place. It would be important to identify the production standards for this task (e.g., how many boxes are to be packed in a shift; whether pay is based on the number of boxes packed). The weight of the box both empty and packed, and the height, width, and depth of the box all must be noted. The weight of the filled cobbler cups and the dimensions of each cup must be determined. These measurements, which affect the physical function, are the beginning steps in looking at the worker (see Appendix 13-1).

The Worker

In evaluating the workers in a workforce, variables such as age, size, and experience must be considered. Studies have shown that younger workers often have a higher rate of injury than do older workers (Brough, 1991). Several theories have been offered to explain this finding. Frequently, younger, more inexperienced workers are placed in the harder, higher-risk positions. Younger workers have not yet learned to efficiently use movement patterns. The poultry industry has determined that more experienced workers use fewer motions to debone poultry, thereby reducing their risk of work-related MSDs from to cumulative trauma. Knowledge of the work activity and adherence to safety procedures through experience are also believed to play a role in the reduction of injury rates.

It is important to look at the workers as a group to determine the general characteristics of the group. Examples of worker population changes may include shifts in the ethnic population of the workforce. This may mean changes in anthropometric measurements and may require changes in workers' tools and equipment. An aging workforce could introduce a new group of problems related to older workers. The introduction of women into nontraditional positions may present different problems in a particular worker population.

In evaluating the workers in particular jobs, the therapist uses factors descriptive of activity. For example, the fourth step of the cobbler-packing job requires placing filled cups into the packing box. This function requires standing at the conveyor table, reaching for the cups, and handling the cups to lift and place them into the box. Vision would also be an important factor in this step.

Anthropometric measurements are used to evaluate individual workers or to gather data about a group of workers. The following are the most frequently used measurements, with their relevance to the worker (Pheasant, 1986) (see also Chapter 11).

- Stature: vertical distance from floor to vertex (standing clearance)
- Shoulder height: vertical distance from floor to acromion process (zone of reach)
- Elbow height: vertical distance from floor to radius (work surface height)
- Hip height: vertical distance from floor to greater trochanter (functional leg length)
- Knuckle height: vertical distance from floor to third metacarpal (optimal height for heavy lifting)
- Fingertip height: vertical distance from floor to top of middle finger (lowest acceptable level of finger control)
- Sitting height: vertical distance from sitting surface to crown of head (clearance required between seat and overhead)
- Elbow rest height: vertical distance from sitting surface to underside of elbow (armrest and desktop height, work surface with respect to seated surface)
- Thigh clearance: vertical distance from sitting surface to top of one uncompressed thigh at thickest point (clearance required between seat and underside of work surface)
- Buttock-to-knee length: horizontal distance from the back of the uncompressed buttock to the front of the kneecap (clearance between seat back and obstacles in front of the knee)
- Popliteal height: vertical distance from floor to popliteal angle (acceptable seat height)
- Hip breadth: maximum horizontal distance across the hips in a seated position (acceptable seat width)
- Chest depth: maximum horizontal distance from the vertical plane to the front of the chest (clearance)
- Abdominal depth: maximum horizontal distance from the vertical plane to the front of the abdomen (clearance)
- Elbow-to-fingertip length: distance from back of elbow to the tip of the middle finger (forearm reach, defining normal work area)
- Shoulder-to-grip length: distance from the acromion to the center of an object gripped in the hand (zone of convenient reach)
- Hand breadth: maximum breadth across the palm of the hand (clearance required for hand access)
- Hand span: maximum horizontal distance between the fingertips when both arms are stretched out to the sides (lateral reach)
- Elbow span: distance between tips of elbows when both elbows are fully flexed, fingertips touching at the chest (elbow room)

Anthropometric data must be used judiciously in making assumptions about a group of workers. Averaging worker measurements may provide data that do not fit the worker group, since a wide disparity in size exists. This could lead to inappropriate and ergonomically incorrect workplace design.

The Workplace

As described, evaluating the workplace requires examining space and accessibility, equipment, tools, lighting, temperature, vibration, noise, air quality and general environment, and aesthetics. One must measure the space assigned to various work tasks, clearances between equipment, aisle width, distance from one work area to another, and accessibility to various work areas. Equipment evaluation may necessitate measuring the weight to be lifted, the reach, the height of the work surface, seating heights, widths, and depths, the height of sighting devices, placement of controls, and force necessary to operate controls. The tools used by the worker in the performance of the work should be measured, weighed, and evaluated for the force required in their operation. Lighting and visual requirements must be observed and noted for the effect they have on the workplace.

Similarly, temperature considerations, such as exposure to high heat, humidity, or extreme cold, are documented. Prolonged exposure or intermittent movement between extreme temperatures would be important to note. If a worker is frequently or consistently exposed to direct temperature extremes (e.g., cold running water on the hands and forearms), a measurement of this factor would be appropriate.

The general environment, including cleanliness, color, and aesthetic appearance, should be noted. Individual perception about one's work environment may affect efficiency, attention to detail, and overall satisfaction.

Once the data are gathered and organized, there is a detailed, step-by-step description of the work being performed. Observations of the workforce will provide information about the workers. This may include documentation regarding gender, stature, age, skill level, experience level, work stress, and problem tasks. Information about the workplace will include measurements and observations about the environment (Ellexson, 1995).

Job analysis can identify those tasks that are of greater risk by identifying forces, postures, and repetitions. It can lead to the development of alternative methods of activity to lower risk of injury and increase productivity.

ERGONOMIC ASSESSMENT: THE BASIC PLAN

Development of technology has led to less physically strenuous jobs. At the same time, psychologic stress has increased as the demand for greater proficiency and efficiency has increased. Subsequently, these developments have created greater risk of repetitive activity and the associated physical degeneration and possibility of injury.

Although work environments are often described in terms of the technical and physical factors, the psychosocial aspects of the work environment must be considered as part of the broad scope when assessing the workplace (Elmfeldt, Wise, Bergsten, & Alsson, 1983; Rodgers, 1988).

Ergonomics, like occupational medicine and rehabilitation, is a multidisciplinary approach encompassing epidemiology, biomechanics, physiology, and psychology. Epidemiology identifies the incidence and distribution of illnesses and injury. OSHA requires most employers to maintain records of work-related injuries and illnesses. Biomechanics concentrates on the physical stresses p laced on the musculoskeletal structure of an individual when he or she is performing various tasks. Physiology is concerned with a person's metabolic and cardiovascular response to various tasks. Research addressing the expenditure of calories and consumption of oxygen during work activity has been well publicized.

A worker's psychologic response to physical stress, productivity standards, work environment, and other life pressures has more recently been recognized as a contributing factor to workplace safety. Such response requires assessment and control.

Ergonomic assessment of the worksite requires a job analysis that examines the work, the worker, and the workplace within the context of ergonomic risk factors. A simple seven-step guide will assist the rehabilitation professional in completing an efficient, cost-effective ergonomic worksite assessment.

1. *Job analysis:* Assess the job. Management and employee involvement in this assessment is critical to the accurate documentation of specific job function.
2. *Problem identification:* Identify the problems and obstacles that require change or adaptation. Again, it is important not to overlook the suggestions of the workers; these are often the most accurate reflections of the work situation.
3. *Problem assessment-solutions:* Assess each problem and research solutions. Each problem must be examined, and possible solutions must be developed. Technical and economic factors affecting the implementation of each possible solution must be investigated. Any outside sources of funding should be identified.
4. *Plan development and action:* Devise a plan of action. This plan should describe what measures can realistically be achieved by the team, detail the time frames for the start and completion of each solution, and document the methods by which the plan can be carried out.
5. *Implementation:* Implement the plan. Management and workers must be aware of what is to be changed, why the changes are being made, and what results are anticipated. Worker cooperation and participation are necessary for this step to work smoothly and effectively.
6. *Problem reevaluation:* Determine what value has been obtained by implementing the plan of action. A decision to continue current activity, to change the activities, or to alter the direction of ergonomic control must be made.
7. *Plan revision:* Take corrective action to alter the plan or to add to the ergonomic management approach in an effort to achieve ongoing utility.

BIOMECHANICAL ASPECTS OF ERGONOMIC JOB ANALYSIS

Job analysis requires identifying essential job tasks, describing those tasks, and determining basic physical requirements. Step two of our ergonomic worksite guide requires identification and assessment of problem areas. Biomechanics is one frame of reference that analyzes human activity effectively. The rehabilitation professional must relate the activity to the work environment and to the cognitive, emotional, and social aspects of function.

Biomechanical analysis can be quite complex and can include concepts of physics, linear motion, gravity, torque, and equilibrium. The rehabilitation professional must have a working knowledge of biomechanical principles in assessing ergonomic problems. Biomechanical factors include force, posture, position, repetition versus static posture, vibration, and the environment (see Chapter 10 for a complete discussion on biomechanical risk factors). Once a problem has been identified, one can begin the assessment by evaluating the factor of movement to find ergonomic solutions. The body requires the right amount of movement to operate efficiently. Too much movement may cause dynamic fatigue; too little movement may cause static fatigue. Each essential task should be analyzed for frequent repetitive motions or too little motion (Roberts & Falkenberg, 1992).

Some tasks can involve both static and dynamic movements. An example is the act of sawing a board. The person holds the board in place with one hand; this is static motion. The hand sawing the board is involved in dynamic movement. In this example, the static motion creates greater fatigue because of the force exerted to hold the board in place by the extension of the arm away from the body.

Force and distance from the body are two of the components that affect movement. Others are twisting and time spent on the activity. Force is defined as something that causes an object to be moved. Normal forces push surfaces together or pull them apart. In the preceding example, the upper extremity holding the board pushes together the surfaces of the glenohumeral joint. This compressive force pushes together tissue and causes muscle to shorten and thicken. If the saw were to bind or get caught up in the sawing process, causing the arm in motion to pull against resistance, the anatomic structures would get longer and narrower. This reaction is called tensile force. Normally, structures return to their original shape; this ability is called elasticity. If elasticity is exceeded, injury may result. Ergonomic assessment requires careful examination of forces acting on the body during movement (Roberts & Falkenberg, 1992).

It is important to assess the worker's movement to determine where activity occurs in relation to the body. Generally, an activity that takes place away from an individual center of gravity creates greater risk. Certain questions must be asked in evaluating movement.

- Is the task necessary?
- Are certain muscle groups overused?
- Can the work be done by calling on a larger muscle or group of muscles?
- Can a variety of motions be introduced into the task?
- Can either the right or the left hand be used?
- Can adjustments be made to the work task or to the work surface to reduce static or dynamic fatigue?
- Is alternating the task or job rotation a possibility?
- Is there a jig or fixture that could add support?
- Is the frequency of the task caused by machine pacing?
- Is the frequency of the task caused by an incentive plan?
- Is overtime involved?
- Are there adequate rest periods between activities?

In the board-sawing example, one ergonomic solution would be to fix the board to the work surface with a jig or a C-clamp. This would eliminate static movement of the worker's upper extremity. Generally, a variety of movements within a task or group of tasks creates less fatigue than does the same movement repeated several times. Proper work-rest cycles are important elements for ergonomic control. Muscles respond better to frequent short breaks than to less-frequent long breaks. Precaution must be taken to ensure that job rotation does not move workers from one task to another with similar motion requirements.

Positional Posture

Position as an ergonomic factor must be looked at in two separate ways. First, it is important to examine the position of a load both before and after it is moved. Critical factors to observe are the angle of the back, extension of the arms, and bending of the legs. For example, picking up and moving a 4-pound object at arm's length places more force on the back than does holding or carrying a 40-pound object close to the body at waist level. The second element to be examined is the body position through the task. If the worker maintains one position for long periods, the body will fatigue faster than if it is moving periodically. Soldiers at parade rest often complain of fatigue greater than that experienced while marching. Shoulder position is also important. Stress on the shoulder is reduced when the elbow is kept close to the body. The optimal angle between the upper arm and forearm depends on the task to be accomplished. For light and fine motor tasks, the optimal angle is 90 degrees. As the weight of the object being manipulated increases, the angle also increases. Carrying a suitcase is easier with the arms straight down at 180 degrees. Wrist position is also important (Rodgers, 1988). The wrist in neutral position allows for greatest strength. Wrist flexion to 60 degrees reduces strength by more than 50%. Extension to 60 degrees reduces wrist strength to approximately 60%. Ulnar and radial deviation also reduces strength of grip (Rodgers, 1988).

Other questions the health care practitioner may ask include the following.

- Is the position used for performing the task necessary?
- Can the object's shape, size, or placement be changed?
- What keeps the load from being held close to the body?
- Is there room for the feet and legs to move?
- Is it possible to keep the back straight?

- Is there a mechanical device that could do the job?
- Can the task be modified to allow the elbow to be kept close to the body?
- Is there a way to support the arms?
- Can the objects to be manipulated be supported with a counterbalance, jig, or brace?
- Can the person use either hand to perform the task?
- Can the work surface be adjusted for better position?
- Can handles be added or changed to improve position?

Position solutions might include designing workstations to provide as much flexibility as possible. Foot and armrests can be added for support. Periodic stretch breaks allow muscles to move through their entire range of motion. This allowance is particularly important when tasks require static positions or very little movement. Avoiding overhead work by raising the person or lowering the work not only avoids muscle fatigue but reduces strain on the heart, which must pump blood to elevated areas. The ideal arm position is with the elbows as close to the body as possible. For fine motor activity, the forearms should be kept at approximately 90 degrees to the upper arm. Support should be considered if the arms must be extended for longer periods. Supports must not restrict movement or place stress on the arms or wrists. Whenever possible, workstations should be designed to allow workers to complete tasks at positions of greatest strength.

Force (Weight)

Weight is another factor to be considered in finding ergonomic solutions. Logic tells us that the greater the weight of the object to be manipulated, the higher the risk of injury. Age, weight, height, gender, and physical condition also affect how heavy an object feels to a particular person (Rodgers, 1992). In the board-sawing example, the saw represents a variable weight. To some the saw may seem heavy, whereas to others the weight is insignificant.

These are some questions to consider when examining weight.

- Is the task necessary?
- Can the item to be moved be broken down into smaller components?
- Can the object be handled mechanically?
- Are there other people available to assist with the task?
- Is employee rotation possible?
- Are there mechanical aids that could be modified or adapted to reduce the physical demands of the lift?

It is important to remember that the force on the body during a lift is a combination of the weight of the upper body, the weight of the object, and the distance of the object from the body. Simply reducing the weight of an object may not reduce the force on the back to the degree expected. Reducing an object's weight may increase repetitions of a task and add to fatigue. In general, the advantage of changing body position will be greater than that of reducing the weight of the object.

Grip Force

Another important ergonomic factor is force as related to grip. The human hand is a nearly perfect processor or end receptor. It can be positioned at desired places, exert force to hold or move objects, provide tactile information about the environment, and provide feedback for the control of force and movement. In gripping action, parts of the hand are used in mechanical opposition to each other to exert force on an object and hold it in place.

Gripping actions may be divided into three main categories: (1) a power grip requires the fingers to flex around an object and hold it against the palm, (2) a precision grip is used to hold an object between the tips or pads of the thumb and fingers, and (3) an open grip is used when an object rests on the hands. This grip is used in carrying large objects without handles. The grip used for work activity depends on the objects to be manipulated and the demands of a particular task. Some tasks allow for gripping in only one way. An example of this limitation is holding a hammer, which requires a power grip. The amount of force necessary to hold the hammer depends on hand strength and size, the density of the material being hammered, and the speed used in the activity. Holding the nail would require a precision grip, and force would be related directly to the size of the nail and the position of the hand in relation to the body. Pounding a nail into something that is well above shoulder height generally would require more forceful exertion in gripping the nail. The tendons that connect the finger to muscle in the forearm pass through the carpal tunnel of the wrist. If the wrist is bent, grip strength is lost (see Chapter 11 for further discussion).

Gloves also influence the amount of power available. Gloves without seams between the fingers interfere the least with grip force. Thick gloves with seams can reduce grip strength by 40%. If barehanded grip strength is rated as 100% of available power, wearing rubber gloves reduces strength by 25%, and heat-resistant gloves reduce strength by approximately 40% (Rodgers, 1988).

It is important to remember that the greater the force required for a grip, the shorter the period of time a grip can be maintained. Recovery time, or the time required for muscles to be able to perform at maximum, also increases with the grip force required for an activity (Rodgers, 1988).

Certain questions should be asked when evaluating grip force.

- Is the task necessary?
- Are objects as light as possible?
- Can supports be added to reduce the force required?
- Is the body in the best position for the activity?
- Can the activity be performed with the wrist in neutral?
- Are there available tools that would reduce the amount of force required?

The amount of force a person must exert depends on body position. Workplaces should be designed to allow for maximum flexibility in moving the body into positions best suited to the individual. Objects to be gripped should be clean and free of grease or oil. Slippery surfaces require greater force to grip. If gloves are used for work activities, they should fit properly and allow for optimal grip. Tools should fit the hand of the user. Mechanical devices for holding, stabilizing, or assisting with activity will decrease the force required and will reduce fatigue.

Vibration

The body's response to the ergonomic factor of vibration will vary with frequency and duration of time spent on the task. Vibration may cause tissue and nerve damage and can cause small blood vessels to close. Vibration makes muscles contract, thereby adding to fatigue. The use of certain hand tools, machinery, and equipment may cause muscles to tire as they absorb vibration. Also, vibrating tools require a tighter grasp.

Certain questions must be asked when assessing vibration.

- Is the task necessary?
- Have tools been properly maintained?
- Are new tools available that are designed to reduce shock and vibration?
- Can the tool be mounted in a fixture that will absorb the shock or vibration?
- Can the tool be counterbalanced to help reduce the force required?
- Can the worker assume a position for maximum benefit?
- Can the tool be used (or the activity performed) with the wrist in a neutral position and the arms close to the body?
- Can the tool or work area be modified to fit the worker?
- Can the work area be isolated from vibration?

Hand tools are common sources of vibration in the workplace. As new tools are designed to reduce or eliminate vibration, replacements should be considered. Although padded handles and shock-absorbing gloves may reduce vibration, they may require a person to use greater force in gripping. There is a natural tendency to grip vibrating tools harder, so hand tools should not be in awkward, end-range positions because the effects of vibration will increase (see Chapter 10 for further discussion about vibration).

Environment

The final biomechanical factor to be considered is the environment. The human body works best with certain temperature ranges, generally between 65° and 75° F (Battié et al., 1989). More specifically, the optimal temperature for mental work is 70° F, with 65° F being the most comfortable for physically active people. Sedentary workers will be most comfortable at approximately 72° F (Pheasant, 1992).

When combined with heavy physical work and high humidity, high temperatures can cause increased fatigue, dehydration, abnormal cardiac function, and even collapse. Perspiration can make the hands slippery, requiring added exertion to maintain grip on tools and equipment. Cold can cause joints to stiffen because of reduced blood supply. This condition may decrease productivity and can cause hypothermia if workers are inactive. Wearing gloves for protection from cold will increase the force necessary to grip. Extra or bulky clothing may increase fatigue.

The following questions should be asked when evaluating environmental conditions.

- Is the task necessary?
- Can drafts be controlled?
- Can cooling fans be added?
- Can warm or cool air be supplied?
- Is heat adequate?
- Can areas be fully or partially enclosed?

Certain materials, such as steel, transfer heat and cold faster than do wood or rubber. Tool handles should be covered or wrapped to prevent exposure. For the safety of the workers, production schedules may have to be altered during periods of extreme heat or cold. Increased rest periods may offer a measure of safety by reducing fatigue. The effects of the environment may be reduced by work schedule changes that allow for the most physically demanding work to be done at the most optimal time.

PSYCHOSOCIAL ASPECTS OF ERGONOMIC JOB ANALYSIS

Information regarding employee turnover, job satisfaction, or labor action may be valuable in identifying psychosocial stress (Ellexson, 1995). These psychosocial factors can be assessed by looking at the degree of control the worker has at a particular job site. The following questions may be asked relative to psychosocial influences on the work.

- Does the worker control the pace of the work?
- Does the worker have variety in his or her job?
- Does the worker have a positive relationship with his or her boss and co-workers?
- Does the employee give input as to the workings of the job?
- How are productivity standards determined?
- Does the worker have incentives to work faster or harder?
- Can the worker take a bathroom break at will?
- Can workers ask for and receive assistance when needed?
- Are workers able to set up their work station as they want?

Answers to these questions, and others, will often provide information regarding the flexibility and related control one has at work and the degree to which recommendations may be implemented (see Chapter 8 for further discussion).

CONCLUSION

Job analysis must identify the essential tasks and describe in detail the work to be accomplished, the physical requirements of the worker, and the work site measurements. Job analysis can identify those tasks that are of greatest risk by identifying force, postures, and repetitions. It can lead to the development of alternative methods of activity to lower risk of injury and increase productivity. Job analysis is a requirement in identifying which worker is best suited for a job and for making any reasonable accommodation necessary when employing individuals with disabilities.

Job analysis will identify which skills and functions require training through formal education or on-the-job activity. Similarly, job analysis assists in the development of rehabilitation programs, which incorporate work simulation practice. Through observation, demonstration, participation, documentation, and analysis, a clear and complete picture of a specific job can be developed.

REFERENCES

Battié, M. C., Bigos, S. J., Fisher, L. D., Hansson, T. H., Jones, M. E., & Wortley, M. D. (1989). Isometric lifting strength as a predictor of industrial back pain reports. *Spine, 14*(8), 851-856.

Brough. (1991). *Evaluating your workplace.* Washington DC: Brough & Associates.

Ellexson, M.T. (1995). *Job analysis and ergonomic assessment: A continuing education manual.* Memphis, TN: Physiotherapy Associates.

Ellexson, M.T. (1997). Job analysis and work-site assessment. In M. J. Sanders (Ed.), *Management of cumulative trauma disorders.* Boston, MA: Butterworth-Heinemann, 195-213.

Ellexson, M.T. (2000). Job analysis. In B. L. Kornblau & K. Jacobs (Eds.), *Work principles and practice* (Lesson 5). Bethesda, MD: American Occupational Therapy Association.

Elmfeldt, G., Wise, C., Bergsten, H., & Alsson, A. (1983). *Adapting work sites for people with disabilities: Ideas from Sweden.* Sweden: The Swedish Institute for the Handicapped.

Federal Register (July 26, 1991). Part V: Equal Employment Opportunity Commission 29 CFR part 1630, *Equal Employment Opportunity for Individuals with Disabilities,* Final Rule (p. 35736).

Kirkland, M., & Robertson, S. C. (1985). The evolution of work-related theory in occupational therapy. In M. Kirkland & S. C. Robertson (Eds.), *PIVOT: Planning and implementing vocational readiness in occupational therapy*. Rockville, MD: American Occupational Therapy Association.

Kornblau, B. L., & Ellexson, M.T. (1991). Hiring employees under the Disability Act. *Risk Management, 38,* 46-51.

Larson, B.A. & Ellexson, M.T, (2000). Blue print for ergonomics. *Work, 15*(2), 107-112.

Pheasant, S. (1986). *Body space: Anthropometrics, ergonomics and design.* London: Taylor & Francis.

Pheasant, S. (1992). *Ergonomics, work and health.* Rockville, MD: Aspen.

Roberts, S. L., & Falkenberg, S.A. (1992). *Biomechanics: Problem solving for functional activity.* St. Louis: Mosby.

Rodgers, S. H. (1988). Matching workers and work site ergonomic principles in work injury—management and prevention. In S. J. Isernhagen (Ed.), *Work injury management and prevention.* Rockville, MD: Aspen.

Rodgers, S. H. (1992). A functional job analysis technique. In J. S. Moore & A. G. Garg (Eds.), *State of the art reviews, occupational medicine, ergonomics: Low back pain, carpal tunnel syndrome, and upper extremity disorders in the workplace*. Philadelphia, PA: Hanley & Belfus, Inc.

APPENDIX 13-1

Work Activity Analysis

COMPANY: Boing & Boing Inc.
March 20, 2000
2121 West Nile Boulevard
Hartman, Kentucky
POSITION: Spring Grinder

The essential functions of this position were determined to be as follows:

1. Place springs for grinding and tend machine
2. Test for specifications
3. Place and move bins

Essential Function Analysis:

1. Place Springs for Grinding and Tend Machine:

The spring grinding machines are set to grind springs of varying sizes. Three sizes of springs, ranging from very small to the largest size spring manufactured at this facility, were observed in the grinding process. Springs may vary in size and in the gauge of the wire used to produce the spring. The operation for all grinding is basically the same. The operator sits on a high stool or stands, depending on preference and fit with the particular grinding machine. The operator sits or stands on a platform that averages 9 in to 13 in from the floor. The working surface of the machines averages 33 in to 36 in from the platform. The worker sits or stands at the center of the turntable and works with approximately 90 degrees of the turntable at one time. Springs come down a gravity-fed center funnel, and the worker may palm several springs and then use a three-point pinch and place them into holes in the "knock out blocks" set in the turntable. Pinch grip varies from approximately ¼ in to 3 in, depending on the size of the springs. The heaviest spring observed weighed approximately 6 ounces. The springs slowly move from right to left into the grinder and are expelled from the grinder and fall into large square bins on wheels. The bins measure 33 in × 33 in × 33 in and require 50 lb of forward push to move when three-fourths full of medium-size springs. The operator must make minor adjustments to controls located under the turntable at an average height of 24 in to 30 in above the platform. Occasionally, the operator must adjust machine parts to the right or left of the center operating area and remove "clinkers" and debris. The turntables move at various speeds from 30 degrees per 15 seconds for larger springs to 30 degrees per minute for smaller springs. Small springs are placed on average at a rate of 30 in each knock out block every 20 seconds, medium springs are placed on average at a rate of 24 in each knock out block every 20 seconds, and the larger springs are placed on average at a rate of 1 every 5 seconds with 3 in each knock out block. Occasionally, the worker removes the knock out blocks using a piece of wire to pry up one end, wipes them off, and replaces them.

Physical Requirements:

Climbing: to step up onto the platform
Sitting: to operate machine
Standing: to operate machine
Handling: knock out blocks, parts, springs
Fingering: springs

Seeing: holes in knock out blocks, machine operations, work orders
Bending: to reach machine parts for adjustment, to reach controls
Twisting: to reach machine parts
Reaching: to place springs, to reach machine parts and controls

Measurements:

Walking distance: 10 in
Climbing: 9 in to 13 in
Small springs: (approximate size range in inches) $\frac{1}{4}$ to $\frac{1}{2} \times \frac{1}{2}$ to 1
Medium springs: (approximate size range in inches) $\frac{1}{2}$ to $1\frac{1}{2} \times 2\frac{1}{2}$ to 4
Large springs: (approximate size range in inches) $2\frac{1}{2}$ to 3 to $4\frac{1}{2}$
Knock out blocks: range in size from 6 in × 10 in to 10 in × 13 in; there is one block approximately every 6 in
Controls: located 24 in to 30 in from the platform
Platforms: 9 in to 13 in from the floor
Work surface height (turntable): 33 in to 36 in from the platform
Turntables: move at an average rate of between 30 degrees per 15 seconds to 30 degrees per minute for those observed
Reach: to place springs 9 in to 15 in; to adjust machines and remove debris is 9 in to 36 in

2. Testing:

The worker tests five springs per hour on computerized equipment located throughout the work area. The spring grinder operator stands in front of the machine and sets a spring in place at a height of 48 in from the floor.

Two buttons, left and right, located at 52 in from the floor, are pushed to compress the spring and take measurements. The worker takes readings from an 8-in screen. The top edge of the screen is 58 in from the floor and the bottom edge is 50 in from the floor. Occasionally, a worker may be required to test more springs at one time. The number usually does not exceed 30.

Physical Requirements:

Walking: 10 feet to 15 feet from spring grinder to computer station
Standing: to test springs
Handling: to place and remove springs
Reaching: to place springs and operate controls
Seeing: to observe measurements, to inspect the springs

Measurements:

Computer station work surface: 48 in from the floor
Computer screen: 50 in to 58 in from the floor
Control button: 52 in from the floor

3. Place and Move Bins:

The worker must place square bins measuring 33 in × 33 in × 33 in using either a hand forklift or a forklift truck. The bins are on casters. The empty bins are brought to the area and must be pushed into place at the spring grinding machine to catch the springs as they come out of the machine. The operator pushes the bins into the proper position using an average push force of 50 lb. When the bins are full, they are removed to a holding area using the same forklift equipment. Travel distance to obtain empty bins and store full bins does not exceed 25 feet on average. Frequency for placing and removing bins depends on the size of the springs, but usually occurs every 4 hours. Workers report this occurs less than one time per hour on average.

Physical Requirements:

Walking: to obtain and remove bins
Handling: to move bins and operate forklift equipment
Pushing: to place the bins
Seeing: to determine placement of bins and appropriate area for storage

Measurements:

Bins:	33 in × 33 in × 33 in; average of 50 lb force to push
Walking distance:	does not exceed 25 feet on average

Frequency:

Small springs:	placed at an average rate of 30 per 20 seconds
Medium springs:	placed at an average rate of 24 per 20 seconds
Large springs:	placed at an average rate of 3 per 15 seconds

There are breaks every 3 to 5 minutes to adjust the machine, wait for the grinder to process the springs, and check the springs as they come out of the machine.

Time Spent:

This job works 8 hours with one 15-minute break and one 20-minute lunch and a 5-minute clean-up at the end of shift as designated by labor union agreement.

Skills or Specialization:

The spring grinder position requires on-the-job training; however, experienced workers are employed whenever possible.

Physiologic Considerations:

There is little static positioning with ample opportunity to change position.

Workers are able to take bathroom breaks as needed.

There is no overhead work.

Environmental Considerations:

The environment is free of clutter.

There are no significant fumes or odors.

Hearing protection, safety goggles, and hard hats are provided.

Heat-resistant gloves coated with a nonslip material are provided.

Cognitive Considerations:

Workers must be able to read work orders and process control plans.

Workers must be able to recognize measurements.

Workers must solve problems and implement solutions to adjust equipment.

Workers must be able to communicate with co-workers and supervisors regarding problems, work to be completed, and the need for tools, parts, and equipment.

Comments:

This job does require repeated activity; however, there is adequate recovery time to significantly decrease any risk from repetition. The workers move from one grinder to another, providing for change in required pinch grip. There is adequate lighting and work space. The push/pull requirements are within accepted NIOSH guidelines. There is no lifting required for this operation. There are acceptable rest breaks and frequent opportunities to change position. There are no static postures or awkward postures required and workers are given the option to sit or stand to operate the spring grinder. Twisting and/or bending was observed occasionally and could be controlled by proper positioning.

Job Analysis Completed: 4/10/03

Melanie T. Ellexson MBA, OTR/L, FAOTA

________________ Date: ________________

R. Band

Plant Manager

Boing & Boing Inc.

________________ Date: ________________

CHAPTER 14

Reducing Injuries, Claims, and Costs

Donald Clark

INTRODUCTION

This chapter directs attention to practical strategies designed to minimize or eliminate predisposing factors that can cause or aggravate work-related musculoskeletal disorders (MSDs). Attention is also directed toward optimum management of employee injuries in order to facilitate expedient recovery, high morale, and return to work. The first goal of this chapter is to provide the reader with practical recommendations to prevent gradual onset of musculoskeletal injuries. Second, employers will appreciate bottom-line savings achieved through effective handling of injury claims. Six real-world case histories will serve to acquaint the reader with both the obvious and subtle complexities that characterize the phenomenon known commonly as ergonomic injuries. Included are work demands requiring sustained sitting or standing, repetitive use of the arms and hands, material handling, and special physical tasks experienced by health care providers, particularly those who must routinely provide physical assistance to patients.

The primary biomechanical risk factors implicated in the genesis of work-related musculoskeletal disorders (MSDs) are *repetition*, *force*, *awkward posture*, *vibration*, and *contact stress* (see Chapter 10 for a complete discussion). The forthcoming discussions will demonstrate that successful prevention strategies arise from a broader appreciation of additional psychosocial factors impacting workers' compensation claims. Such elements include organizational supervision and job design, inadequate rest, poor fitness and physical conditioning, mental and emotional stress, age, sex, health history, lifestyle activities away from work, and poor morale on the job. A holistic prevention plan necessarily includes a comprehensive consideration of all the heretofore noted physical, psychophysical, and attitudinal dimensions that juxtapose to produce injuries and claims.

Let us first consider important aspects of the injury response and management process within the workers' compensation system. It is essential to achieve an understanding of both management and employee perspective regarding work-related injuries.

ISSUES IN DETERMINING AND MANAGING WORK-RELATED INJURIES

Determining Whether a Claim Is the Result of a Work-Related Injury

An assembly worker walks hurriedly, unaware of a recent oil leak; the slip and fall result in a fractured ankle requiring surgical treatment and immobilization. Another employee comes forward with a chemical burn incurred on the job while mixing solutions. A computer programmer presents with gradual-onset neck pain and numbness in the fingers. The fracture and chemical injury were obvious traumatic incidents that occurred during the course of work. There can be no question in the supervisor's mind that these injuries were job related and compensable. In the case of the worker complaining of finger numbness, the employer is not certain that this problem was caused by work demands.

Many types of musculoskeletal injuries can and do arise during the course of work. Obvious, irrefutable claims include slips and falls, burns, lacerations, and objects in the eyes, to name a few. The insidious, work-related injuries such as muscle aches, tendinitis, numbness, and vague strains, however, are difficult to verify, since there is only *invisible* damage that doesn't produce the basic signs and symptoms of injury. The worker's subjective complaints of pain and inability to function normally are the basis of the documentation. Determination of cause and mechanism of injury may require a comprehensive investigative effort involving the injured worker, medical provider, supervisor, safety official, and workers' compensation insurance specialist. A growing number of such claims have become compensable, with a concomitant increase in attention and research directed to this important modern-day problem.

The Worker's and Supervisor's Perceptions of a Job-Related Injury

An employee who sustains a laceration or burn during the customary course of duty will view such an injury as a simple cause-and-effect incident wherein fault lies solely with the worker, the employer, or some combination of both. For the worker who develops tendinitis or nerve damage over a long period, perceptions of cause and responsibility become more complex among a greater number of involved people (i.e., supervisor, co-workers, medical provider, workers' compensation insurer, and attorney).

To illustrate, we can draw some similarities and distinctions between a typical worker (sometimes termed an *industrial athlete)* and a professional athlete. Although both the competitive athlete and the worker use physical abilities to undertake a sport or paid job, their psychosocial experiences surrounding the injury differ greatly. Consider a worker who presents with rather nondescript pain and numbness in the upper limbs and an athlete who severely sprains an ankle. Both are carrying out specified activities under the direction of either a coach or a supervisor. In the case of the athlete, the injury was witnessed by all, thus establishing legitimacy. The victim takes on all the empathy, support, and care deserving of a wounded, highly regarded member of the team. The player rests in confidence that the coach, medical provider, and coplayers will direct extraordinary efforts to encourage and resolve the incident until full restoration to the team is achieved. Throughout the entire course of events, the injured athlete receives the strong message, "I am a valuable and essential part of the team. My absence is a loss, and everyone wants me back on the job (field) as soon as possible."

Contrast this scenario with that of the assembly worker and the telecommunications operator who report neck and shoulder pain with finger numbness. Because the demands of their jobs require constant sitting and repetitive use of the hands, it is their belief that symptoms were caused by excessive demands of work. These so-called industrial athletes suffer pain and debility just as real and significant as that of the injured competitive athlete.

Instead of receiving validation, these workers may get the clear message from their supervisor and co-workers that their ailments are not real injuries but, rather, that they are either falsifying or magnifying their problem to access workers' compensation. In the face of critical suspicion, the suffering employees approach the supervisor (coach) and sense the disbelief and suspicion. Humbly, the workers quietly slip back to their assignments. Even they are unsure of themselves; after all, their co-workers do not seem to be having any problem.

This situation may play itself out until symptoms and frustration escalate to the point at which medical intervention becomes necessary. The medical examination is essentially negative; there are no remarkable objective findings, and the doctor provides the usual medications and tells the workers to return to the job and "take it easy." In the workers' eyes, this is a rather cursory response that results in additional erosion of self-worth. Ultimately, the workers have become angry with their supervisor and unsatisfied with medical attention and the prevailing lack of regard for their plight. It is not uncommon for individuals in this state of mind to seek legal counsel in anticipation of an adversarial response to their call for an appropriate response to their injuries. Enmity has been established between these workers and their employer.

These illustrations readily underscore important considerations that the employer must become aware of when dealing with MSDs. Slow-onset musculoskeletal ailments do not reveal obvious signs and symptoms, as in the case of an injured competitive athlete. It is vitally important for supervisors to become aware of both the physical and the psychosocial impact of gradual-onset MSDs that usually originate as chronic fatigue and intermittent discomfort.

The foregoing illustration brings to light the significance of injury claims policies and procedures. The injured worker who is not properly acknowledged and respectfully treated will likely become frustrated in an atmosphere of suspicion and poor injury-management practice. Unlike the competitive athlete whose injury is comparatively heroic, the industrial athlete may suffer alone without the open support and assistance necessary to promote a positive attitude and successful resolution. Critical and judgmental behavior on the part of managers and supervisors will most assuredly drive many injured workers to their attorneys. Adversarial relationships are created thus leading to excessive workers' compensation costs and damaged lives.

Relationship of Costs to Injury Severity

An on-the-job injury may or may not produce a workers' compensation claim. Principle costs of a claim arise from time out of work, medical expenses, and insurance indemnity payments. Additional costs to the employer include all indirect expenses, such as overtime for other workers to cover the injured employee, cross-training, hiring temporary replacements, and so forth. Additional expenses increase when litigation enters the picture. The direct cost of a properly handled claim for a simple nonsurgical elbow tendinitis may be as little as $150 to $300 for medical treatment, medication, and only several hours of lost time. A mismanaged, adversarial claim for the same diagnosis may result in more than $100,000 of direct and indirect expenses if medical treatment is unsuccessful and significant disability results (see Chapters 4 and 17 for a complete discussion).

Thus far, we have demonstrated an important link between injury management policies, the worker's perception of injury, the prevailing attitude of the employer and costs. Those who wish to enlarge their understanding and to uncover cost-saving strategies must give consideration to the foregoing medical, social, and legal influences on costs. Injuries, claims, and costs are separate but related entities. Employers who endeavor to maximize productivity, prevent injuries, and promote good relations must treat each of these segments uniquely to establish successful safety and injury prevention programs.

NATIONAL STRATEGIES FOR ERGONOMICS AND INJURY PREVENTION PROGRAMS

With the rise in the incidence of MSDs, increasing attention has been directed to workplace factors that can contribute to or cause such injuries. At the forefront of ergonomic research and problem-solving strategies is the Occupational Safety and Health Administration

(OSHA), which continues to pursue development of a nationwide ergonomics program. The newest voluntary guidelines are a valuable resource to industry. The National Institute of Occupational Safety and Health (NIOSH), which functions as the research arm of OSHA, has contributed substantially to our understanding of ergonomics as it applies to workplace safety.

NIOSH has proposed definitions of the terms *ergonomic hazards* and *ergonomic disorders. Ergonomic hazards* relative to work-related MSDs refer to physical stressors and workplace conditions that pose a risk of injury or illness to the musculoskeletal system of the worker. Ergonomic hazards include repetitive and forceful motions, vibration, temperature extremes, and awkward postures that arise from poorly designed workstations, tools and equipment, and improper work methods. The effects of ergonomic hazards may be amplified by extreme environmental conditions. In addition, ergonomic hazards may arise from poor job design and faulty organizational factors, such as excessive work hours, external pacing of work, shiftwork, imbalanced work-to-rest ratios, demanding incentive pay or work standards, restriction of operator body movement and confinement of the worker to a workstation without adequate relief periods, electronic monitoring, and lack of task variety. The term *ergonomic disorders* has fallen into disfavor and now is being replaced by the concept embodied in the phrase *work-related musculoskeletal disorders.* Such disorders are those diseases and injuries that affect the musculoskeletal, peripheral nervous, and neurovascular systems and are caused or aggravated by occupational exposure to ergonomic hazards.

In light of the foregoing definitions, consider the implications in the case of a meat cutter who complains of wrist pain and abnormal sensation in the fingers. According to the NIOSH definitions, this worker has sustained a work-related musculoskeletal injury because an ergonomic hazard exists. In this case, the primary hazards are highly repetitive motions, excessive force, and awkward posturing of the upper limb, particularly the wrist and fingers. This model would direct us to an *ergonomic solution*—that is, some type of engineering remedy that reduces or eliminates known hazards. The elements of force and awkward positioning of the upper limb are addressed through redesign of cutting tools that will permit the operator to work with the wrist closer to neutral position or midposition. Such tool modification also provides for better leverage of the entire upper limb, thereby reducing average force. This relatively simple sequence, wherein an ergonomic (engineering) fix has resulted in an ergonomic solution, partially fulfills the definition of ergonomics by adjusting work to fit the capabilities of the worker.

Despite such engineering interventions intended to reduce risk factors, workers may still incur progressive stress and fatigue as a result of other factors, such as habitual work style, poor work-to-rest ratios, piecework, and excessive work hours. Commonly, individuals will suffer persistent musculoskeletal ailments caused by intrinsic health problems, poor fitness, psychosocial stress, and habitually strenuous posture and body mechanics. The forthcoming discussions stress the importance of ergonomic corrective strategies that complement engineering solutions by attending human performance and psychosocial factors fully.

OSHA activities that have contributed to our understanding and approach to work-related musculoskeletal injuries include the Occupational Safety and Health Act of 1970, mandating that it is the general duty of all employers to provide a workplace free from recognized serious hazards, including the prevention and control of ergonomic hazards. In January 1989 OSHA published voluntary *General Safety and Health Program Management Guidelines*, which are recommended to all employers as a foundation for their safety and health programs and as a framework for their ergonomics programs. Later, OSHA developed *Ergonomic Program Management Guidelines for Meatpacking*

Plants (August 1990). These voluntary guidelines marked the beginning of a nationwide effort by OSHA to help reduce or eliminate worker exposure to ergonomic hazards that lead to MSDs and related illnesses and injuries. The suggested program included a coordinated effort involving enforcement, information, training, cooperative programs, and research. The reader is directed to *www.osha.gov* for more detailed information about OSHA's early ergonomic guidelines.

OSHA established a new Ergonomics Program Standard *(Federal Register*, New Subpart W of 29 CFR Part 1910 is added to read as follows: Subpart W-Program Standards, 1910.900, Ergonomics Program Standard) that became effective on January 16, 2001, and was nullified on March 20, 2001, through a joint resolution of Congress. On March 22, Senator Breaux (D-LA) introduced legislation requiring OSHA to issue a new ergonomics rule within 2 years. Although the Congressional Review Act that gave Congress the authority for the joint resolution of disapproval does not permit reissue in substantially the same form, it does not forbid reissue as guidelines or other form or rulemaking.

A substantial body of scientific and empirical evidence supports the efficacy of ergonomics programs. In 1998, the National Research Council/National Academy of Sciences found a clear relationship between MSDs and work and between ergonomic interventions and a decrease in the number and severity of such disorders. According to the Academy, "Research clearly demonstrates that specific interventions can reduce the reported rate of musculoskeletal disorders for workers who perform high-risk tasks" (National Academy Press, 1998).

Although the OSHA Ergonomics Standard is withdrawn in its present form, certain key components of this program are critically essential to the organization and implementation of successful ergonomics programs. The cornerstones of OSHA's most recent initiative are essentially the same as those put forth in the original *Meatpacking Guidelines,* noted earlier: namely, management leadership, employee participation, management of MSDs, job hazard analysis, hazard reduction and control, and training. These are the six building blocks of an ergonomics program focused on eliminating work-related musculoskeletal injuries.

For our purpose, we will establish a firm foundation for injury prevention through applications of *Engineering, Administrative,* and *Work Practice* Controls, as defined in the New Ergonomics Standard noted previously *(Federal Register,* 11/14/00, Vol. 65, No. 220).

Administrative Controls

The word *administer* can be defined as to manage, have charge of, or to bring into use. An *administrator* refers to a person who manages affairs of any kind. In the context of ergonomics, administrative controls are changes in the way that work in a job is assigned or scheduled that reduce the magnitude, frequency, or duration of exposure to ergonomic risk factors. Examples of administrative controls for MSD hazards include employee rotation, job task enlargement, alternative tasks, and alteration of work pace. Administrative policies and strategies can be a powerful deterrent to work-related injuries.

One may enlarge the concept of administrative controls to include the following categories of consideration.

- Sociopolitical atmosphere and employee morale
- New employee orientation and training
- Injury reporting and the accident investigation process
- Early return to work and modified duty
- Productivity standards and paced work

Sociopolitical Atmosphere and Employee Morale

Prevailing employee attitudes and morale derive primarily from human relations policies and the example set by leaders. Managers, supervisors, and others in authority must set a good role model for fair and equitable leadership to promote employee loyalty and enthusiasm. With regard to the management of MSDs, the company's general policy should be objective and indiscriminate. Workers with early signs and symptoms of slow-onset musculoskeletal ailments should be encouraged to avoid delays in reporting such problems to management. If employees perceive that their supervisors regard such maladies as griping and complaining, injured workers will be reluctant to come forth early, when symptoms first appear. Prolonged silence paves the way for ongoing discomfort culminating in more serious injury. Such mismanaged injury claims may produce excessive costs to the company and hardship to the injured worker in the long term.

Management can take the following practical steps to establish optimal attitudes and a positive culture of injury prevention among the workforce.

- Establish uniform policies and procedures for the management of MSDs. This procedure connotes management's position that such conditions deserve the same attention as the more obvious traumatic injuries exhibiting overt symptoms.
- Educate management-level personnel about work-related MSDs, thereby instilling an appreciation for the broad implications of this significant industrial health and safety issue.
- Educate the employee about MSDs, early signs and symptoms, risk factors (at work and home), individual responsibility for health and safety, and reporting procedures.
- Include employees in problem solving, policy making, and the development of action plans.

These recommendations are only a few of the many initiatives a company can develop to improve morale and the general positive social atmosphere. Management attitude and leadership style are among the most important determinants of a successful injury abatement program.

New-Employee Conditioning and Training

In the context of our characterization of the worker as an industrial athlete, employees who engage in physically demanding jobs will be at less risk for injury if provision is made for physical and procedural adaptation to the task. Just as a competitive athlete must become trained, conditioned, and skilled at a particular sport, the new employee should gradually adjust to new demands physically, procedurally, and psychosocially (APTA, 1991; Goidi, 1964; Thompson, Plewes, & Shaw, 1951; Wilson & Wilson, 1957). Even veteran workers who are transferred to another job assignment should be given an appropriate transition period in which to make adjustment. These new employees or those with significant changes in work assignments should be given the opportunity to observe, learn, and practice new skills through a progressive adjustment process.

It is important to understand that *physically demanding* does not simply apply to such hard labor as heavy manual work. Jobs that demand constant sitting to perform highly focused, repetitive tasks can and do produce significant human effort, fatigue, and injury. More physical stress and less economy of motion occurs during early adaptation to new tasks. As the worker becomes more proficient, skill increases, as does higher productivity via more economical technique. These factors justify establishing a new-employee conditioning or break-in period, which should occur over two or more weeks, depending on an individual's learning curve and physical tolerance. Close monitoring should ensure that acceptable adjustment and performance is being achieved. Also, policies and procedures should exist to evaluate, monitor, and administrate the process by which this transition period is being managed. Further, provision for employee feedback is essential.

Injury Reporting and the Accident Investigation Process

Timely reporting of an incident, accompanied by a full explanation of cause, is a critical component of injury prevention and cost-saving strategy. Such obvious traumatic injuries as contusions, lacerations, burns, and the like routinely are reported immediately. The follow-up investigation usually reveals a straightforward cause that can be remedied easily. Uncovering the causes of cumulative trauma-based musculoskeletal injuries is not as exact and becomes subject to diverse opinion. The OSHA Illness and Injury log can be a starting point for understanding the root causes of the incident.

The term *mechanism of injury* is important in exposing the fundamental cause of acute and insidious injuries. In the case of a simple laceration, the injured worker will report that the cut resulted from a slip while using a hand knife to open cardboard boxes. The investigation of this incident reveals that the individual was not following proper procedures (i.e., wearing a protective glove on the hand receiving the injury). In this case, the mechanism of injury is straightforward and obvious to all. In another claim, an employee comes forward reporting gradual-onset pain in the left thumb. As a product "picker," this worker continuously holds a standard clipboard in the left hand and a marking pen in the right hand. The clipboard serves a dual purpose: to hold the invoices and as a platform on which multiple small products are carried. On initial reporting of this problem, the supervisor may logically ask when the injury occurred (anticipating a single incident with a date of occurrence). The employee is uncertain of how or when the injury was born but feels the problem is work related. The worker is also seeking the satisfaction of a single, explainable cause that can account for the symptoms. In this case, the mechanism of injury—the exact series of events that contributed to this problem—is unclear to both the investigator and the claimant, because neither of them have the knowledge to ask the types of questions that will yield a reasonable explanation of how this injury developed over time.

By conducting an injury review process (IRP), an investigative group can effectively identify multiple factors giving rise to cumulative wear and tear, producing damage to neuromusculoskeletal structures. The IRP becomes most effective when participants include the injured employee, the supervisor, and a health professional knowledgeable in ergonomics and MSDs. In the previously mentioned case of the thumb injury, medical evaluation produced a diagnosis of de Quervain's tendinitis. A basic understanding of this diagnosis, its pathology, and the mechanism of injury will be invaluable to the injury review group as it details the events leading to this injury. A careful historical account will acknowledge the importance of such factors as size, weight, and configuration of the clipboard; how the worker must grasp the board; the length of time the board is held without a pause; duration of rest periods; how much weight is placed on the board; in what position the clipboard is held most of the time; and pressure points against parts of the hand. These factors are some of the important issues that play a contributory role in fatigue and progressive damage. Such an in-depth examination provides the IRP members with the necessary data to establish fundamental cause. The knowledge accumulated by this process generates recommendations for corrective actions and other injury prevention measures.

At first glance, an injured employee may be apprehensive about sitting down with the supervisor, the company health provider, a safety committee designate, and possibly a workers' compensation loss control consultant. The group facilitator should take careful steps to inform the injured worker that the purpose of the IRP is not intended to be individually punitive or judgmental. The essential function of this meeting is twofold: to apply an objective systems approach to uncover the fundamental cause of a reported injury and to implement corrective actions to prevent reoccurrence of such injuries.

Properly administered, the IRP is a powerful problem-solving tool that yields benefits beyond its primary directive. The process of inquiry, interpretation, and resolution is enhanced greatly when multiple contributors provide increased understanding and clarification. It is not uncommon to discover that successful problem solving in one area transfers value to other applications. In the case of the de Quervain's tendinitis, much more attention will be directed to other operations and manual tasks that may pose a risk for injury to wrists and fingers.

Important features and outcomes of the IRP include the following.

- A positive, fact-finding, nonpunitive process. This meeting is not the appropriate occasion for reprimands associated with noncompliance with safety rules.
- An analysis of injury causes and corrective strategies.
- Valuable information and understanding through a formal group process.
- A powerful tool in reducing frequency and severity of injuries, thus lowering workers' compensation costs.
- Establishment of company's commitment to safety and injury prevention.
- Increased company wide safety awareness and participation.
- Strengthened communication throughout the ranks of management and workers.
- Increased accountability for safety and follow-up action.
- Reduced instances of malingering and fraudulent claims.
- A valuable educational and brainstorming opportunity.

Relevant to this discussion is *lag time,* the time between the onset of injury and notification of the workers' compensation claims representative. Ideally, a *first report of injury* reaches the company personnel office immediately following the incident. This report should be transmitted to the insurance claims representative on the very same day. Such timely communication establishes the best opportunity for obtaining accurate information concerning all circumstances surrounding the incident, for understanding the nature of the injury, and for a resolution satisfactory to both the injured employee and the employer. The longer the lag time, the more cost is incurred by both the employer and insurer. Lag time tends to be much shorter for traumatic types of injuries, whereas many workers tend to put off their complaints of gradually progressing aches and pains. Common consequences of excessive lag time are:

- Increased errors, omissions, and inaccuracy.
- Impaired effectiveness of accident investigation process.
- Erosion in employee's motivation to return to work or engage in modified duty.
- Degeneration of trust and good will between management and worker.
- Increased medical costs secondary to late intervention and subsequent reduced effectiveness of treatment.
- Increased tendency for fraud and litigation.
- Increased potential for additional claims from other workers exposed to similar hazards.

It is vitally important that management provide for the early recognition, investigation, and treatment of MSDs. Employees should be encouraged to come forth as soon as significant symptoms become apparent. This policy may initially lead to a higher than normal volume of reporting. Management should not fear this because early intervention has proven to yield positive cost-saving outcomes.

Early Return to Work and Modified Duty

Considering the costly consequences of poor injury claims handling and excessive lag time, it is to everyone's advantage to bring the injured worker back into appropriate employment as soon as possible. Not uncommonly, absence from work of three or more weeks significantly reduces the chances that an injured worker will successfully return to the workforce. Employers who have committed themselves to a comprehensive injury prevention and management program will discover the value of a strong modified duty opportunity for their injured employees.

The designation *light duty* often carries a negative connotation, as it may stereotype certain workers as lazy and malingering. This connotation has given way to the more objective expressions, *modified* (or *alternative) duty*, which do not carry implicit judgmental inference. A well-thought-out modified duty program reflects a company's commitment to cost containment and workers' welfare.

A successful modified or restricted duty program will meet legitimate needs, (i.e., the alternative work is justifiable in everyone's eyes). Such special work assignments fill an important niche that will benefit both the company and injured worker. Ideally, the worker enters alternative duty with the understanding that this duty is essential to the employer. Moreover, the employee's continued presence on the job and participation with coworkers is vital to everyone's interest. Managers who hastily fabricate alternative duty assignments with the mindset of light duty are likely to set themselves up for resentment and poor morale from the workforce.

In summary, a productive program of modified duty will reflect the following guidelines.

- Duty assignments should meet a valid need, not senseless busywork.
- Alternative work tasks should be accompanied by written physical demand requirements.
- The injured worker's physical limitations and work capacity should be elucidated clearly and fully by proper medical authority.
- The modified duty assignment should be analyzed to assure that the demands of this job are within the stated restrictions of the worker.
- The designated manager or overseer of the modified duty should be trained fully to observe and monitor a worker's adjustment and tolerance to work tasks.
- Policies and procedures and the mission of the alternative duty program should be communicated to all staff, with emphasis directed to positive attitude and conduct toward injured workers on temporary assignment.
- The duration of the modified duty should be established via objective criteria that apply uniformly to anyone who should become a candidate.
- The employee's progress in this program should be documented carefully via systematic communication between the company, worker, insurer, health provider, and any other relevant parties.

The focus of this program is to maintain the employee in a productive capacity while facilitating progressive recovery. The entire process should be directed to restoration of unrestricted work performance that includes return to customary duty.

Productivity Standards and Paced Work

A worker's level of energy expenditure and physical effort is linked directly to such influences as the job's physical demands, incentives, and enforcement policy. Incentives include pay rate, bonuses, special recognition, gifts, benefits, and so forth. Enforcement may be executed through goal setting, performance appraisal, and other administrative controls. Establishing productivity standards and the supportive human output necessary to meet quotas necessitates a thorough understanding of human capacity, physically and psychosocially.

Consider the experience of running at race pace on a treadmill. Speed and rhythm are dictated by a mechanical standard outside human control and choice. If the accelerated pace continues, the runner (industrial athlete) surely will fatigue and eventually will fall off. This scenario is analogous to production workers who must maintain a preset standard for speed and units per hour of production, or those who work faster and harder to earn incentive pay. Not infrequently, workers who must perform highly repetitive tasks under external controls for speed are subjected to excessive physical demands, increasing risk for MSDs (Arndt, 1987).

WORK PRACTICE CONTROLS

Work practice controls are changes in the way an employee performs the physical work activities of a job such as postural improvement, proper body mechanics, pacing, timely rest stops, use of personal protective equipment, economizing of movements, getting assistance from others, and on-the-job stretching exercises. The design of a job and associated processes often dictate how the worker will physically orient themselves and define functional motions to carry out necessary tasks. These areas tend to be the responsibility of the employee once proper training and engineering controls have been put in place. On-the-job stretching can be an important preventative strategy; therefore, more discussion is provided.

On-the-Job Stretching Exercises

There is general agreement in the world of athletics that warm-up and stretching are advisable. Stretching is considered to be an injury prevention measure that should be included in every athlete's training program (Allers, 1989; Anderson, 1980; Hansford, Blood, Kent, & Lutz, 1968; Jacobsen & Sperling, 1976; Sawyer, 1987). Although evidence is lacking to demonstrate the absolute preventive value of stretching, when performed correctly, people have more to gain than lose from systematic stretching (Hess & Hecker, 2003; Amako, Oda, Masuoka, Yokoi & Campisi, 2003).

The theoretic basis for periodic stretching on the job lies with an understanding of the basic physiology of tissue nutrition and pathology of tissue injury. In short, working tissues require oxygen and nutrients if they are to remain healthy. When physical demands or other events result in diminution of blood supply to working structures, fatigue, inflammation, and destructive changes ensue. Some researchers have stated that tendinitis and carpal tunnel syndrome are not so much problems of repetitive motion, or friction wear, as they are a lack of tissue perfusion (Jacobsen & Sperling, 1976). In practical terms, is carpal tunnel syndrome derived from high repetition and friction-wear occurring within the carpal tunnel? Does another contribution possibly emanate from restriction of blood flow from more proximal regions, such as the cervicobrachial area, wherein vessels can be restricted by the scaleni muscles and other compressive elements in this forest of musculature? This so-called cervicobrachial explanation appears to have merit, particularly when one considers the anatomical positions of tissues and joints when the head is thrust forward, the scapulae are protracted, and the anterior trunk musculature is tight.

In light of these fundamental concepts of physiology, anatomy, and function, we can justify that blood supply and tissue perfusion can be enhanced through optimal postures and systematic stretching. Opinions vary widely on the recommended type and frequency of stretching.

Selection and prescription of on-the-job stretching exercises should take the following considerations into account.

- Exercises should target specific muscles and tendons that incur the most stress and wear during work activity.
- Consider what tissues are being stretched and the impact on associated joints.
- Proper exercise technique is essential to achieve desired goals.
- The primary purpose of stretching is to increase blood flow and tissue perfusion, not joint flexibility.
- The duration of each stretch should be 5 to 10 seconds.
- Stretching should not cause pain or pose risk of injury to joints.
- Selected stretching should not be conducted where it is contraindicated medically.
- Instruction in stretching should be conducted by a qualified health professional, such as a physical or occupational therapist, certified personal trainer, athletic trainer, or exercise specialist.
- The frequency of stretching should match intensity of effort. Generally, hard-working tissues should receive a stretch respite at least every hour. If six strategic exercises were selected, they would consume only 1 minute per hour.

Although numerous exercise choices are available, I support the following group of stretching movements that target the most needy body areas often implicated in work-related musculoskeletal ailments.

- *Chin tuck:* This is a backward-gliding motion of the head with the chin positioned slightly downward. The head remains level as it retracts backward. This movement reduces forward head posture by improving alignment of the cervical vertebrae and reestablishing a better length-tension relationship among the cervical and upper-thoracic musculature.
- *Neck side-bending:* The neck is gently tilted sideways while keeping the shoulders level. The head can be held in various degrees of rotation to select specific neck muscles for stretching.
- *Wrist flexor stretch:* Bending the wrist and fingers backwards. This can be done with the elbows bent or fully extended.
- *Wrist extensor stretch:* One of the most effective techniques is referred to as the *Mill's stretch.* To stretch the right wrist extensors, fully extend the elbow, make a tight fist, fully rotate the right shoulder internally, and then flex the wrist in this position. The other hand may assist to get more wrist flexion.
- *Codman shoulder pendulum exercise:* This seemingly easy movement rarely is performed properly. The purpose of this exercise is to achieve full relaxation of the shoulder mechanism, particularly the shoulder joint. This goal is accomplished by bending forward and supporting the upper body with one hand on a knee or some object. The other arm is left to hang totally passive. The passive, dependent arm can now be made to move passively by first moving the trunk while concentrating on dangling the dependent arm with no muscular splinting or guarding from the shoulder. The hanging arm can be made to move back and forth or to circumscribe clockwise and counterclockwise circles.
- *Statue of Liberty stretch:* This author-coined term describes a standing stretch that addresses multiple body areas simultaneously. The individual stands with one foot approximately 18 to 20 inches in front of the other, measuring from the large toe of the rear foot to the heel of the forward foot. The feet are placed approximately shoulder width apart. The hands are clasped together, reaching fully above the head while gently flexing the forward knee and hip, keeping the rear knee straight. This movement provides a comfortable stretch to the muscles of the upper thorax and the hips as well as providing a lumbar hyperextension stretch to offset prolonged kyphotic posturing of the spine.

These stretches can be a valuable adjunct to the other exposure reduction recommendations outlined earlier. Note that not every exercise stretches muscles and tendons. For example, the Codman pendulum movement functions more as a passive relaxation technique for the shoulder joint. It also provides a rest for frequently compressed and irritated suprahumeral structures (i.e., the supraspinous portion of the rotator cuff).

ENGINEERING CONTROLS

Engineering controls include design of workstation, tools, proper maintenance, environmental layout, mechanical assist for material handling, and alterations in processes. The first line of defense in reducing risks of injury in the workplace is to start with proper design of the working environment, tools, and processes. The goal is to "design out" known ergonomic hazards. Recent times have seen increased mechanization, automation, and intensive safety campaigns that have produced increased general safety in the workplace. Although risk of traumatic injuries is reduced, MSD conditions continue to be problematic. The human interface with this sophistication has produced work demands characterized by fixed positions, body stasis, intense concentration, and highly repetitive movements using the same anatomic structures. These physical and mental stresses are well recognized and merit a strategic position in our concept of ergonomics. For illustration, we may conceptualize an *ergonomics equation* as follows.

Demands of job = Human functional capacity

When the psychophysical demands of work are balanced with human psychophysical capacity, efficient productivity and outcomes are realized. The goal of ergonomics is to achieve an optimum "fit" between work and worker. This balance is best achieved by adjusting the left side of this equation (through engineering improvements) rather than expecting the worker to make all the adjustments on the right side of the equation (through work practice changes). The structure of the work environment, design of tools, and physical demands of the job will directly influence how the worker uses his or her physical and mental resources. Additional examples of engineering considerations include mechanization, hoists, lifts, conveyors, robotics, air quality, noise, temperature, lighting, walking surface, and so forth.

Although it is true that strictly engineering interventions (left side of the equation) can remedy existing hazards immediately, it also has been realized that expensive changes in the workplace may not improve injury statistics. One must realize that the right side of this ergonomics equation presents many opportunities to affect workers' health and productivity as discussed previously, sometimes with comparatively less expense associated with engineering changes. The following discussion highlights considerations in engineering controls.

Seating, Standing, and Posture Considerations

Working postures and movements vary widely depending on the task and environmental factors. Engineering controls for seated and standing work should be designed to minimize ergonomic hazards by optimizing body and joint position and patterns of motion.

Seating

Seating considerations include adjustability, shape and size of the seat pan and backrest, armrest, mobility, provisions for foot placement, lower limb positioning, and sit-stand options.

The decision to purchase high-quality ergonomic seating should be accompanied by employee education directed to proper use and adjustment. All too often, workers can be observed sitting on their expensive office chairs as if they were sitting on stools. Not uncommonly, quick fixes by throwing money into high priced chairs will not reduce ergonomic hazards associated with sitting work.

Adjustability

This feature is needed most when a worker is committed to continuous sitting to perform intense, focused work during which body movements are minimal. Sitting height, angle of the seat pan, backrest, and armrest should be easy to adjust without getting out of the chair. Workers are commonly unfamiliar with the features of a high-quality chair and therefore do not take advantage of the benefits available. Altering positions can provide much needed relief from static work in a confined posture.

Seat and Backrest

The shape, contour, size, and covering of the seat and backrest are important details in matching seating to individuals. Certain flashy chairs may initially look attractive but soon reveal their functional inadequacy. For example, a seat pan may be too large, have an excessively deep depression, or exaggerated sloping. Such features may limit the chair to few users.

Armrests

Armrests should provide comfortable support for the forearms. Fully adjustable armrests can be moved to the proper height and width to accommodate the user. Many chairs have fixed armrests that are typically too low; thus the worker is commonly seen slouching to rest on one or both elbows. Armrests may also limit one's ability to get close enough to the keyboard.

Mobility

Seated work may require that the worker roll from one location to another. Higher quality chairs have five castors with good stability and swiveled wheels. Floor condition and covering should be sufficient to permit easy mobility about the work environment. A surface that is not level and smooth, or has carpeting, can impede mobility and ruin wheels and bearings.

Foot Placement and Lower Limb Positioning

The position of the legs and feet will dictate how the worker aligns the upper body. For example, a work task may require that a short operator sit with the seat adjusted high such that the legs are essentially dangling. The worker will habitually place the feet with the ankles interlocked onto the wheel base. The worker compensates by sitting at the forward edge of the seat. This is akin to "sitting on a stool," without back support. Also, barriers to the knees that cause excessive forward bending to access work tasks on a desk or bench need to be avoided. Proper foot support provides for adequate space under the thighs and permits the worker to sit fully back against the backrest.

Sit-Stand Options

Modern seating designs provide for highly adjustable options to work from sitting in a semi-standing position. This type of seating is useful in situations in which customer service providers must routinely move about and perform duties at a high counter.

Standing Considerations

Workers who must stand constantly may also incur chronic fatigue, postural stress, and musculoskeletal pain. Important factors to consider include footwear, standing surface, extent of body movement, predominant posture of the neck and trunk, and nature of the work activity. For example, a worker whose job task permits a broad choice of unrestricted lower-extremity movements will very likely become less fatigued than will an individual who must stand with both feet confined to one position, as in the case of foot pedal operation. A hard standing surface (e.g., cement) contributes to joint fatigue because there is minimal shock attenuation. Inappropriate footwear may further contribute to compressive and postural stresses to the feet and knees. Job tasks may demand substantial and prolonged deviations from neutral working alignment through the trunk, neck, and shoulder girdles. Sustained forward bending and reaching, with forward head posture, is a common contribution to painful syndromes in the stressed anatomic regions (see Chapter 6).

Here are some helpful tips to reduce fatigue and injury risks associated with prolonged standing.

- Install shock-attenuating pads or mats. If this is not possible, provide workers with access to acceptable footwear or suitable shock-absorbing materials.
- Provide opportunity for changes in foot position, such as a "bar rail."
- Check for barriers in front of the worker's feet. The operator should be able to work as close to a task as possible; even several inches of restriction in front of the toes can result in sustained forward leaning or excessive forward positioning with the upper limbs.
- Consider a "belly rest" or any suitable form of trunk rest against which the operator can take momentary breaks to lean and relax.
- Set work height and task access to permit neutral trunk positioning.
- For individuals with lower-limb circulatory insufficiency, consider pressure-gradient, leg-length socks to promote venous return.

A Summary List of Engineering Controls

Industrial positioning and transport devices:

- Rollers, conveyors, reduced-friction surfaces
- Mechanical holding, turning, and counter-balancing devices
- Powered hoists

Automation:

- Robotics
- Automated assembly technology

Tools and adaptations for worker comfort and protection:

- Ergonomic tools of specific design
- Shock-absorbing materials for the hands and feet
- Proper footwear and gloves for specified work
- Hearing and eye protection devices
- Protective clothing and barriers to hazardous materials and chemicals
- Provisions for protection of respiratory health
- Counterbalanced sling suspension for upper-limb support
- Elasticized supports for the trunk and limbs
- Ergonomic writing implements and accessories
- Vision aids and antiglare devices
- Provisions for ease of communication, (e.g., telephone headset, hands-free devices, etc.)
- Document holders, keyboard, and mouse designs
- Voice-activated computer technology

The work environment:

- Workstation design to facilitate optimal positioning, movement, and efficiency
- Fully adjustable features where needed
- Lighting, temperature, and humidity controls
- Floor surface
- Ambient noise control
- Workstation design to provide adequate space for all operations

In summary, the basic framework for an ergonomically based injury-prevention program consists of administrative, work practice, and engineering controls. Two additional key components of a comprehensive program are the safety committee and ergonomics team.

Safety Committee

The costly rise in work-related MSDs over the past several decades points to increased urgency to define effective safety and injury prevention programs. Safety committees and their policies and procedures should not be just paper-bound; they should be functionally strong. A company's philosophy toward production can be in conflict with its position on safety. If safety is regarded as inferior to manufacturing, priority will be directed to productivity, with a comparatively weaker commitment to the prevention of work injuries. In light of workers' compensation costs associated with MSDs, industry is appreciating the need to harmonize production needs with preservation of employee health and well-being (see Chapter 16 for further discussion).

The concept of process safety management is one way of addressing the possible conflict between manufacturing goals and injury prevention. Process safety management is reflective of a company's total plan to integrate safety seamlessly with all operations. Safety committees alone, as isolated entities, do not necessarily create the highest possible level of safety. It is a comprehensive means of managing process safety by recognizing and understanding the risks of production and by operating in a safe manner, reducing injury risks. In this broader context, the following recommendations are presented for those managers who wish to construct or improve safety committees and programs.

- Give safety the same priority as that given production.
- Establish management safety commitment with employee participation.
- Include a representative on the safety committee from all departments.
- Develop comprehensive policies, procedures, methods, and incentives.
- Define a system for collection and analysis of injury data.
- Organize appropriate subcommittees (e.g., for plant operations, maintenance, safety education, hazardous materials, accident investigation, ergonomics team).

- Delegate appropriate authority and responsibilities and provide necessary resources.
- Provide for necessary education and training of management and staff.

Safety committees alone do not ensure safety. Employee well-being and injury prevention is everyone's job. Company injury statistics will improve when safety planning becomes tightly woven into the matrix of a comprehensive plan that blends manufacturing goals with safety necessities.

Ergonomics Team

An ergonomics team may be a subcommittee of the safety committee or a stand-alone task force given the imperative to undertake all issues pertaining to ergonomics and MSDs. Because of the multifaceted nature of ergonomic science, an ergonomics team should be composed of representatives from management, labor, engineering, maintenance, human resources procurement, health care, safety personnel, union, and consultants (if necessary). Production workers should play a prominent role in decision making because they are the key players who must live and work with the final outcomes.

The mission of an ergonomics team should be to recognize ergonomic hazards and solve problems that are predisposing or causing work-related injuries arising from cumulative trauma. Such a task force will become most effective when it becomes educated and skilled in problem analysis, abatement planning, medical management, surveillance, and training. Not infrequently, it becomes necessary for some companies to contract the services of a consultant with expertise in ergonomics to provide the initial start-up team training and organizational layout (Klafs & Arnheim, 1973).

The reader will now discover how effective teamwork and controls led to successful outcomes in six real-world case histories. Varied circumstances and events are depicted, thus calling for unique strategies in selecting corrective actions from our three-pronged framework.

CASE NUMBER 1: SOLDER TECHNICIAN

A 45-year-old, highly skilled assembly operator has 15 years of experience as a veteran solder technician. An increase in demand for product necessitates a mandatory change in work schedule from a 5-day, 40-hour week to a 6-day, 60-hour week.

The essential physical demands of this job (67% to 100% of the work shift) are constant sitting; constant elevation of one or both upper limbs such that hands and elbows are non-weight-bearing (unsupported) during task; constant highly focused visual attention for viewing small parts and maintaining fixed positions of minute items and hand tools; and occasional walking (1% to 33% of work shift). Specifically, as part of a group of assembly functions, this position calls for the ability to execute rapid and forceful bilateral pinching, grasping, and highly coordinated manipulatory activity with cables, plugs, and other assorted accessories, machinery, tools, and hardware. Shoulders, forearms, wrists, and hands are frequently (sometimes constantly) postured in extremes of joint position to carry out job tasks. Tools used include small and large cutters, pliers, screwdrivers, hammers, calipers, micrometers, special knives, solder guns, picking tools, and solder holders.

A soldering specialist uses both hands in a very precise and highly coordinated fashion to properly position and stabilize multiple small wire leads in readiness for the soldering process. Typically, such workers sit in nonadjustable metal chairs. Foot support consists of metal cross bars under the work table or empty spools that have been appropriated for such use. The work surface is also nonadjustable and provides space for all necessary tools and working materials, including solder vise, tin dip heater, heat gun, and so on.

Several weeks of extraordinarily intense work left the solder operator fatigued, complaining of discomfort in the neck, shoulders, and hands.

The left shoulder became so painful that this worker took nonprescription medicine to reduce pain so as to tolerate the long workday. Symptoms persisted even off-duty, placing a serious constraint on this individual's ability to engage in normal activities of daily living.

By the end of the fourth week, this worker's left shoulder was so painful that self-medication was ineffective. Because of the imperative for accelerated productivity and the department's prevailing urgency, this operator initially did not approach the supervisor with a complaint. Also, this division's particular supervisor was generally regarded as unsympathetic, dictatorial, and insensitive to employee needs. Tentatively, the injured worker finally approached the supervisor, who responded in a suspicious and disbelieving manner. Reluctantly, the supervisor directed this worker to fill out a first report of injury, then ushered the operator off to the company nurse. At the first-aid office, this worker received basic medical attention. There were, however, no outward, classic signs of injury such as edema, redness, or bruising; the only evidence was this individual's subjective report of pain and disability. The recommendation was made for this person to be evaluated by the company physician.

The physician issued a diagnosis of severe tendinitis of the left shoulder (rotator cuff), administered an injection, and wrote a prescription for antiinflammatory and analgesic medicine. The doctor ordered the employee back to work with restricted duty for a 2-week period. Medical work restrictions of the modified duty assignment were: no lifting above shoulder level, no lifting in excess of 5 pounds, no repetitive motion with the hands, and no standing or sitting for more than an 8-hour work shift.

On return to work, the impaired worker was hustled off by the supervisor to another department, the manager of which tried to find something for the injured worker to do. The modified duty assignment was to collate and classify reams of files 8 hours per day. This task required constant sitting and handling of files and stacks of paper.

It is revealing to consider in more depth the details of this modified-duty work environment and its physical demands. The worker was sitting in an old swivel chair with a deep and wide seat pan, nonadjustable armrests with loose forearm supports, and faulty controls for tilt, backrest, and seat height adjustment. It was necessary to sit toward the front edge of this chair to keep from falling backward, and the high armrests prevented positioning close to the table. This inappropriate and defective chair did not allow the individual to use the backrest; therefore, work was being carried out in the presence of excessive loading and tension of the trunk postural muscles. The work table was of the folding conference type, measuring 3 × 6 feet. On the table were cardboard file boxes filled with thick folders. The task was to remove selected folders and to separate designated paper material for reorganization. Although this worker may opt to stand, the choice was made to remain sitting to carry out this work. An observer readily can note the frequency of forward reaching and fingering, making for awkward retrieval of bulky paper material that is difficult to handle. The shoulders are elevated to eye level much of the time, allowing minimal weight-bearing rest.

Within 8 hours of this so-called "light duty," the worker's left shoulder pain intensified. Why did this happen? At this point it is necessary to consider all the factors that originally caused or contributed to this injury. Furthermore, attention should be directed to additional circumstances that were associated with the modified duty program that further aggravated this employee's shoulder problem.

- Significant increase in daily and weekly work hours
- Increased work pace and intensity, fewer rest intervals
- Lack of task differentiation
- Late symptom reporting
- Late medical intervention
- Adversarial relationship between employee and supervisor
- Sustained and prolonged static posturing of trunk and upper limbs

- Minimal upper-limb weight bearing; prolonged, sustained elevation
- Ill-defined modified duty program; poor supervision and duty assignment
- Supervisor and manager uneducated about injury management
- Poor medical specification of appropriate modified duty

This employee was suffering from a severe pathology of the rotator cuff caused primarily by the impact of job physical demands. The modified-duty work failed to significantly reduce stress to the injured structures of the left shoulder (i.e., tendons of the rotator cuff and contents of the suprahumeral space). This person continued to work with the shoulders elevated into the "impingement zone," and stress was intensified by efforts to handle awkward, bulky file folders and papers from a sitting position. Many of the factors that predisposed this operator to injury on regular duty remained in effect during the alternative work assignment. The story does not have a happy ending; this highly productive and valued employee went on to surgery and extensive rehabilitation, unable to return to regular duty for 6 months.

Selected Corrective Workplace Recommendations

The injured solder operator's experience typifies events and shortcomings so common to work-related MSDs. Recommendations follow that may have reduced the risk of such injuries.

Administrative Corrective Actions

- Adjust work hours or staffing to meet production goals and preserve the health of operators.
- Adjust the work-rest cycle within acceptable established parameters to prevent injuries.
- Report signs and symptoms early; minimize lag time.
- Modify attitude of supervisor to eliminate employee fear of reprisal.
- Medical evaluation and initial treatment should be prompt.
- Establish appropriate modified duty that would not aggravate the existing injury.
- Monitor the injured worker's progress and adjust the program as necessary.
- Provide rotation to another job requiring significantly varied physical demands.

Work Practice Actions

It was emphasized earlier that the architecture of the work environment and design of the process may limit how the operator can physically carry out necessary job functions. In the absence of engineering changes for this solder technician, some improvements in work practice are as follows.

- Adjust the work-rest cycle (an administrative change will result in a work practice change).
- Where feasible, provide a way to perform work from both standing and sitting position.
- Provide timely brief stretch breaks, focusing on the working tissues at most risk of injury.

Engineering Actions

- Create adjustable-height work stations.
- Design the job so that it can be done with improved postural positions and movements.
- Obtain tools that provide for optimum handling, minimizing extremes of joint posturing and force.
- Provide a suitable cushion for intermittent weight-bearing to unload the shoulder girdles, neck, and spine.
- Select adjustable seating to provide for comfort and variations in working position.
- Provide for adequate placement of the feet with variations.

CASE NUMBER 2: TWO ASSEMBLY WORKERS ATTENDING A MECHANIZED CONVEYOR

A typical example of paced work with predetermined external speed is illustrated by two assembly operators positioned facing each other on opposite sides of a conveyor belt. These assemblers are sitting in nonadjustable, high metal chairs without backrests. The hardwood seats are contoured slightly, and brackets connecting the legs serve as foot supports. Each worker is free to sit or stand and face the conveyor line at any angle desired while carrying out the job task. When sitting, space for alternative foot positioning is minimal because of barriers below the conveyor unit. In this scenario, 55-year-old Operator 1 is sitting directly facing the conveyor belt, whereas 23-year-old Operator 2 is sitting at an oblique angle, facing the oncoming belt. Each worker performs identical functions: inserting a 12-space partitioned divider into a pint-sized container made of cardboard; inserting the sales product into each of the 12 spaces; and closing and securing the side flaps and lid of the container with labeled packing tape.

Close observation of the habitual work style of these operators reveals important distinctions that bear significance on work-related injury risks. As noted previously, Operator 1 is sitting with the trunk and arms facing the moving assembly line, whereas Operator 2 is positioned at an angle of 45 degrees facing the oncoming belt.

The details of Operator 1's work history and work behavior are as follows.

- Has been on the job for 15 years
- Sits forward on the front portion of seat with feet supported
- Sits upright and maintains normal spinal curves
- Head and neck remain in midline during course of work
- Minimizes trunk twisting during packaging procedure
- Product supply located 16 in from worker's right side in forward-tilted box
- Conveyor line set at operator's elbow height when sitting
- Conveyor belt speed provides ample time to complete task without rushing
- Operator patiently waits for all material to arrive in front of torso before assembly
- All motions are rhythmic, coordinated, and synchronized with conveyor
- Good interpersonal relations with supervisor

Operator 2 is working at the same pace, but significant differences become apparent, as follows.

- Has been on the job for 1 year
- Sits leaning forward, with trunk obliquely facing oncoming conveyor
- Holds head forward, with trunk rotated
- Holds slumped posture, with prominent loss of normal spinal curves
- Sustains shoulder-scapular elevation in "hurry-up" posture
- Makes frantic, jerky movements, as if trying to outrun machine pace
- Is impatient, reaching ahead for products instead of waiting for products to arrive
- Frequently fumbles, dropping items
- Frequently complains of fatigue
- Criticizes work layout and physical demands
- Has poor interpersonal relations with supervisor

The younger, less-experienced Operator 2 approaches the supervisor with complaints of pain in the neck, midback, and shoulders. The worker is convinced that this discomfort is caused by the job's physical demands. The older, more-experienced operator is not reporting fatigue problems or criticism of work layout.

These are the questions that now loom before the supervisor or medical provider.

- Is this worker truly incurring excessive stress because of the design and demands of the job?
- Why is only one of many such operators sustaining undue fatigue and discomfort?
- Are *ergonomic hazards* or worker behaviors precipitating this worker's *ergonomic injury?*
- Are this worker's problems exclusively ergonomic problems that call for ergonomic interventions (purely engineering changes)?
- Are this operator's problems the result of work stressors that obligated this individual to a restrictive, overly laborious work style or, perhaps, was this person exerting excessive, unnecessary effort as a result of habitual, voluntary activity?

This practical work example serves to highlight important considerations applicable to the design of work as it interfaces with human performance and attitudes. The assembly job did have an externally set pace that was satisfactory and acceptable to 99% of the workforce. The solution to injury prevention in this illustration lies less with *engineering* intervention and more with appropriate *administrative* and *workplace practices* (e.g., job-specific training, allowance for a conditioning-adaptation period, close monitoring and communication with the less-experienced operator; and learning to pace oneself).

CASE NUMBER 3: WIRE-PLUG ASSEMBLER

This illustration demonstrates how financial incentive can be a contributory factor to the genesis of work-related cumulative trauma injury. As a highly experienced, veteran employee of a wire and cable manufacturer, the operator had the arduous task of inserting 10-lead, color-coded wires into small plastic plugs similar to a common telephone jack plug. The physical demands of this job require constant forceful pinching and finger manipulation, prolonged sitting, and highly focused visual attention for viewing very small parts. Because of exceptional proficiency at this task, this operator consistently produced 50% more units per hour than did co-workers, thereby earning a significantly higher wage because productivity was linked with wages. Over time, this worker began to experience chronic fatigue and increasing discomfort in the arms and wrists. Symptoms advanced to include numbness and decreased ability to maintain high level of output.

This worker was reluctant to report symptoms, knowing that lost work time or a modified duty assignment would result in reduced wages. Also, a negative stigma was associated with claims for "aches and pains" discomfort. This individual persevered until severity of symptoms intensified, resulting in loss of physical ability to participate in regular duty. The long delay and chronicity of symptoms eventually led to severe pathologic problems requiring surgical treatment and extensive rehabilitation. It is evident here that piecework—equating wages with work output—can be a contributing factor to increased risks for MSDs (Arndt, 1987; Lanfear & Clark, 1972; Levi, 1972; Welch, 1972).

It is important to distinguish between whole-body energy expenditure and local muscle fatigue in discussing work pacing and rest periods. With reference to our previous illustration, attention is best directed to the work-rest cycle of the upper limbs, particularly the muscles of the forearms and hands. Historically, work site experience indicates that incidence of upper-limb MSDs is linked most closely to the work-rest cycle of the forearms and hands and less so with overall body energy expenditure (Arndt, 1985; Borg, 1982; Rodgers, 1987; Putz-Anderson, 1992; Rohmert, 1973). Guidelines are available for estimating rest pauses for repetitive jobs involving various levels of effort, based on maximum voluntary contractions (Arndt, 1987).

From an administrative design, deterrents to injury claims associated with work pacing and piecework must address the influence of incentives or penalties associated with job performance and productivity. Helpful *administrative* strategies to curb work-related injuries in this case include the following.

- Set work pace at a level that meets workers' physical capabilities safely.
- Establish appropriate work-rest cycles.
- Apply piecework incentives cautiously, with safeguards to minimize injury risk.
- When feasible, create job rotation to diversify physical demands.
- Provide incentives for safety and injury prevention and productivity.

CASE NUMBER 4: SEWING OPERATOR

The sewing operator must sit constantly, allowed only two 10-minute breaks and 30 minutes for lunch. This operator is sitting on an all-metal, nonadjustable chair with a fixed backrest and flat, noncontoured seat. Both the seat and backrest have been cushioned with personally acquired padding. On either side of this worker are large, wheeled laundry bins containing bundles of fabric. The work requires that the operator periodically reach into these bins to grasp a bundle and place it on the flat work surface for accessibility. Some workers choose to remain sitting when they are acquiring their bundles, whereas other operators will get out of their chairs to reach into bins. Those individuals who remain seated while removing fabric bundles are observed to twist, lean, and stretch awkwardly as they extend one hand over the rim of the basket, often groping to grasp and remove the loosely tied material. During the sewing operation, the worker is relatively confined because of the necessity of keeping both feet in fixed positions on controls; also, the right knee is used to activate a lateral switch pad used during the procedure.

A scan of the workplace reveals that other operators carry out similar tasks. However, many individuals are sitting in upholstered swivel chairs from which the wheels have been removed to provide stability. These operators claim more satisfaction and comfort with their modified office chairs because they have less restricted mobility, a more comfortable seat surface, and a broader back support. Closer scrutiny of workers' sitting postures discloses that most individuals are sitting forward in their chairs, seldom using backrests during actual sewing procedures. Reclining backward only occurs during momentary pauses. The forward-sitting position provides for less total contact with the supporting surface underneath thighs, thus enabling greater freedom of movement of the lower limbs. This positioning also facilitates fewer restrictions to pelvic mobility, making it seemingly easier to pivot or tilt the pelvis while remaining seated to work.

Why do some workers cling tenaciously to the old metal, nonadjustable chairs that have been padded selectively to meet their needs? An explanation for this phenomenon is forthcoming simply by observation. It is important to consider how very important are the elements of mobility and positioning choice. Prolonged postural stasis is fatiguing, particularly during focused work, and this is especially applicable during confined sitting wherein minimal opportunity for diversified positioning changes is available. The fixed, static posturing of the head and trunk demands sustained tension from all the axial postural maintenance musculature.

Workers committed to such limited options will seek ways to incorporate as much movement and position choice as possible while maintaining a productivity standard. Sitting far forward in a seat and supplying padding provide one mechanism for operators to exercise more options for body posturing and general mobility while working. Asking such a worker to sit fully back in the seat with the spine pressed upright against the backrest is restrictive and confining.

Still another consideration that has an impact on posturing and freedom of movement is vision or visual access to task. Head positioning is determined by a person's ability to visualize the task adequately. Some workers are observed to work with the eyes only several inches away from the task, whereas other individuals will find it satisfactory to work at a comparatively greater distance from the work object.

This brief illustration points to the importance of proper seating. In this case risks for injury include prolonged sitting, frequent awkward bending and twisting to retrieve fabric bundles, and highly repetitive use of the hands to carry out sewing functions. Self-imposed commonsense ergonomics interventions were primarily *work practice* changes achieved through *engineering* modifications. Such engineering changes included removal of wheels from swivel chairs and addition of personalized padding. These simple adjustments made it possible to improve mobility, thus reducing fatigue associated with constant positioning.

CASE NUMBER 5: TELEMARKETING ASSOCIATE

A telemarketing associate spends hours sitting in front of a computer workstation. This job demands constant combined use of the telephone and calculator, writing notes in longhand, and keying while handling data from the video display terminal. Although this individual already possesses a fully adjustable office task chair with armrests and a footrest, the chair is adjusted too high to position the armrests under the desktop. The operator has adjusted the seat to this height because of other constraints in the workstation. Additional inspection of the work area reveals the presence of numerous personal items, such as pictures, small plants, and decorations placed at arm's reach within the work space.

Observation of this individual executing work tasks demonstrates the factors underlying his complaints of fatigue and discomfort. This person holds his telephone between the neck and left shoulder, fingering the calculator with the left hand and alternately keying and note taking with the right hand, all the while keeping the pencil in readiness in the right fingers. He maintains an elevated shoulder girdle throughout the observation. There is highly repetitive reaching over and around numerous items throughout the work area. Many obstacles in the work space prevent comfortable positioning and weight bearing of the upper limbs.

In this context, selection of seating should take into account far more than the singular goal of establishing an artificial concept of good posture—that is, sitting totally upright, with knees and hips at 90-degree angles and the back in full contact with a backrest. Also, one must assess whether the worker's body positions and movements are obligatory, habitual, or some combination of both. *Obligatory* suggests that the worker is mandated to assume a particular position and move in specific patterns to accomplish the job task. *Habitual* implies that the worker has choices and has elected to adopt certain anatomic positions and functional motions for reasons that may be either obvious or obscure. For the individual who habitually sits with pronounced forward head posture and a slumped, kyphotic spine, a new ergonomic chair may not result in desired behavior changes. Most often, ergonomic offerings should be accompanied by appropriate employee education about the justification for the changes and how best to take advantage of such ergonomic improvements.

Engineering corrective recommendations for this scenario include the following.

- Adjust the height of the desktop to accommodate the height at which the operator must sit.
- Provide wider foot support to permit variable foot positioning.
- Remove extraneous items from the immediate work area to provide for complete freedom of movement.
- Provide a suitable telephone headset to eliminate crimping the desk phone into the neck area.
- Arrange all desktop items for maximum accessibility.
- Adjust VDT, mouse, and keyboard to optimum positions for easy access and working in neutral joint positions.
- Optimize lighting and visual access to the VDT and work area.

Work practice suggestions include the following.

- Adjust work-rest cycle; take mini-rest-stretch breaks.
- Be conscious of maximizing all of the chair's features—that is, establish body position for easy access to all tasks while being fully supported by the backrest, feet well supported in good position. Adjust and use the armrests to unload the shoulders and spine.

CASE NUMBER 6: NURSING AIDE

Jane Doe is a veteran certified nursing assistant (CNA) who has been working in the same skilled nursing and rehabilitation center for the past 10 years. Her daily routine is to provide care and assistance for a group of permanent, long-term residents. Job duties include attending to all physical needs, including bathing, grooming, hygiene, dressing, physical assistance with bed mobility, positioning, transfers and ambulation, cleaning bed frames and mattresses, changing linen, executing the rehab restorative program (range of motion, feeding, ambulation activity, and so on), and transporting to various locations for selected programs. Jane is responsible for the safety, comfort, and general well-being of each resident under her care. This means that she must be vigilant to answer call lights, be proactive to meet clients' needs, and maintain proper communication with her supervisor and all members of the health care team.

Jane's work duties and responsibilities are demanding physically, mentally, and emotionally. She is constantly on her feet, moving quickly from one task to the next. Constant or prolonged repetitive forward reaching, bending, and twisting are routine. Lifting and handling clients from awkward positions, either by habit or circumstance, is standard fare on any given day. Jane's neck, shoulders, and low back are tired, but she is devoted and stoic and not given to complaints.

Jane's fatigue and general discomfort are intermittent at first, typically worse by the end of the work week. She fully recovers on her days off and returns to duty refreshed. During the weeks that follow, Jane's caseload expands with more than half of her clients being very ill and needy. There comes a time when Jane's fatigue becomes constant and physical distress limits her ability to move freely. She can no longer tolerate bending forward for more than a brief moment, so she compensates by keeping her spine rigid and seeking ways to minimize the stress. Job performance begins to erode because she becomes less mobile, must work slower, and take more minibreaks. Finally one day Jane is assisting her client with a transfer from wheelchair to bed. This particular resident is known for her fearful, panicky behavior and unpredictable reactions. She is recovering from surgical hip repair and is ordered to be non–weight-bearing on the involved leg. Jane sets the stage properly, uses a waist transfer belt on the patient, and begins to execute the procedure flawlessly. Halfway through the transition, the client panics and lunges off-balance. Jane is violently pulled off her position of control and reacts quickly to complete the transfer, guiding the fearful resident to the bed. In so doing, Jane is forced into an extreme position of forward bending and twisting while exerting maximum force to hold, guide, and protect the client. Jane immediately grimaces with a stabbing pain in her right low back. Her stoicism no longer conceals the obvious injury. Reluctantly, Jane enters the workers' compensation arena by reporting this incident to her supervisor and completing the necessary form.

A close study of Jane's history reveals significant trends and milestones that paved the way for Jane's traumatic injury. Her problem first began with intermittent fatigue. Soon she noticed that her low back was always tired. Then came the onset of episodic discomfort, mostly in her right low back. The incident with the panicky client was the "straw that broke the camel's back." Important events that triggered Jane's final demise were an increase in the size of her client population and a disproportionate increase in the percentage of very dependent individuals. Although Jane followed proper principles of body mechanics, both the cumulative sequence of risks and the last unforeseen occurrence were enough to cause this incident.

Was Jane's injury acute, or should it be regarded as a cumulative trauma event? Perhaps the answer lies in both her history of progressive stress and the precipitating event. In other words, would this injury have occurred if Jane's workload, and associated increased physical demands, had not expanded? This scenario will challenge the safety committee to uncover all factors and circumstances that led to this employee injury claim. Let us now consider preventive steps that would have reduced exposures and subsequent risk for injury.

Administrative actions include the following.

- Staffing adjustments should be made to provide extra help when needed.
- This client should be identified as high risk with handling precautions.

- Signs and symptoms of impending MSD should be reported early.
- Early preinjury management, before onset of functional impairment, should be put in place.
- Client-handling policies and procedures to minimize exposures to injury should be established.

Work practice actions include the following.

- Jane should have taken the initiative to seek assistance, knowing this client was a two-person transfer.
- In the absence of another helper, Jane should have used a suitable mechanical hoist to transfer this client from wheelchair to bed. This is applying an engineering tool to achieve safer work practice.
- The immediate setting should have been assessed more carefully—for example, the position of the wheelchair relative to the bed, position of the client just prior to the transfer, and so on.
- Jane should have taken extra precautions with body mechanics and positioning of the waist transfer belt.
- Jane should communicate more effectively with the client and set the stage to best facilitate patient participation in the transfer.

Engineering actions include the following.

- The facility should have appropriate mechanical patient-handling equipment that is readily accessible.
- Additional engineering options include transfer sliding boards, various designs of looped transfer belts, wheelchairs with removable armrests and leg rests to facilitate less restrictive exit, and grab bars.

The preceding are specific ergonomic applications relative to real-world case histories. The following are some additional important factors to consider.

PHYSICAL COMFORT AIDS

The ergonomics market has seen a proliferation of paraphernalia and gadgets directed at the comfort and safety of the workforce. Such items include elasticized back supports, shock-attenuating insoles, vibration-dampening products, wrist and elbow bands, and the like.

It is useful to distinguish a splint from a support. A *splint* is a therapeutic device commonly used to support, restrict motion, or substitute for weakened muscles (Coppard & Lohman, 1996). Thus, splinting limits motion (e.g., a wrist splint restricts normal excursions of flexion and extension; likewise, a torso brace will prevent flexion and extension of the lumbosacral spine). A flexible *support* may sustain or provide a basis for continued function while stabilizing the limb.

It is not uncommon in the workplace to see workers wearing elasticized bands around upper forearms or using garments to restrict wrist motions. Such compression bands and splints are more likely to be seen in work settings that require highly repetitive upper-limb tasks. Such products are in response to the injury claims for elbow tendinitis and wrist-hand problems, particularly carpal tunnel syndrome.

The definition of splint as a device that limits motion of a joint is important to consider when, for example, a wrist splint is worn by a laborer who must carry out repetitive hand functions that demand a full range of motion with the forearm, wrist, and fingers. When the splint is applied, normal flexibility of the wrist is no longer available; therefore, the individual will compensate for the lack of wrist motion by expanding range of motion from other joints that are not limited. Commonly, the limited wrist motions will demand extra effort from the shoulder. This can create a risk for shoulder strain or tendinitis through repeated elevation and stress in the "impingement zone." Once again, when any device is worn on the body, both advantages and consequences must be taken into account. Just as prescription medicine has indications, contraindications, precautions, and side effects, so do splints, braces, supports, and garments worn by workers. Selection and use of comfort aids must satisfy reasonable indications if the anticipated benefits are to be realized.

The use of splints and supports should be judicious. Compressive, elasticized supports can provide comfort and retention of heat in underlying tissues. This is particularly true when a support is constructed from closed-cell material such as neoprene. Caution should be used to ensure proper fit and stability of position. For example, a tennis elbow band should not be so tight as to reduce circulation and not so loose that it slides down the forearm. Precautions should also be taken when any garment is susceptible to being caught in machinery or impeding work performance in any way. Motion-restricting splints may pose a more serious consideration, as noted earlier. In work that demands highly mobile wrist-hand motions, the restrictions imposed by a wrist band, for example, may force accommodation by substituting more forceful finger motions, with concomitant increase in motion and stress to the shoulder. It is necessary to carefully evaluate the need and weigh the benefits and precautions when donning a splint during work. Usually, a medical consultation and authorization are indicated before an employee is directed to wear a joint-limiting device; a medical prescription will specify when and how long the user should wear the splint.

IMPORTANCE OF MANAGEMENT-EMPLOYEE TRAINING

Management-Employee Education and Training

The incidence of MSDs in the workplace presents one of the greatest challenges for problem solving in U.S. industry. Determination of root causes and mechanisms of injury is even more difficult. The complexity of these disorders, some of which may be clearly work related, demands a level of knowledge and problem-solving skills higher than that necessary for the former, more obvious maladies. Abatement strategies, medical management, and prevention programs directed to the elimination of work-related MSDs demand that both management and employees become educated about this subject. Greatest success derives from a collaborative effort between fully informed managers, supervisors, safety personnel, employees, and health care providers.

Because managers have the authority to establish policy and to exercise leadership, it is incumbent on them to become informed and to assign responsibilities, with the appropriate resources, to key players who will implement prevention programs. Suggested objectives for management level training are as follows.

- Develop a practical knowledge of common work-related musculoskeletal injuries and their causes, symptoms, and treatments.
- Learn to recognize and distinguish risks associated with job tasks, worker behaviors, and companywide attitudes.
- Learn how to analyze and interpret injury data (e.g., OSHA 300 logs, insurance loss runs).
- Develop a methodology of worksite analysis (e.g., study of trends, ergonomic assessment).
- Develop a broad understanding of all issues that contribute to injuries, worker compensation claims, and costs.
- Acquire essential knowledge and resources to define, document, and implement fully a comprehensive plan for the prevention of job-related musculoskeletal disorders (i.e., an ergonomics program).
- Learn how to establish, organize, and conduct an *ergonomics team* with supplemental training to address this specialty.

Employees have the primary responsibility to follow safety procedures and care for their health. Working individuals should participate in decision making that will have an impact on their performance and well-being on the job. Employee feedback without reprisal is an essential prerequisite to good relations and optimal success. Employees who undertake training directed to the prevention of musculoskeletal problems should achieve the following objectives.

- A fundamental knowledge of common musculoskeletal ailments most frequently encountered in their industry.
- Knowledge of how to participate in a total system of health surveillance with procedures for reporting symptoms.
- Recognition of inefficient and overly stressful work habits.
- Techniques of improving posture and body mechanics, on and off the job.
- Strategies to work with more energy conservation and less fatigue.
- Procedures for self-management and symptom relief from common, uncomplicated types of soft-tissue discomfort.
- Techniques to carry out on-the-job stretching and relaxation exercises.

It is my intention that the reader will appreciate the complexity of science and opinion surrounding the field of ergonomics as it relates to the prevention of work-related MSDs. Within this maze of diverse opinions representing numerous intellectual specialties, common sense surfaces as an anchor on which reasonable people can identify ergonomic hazards and achieve lasting solutions.

REFERENCES

Allers, V. (1989). Work-place preventive programs cut costs of illness and injuries. *Occupational Health and Safety, 58*(8), 26-29.

Anderson, B. (1980). *Stretching.* Bolinas, CA: Shelter Publications.

APTA News Release. (1991) Physical therapists say most carpal tunnel syndrome injuries preventable through education. *Orthopedic Practice 3*(4).

Arndt, R. (1985). *A prospective study of the psychological and psychosocial effects of machine-paced work in the US Postal Service.* Cincinnati: NIOSH (Contract 210-79-0072), 1-40.

Arndt, R. (1987). Work pace, stress and cumulative trauma disorders. *Journal of Hand Surgery [Am], 12*(5, Pt 2), 866-869.

Borg, G.A.V. (1982). Psychophysical basis of perceived exertion. *Medicine and Science in Sports and Exercise, 14,* 377-381.

Coppard, B.M. & Lohman, H.L.(2001). *Introduction to splinting* (2nd ed.). St. Louis: Mosby.

Goidi, I. (1964). Epicondylitis lateralis humeri: A pathogenic study. *Acta Chirurgica Scandinavica Supplementum, 339,* 119.

Hansford, T., Blood, H., Kent, B., & Lutz, G. (1986). Blood flow changes at the wrist in manual workers after preventive interventions. *Journal of Hand Surgery [Am], 11*(4), 503 508.

Hess, J. A., Hecker, S.(2003). Stretching at work for injury prevention: issues, evidence, and recommendations, *Applied Occupational and Environmental Hygiene, 18*(5), 331-338.

Jacobsen, C., & Sperling, L. (1976). Classification of the handgrip. A preliminary study. *Journal of Occupational Medicine, 18,* 395-398.

Klafs, C., & Arnheim, D. (1973). Scientific basis for conditioning and training. In D. D. Arnheim (Ed.), *Modern principles of athletic training*. St. Louis: Mosby.

Lanfear, R., & Clark, W. (1972). The treatment of tenosynovitis in industry. *Physiotherapy, 58*(4), 128-129.

Levi, L. (1972). Stress and distress in response to psychosocial stimuli. *Acta Medica Scandinavica, 528*(suppl), 191.

National Academy Press (1998). *Work-related musculoskeletal disorders: A review of the evidence.* Washington, DC: National Academy Press.

Amako, M., Oda, T., Masuoka, K., Yokoi, H., & Campisi, P. (2003). Effect of static stretching on prevention of injuries for military recruits. *Military Medicine, 168,*(6), 442-446.

Putz-Anderson, V. (1992). *Cumulative trauma disorders: a manual for musculoskeletal diseases of the upper limbs.* London: Taylor & Francis.

Rodgers, S. H. (1987). Recovery time needs for repetitive work. *Seminars in Occupational Medicine, 2*(1), 19-24.

Rohmert, W. (1973). Problems in determining rest allowances: Part I. *Applied Ergonomics, 4*(2), 91-95.

Sawyer, K. (1987). An on-site exercise program to prevent carpal tunnel syndrome. *Professional Safety, 5,* 17-20.

Thompson, A., Plewes, L., & Shaw, E. (1951). Peritendinitis crepitans and simple tenosynovitis: A clinical study of 544 cases in industry. *British Journal of Industrial Medicine, 8,* 150-160.

Welch, R. (1972). The causes of tenosynovitis in industry. *Indiana Medicine, 41*(10), 16-18.

Wilson, R., & Wilson, S. (1957). Tenosynovitis in industry. *Practitioner, 178,* 612-625.

CHAPTER 15

Employment Examinations

James W. King

Most individuals use their hands to perform the tasks that provide their livelihood. Surgeons, carpenters, butchers, and seamstresses are among many workers whose primary service or product comes directly from the countless simple and complex functions of the hand. Littler (1960) eloquently stated, "With any degree of incapacity of the hand, man's potential is diminished. Function of this unique part is dependent upon its structure, its strength, its critical sensation, and its integration with the mind and the eye" (p. 259). With their concern for the functional ability of humanity, therapists perform many activities to prevent and rehabilitate hand dysfunction.

Gilbreth and Gilbreth (1924) identified specific elements of hand function, such as search, grasp, move, position, reach, and hold, to describe workers' activities. Barnes, as described by Armstrong, Radwin, Hansen, and Kennedy (1986), modified these elements to include another function: rest, to overcome fatigue. When used repeatedly following the onset of fatigue, the soft tissues of the upper extremities undergo stress. Daily stress may occur when the job exposes a person, either on an intermittent or on a continuous basis, to certain high-risk activities. If the accumulating stress exceeds the body's normal recuperative ability during rest cycles, inflammation of the tissue may follow. Chronic inflammation can lead to the development of musculoskeletal disorders (MSDs). The results of MSDs may be medical costs, indemnity costs, and difficulty meeting production demands (see Chapters 4 and 17 for a complete discussion of costs related to MSDs).

There are several methods to reduce the costs of MSDs, including decreasing workers' exposure to environmental risk factors, training workers to recognize symptoms, initiating early intervention programs for symptomatic workers, and minimizing the placement of individuals with existing or developing abnormal conditions in high-risk jobs. This chapter addresses job placement and monitoring of MSDs through the development of an objective, accurate, valid, and reliable assessment of upper-extremity function as a means of minimizing MSD-related costs.

Proper job placement can benefit both the worker and the company. Certain individuals may be unsuitable for jobs having one or more environmental risk factors because of their current hand function, which may be influenced by past exposures at work and at home. Placement in a job with additional risk could lead to the development or exacerbation of the symptoms of an MSD. An objective assessment would assist in the following work-related situations.

1. An initial screening with a standardized, accurate test may identify existing MSDs in applicants. Consequently, an employee would be matched with an appropriate job.
2. An ongoing assessment that is sensitive to early changes in hand function could identify

an early MSD. Monitoring in this way would clarify the point at which switching the worker from the high-risk job to a lower risk job or referral for medical management would be appropriate.

3. Finally, an objective assessment would identify the point at which previously injured workers have the physical capacity to return to varying levels of hand-intensive work.

This chapter addresses a history of employment examinations and the typical components of these assessments, the factors to consider in the development and analysis of employment examination accuracy, including the effect of the Americans with Disabilities Act (ADA) on the application-testing-placement process, and a suggested examination, called the Upper Extremity Fitness for Duty Evaluation (UEFFDE).

SUPPORT OF MEDICAL EXAMINATIONS IN INDUSTRY

Medical examinations that can identify current symptoms or reliably identify a combination of personal and environmental risk and classify an individual accurately will be paramount to long-term management of workers in hand-intensive jobs. Although not all individuals exposed to risk factors in their job will develop MSDs, many risk factors contribute to their development. Biomechanical risk factors for this disorder in work environments include repetition, abnormal postures of the hand, resistive hand motions, exposure to vibration, and, to a lesser degree, exposure to extremes of temperature (see Chapter 10).

Those who study the incidence of MSDs initially proposed that there is a predisposition in some individuals to these types of disorders. Bleecker (1987) has identified carpal canal size as a risk factor associated with carpal tunnel syndrome (CTS). Castelli, Evans, Diaz-Perez, and Armstrong (1980) studied the morphology of the median nerve vasculature within the carpal tunnel in cadavers. They identified excessive carpal canal pressure as a factor that could lead to the development of anoxia and secondary destruction of nerve fibers. Szabo and Gelberman (1987) also identified differences in individual response to laboratory-induced pressure in the carpal canal.

Other theorists believe that work conditions are largely responsible for MSD development, because the soft tissue of the hand and wrist is susceptible, particularly in certain individuals, to the stress of excessive working conditions. Kazarian (1975) has identified a creep effect (viscoelastic deformation of the tissue) related to the duration of loading of musculotendinous units. Chu and Blatz (1972) identified microdamage, leading to the same viscous deformation, from failure on a molecular level of the links between the tissue matrix and filler material in muscle. Additional studies have identified the frequency of these disorders (Armstrong & Chaffin, 1979; Hartwell, Larson, & Posch, 1964; Hymovich & Lyndholm, 1966; Masear, Hayes, & Hyden, 1986). The question still remains as to why some workers develop MSDs and some do not.

Some clinicians suggest that individuals who do not develop MSDs have developed greater than average strength. An assessment that could identify the unique genetic physical characteristics or potential of such workers could lead to future research in predicting workers best suited for high-risk work.

Many industries are likely to hire workers who have experience in hand-intensive production work. However, these are the very individuals who may already have developed MSD symptoms. This set of circumstances has been described as "cumulative trauma roulette" (King, 1990). In this scenario, workers who may have developed hand problems during previous work are hired or transferred to high-risk jobs. When a worker with a previously subclinical problem becomes symptomatic, the current employer is liable for the worker's medical care. An objective test to screen for this may eliminate longer-term liabilities.

Finally, following medical care, injured workers often return to the same job with little or no objective measurement of their readiness to perform their jobs. This practice may result in reinjuries; additional lost time; and increased morbidity and antagonism among the injured workers, their employer, and the medical treatment team. One of the best reasons to perform testing is to establish the presence or absence of medical problems or physical limitations in the event that an injury occurs on the job.

HISTORY OF EMPLOYMENT EXAMINATIONS

Medical History

Preemployment examinations have traditionally been used for assessment of the spine. As early as 1947, Stewart described preemployment examinations of the back that included x-rays. However, research later indicated that the correlation between most of the radiographic abnormalities identified on x-rays and the risk of low-back pain is weak. In 1973, the American College of Radiology and the American Occupational Medicine Association joined in a conference to evaluate the effectiveness of such x-rays in comparison with the potential radiation hazards. They concluded that the use of x-rays as the sole criterion for selection of workers was not justified and that more concern was needed to protect workers from unnecessary radiation in such examinations. The use of x-rays has subsequently been refuted and now is obsolete as a reasonable predictor of successful job performance. This is an example of how employment tests based on medical history alone have been discriminatory.

Chaffin et al. (1978) found strength testing to be a better indicator of worker performance in heavy-lifting jobs. Medical history has also been identified and used as a factor in screening workers. The literature makes a strong case for the association of certain conditions with the later development of MSDs, and medical screening often includes a review of medical history.

Several authors have presented the incidence of median nerve injuries in fractures of the distal end of the radius, particularly Colles' fractures. Abbott and Saunders (1933) identified a risk of median nerve compression in fractures of the distal radius. Meadoff (1949) noted median nerve injuries in many fractures in the region of the wrist. Cooney, Dobyns, and Linscheid (1980) identified median nerve entrapment as one complication of Colles' fractures.

Phalen (1966) described diabetes as a risk factor for MSDs. Michaelis (1950) described compression of the median nerve through stenosis of the carpal tunnel and flexor tendon sheath associated with rheumatoid arthritis. In Phalen's study (1966), 49 of the 654 hands studied had rheumatoid arthritis. Forceful gripping and repetitive use of the hand would exacerbate the active synovitis of rheumatoid joints.

Previous surgery for traumatic conditions may inherently impair hand function. Included are limitations from the surgery or trauma itself, the presence of scar tissue, or the residual presence of foreign bodies in the hand (e.g., surgical fixation devices). There is significant literature that correlates development of multiple MSDs. Phalen (1966) reported the following diagnoses occurring with MSDs in his subjects: trigger finger or thumb in 34 hands, de Quervain's disease in 10 hands, and the presence of ganglion cysts in several patients.

Although Phalen (1966) reported that surgical carpal tunnel releases are not necessary in most cases, a case severe enough to need surgery may have sustained permanent vascular changes (Gelberman, Hergenroeder, Hargens, Lundborg, & Akeson, 1981). In the author's experience, there has generally been a small permanent impairment following carpal tunnel release, based on weakness of grip, occasional loss of range of motion, and loss of sensibility.

Analysis of Accuracy in Medical Screening Examinations

In the process of standardization, establishing reliability and validity of an evaluation is a foremost priority. Fess (1986) defines reliability as "...an instrument's ability to measure consistently and predictably" and validity as "...the truthfulness of an assessment tool...to measure that which it purports to measure."

Chaffin and Andersson (1984) identified four measures of an instrument's ability to select workers appropriately: accuracy, sensitivity, specificity, and predictive value. *Accuracy* is "a measure of a screening test's ability to provide a true measure of a quantity or quality." *Sensitivity* is "a measure of a test's accuracy in correctly identifying persons with a certain condition. [It is] the fraction or percentage of all persons with a condition who will have a positive test." Chaffin and Andersson used the following equation to describe sensitivity.

$$\frac{\text{True positives}}{\text{True positives} + \text{False negatives}} \times 100$$

They defined *specificity* as "a measure of a test's accuracy in correctly identifying persons who do not have the condition. It can be expressed as the fraction or percentage of negative tests in persons free of a condition." For this measure, the following equation was proposed.

$$\frac{\text{True negatives}}{\text{True negatives} + \text{False positives}} \times 100$$

Predictive value refers to the test's ability to predict the presence or absence of a specific condition. The predictive value is influenced by the prevalence or base rate of a condition in the general population.

Typical Components of Medical Screening

Although we ultimately strive to design a workplace that "fits" most workers, the concept of job-worker matching is well accepted in our society. Industry uses standard qualifications to screen applicants who should be assessed for material-handling or excessively hand-intensive jobs. Assuring the applicant's fitness for duty before he or she enters the workplace is paramount in reducing the number of sudden-onset disorders and MSDs that a company experiences. In addition, thorough physical and functional testing can establish a baseline by which to compare subsequent tests for changes in functional ability or fair impairment ratings in the event of an injury.

Many factors contribute to successful job performance. Strength, flexibility, endurance, and job skill techniques all have been used to establish work readiness. However, the increasing cost of MSDs in industry has brought some urgency (and in many cases, discriminatory methods) into the employment examination picture.

Such general assessments of hand function as grip and pinch-strength testing have the benefit of establishing "normalcy" of the applicant; however, they can be used only individually as a factor to screen out potential workers if the amount of strength required by the job has been established clearly. To establish this criterion, the following two methods can be used: measuring with sophisticated torque gauges the force needed to perform the job and measuring incumbent worker's strength.

Other, more sophisticated measures of hand function, such as vibrometry, sensibility, and nerve conduction, are being used to establish pass-restrictive criteria (as opposed to pass/fail criteria, which are not appropriate for ADA-acceptable exams) for applicants. The sensitivity of examinations for early MSDs was established by Szabo and Gelberman (1987) in the following order: vibrometry, Semmes-Weinstein Monofilaments (SWMFs), sensory nerve conduction velocity (NCV), moving two-point discrimination, static two-point discrimination, and motor NCV. These components of hand function must not be used randomly or without consideration of the implications of discrimination when they are used only to eliminate a certain class of potentially disabled individuals.

Constraints on the Use of Employment Examinations: The Americans with Disabilities Act

The ADA of 1990 (Public Law 101-336) mandates equal treatment of individuals with disabling conditions and the rest of the nation's citizens. The act became effective for most employers in

July 1992. The ADA mandates accessibility and equality in four primary subtitle areas: Title I, employment; Title II, public services; Title III, public accommodations and services operated by private entities; and Title IV, telecommunications. The directives of Title I affect the use of the employment examinations.

Under the ADA's provisions, applicants to industry can be screened appropriately by the use of standardized medical tests. In such testing, the results are interpreted, and decisions regarding the appropriateness of placement are made on the basis of preestablished criteria. To be effective in disqualifying, without discriminating against, applicants who do not meet physical criteria, such tests must establish appropriate, defensible criteria before examination begins; each applicant for the position must be screened; and interpretation must be made on a pass/fail basis (i.e., the stronger of two applicants—if both meet the criteria established—cannot be chosen on the basis of strength alone).

Employment evaluations can be used to match workers with their jobs but cannot be discriminatory. Examinations can establish the presence of abnormal conditions, but specific portions of the test cannot be interpreted as showing a higher or lower risk for injury. A significant risk—not a nominal risk—of substantial harm must be established. Clearly, workers who are placed in jobs that do not exceed their physical capacity are less likely to become injured. Incumbent workers (those who have been working for the company) also are good candidates for screening once criteria are established. Testing can identify symptomatic and presymptomatic employees, and appropriate intervention can be initiated.

The Americans with Disabilities Act Guidelines and the Definition of Discriminatory Testing Methods

The goal of the ADA is to minimize discrimination in the hiring process. Section 102 of the ADA sets forth this standard, providing "No covered entity shall discriminate against a qualified individual with a disability because of the disability of such individual in regard to job application procedures, the hiring, advancement or discharge of employees, employee compensation, job training, and other terms, conditions, and privileges of employment."

The *Texas Employment Law Handbook* defines different types of discrimination. The following are prohibited by the ADA.

- Opportunity status discrimination based on classification
- Participation in a contract or other arrangement or relationship having a discriminatory affect
- Use of standards, criteria, or methods of administration that have the affect of discrimination on the basis of disability or that perpetuate the discrimination of others who are subject to common administrative control
- Discrimination based on a qualified individual's known association or relationship with disabled individual
- Failure to reasonably accommodate, or denial of opportunity due to need to reasonably accommodate
- Use of qualification standards, employment test, or other selection criteria that tend to screen out disabled individuals, unless the criteria are shown to be job related for the position in question and consistent with business necessity
- Failure to select and administer tests concerning employment in the most effective manner to ensure that tests measure only necessary skills and aptitude rather than reflecting the disability

Medical history inquiries are prohibited in the preoffer stage. With regard to employment physicals (and examination of injured workers who may be covered under ADA), employers may require medical examinations only if they are job related and consistent with business necessity and only after an offer of employment has been made to a job applicant. The physical examination may be given after the conditional job offer and before the commencement of employment duties. An offer of employment, however, may be conditioned on the results of examination only if all employees are subjected to examinations and such information is kept confidential and maintained in separate medical files.

Determining What Constitutes a Disability

To qualify as a disability covered by the ADA, an impairment must limit substantially one or more of the following examples of major life activities.

- Walking
- Speaking
- Breathing
- Caring for oneself
- Performing manual tasks
- Sitting
- Standing
- Seeing
- Hearing
- Learning
- Working
- Lifting

It is not necessary to consider if a person is substantially limited in the major life task of working if the person is substantially limited in any other major life activity.

Employers may not make inquiries of a job applicant as to whether the applicant has a disability or as to the nature or severity of the disability. Employers may ask, however, whether an employee can perform job-related functions and then can evaluate the worker for physical capacity to confirm his or her capabilities.

The ADA defines a qualified individual with a disability as a disabled individual who meets the skill, experience, education, and other job-related requirements of a position held or desired, and who, with or without reasonable accommodation, can perform the essential functions of a job. Therefore, employers evaluate the individual solely based on the ability to perform the essential functions with or without a reasonable accommodation.

When Testing Should Be Done

Examinations may be performed when they are necessitated by business. The ADA's interpretive guidelines state that if a test excludes a person with a disability *because* of issues inherent to the disability and does not relate to the *essential functions of the job,* it is not a business necessity.

Testing may also be done when the test is job related. Interpretive guidelines state that if a qualification test results in screening out an individual with a disability, it must be a legitimate qualification for the *specific* job for which it is being used.

The key to restricting placement of an individual with an MSD on the basis of the medical examination is to establish the significant risk of substantial harm.

Summary: Examinations Allowed Under the Americans with Disabilities Act

Key concepts of the preoffer stage:

1. Coordination or agility test related directly to the essential functions of the job
2. Must offer accommodation
3. Disqualification based on inability to meet critical job tasks' requirements with or without accommodation

Key concepts of postoffer stage:

1. Medical history and related examinations acceptable
2. Must offer accommodation
3. Disqualification must be based on significant risk of substantial harm when performing essential job function

Testing allowed by ADA:

1. Only after an offer of employment has been made
2. Only if all applicants for the position are subject to the examination
3. Only if disqualification is based on job-related and business necessity or placement would pose a significant risk of substantial harm
4. Only if results are kept confidential

Testing prohibited by ADA:

1. Use of standard, criteria, or methods of

administration that have the effect of discrimination
2. Use of qualification standards, unless job related or of business necessity
3. Medical examinations in the preoffer stage
4. Decisions based on physical appearance alone

SUGGESTED ASSESSMENT WITH EMPIRIC EVIDENCE OF ITS ACCURACY IN BOTH NORMAL AND ABNORMAL POPULATIONS

The UEFFDE and its component evaluations suggest a process to establish other groups of assessments that are accurate, reliable and legally defensible. An initial general description is followed by the specific components of the evaluation. Point values and scoring are described in the earlier edition of this chapter (King, 1997).

General Description

The UEFFDE measures hand function to identify those individuals who have symptoms of MSDs. The physical examination uses clinical signs and observations of actual activity. The UEFFDE includes a stress test that uses certain tools with work-simulation equipment. This specific test used the work simulator manufactured by the Baltimore Therapeutic Equipment (BTE) Company, in Baltimore, Maryland. Stress testing occurs before sensibility testing, nerve conduction testing, and observations for Raynaud's phenomenon, triggering finger or thumb, and the presence of edema. This allows for measuring the influence of resistive and repetitive activity on the hand and would better detect the presence of any dynamic pathologic processes (Braun, Davidson, & Doehr, 1989).

Item Development

The subtests of the UEFFDE presented in this chapter are included because of the significant research used to support the rationale and weighting for each test as an indicator of the presence of MSDs. Several authors (American Society for Surgery of the Hand, 1983; Hartwell et al., 1964; Hymovich & Lindholm, 1966; Kuorinka & Koskinen, 1979) have described the value of physical examinations in identifying MSDs. Weighting for the subtests of the UEFFDE have been based on three factors.

The first factor was the relative subjectivity of the examination. Deficits noted in objective measurements of hand function are weighted more heavily in the UEFFDE than are subjective responses. The second consideration was the strength of support and number of citations in the medical literature for the test as a valid measure of the condition. The third consideration was the results of a survey of certified hand therapists who were members of the American Society of Hand Therapists' Occupational Injuries Prevention and Rehabilitation and Clinical Assessment committees.

The therapists were surveyed regarding their opinion on the relative value of the different examinations in accurately determining the diagnosis of an MSD. What follows are the subtests with definitions, methodology, and literature support.

Intrinsic Atrophy

Phalen (1966) described atrophy of the abductor pollicis brevis muscle as one sign of CTS. Over 17 years, 47% of his patients with CTS had this condition. He stated that often this muscle is the first affected by compression of the median nerve. Loong (1977) found a sensitivity of 53% in CTS patients. Feldman, Travers, Chirico-Post, and Keyserling (1987) identified motor weakness of the hand and atrophy of the abductor pollicis brevis muscle in their description of the last stage of CTS. Muscle atrophy involvement has been noted at lower sensitivity by other researchers (Golding, Rose, & Selvarajah, 1986; Shivde & Fisher, 1981). MacDermid (1991) speculated that Phalen's group of subjects presented much later for clinical examination than did those of other researchers. This test is based on visible atrophy and is, thus, an objective measure.

Atrophy or weakness of thenar muscles, if not obvious, can be assessed best by comparison with the contralateral side. The abductor pollicis brevis muscle produces the rounded appearance of the thenar muscle group on the radial aspect of the first metacarpal. Flattening or actual depression indicates atrophy (Figure 15-1). This indication can be confirmed by brief muscle testing (the client points the thumb toward the ceiling while placing the dorsum of the hand and fingers flat against a table surface). For testing of ulnar nerve innervated muscles, the dorsum of the hand is observed for atrophy in the interosseous spaces. If atrophy is not obvious, muscle testing of the dorsal and palmer interossei muscles can be performed by resisting abduction and adduction of the fingers.

Ganglion Cysts

Common sites for development of these cysts are the tendon sheaths, the dorsal wrist in the area of the scapholunate joint, and the volar wrist in the region of the flexor carpi radialis insertion (Figure 15-2). Mathews (1973) described the effects of the ganglia on the flexor tendon sheath in the hand. Ganglia that have developed enough to be palpable can become symptomatic and cause pain (American Society for Surgery of the Hand, 1983). Phalen (1966) identified a correlation between ganglion cysts and other MSDs. Chaffin and Andersson (1984) have noted ganglia as a risk factor for preventing successful performance in high-risk jobs.

Thus, in the literature it is accepted widely that ganglion cysts can be precipitated and worsened by hand-intensive work. The Texas Worker's Compensation Commission has recognized ganglion cysts as a compensable disorder when the worker has acute trauma or cumulative trauma. Failing to note this as an abnormal condition would not protect employers when a cyst was identified in the preplacement setting. Likewise, failure to identify the cyst as an abnormal condition in a follow-up to baseline testing would prevent workers from making a claim for medical and other appropriate compensation. Palpable ganglia either are present or are not and, thus, represent an objective measure.

Sensibility Loss

Feldman et al. (1987) described paresthesia in the median nerve distribution as early as Stage 1 of CTS and identified elevated touch threshold as early as Stage 2. Because of its importance in diagnosis of CTS, sensibility testing has received a large share of attention in the literature (MacDermid, 1991).

Two common clinical examinations used to measure a subject's sensibility are described frequently in the literature: two-point discrimination (both static and moving) and the SWMFs. The SWMFs have been shown to correlate well with reported sensibility impairment by the

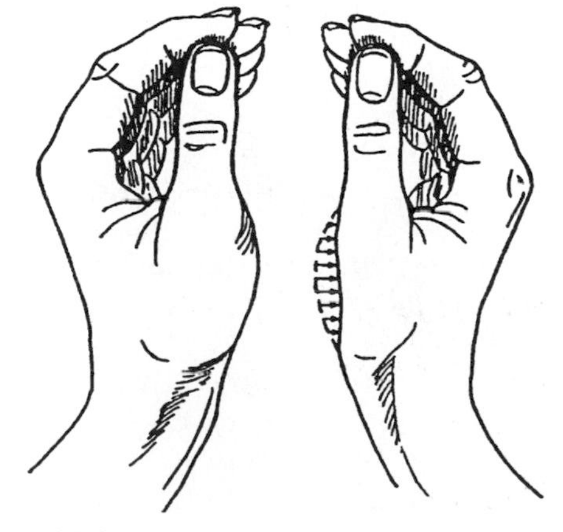
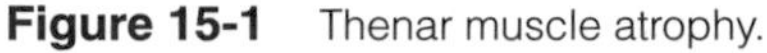

Figure 15-1 Thenar muscle atrophy.

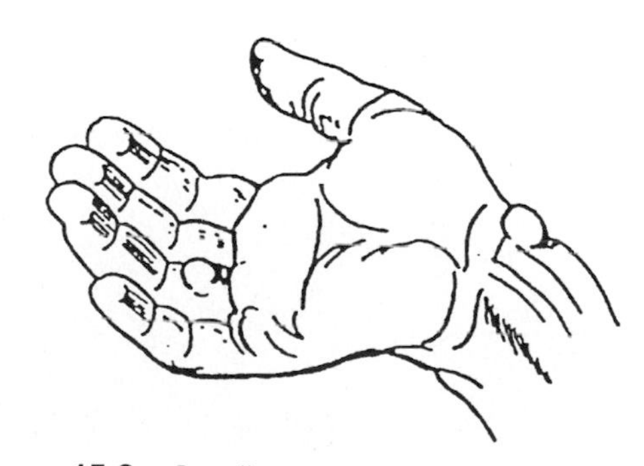

Figure 15-2 Ganglion cysts.

client and sensory nerve conduction tests (Breger, 1987). Dellon (1978) reported that significant areas of peripheral nerves and the brain are devoted to discriminative touch of the hand and that the maximum information on nerve function could be obtained with the two-point discrimination test. Gellman, Gelberman, Tan, and Botte (1986) reported 71.4% sensitivity and 80% specificity for sensibility impairment in 67 electrodiagnostic-positive CTS clients compared with 50 normal controls.

Testing vibration-sense threshold changes with commercially available vibrometers has been advocated (Gelberman, Szabo, Williamson, & Dimick, 1983). However, vibrometry protocols require a subjective response by the individual being tested.

In 1983, Gelberman et al. found a high sensitivity of the SWMFs in identifying CTS. In their research, artificially induced CTS was produced by injecting saline solution into their subjects' carpal canals and was measured with a wick catheter. Their subjects first complained of numbness and tingling leading to loss of vibratory sense. Subjects subsequently experienced loss of perception as measured by the SWMFs, loss of moving two-point discrimination, impairment of sensory nerve conduction, diminished static two-point discrimination, and finally, slowing of motor NCV.

Later, Szabo et al. (1984) compared vibrometry, two-point discrimination, and the SWMFs to evaluate nerve compression. Vibrometry and the SWMFs had a similar sensitivity rate (87% and 83%, respectively) in symptomatic hands. Two-point discrimination had a sensitivity rate of 22%.

For the UEFFDE sensibility test, the SWMFs were used (Figure 15-3). Two-point discrimination and vibrometry were not included in this initial assessment because of its time restraints and to limit the number of subjective sensibility tests.

The monofilaments are nylon filaments of descending thickness attached to lucite rods. Their gradation is based on the force required to bend them when they are placed against the

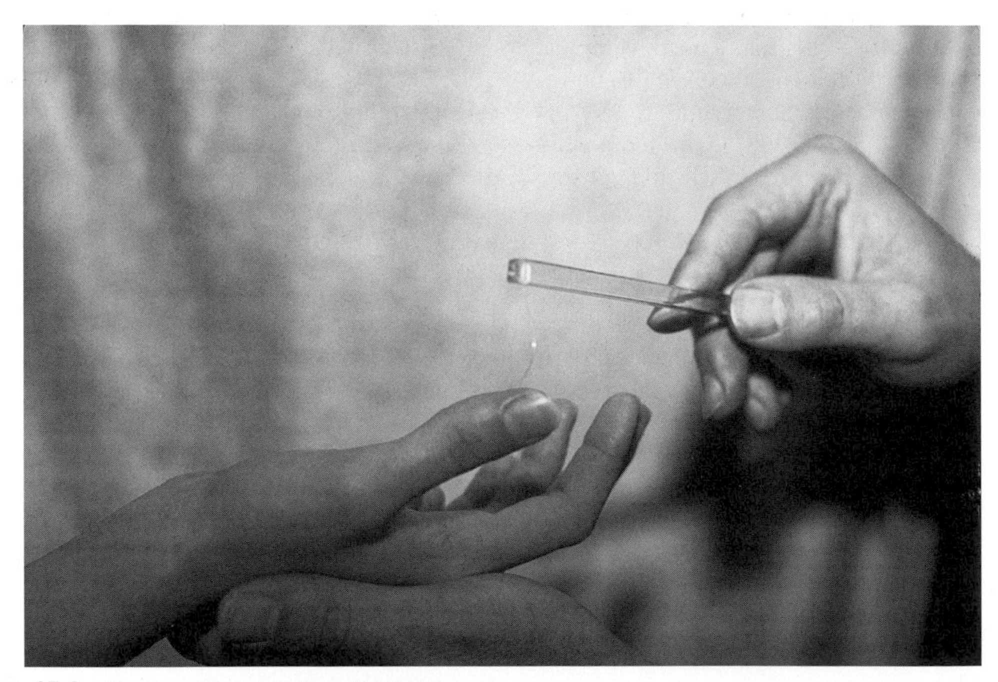

Figure 15-3 Semmes-Weinstein monofilaments.

skin. The monofilament is applied perpendicular to the finger until it bends. The measure of normal sensory threshold is based on the individual's ability to feel and identify the touched finger.

Bell-Krotoski (1987) has verified the test's repeatability and has provided a standardized format for testing with the SWMFs. The 2.83 monofilament is normal for most individuals. Failure of this section would be a sensibility threshold below perception of the 2.83 monofilament in the median or ulnar distribution of the hand. Even though reliable instruments and methods are used, careful interpretation of the results of this examination is required. Many factors, such as calluses on the subject's fingertips, can influence the examination. Because it requires response from the subject, the test is subjective; however, its interpretation is objective because of the validity of the SWMFs.

Triggering

Triggering can be very painful and can impair hand function significantly (American Society for Surgery of the Hand, 1983). This disorder can be identified by placing the examiner's fingers over the volar, proximal surface of the metacarpophalangeal joints of the fingers and asking the person to open and close the hand slowly and completely. The thumb is examined in the same manner (Figure 15-4). Snapping or locking of a finger would be a positive response and is measured objectively.

Triggering is one sequela of finger tenosynovitis strongly correlated with repetitive forceful motion, excessive contact, and vibration exposure over the volar surfaces of the metacarpophalangeal joints of the hand (Chaffin & Andersson, 1984). Similar to ganglion cysts, triggering has been identified as a compensable disorder in workers who perform high-risk activities. For the same rationale as noted earlier to protect employer and worker, the presence of triggering is identified as an abnormal condition in the UEFFDE. Triggering is an objectively measurable phenomenon.

Raynaud's Phenomenon

If present, Raynaud's phenomenon would be observed most readily following stress testing. It occurs as blanching or coldness in one or more of the fingers (Taylor, 1982). For this test, the examiner palpates the fingers to feel for coldness. Each fingernail is pinched to observe capillary refill. In the presence of Raynaud's phenomenon, sensibility may be affected as well. Brown (1990) reported this phenomenon as a significant MSD in industry.

Epicondylar Pain

Epicondylar pain is identified as expressed tenderness over the lateral or medial epicondyle and is isolated via palpation of the area during pronation and flexion of the wrist. Lateral epicondylitis is assessed best during the examination for Phalen's test (described later). It is a subjective test.

While the subject is in the position for the Phalen's test, the examiner palpates the region of the lateral and medial epicondyle of the humerus from 1 inch above to 3 inches below the

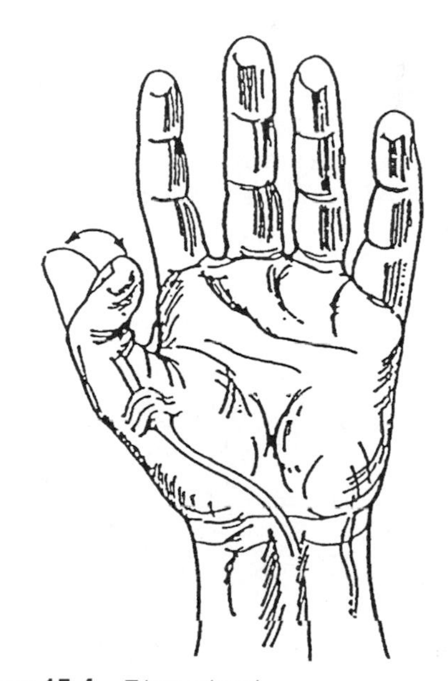

Figure 15-4 Trigger thumb.

elbow crease. A positive sign is tenderness or wincing by the subject. Epicondylitis also likely would manifest itself as weakness of grip or pinch.

Tinel's Sign

Tinel's sign is recorded as positive when symptoms of tingling occur on tapping over the anatomic distribution of the nerve. As early as 1946, Weddell and Sinclair identified "pins and needles" with mechanical compression of a nerve. In 1966, Phalen described a positive Tinel's sign from percussion of the median nerve at the carpal tunnel in many of his CTS patients (Figure 15-5). A Tinel's sign of the anatomic distribution at the elbow may be present with cubital tunnel syndrome or at the wrist on the ulnar side with Guyon's canal syndrome (American Society for Surgery of the Hand, 1983). The test for Tinel's sign requires a subjective response.

A Tinel's sign is not always indicative of a disease process, however, because it may be present in the normal population as well. Although LaBan, Friedman, and Zemenick (1988) reported a sensitivity of 100% in a small population of chronic carpal tunnel clients, in 1990 de Krom, Knipchild, Kester, and Spaans (as reported by MacDermid (1991) found 25% sensitivity and 59% specificity in 715 randomly chosen persons. Gellman et al. (1986) reported 43.9% sensitivity and 94% specificity for Tinel's sign. The relatively low specificity and sensitivity rates given by de Krom et al. (1990) and Gellman et al. (1986), as well as the level of subjectivity of the response by tested individuals, would favor weighting Tinel's sign lower.

Finkelstein's Test

Finkelstein's test is performed by having the individual grasp the thumb with the fingers (thumb in palm) and ulnarly deviate the wrist (Figure 15-6). This is the recommended method for evaluating de Quervain's disease; if the maneuver reproduces or exacerbates the pain at the base of the thumb, the test is positive (American Society for Surgery of the Hand, 1983). Stenosis, or catching of the tendon, in this area is palpable by the examiner. The test requires a subjective response, and no sensitivity or specificity data have been found in the literature.

Phalen's Test

In 1966, Phalen described for CTS a wrist flexion test that is positive when numbness and paresthesia in the median nerve distribution is reported by the subject following the wrist held in complete flexion for 30 to 60 seconds. Sensitivity for Phalen's test in CTS clients has been reported as high by LaBan et al. (1988) and moderate by de Krom et al. (1990). It requires a subjective response.

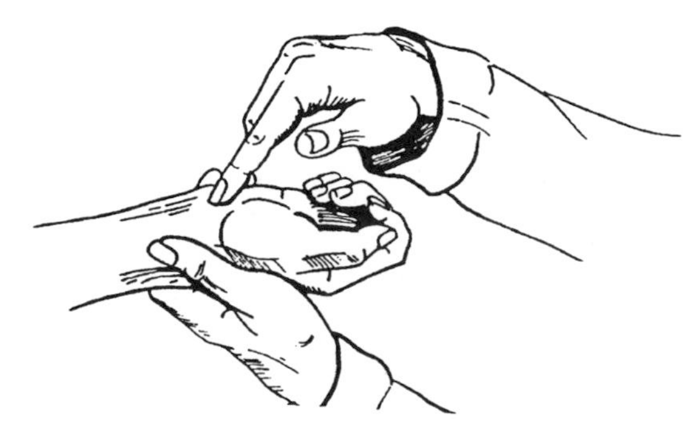

Figure 15-5 Test for Tinel's sign: median nerve at the wrist.

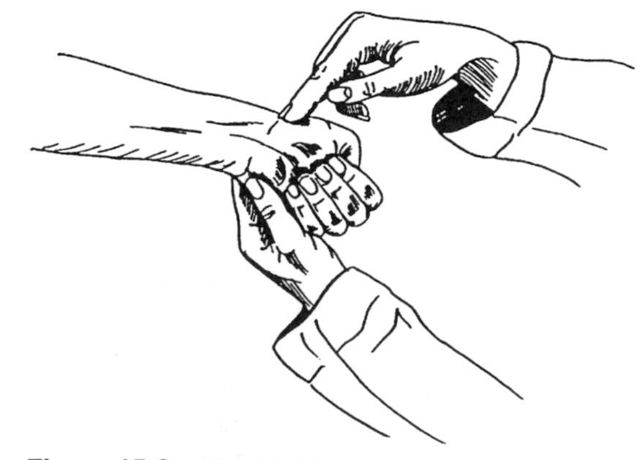

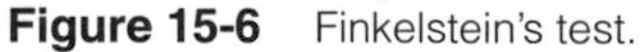

Figure 15-6 Finkelstein's test.

Smith, Sonstegard, and Anderson (1977) described a modified Phalen's test (Figure 15-7) wherein the fingers are pinched in addition to flexion of the wrist. The protocol for this test instructs the subject to hold the modified Phalen's test for 1 minute, with expressed numbness, tingling, or other paresthetic sensory phenomena judged as a positive response. The test is known as being sensitive to median nerve compression.

Weakness of Grip or Pinch

Mathiowetz, Weber, Volland, & Kashman (1984) have shown that grip and pinch strength evaluations performed in standardized positions are reliable and valid. Mathiowetz et al. (1986) presented norms for pinch and grip strength in adults. The instruments used for this portion of the evaluation are the Jamar dynamometer (TEC, Clifton, NJ) and the pinch gauge (Figure 15-8).

Both Feldman et al. (1987) and Phalen (1966) have identified individuals with CTS having decreased grip and pinch strength. Loong (1977) has reported 53% sensitivity for pinch weakness in CTS clients. Although it requires effort by the individual, grip and pinch testing generally is considered objective.

Abnormal Nerve Conduction Velocity

Feldman et al. (1987) identified slowed motor latency of the median nerve as early as Stage 3 CTS. A portable electroneurometer (Figure 15-9) manufactured by Neurotron Medical (Lawrenceville, NJ) was used in the UEFFDE to screen the median nerve motor latency at the wrist. Rosier and Blair (1984) described the electroneurometer as providing less information than does standard NCV equipment. However, they reported that it served as a diagnostic adjunct for median and ulnar compression

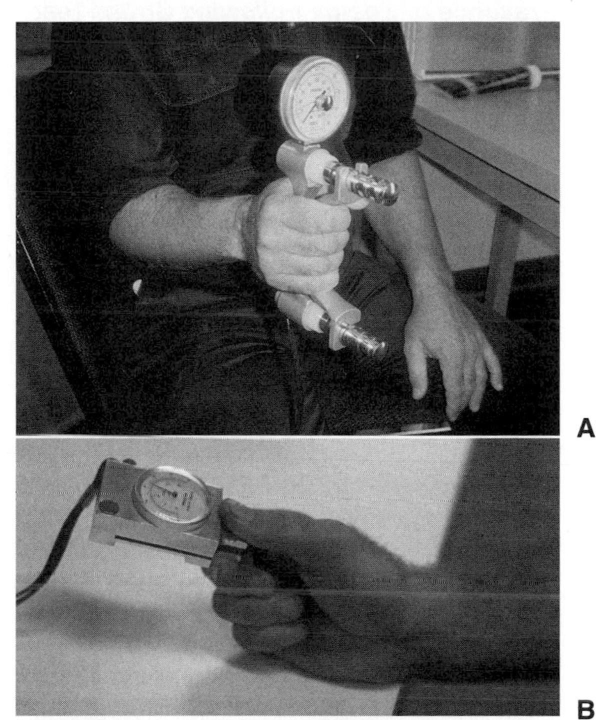

Figure 15-8 **A,** Dynamometer. **B,** Pinch gauge.

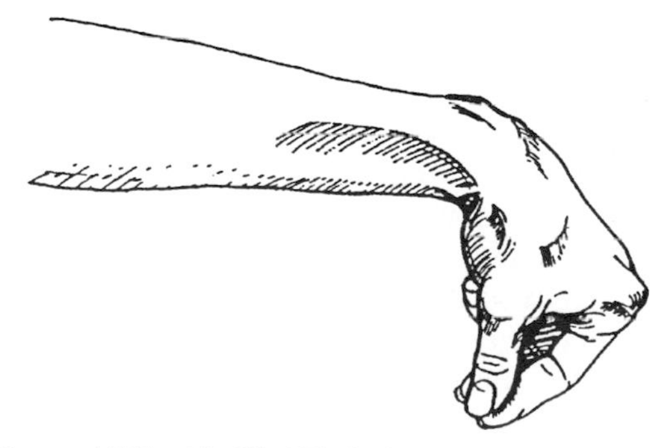
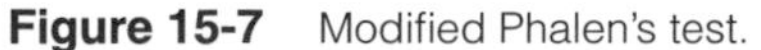

Figure 15-7 Modified Phalen's test.

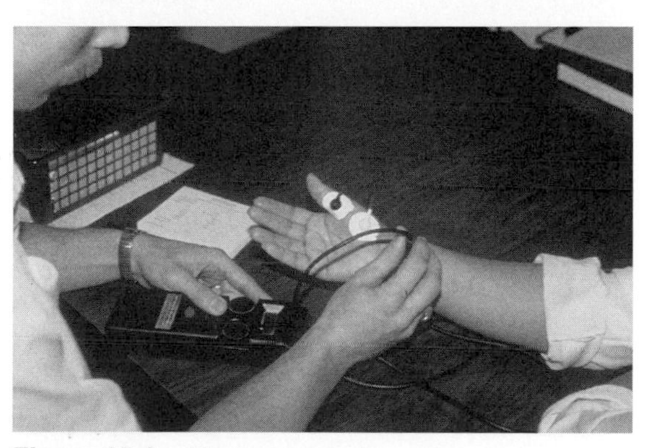

Figure 15-9 Electroneurometer.

neuropathy. Their study supported excellent correlation between diagnoses made with the electroneurometer and standard techniques of nerve conduction. They determined NCVs of 4.40 milliseconds or greater in the median nerve at the wrist measured with the electroneurometer as abnormal.

Presence of Edema Following Stress Test

Edema is a symptom of inflammatory disorders. Braun et al. (1989) stated that provocative testing measures, such as those proposed, would better identify dynamic pathologic conditions of the hand. The presence of edema following exercise similar to the person's work (stressing) can be measured with a commercially available volumeter.

Waylett-Rendall and Sibley (1991) found the volumeter (Figure 15-10) to be accurate within 1%. They recommended consistent placement of the volumeter, careful filling of the tank, and standardized instruction to increase the instrument's accuracy.

In the UEFFDE, the worker undergoes a stress test using tools of the BTE work simulator. Curtis and Engalitcheff (1981) described the work simulator as a way to perform many functional activities in the clinic. The simulator has an adjustable isotonic force-producing mechanism that can be used to alter the amount of resistance to turn a tool in a shaft. Workers performed at 30% of maximum isometric torque, moving the chosen tool one repetition per second for 90 seconds. Three tools were used; the BTE No. 701 (wrist flexion and extension), the No. 302 (wrist ulnar-radial deviation), and the No. 162 (finger flexion and extension) (Figure 15-11).

To determine an acceptable percentage of volumetric change, the author reviewed the results of McGough and Zurwasky's study (1991) that assessed volumetric change following activity. In a pilot study, they reported that the normal increase in volume, measured 5 minutes following similar activities proposed for the stress test, was 3.6% for women and 5.4% for men (mean of total group = 4.5%).

Because the goal was to measure for and identify edema, a 5-minute rest period was taken before the poststress test volumetric measurements were taken. During that time, the individuals participated in the poststress portions of the evaluation. With this stress test and the accurate measure of hand volume before and after, an objective measure indicating 5% change or greater would represent a positive sign and a failing score for that subtest.

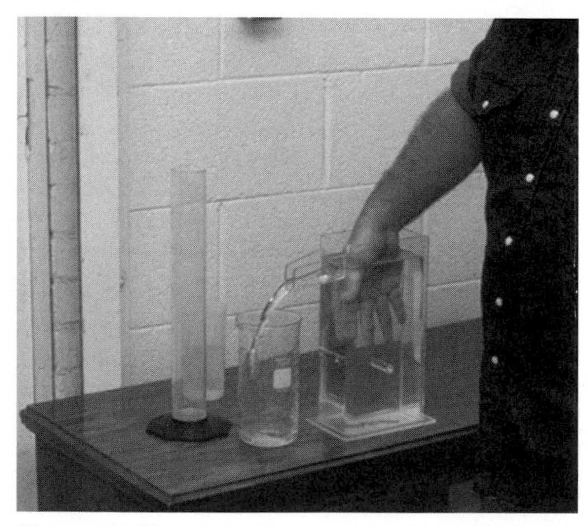

Figure 15-10 Volumeter.

UPPER-EXTREMITY FITNESS-FOR-DUTY EVALUATION ACCURACY

The UEFFDE was used to assess 30 injured participants (group A) with a total of 43 affected hands and a total of 60 hands from 30 normal participants (group B). Following the evaluation, each of the person's hands was scored independently and, on the basis of the score, categorized as within acceptable limits, suspect, or abnormal condition identified. Classification for each hand tested in the two groups and subsequent analysis of accuracy by sensitivity and specificity equations was based on these categorizations (see King [1997] for specifics of subject demographics and scoring). Analysis of UEFFDE results indicated high sensitivity and

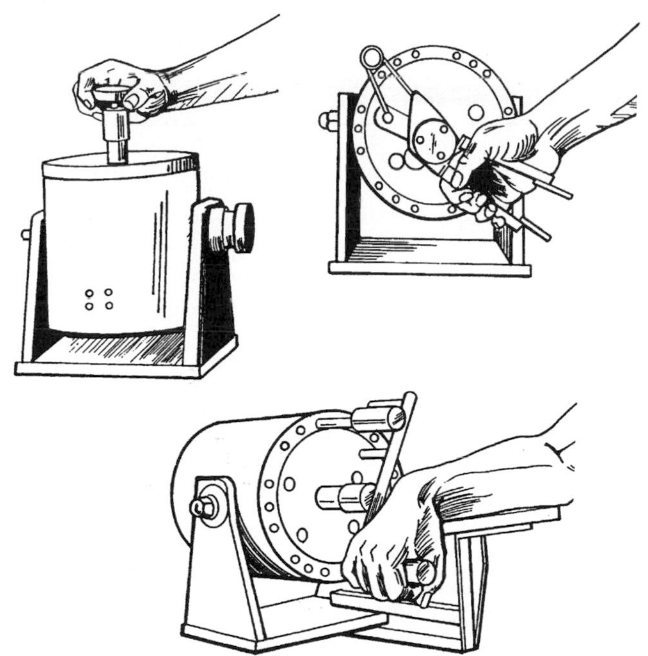

Figure 15-11 Tools in the Baltimore Therapeutic Equipment Work Simulator.

specificity rates for abnormal and normal hands tested. Sensitivity and specificity of the subtests are detailed in Table 15-1.

The findings support the hypothesis that analysis of accuracy of the UEFFDE would reveal a high percentage of sensitivity in a population of subjects with known MSDs. They also support a high percentage of specificity in a population of normal participants who have not been exposed to high-risk jobs and have no history of hand disorders. Percentages for both sensitivity and specificity have exceeded the hypothesized percentage of 90%. It is concluded that the UEFFDE, as a clinical assessment, has been an accurate measure for the presence of MSDs in this population.

Use of the Upper-Extremity Fitness-for-Duty Evaluation in Industry

It is recognized that, in addition to identifying personal risk factors in applicants in preplacement examinations, the UEFFDE would be useful in establishing a baseline level of function and then following up for threshold changes in workers in high-risk industries. The UEFFDE could also be used to assess individuals with diabetes or other central nervous system problems.

Significant changes in hand function could be indicative of systemic diseases other than an MSD. The UEFFDE is a screening test and cannot be substituted for thorough medical examinations. It does have value in its ability to correctly classify individuals who have hand disorders. Within the guidelines of the ADA, the UEFFDE's results are suggestive and useful as a measure of who will need reasonable accommodation.

As a baseline, follow-up examination and routine screening could be used with workers to identify threshold changes and lead to either changing the job or removing a worker periodically or permanently from such work. Recommended time frames for reevaluations would be 3 months for newly hired individuals placed in high-risk jobs and 6 months for less-

Table 15-1
Sensitivity and Specificity of Subtests

Subtest	Diagnosis	Sensitivity (%)	Specificity (%)
Atrophy	CT	23.8	100.0
Ganglion	GC	100.0	100.0
Sensibility	CT	61.9	100.0
Triggering	TF	100.0	100.0
Raynaud's phenomenon	CT	0.0	100.0
Epicondylar pain	EP	100.0	96.6
Tinel's sign	CT, C	61.9	95.0
Finkelstein's test	DQ	100.0	98.3
Phalen's test	CT	52.4	98.3
Weak grip, pinch	All	72.1	98.3
Abnormal nerve conduction velocity	CT	61.9	100.0
Edema	All	23.8	100.0

C, Cubital tunnel syndrome; *CT*, carpal tunnel syndrome; *DQ*, de Quervain's syndrome; *EP*, epicondylitis; *GC*, ganglion cyst; *TF*, trigger finger.

hand-intensive work. After that, yearly analysis would be recommended.

Threshold Changes

If threshold changes were noted from baseline function, the worker could be retested within 2 days to confirm the results. Medical treatment or removal from risk factors (depending on the severity of the problem) would be indicated if the follow-up and repeat test indicated a significant change in hand function. A concern is that the UEFFDE may not identify changes until symptoms are present.

Use of the Upper-Extremity Fitness-for-Duty Evaluation as Part of an Overall Prevention Program

Early use of the UEFFDE to follow up on injured workers would assure job-worker matching when such individuals return to work following an injury. As part of an overall program of ergonomic job analysis and changes and of identification of early symptoms to facilitate treatment, the UEFFDE has been shown to be sensitive and specific enough to clearly identify those individuals with problems that should be treated.

ETHICAL AND LEGAL RIGHTS OF EMPLOYERS AND EMPLOYEES

Prior to employment, identification of any hand impairment would be beneficial to employers in the event that an injury occurred later. For example, if the UEFFDE determined sensibility impairment of 25% to one finger in an applicant, and that worker subsequently had an injury leading to amputation of the finger, the employer would only be liable for 75% of the final impairment.

Another use of UEFFDE information in relation to workers would be to help resolve the question of whether hand-intensive work leads to the development of MSDs. In the past, physicians and therapists have relied on "reasonable medical probability" to make the determination of causation. The incidence and prevalence rates of MSDs in a given population of workers could be established by use of the UEFFDE.

If the prevalence of the disorder in any given group did not exceed that of the average population, any developing disorders would not be compensable under workers' compensation laws. Likewise, the employee would have a claim if the rate exceeded the average population. This arrangement would remove the burden of proof from any one source and would provide a legal definition of financial responsibility.

REFERENCES

Abbott, L. C., & Saunders, J. B. (1933). Injuries of the median nerve in fractures of the lower end of the radius, *Surgery, Gynecology, and Obstetrics, 57,* 507–516.

American Society for Surgery of the Hand. (1983). *The hand examination and diagnosis* (2nd ed.). New York: Churchill Livingstone.

Americans with Disabilities Act. (1990). Public Law 101-336, S. 933.

Armstrong, T. J., & Chaffin, D. P. (1979). Carpal tunnel syndrome and selected personal attributes. *Journal of Occupational Medicine, 21,* 481–486.

Armstrong, T. J., Radwin, R. G., Hansen, D. J., & Kennedy, K. W. (1986). Repetitive trauma disorders: Job evaluation and design. *Human Factors, 28,* 325–336.

Bell-Krotoski, J. (1987). The repeatability of testing with the Semmes-Weinstein monofilaments. *Journal of Hand Surgery (Am), 12,* 155–161.

Bleecker, M. L. (1987). Medical surveillance for carpal tunnel syndrome in workers. *Journal of Hand Surgery (Am), 12,* 845–848.

Braun, R. M., Davidson, K., & Doehr, S. (1989). Provocative testing in the diagnosis of carpal tunnel syndrome. *Journal of Hand Surgery (Am), 14,* 195–197.

Breger, D. (1987). Correlating Semmes-Weinstein monofilament mappings with sensory nerve conduction parameters in Hansen's disease patients: An update. *Journal of Hand Therapy, 1,* 33–37.

Brown, A. P. (1990). The effects of anti-vibration gloves on vibration-induced disorders: A case study. *Journal of Hand Therapy, 3,* 94–100.

Castelli, W. A., Evans, F. G., Diaz-Perez, R., & Armstrong, T. J. (1980). Intraneural connective tissue proliferation of the median nerve in the carpal tunnel. *Archives of Physical Medicine and Rehabilitation, 61,* 418–422.

Chaffin, D. B., & Andersson, G. B. J. (1984). *Occupational biomechanics.* New York: Wiley.

Chaffin, D. B., Herrin, G. D., & Keyserling, W. M. (1978). Pre-employment strength testing: An updated position. *Journal of Occupational Medicine, 20,* 403–408.

Chu, B M., & Blatz, P. J. (1972). Cumulative microdamage model to describe the hysteresis of living tissue. *Annals of Biomedical Engineering, 1,* 204–211.

Cooney, W. P., Dobyns, J. H., & Linscheid, R. L. (1980). Complications of Colles' fractures. *Journal of Bone and Joint Surgery (Am), 62,* 613–619.

Curtis, R. M., & Engalitcheff, J. (1981). A work simulator for rehabilitating the upper extremity—preliminary report. *Journal of Hand Surgery, 6,* 499–501.

de Krom, M. C., Knipchild, P. G., Kester, A. D. M., & Spaans, F. (1990). Efficiency of provocative tests for the diagnosis of carpal tunnel syndrome. *Lancet, 335,* 393–395.

Dellon, A. L. (1978). The moving two-point discrimination test: Clinical evaluation of the quickly adapting fiber/receptor system. *Journal of Hand Surgery, 7,* 252–259.

Feldman, R. G., Travers, P. H., Chirico-Post, J., & Keyserling, W. M. (1987). Risk assessment in electronic assembly workers: Carpal tunnel syndrome. *Journal of Hand Surgery (Am), 12,* 849–855.

Fess, E. E. (1986). The need for reliability and validity in hand assessment instruments. *Journal of Hand Surgery, 5,* 621–623.

Gelberman, R. H., Hergenroeder, P. T., Hargens, A. R., Lundborg, G. N., & Akeson, W. H. (1981). The carpal tunnel syndrome: A study of carpal canal pressures. *Journal of Bone and Joint Surgery (Am), 63,* 380–383.

Gelberman, R. H., Szabo, R. M., Williamson, R. V., & Dimick, M. P. (1983). Sensibility testing in peripheral nerve compression syndromes. *Journal of Bone and Joint Surgery (Am), 65,* 632–638.

Gellman, H., Gelberman, R. H., Tan, A. M., & Botte, M. J. (1986). Carpal tunnel syndrome: An evaluation of the provocative diagnostic tests. *Journal of Bone and Joint Surgery (Am), 68,* 735–737.

Gilbreth, F. B., & Gilbreth, L. M. (1924). Classifying the elements of work. *Manage Administration, 8,* 151.

Golding, D. N., Rose, D. M., & Selvarajah, K. (1986). Clinical tests for carpal tunnel syndrome: An evaluation. *British Journal of Rheumatology, 25,* 388–390.

Hartwell, S. W., Larson, R. D., & Posch, J. L. (1964). Tenosynovitis in women in industry. *Cleveland Clinic Quarterly, 31,* 115–118.

Hymovich, L., & Lyndholm, M. (1966). Hand, wrist, and forearm injuries—the result of repetitive motions. *Journal of Occupational Medicine, 8,* 573–577.

Kazarian, L. E. (1975). Creep characteristics of the human spinal column. *Orthopedic Clinics of North America, 6*(1), 3–18.

King, J. W. (1990). An integration of medicine and industry. *Journal of Hand Therapy, 3,* 45–50.

King, J. W. (1997). Employment examinations. In M. Sanders (Ed.), *Management of cumulative trauma disorders.* Woburn, MA: Butterworth-Heinemann.

Kuorinka, I., & Koskinen, P. (1979). Occupational rheumatic diseases and upper-limb strain in manual jobs in a light mechanical industry. *Scandinavian Journal of Work, Environment, and Health, 5,* 9–47.

LaBan, M. M., Friedman, N. A., & Zemenick, G. A. (1988). "Tethered" median nerve stress test in chronic carpal tunnel syndrome. *Archives of Physical Medicine and Rehabilitation, 67,* 803–804.

Littler, J. W. (1960). The physiology and dynamic function of the hand. *Surgical Clinics of North America, 40,* 259–266.

Loong, S. C. (1977). The carpal tunnel syndrome: A clinical and electrophysiological study in 250 patients. *Clinical and Experimental Neurology, 14,* 51–65.

MacDermid, J. (1991). Accuracy of clinical tests used in the detection of carpal tunnel syndrome: A literature review. *Journal of Hand Therapy, 4,* 169–176.

Masear, V. R., Hayes, J. M., & Hyden, A. G. (1986). An industrial cause of carpal tunnel syndrome. *Journal of Hand Surgery (Am), 11,* 222-227.

Mathews, P. (1973). Ganglia of the flexor tendon sheaths in the hand. *Journal of Bone and Joint Surgery (Br), 55,* 612–617.

Mathiowetz, V., Kashman, N., Volland, G., Weber, K., Dowe, M., & Rogers, S. (1986). Grip and pinch strength: Normative data for adults. *Archives of Physical Medicine and Rehabilitation, 66,* 69–74.

Mathiowetz, V., Weber, K., Volland, G., & Kashman, N. (1984). Reliability and validity of grip and pinch strength evaluations. *Journal of Hand Surgery (Am), 9,* 222-226.

McGough, C. E., & Zurwasky, M. L. (1991). Effect of exercise on volumetric and sensory status of the asymptomatic hand. *Journal of Hand Therapy, 4,* 177–180.

Meadoff, N. (1949). Median nerve injuries in fractures in the region of the wrist. *California Medicine, 70,* 252–256.

Michaelis, L. S. (1950). Stenosis of carpal tunnel; compression of median nerve, and flexor tendon sheaths, combined with rheumatoid arthritis elsewhere. *Proceedings of the Royal Society of Medicine, 43,* 414–417.

Phalen, G. S. (1966). The carpal tunnel syndrome. Seventeen years' experience in diagnosis and treatment of 654 hands. *Journal of Bone and Joint Surgery (Am), 48,* 211–228.

Rosier, R. N., & Blair, W. F. (1984). Preliminary clinical evaluation of the digital neurometer. *Proceedings of the Twenty-First Annual Rocky Mountain Bioengineering Symposium and Twenty-First International ISA Biomedical Sciences Instrumentation Symposium,* Boulder, CO.

Shivde, A. J., & Fisher, M. A. (1981). The carpal tunnel syndrome: A clinical-electrodiagnostic analysis. *Electromyography and Clinical Neurophysiology, 21,* 143–153.

Smith, E. M., Sonstegard, D. A., & Anderson, W. H. (1977). Carpal tunnel syndrome: Contribution of flexor tendons. *Archives of Physical Medicine and Rehabilitation, 58,* 379–385.

Stewart, S. F. (1947). Pre-employment examinations of the back. *Journal of Bone and Joint Surgery, 29,* 215–236.

Szabo, R. M., & Gelberman, R. H. (1987). The pathophysiology of nerve entrapment syndromes. *Journal of Hand Surgery (Am), 12,* 880–884.

Szabo, R. M., Gelberman, R. H., Williamson, R. V., Dellon, A. L., Yaru, N. C., & Dimick, M. P. (1984). Vibratory sensory testing in acute peripheral nerve compression. *Journal of Hand Surgery (Am), 9,* 104–109.

Taylor, W. (1982). Vibration white finger in the workplace. *Journal of the Society of Occupational Medicine, 32,* 159–166.

Waylett-Rendall, J., & Sibley, D. S. (1991). A study of the accuracy of a commercially available volumeter. *Journal of Hand Therapy, 4,* 10–13.

Weddell, G., & Sinclair, D.C. (1946). Pins and needles: observations on some of the sensations aroused in a limb by the application of pressure. *Journal of Neurology, Neurosurgery, and Psychiatry, 23,* 26–46.

SUGGESTED READING

Amadio, P. C. (1987). Carpal tunnel syndrome, pyridoxine, and the workplace. *Journal of Hand Surgery (Am), 12,* 875–879.

Armstrong, T. J., Fine, L. J., Goldstein, S. A., Lifshitz, Y. R., & Silverstein, B. A. (1987). Ergonomics considerations in hand and wrist tendinitis. *Journal of Hand Surgery (Am), 12,* 830–837.

Arndt, R. (1987). Workpace, stress, and cumulative trauma disorders. *Journal of Hand Surgery (Am), 12,* 866–869.

Arons, M. S. (1987). de Quervain's disease in working women: A report of failures, complications, and associated diagnoses. *Journal of Hand Surgery (Am), 12,* 540–544.

Barrer, S. J. (1991). Gaining the upper hand on carpal tunnel syndrome. *Occupational Health and Safety, 60,* 38–43.

Berryhill, B. H. (1990). Returning the worker with an upper extremity injury to industry: A model for the physician and therapist. *Journal of Hand Therapy, 3,* 56–63.

Bohannon, R. W. (Ed.). (1988). *Measurement of muscle performance.* Washington, DC: American Physical Therapy Association.

Brain, W., Wright, A., & Wilkinson, M. (1947). Spontaneous compression of both median nerves in the carpal tunnel. *Lancet, 292,* 277–282.

Fess, E. E. (1984). Documentation: Essential elements of an upper extremity assessment battery. In J. M. Hunter, L. H. Schneider, E. J. Mackin, & A. D. Callahan (Eds.), *Rehabilitation of the hand.* St Louis: Mosby.

Fine, L. J., Silverstein, B. A., Armstrong, T. J., Anderson, C. A., & Sugano, D. S. (1986). Detection of cumulative trauma disorders of the upper extremities in the workplace. *Journal of Occupational Medicine, 28,* 674–678.

Gilbert, J. C., & Knowlton, R. G. (1983). Simple method to determine sincerity of effort during a maximal isometric test of grip strength. *American Journal of Physical Medicine, 62,* 135–144.

Johnson, S. L. (1990). Ergonomic design of handheld tools to prevent trauma to the hand and upper extremity. *Journal of Hand Therapy, 3,* 86–93.

King, J. W., & Berryhill, B. H. (1988). A comparison of two static grip testing methods and its clinical applications: A preliminary study. *Journal of Hand Therapy, 1,* 204–209.

King, J. W., & Berryhill, B. H. (1991). Assessing maximum effort in upper extremity functional testing. *Work, 1,* 65–76.

Kurppa, K., Pekka, W., & Rokkanen, P. (1979). Paratendinitis and tenosynovitis: A review. *Scandinavian Journal of Work, Environment, and Health, 5,* 19–24.

Lundborg, G., Gelberman, R. H., Convely-Minteer, M., Lee, Y. F., & Hargress, A. R. (1982). Median nerve compression in the carpal tunnel—functional response to experimentally induced controlled pressure. *Journal of Hand Surgery, 7,* 252-259.

Louis, D. S. (1987). Cumulative trauma disorders. *Journal of Hand Surgery (Am), 12,* 823-825.

Matheson, L. N. (1988). How do you know he tried his best? The reliability crisis in industrial rehabilitation. *Industrial Rehabilitation Quarterly, 1,* 11.

Meagher, S. W. (1987). Tool design for prevention of hand and wrist injuries. *Journal of Hand Surgery (Am), 12,* 855-857.

Muffly-Elsey, D., & Flinn-Wagner, S. (1987). Proposed screening tool for the detection of cumulative trauma disorders of the upper extremity. *Journal of Hand Surgery (Am), 12,* 931-935.

Niebuhr, B. R., & Marion, R. (1986). Detecting sincerity of effort when measuring grip strength. *American Journal of Physical Medicine, 66,* 16-24.

Occupational Safety and Health Administration. (1990). *Ergonomics program management guidelines for meatpacking plants.* Washington, DC: US Department of Labor, Occupational Safety and Health Administration.

Pekka, W. (1979). Epidemiology screening of occupational neck and upper limb disorders: Methods and criteria. *Scandinavian Journal of Work, Environment, and Health, 5,* 25-38.

Phalen, G. S. (1972). The carpal tunnel syndrome. *Clinical Orthopaedics and Related Research, 1,* 29-40.

Pinkham, J. (1988). Carpal tunnel syndrome sufferers find relief with ergonomic designs. *Occupational Health and Safety, 8,* 49-52.

Punnent, L. (1987). Upper-extremity musculoskeletal disorders in hospital workers. *Journal of Hand Surgery (Am), 12,* 858-862.

Robbins, H. (1963). Anatomical study of the median nerve in the carpal tunnel and etiologies of the carpal-tunnel syndrome. *Journal of Bone and Joint Surgery (Am), 45,* 953-966.

Schenk, R. R. (1989). Carpal tunnel syndrome: The new industrial epidemic. *Journal of the American Association of Occupational Health Nurses, 37,* 226-231.

Silverstein, B. A., Fine, L. J., & Armstrong, T. J. (1986). Hand, wrist cumulative trauma disorders in industry. *British Journal of Industrial Medicine, 43,* 779-784.

Silverstein, B., Fine, L., & Stetson, D. (1987). Hand/wrist disorders among investment casting plant workers. *Journal of Hand Surgery (Am), 12,* 838-844.

Smith, B. L. (1987). An inside look: Hand injury prevention program. *Journal of Hand Surgery (Am), 12,* 940-943.

Stokes, H. M. (1983). The seriously uninjured hand—weakness of grip. *Journal of Occupational Medicine, 25,* 683-684.

Tanzer, R. (1959). The carpal tunnel syndrome. *Clinical Orthopaedics and Related Research, 41A,* 171-180.

Texas Association of Business. (1991). *Texas Employment Law Handbook,* 21-1-21-6.

CHAPTER 16

Implementing an Effective Injury Prevention Process

Michael Melnick

THE EVOLUTION OF INJURY PREVENTION

This chapter focuses on the evolution of injury prevention as a field, the evolution of the careers of those who provide injury prevention services, and the evolution of programs in companies that choose to undertake such an endeavor. All three of these need to evolve if the concept of injury prevention is to prove truly successful.

Process versus Program

There is a basic difference between a *process* and a *program*. A *program* has a recognizable beginning and end; a *process* has a recognizable beginning but no definitive end. By definition, a process grows and changes. Programs may be 1-hour endeavors, whereas processes are a series of ongoing events that lead to real and permanent change. A back class is a program. The combination of a back class and ergonomics is part of a process.

This chapter addresses the means to implement an injury prevention process. It first introduces the key features of this process (players, money, time) and then discusses how to develop an injury prevention process.

Key Features of an Injury Prevention Process

Successful injury prevention processes rely on a series of fairly basic steps: identifying the problem or problems, implementing effective solutions, and then growing and maintaining this process in the context of the company or business. There are three variables in this equation that can complicate the process: the people who are involved, the money that must be invested, and the time it takes to do injury prevention.

The People

The first and most influential variable in an injury prevention process is the people who will be involved. This includes the consultant, company management, supervisory staff, hourly and salaried employees, union members, the medical community, the legal community, and the entire workers' compensation system. Each of these groups possesses unique talents, personalities, and preconceived ideas of what does and does not work.

Consultants are the provider of the services. Each consultant brings to the workplace a unique set of skills, strengths, and philosophies. When a company calls in an injury prevention consultant, the professional backgrounds of the individuals may be occupational or physical therapists, exercise physiologists, engineers, chiropractors, and so on. Since each provider has a different perspective on how to reduce injuries in the workplace, it is unusual for a company to get all of its injury prevention needs met using the skill set of one particular consultant.

Managers face many challenges. Although managers need to reduce injuries and the associated costs, they are also committed to moving production forward without interruption. Injury prevention is often perceived as an interruption.

Supervisors are most often accountable for the implementation of the injury prevention process. This group is often sandwiched between the expectations of management (production and quality) and the day-to-day interactions with employees. In this group quality and productivity often take priority over safety.

Employees are expected to make the most dramatic changes as a part of the injury prevention process. Many of the employees have existing injuries and preconceived ideas of what the process entails. Many have sat through dozens of back classes, have questioned management's commitment to injury prevention, and have been performing their jobs the same way for the last decade. This creates a very interesting challenge for a consultant who is expected to teach these people how to lift or use their bodies properly.

Unions question the value of this process for its members. If the injury prevention process affects the ways jobs will be performed, how jobs are categorized, the amount of overtime that may be lost because of increased production efficiency, or how the return-to-work process is impacted, the union must be won over.

It is hoped that the *medical community* will support this process and work in concert with the company and the consultant as the process grows. Unfortunately, business and industry still do not use the medical community as a source of injury prevention. Employees still visit a doctor, chiropractor, or therapist if they have musculoskeletal pain but do not invite these professionals to view their specific job and offer solutions. Companies invest significantly more in accident investigation and medical management simply because this is the system that has been institutionalized over the years (see Chapter 3 for more on the medical perspective).

The *workers' compensation system* drives the need for injury prevention. Workers' compensation is often viewed by management as a necessary evil and by employees as a birthright. Although the intent of the system is positive—to pay for employees' medical expenses and wages for injuries occurring in the course of work—the following erroneous assumptions can make the process more complicated.

1. Employers treat all employees fairly and will assist each employee in an efficient return to work.
2. All injured employees want to return to work in an efficient manner.
3. Everyone working within this system has the same goals.

Because most of these assumptions are false, we are left with a system that leads management to believe that employees are dramatizing injuries, employees who believe that workers' compensation and paid time off are a well-deserved benefit, and a legal system that is fed by the antagonism that this system generates.

Why is understanding these varying perspectives so important? It is because a successful injury prevention process requires everyone to work toward a common goal—the reduction of injuries. If everyone prioritizes their professional interests over worker safety and injury prevention, the entire process may be lost, or may become a point of contention. Therefore, it is essential to ask "how do I put in place a process that reduces injuries and invites the participation of all parties?"

The Money Factor

The real expense is taking people away from their work for an hour while they listen to the injury prevention expert. It is important for an injury prevention consultant to recognize that the costs that concern management are the time involved in employee training, the investments to modify work practices, job design, or work flow, and the more subjective perceived and real costs of behavioral change. The consultant must be willing to move the discussion from concern about dollars to concern about change.

The Time Factor

Injury prevention consultants will always find themselves up against time constraints. Companies operate on tight schedules, so anything that remotely appears to conflict with production timelines is considered a costly distraction. Although lack of time is a reality, it does not have to be an obstacle. Although we often think that the length of a training class is directly proportionate to the amount learned by the audience, there are different ways to implement the injury prevention process effectively. A 5-minute shift meeting once a week certainly will have greater long-term impact than a class that loses its audience's attention within the first 5 minutes. A 5-second stretch performed while building a product does not seem to accomplish much, but it does help to ensure that both the quality of the work and the health of the worker are being addressed.

Implementing an effective injury prevention process involves navigating effectively through all the people within a company or system and maneuvering around the issues of money and time. It is important to recognize that companies have priorities, systems, and ideas that are often quite different from the consultant's. If injury prevention is going to become a truly viable and recognized service, the consultant needs to tap into these systems and accommodate the various personalities and issues in order to improve the likelihood of success. An effective injury prevention process is not only about the type and quality of service provided, but about the type of environment established and culture developed to nurture and grow the process.

Further, it is the responsibility of consultants to ensure that the client understands the importance of introducing new and innovative ideas in their process that will move their process to the next level. Just as with quality and productivity, the injury prevention process needs to strive for continuous improvement.

The best example of industries' desire to maintain the status quo is the infamous "back school." Fifteen years ago, I received calls from companies requesting a 1-hour back class for employees. The assumption was that this 1-hour class would transform the audience from a group of at-risk employees into a team of material-handling experts. Each year the companies would call and request a similar class, and the saga would continue. Sometimes injury rates would fall after a class, and sometimes they wouldn't. Finally, after several years of this pattern repeating itself, I decided to alter my approach. When a company called to request a class, I would ask them if they had ever provided this type of class in the past. Then I would ask if this approach had worked well for them. When the response was negative, I would ask why they wanted me to repeat a class that had failed to work for them in the past. This simple question changed the direction of my career from being a provider of back schools to being a provider of solutions. Now, instead of simply agreeing to provide the class, I make it very clear to the client that the class is only one small part of an injury prevention process, and if the client chooses not to do anything else, they must at least understand that I am not claiming that my class alone will reduce injuries.

DEVELOPING THE INJURY PREVENTION BUSINESS

Define Your Niche

An effective injury prevention process includes, at a minimum, the following activities.

- Evaluation of medical and workers' compensation data
- Meetings with management
- Meetings with supervisors
- Meetings with employees
- Preplacement evaluations
- Ergonomics
- Stretching and warming up
- Employee assistance programs
- Safety products

Providing Services

All steps in developing an injury prevention process are important, but a single injury prevention specialist may not provide all services. Some examples of direct services are (1) selling the process, (2) developing the process, (3) meeting with management, (4) meeting with supervisors, (5) meeting with employees, (6) providing ergonomics (employee presentations), and (7) offering stretching and warm-up programs. Other services can be provided by a team of injury prevention consultants. For example, one consultant may work with the client on the overall injury prevention process and present employee training programs, and other consultants on the team provide ergonomic analysis and job redesign. The clients get what they want with the highest quality of service, and the consultants do what they do best and enjoy it.

What Works Best?

What really works in injury prevention? No objective studies can definitively state that a specific method will absolutely reduce or eliminate injuries in all settings. Back schools, stretching programs, preplacement screenings, employee assistance programs, and ergonomics programs all have a place in the injury prevention equation. The key is to recognize that each and every company will introduce different variables into the injury prevention equation. Employee training may have limited use in an environment in which the turnover is 100% in a matter of months. Ergonomic redesign may have limits in an environment in which employees are on the road and changing environments every day. Employee assistance programs help only if one can convince people in a time of need to take advantage of them. Stretching programs have limited impact when a person is required to do a task that is beyond what the human body is designed to tolerate.

Before investing in a single approach for preventing injuries, the consultant needs to acknowledge the limitations of a singular approach. This way, the concerns of a client can be anticipated and addressed in a way that will complement the other important ingredients of a comprehensive injury prevention process.

CRITICAL ELEMENTS TO AN INJURY PREVENTION PROCESS

The following 10 elements are the building blocks for a successful injury prevention process. From the marketing and selling of the service to the implementation and follow-up, the presence (or absence) of these 10 elements impacts the success of the process. It is fairly easy to learn *what* to do in an injury prevention process, but it is much more important to understand *how* to do it. Changing the way these components are developed, introduced, and maintained is more productive than changing the components themselves. These 10 essential elements should be considered during each step.

Commitment

Once a process is started, it cannot stop. It can change, grow, slow down, speed up, or change direction, but the bottom line is that the injury prevention process cannot stop without impacting the perception of the company's commitment. This means companies must start the process at a level of energy that can be sustained over the long haul. Start with low-profile activities and reasonable expectations. This provides the company with the opportunity to exceed expectations. Employees are not going to get fully on board until the company has demonstrated that this process has become part of the normal course of business.

Communication

Lack of communication is one of the main reasons injury prevention processes fail. Injury prevention can be incorporated into whatever internal communication mechanisms already exist in the company. Communication does not have to mean scheduled seminars or videos. It can be 15-second updates on process status or feedback on an idea someone submitted.

Communication can be achieved through shift meetings and toolbox talks, memos, posters, informal conversations, intercom briefings, or whatever other modes of communication currently exist in the facility.

Consistency

For years, companies have told employees in training sessions to wear hard hats and safety glasses. They develop policies and reinforce them in the workplace. Employees learn that there are repercussions if they don't use such protective equipment. Then the company holds a class that instructs the employees on lifting or handling techniques. The employees are told that this is important because people are hurting their backs and wrists and the company cares about their health. However, when the employees leave the classroom and go back to work, they continue to lift or open boxes the same way they have for 25 years, and no one reminds them to use their bodies the way they were instructed in class. Employees perceive that the company is serious about hard hats and safety glasses but is not committed to injury prevention. Messages presented in the classroom, on posters, in shift meetings, and in videos need to be consistent with the messages conveyed by management and supervisors in the work environment.

Accountability

Expectations and repercussions should be made clear and equitable. Responsibility for the process should be delegated to everyone who will be impacted by it. As part of an injury prevention process, the employees should be informed of ways to perform a job that are both more and less demanding. Employees should be involved in writing the policies and procedures that will help them change their habits. Responsibility for developing their own policies not only makes the employees accountable, but also increases the likelihood that they will follow the policies.

Inclusion

People who will be impacted by the process must not be excluded. Exclusion leads to resistance. Inclusion in the process can be achieved by establishing injury prevention teams within departments, conducting surveys that invite feedback (remember to inform people of the survey results), and providing regular memos and updates that keep people abreast of what is going on in the process and ways that they can contribute.

Recognition

The easiest way to recognize people is by simply patting them on the back for working safely. A pat on the back can take many forms, and not all of them have to involve money, time, or an event. Companies are well versed in reacting to things that are done incorrectly. Companies can use recognition to their benefit by expending energy for positive activities. To be effective, a company doesn't need to promise employees a company jacket or color television if they will work safely. Incentives can be as simple as ordering pizza for a department, circulating a memo, or expressing a thanks in passing.

Flexibility

Addressing problems that arise in an injury prevention process is no different than addressing problems that occur regularly on a production line or in a quality process. Periodic problems or obstacles supply valuable information that can be used to improve the process. Companies are constantly searching for problems in quality and productivity so they can improve their product. Problems in the injury prevention process should be regarded as opportunities to grow and change, not as excuses to abandon the process. A company's commitment to sticking with a process despite problems helps demonstrate to the employees that the company is willing to do what it takes to make the process a success.

Respect

Most people are uncomfortable with change. Companies should acknowledge this and provide a grace period for employees to acclimate to change. As a part of an injury prevention process, supervisors should be encouraged to deliver frequent brief messages about safety and injury prevention to their employees. Although most supervisors acknowledge that this is beneficial, many of them do not feel comfortable doing ergonomic training themselves. Therefore, the injury prevention process should include training for the supervisors to improve their skill and comfort level to the point where this can become a more routine part of their jobs.

Creativity

Everyone's workday is already full. The injury prevention professional must find creative ways to make injury prevention part of the normal course of business (there is rarely time for injury prevention if it is viewed as an addendum to productivity and quality). For example, one company wasn't sure how to communicate periodic safety messages to the employees who were out in trucks all day. Since they used the CB radio to contact employees in emergencies, it was recommended that they call the employees on the radio once in a while to remind them to stretch and to be careful. Now the dispatcher gets on the radio every 20 minutes and reminds employees to be more cautious.

Fun

Laughing and injury prevention are not mutually exclusive. People generally are more willing to put energy into those things that make them laugh or feel good. Many people do not want to participate on an injury prevention committee or safety committee because they feel it is going to be energy-draining. The injury prevention professional and those participating in the process development should be willing to laugh, smile, and have some fun.

If each of the above mentioned elements are kept in mind through each step of the injury prevention process, much less time will be spent retracing steps to determine the cause of problems. The elements allow for errors that occur quite naturally and can sabotage a program. Using the elements helps companies anticipate mistakes, and developing the process becomes a learning experience that can serve to improve the process.

SELLING THE PROCESS

Selling is often neglected when discussing injury prevention. If injury prevention isn't sold well, it will not happen. Although it is natural for a consultant to tell a company what he or she can do for them (e.g., teaching a class for employees, evaluating workstations, showing employees the stretches), the injury prevention specialist should first determine the company's goals for the intervention and then devise activities to ensure that the company's risk factors are being addressed.

Sales Approaches and Strategies

Here is a simple list of strategies to keep in mind when selling services to a client.

- Let them speak (don't tell them what you do specifically before they tell you what they have tried before that hasn't worked for them).
- Know what you do, and prepare to do it well. Clients expect a consultant to be as competent and qualified at providing this service as any other professional they hire. Speaking to employee audiences and charging professional fees make consultants professional speakers. Despite this, many consultants regularly go into a company and provide classes without being adequately prepared.
- Have a team together. As stated, it is rare that one person is the best at every aspect of an effective injury prevention process. Clients appreciate a team of highly qualified people who can meet their needs.

- Be flexible. A client may have a unique set of variables that make a consultant's standard way of doing things impractical. Remember that the only way a process will work is if it can be integrated into the organization in such a way that it is well received.

Putting Together a Proposal

Put together a list of proposed activities. This should be the first step in laying out a plan that will work for the company. Then invite the company to modify it to make it a perfect fit for them. If a formal proposal is developed and it does not work (because of price, activities, or other variables), a situation is created in which the company feels it has no choice but to reject the entire proposal. If it is a work in progress, a relationship is being established with the client, and the odds are much greater that the potential client will want to participate in a process that they have had a hand in developing (see Appendix 16-1).

Pricing

What consultants do has a great deal of value. When the process is done well, clients can save thousands, tens of thousands, and quite often even hundreds of thousands of dollars. The question is, what is that worth? My perspective is that if a consultant in any other profession told a company that they could save the company a large amount of money, the consultant would charge professional fees. I determined what the professional fees were in my area for doctors and lawyers and charge this level of fees.

Initial Meetings with Management

Initial meetings are critical. The initial meeting with a client can serve as a very strong marketing opportunity. I use a flip chart to discuss the things that will make a program successful. Go over the 10 essential elements, and ask the client to what level of activity they want to commit. I tell the client that if they choose to move forward, I would like to share their commitment list with supervisors and employees as I take each of the groups through the same exercise.

Alternately, if a client is willing to give me an hour of their time to sell my services, I will ask them if it is okay for me to meet with management for 30 minutes and present a class to a group of employees for another 30 minutes. This allows me to introduce myself to a small group of employees who often will recommend me to co-workers. If a consultant specializes in workstation evaluations, he or she should ask to meet with management for a short time and ask to be taken onto the floor or into the plant and allowed to evaluate a workstation. This demonstrates the consultant's skills, shows the client how he or she interacts with employees, and begins to establish a relationship in a way that is much more effective than a sales meeting in a conference room.

Initiating the Process

Management Meeting

The first step of the process involves a meeting with management. The primary focus of this meeting is to ensure that both the process and the injury prevention specialist will have management support throughout the process. To emphasize this point, remind them that injury prevention is also a business and needs to be run as one. The injury prevention program can either make or cost the client money. Ask management to describe how they commercialize and deliver a product. They typically describe a series of events that includes customer surveys, development of prototypes, focus groups, and quality-assurance programs. All of this leads to a satisfied customer with a high-quality product. Ask them to describe the injury prevention process. They typically say that they conduct a back class once a year and put up some posters. Try to help the client understand the difference between their methods for creating a product and their methods for creating an effective injury prevention process. If they use methods that are working for them in other areas, their injury prevention process is much more likely to succeed.

One of the most critical components of this meeting is to leave the client with some concrete ideas of how they can demonstrate their support. Options include, but are not limited to, the following.

- Financial commitment
- Visual and verbal presence
- Consistent messages (productivity, quality, and safety; lack of productivity; quality versus safety)
- Holding employees and supervisors accountable

In many instances, the client may already be demonstrating the preceding behaviors relative to productivity or quality issues. In this case address ways they can use the same methods to support the injury prevention process. For example, rather than develop an entirely new system for communicating back or upper-extremity care messages to the employees, add a 30-second slot of injury prevention information into an existing toolbox talk or shift meeting. Management must understand its roles and responsibilities in keeping the process alive so that supervisors and employees of all levels will follow with participation.

Supervisor Meeting

Probably the most critical thing to acknowledge with the supervisors is their responsibility for implementing every new program in addition to their many other responsibilities. The injury prevention specialist needs to make clear that he or she understands that they are extremely busy and that the goal is to actually make the supervisors' jobs easier by keeping people on the job and helping them increase their productivity. Supervisors can be involved in the process through both a visual and verbal presence, consistent messages, and communication. During this meeting, ask for feedback and concerns. Remind the supervisors that they have power in this process and that their support is essential to the effectiveness of the process. Clarify that if at any point they feel they are being asked to contribute more than they can, they should let someone know before they undermine the process. Too many times supervisors exert control in ways that sabotage the entire process.

Employee Meeting

Several years ago, a national airline asked me to provide some employee training. They told me it would be several difficult audiences with unique personality traits. I requested the opportunity to present a series of very short (15-minute) introductory classes for these employees to introduce myself, explain my philosophy, and get some feedback. At the end of each of the sessions, I would ask the group if it was all right for me to come back and do a more in-depth class. Each and every group said yes. When I returned for the longer training sessions, I began each class with the statement, "Thank you so much for inviting me back!" This is a rare statement from a consultant to the employee population. Typically, management, not the employees, invites a consultant in. Rarely does the audience know the consultant's philosophy, style, or what he or she personally hopes to achieve. The more groundwork that can be laid before the first class is held, the easier the session will be and the better it will be received by the audience.

The key goal of this meeting is to get the employees involved and motivated. They need the information necessary to actively participate in the process. It is nice to be able to tell the employees what management and supervisors have agreed to.

EMPLOYEE TRAINING AND EDUCATION

Putting Education and Training into Proper Perspective

Employee education plays an important role. It orients employees to the process, gives them tools they need to participate in the process, and provides the inspiration to participate. Unfortunately, some educational programs have been implemented as the only part of the injury prevention process. An injury prevention class does not teach a new technique. A change in deeply ingrained habitual activity cannot be expected with only 1 hour of training. However, an injury prevention class provides basic information and can get workers motivated to participate in the injury prevention process.

Over the past 15 years my employee programs have evolved from 3-hour programs with two carousels of slides, to 1-hour programs with no slides, to 15 to 20 minutes once a month with employees at their workstations. The point is to recognize how people best learn and what they need to know in order to prevent injuries. Now, as I review my presentation, I go through each slide after a class and ask myself, "Why did I make this point? What can someone do with the information I just presented? Did this information add to the program, or did it distract from the more important messages?" Slowly, the amount of information I disseminate has decreased, and the amount of time spent reinforcing specific, useful messages has increased. Now, in my 1-hour program on back injury prevention, I include only essential information.

Everything presented in the 1-hour program should be designed to support these points. Present them in different ways, use a variety of different examples, get the employees on their feet so they can actually feel what is being described, and answer any questions they have about the information. Minimize discussion of specific diagnoses. In this session, do not try to make employees injury experts. Try to motivate them and provide them with usable and practical information that can be put into practice right away.

Since employees have different movement patterns, muscle strength, levels of flexibility, and, often, jobs, only telling them or showing them the "right" way to perform a job often leads to frustration. They must understand that every single job can be done in either a more or a less demanding way. Ask them to take a few seconds and choose the less demanding way. With this approach, every single employee can be complimented for his or her efforts to perform his or her job better or in a less demanding way, even if the technique is not yet perfect. It is important to determine the most critical pieces of information for the audience to absorb and act on, and to emphasize and reemphasize these points in various ways, using different scenarios throughout the class. It does no good to think the audience has been given 100 bits of magnificent information when they can only retain and act on a few points. For this reason, I try to emphasize three or four easily remembered (and easily applied) principles that can make any job less demanding (see Table 16-1).

Supply each of the employees with either a booklet or a handout that supports the emphasized points; each point should be related to specific work activities that are performed on the job. It is important to note that it is not necessary to emphasize the need for an employee to change the technique he or she currently uses to perform his or her work. Truly changing a technique is not unlike trying to get a person to change hand dominance in a 1-hour class. Try to help the employees see the demands that are associated with their choices, and then offer principles that can help them make their techniques less demanding. You may not be able to get a participant to lift loads like a professional weightlifter, but you can teach them the lifting principles that will make the lift physically easier.

Presentation Style

Everyone has a unique presentation style that they must practice and perfect. There are numerous opportunities to improve speaking skills, including with groups such as Toastmasters. One of the best techniques is to tape oneself while speaking. Remember that the art of speaking is not focusing on what is said but on what the audience hears. A consultant may be an expert on a topic, but that does not qualify

Table 16-1
An Example of the Content for a 1-Hour Back Injury Prevention Class

Subject	Points to Make
Background Information	The cumulative nature of most injuries
	The natural curves of the spine and how this natural design complements how we sit, stand, lift, sleep, and so on
	Emphasis on the neutral postures of the body
The Key Principles for Sitting Smart	Move!
	Find two or three ways to perform the same job (e.g., stand and work occasionally, kneel on the chair with one leg, etc.).
	Set up the workstation so it invites neutral postures, and make sure to "check-in" to these neutral postures periodically throughout the day
The Key to Standing for Prolonged Periods	Staggered stance
	Slight bend in the knees
	One foot up
	Move!
The Key to Better Lifting	Keep the load close, and keep the natural curves of the spine
	Build a bridge
	Move with the feet first
	Prepare and compensate (warm up and stretch)
The Role of Stretching	Stretching improves the body's ability to handle the demands of the job

him or her as the best deliverer of that information. Here's a simple exercise. Imagine that it is 3 o'clock in the afternoon. You have been working hard all day, and in the middle of a task you are told to go to the training room for a back class. Now, imagine what *you* would want to hear and how you would want it presented. Putting oneself in the place of the audience will help a speaker get better and better at meeting the needs of the audience.

Finally, the following questions should be considered before a speaker the steps into a training room to conduct a back class.

- How many of the audience members are there by choice?
- How many of the audience members are motivated to be there?
- How many of the audience members are eager to apply the principles they learn to their job?
- How many of the audience members work in an environment that will allow and encourage the types of methods being talking about?
- How much of the material presented will be retained by the audience once the class is over?

The more these issues are addressed before a speaker steps into a classroom, the more effective the program will be.

As the content for the employee training sessions is developed, the 10 critical elements of an effective process should be kept in mind.

- *Commitment:* If information is presented to the employees at only one point in time, what is the company's commitment to helping the employees remember and use this information?
- *Consistency:* Is the information presented in the sessions compatible with what is taking place in the work environment?
- *Communication:* Is a method of presentation (and presenter) chosen based on the needs of the audience? How do people learn best, what information is most essential and most practical, and how is the information communicated on an ongoing basis?
- *Inclusion:* Were the employees involved in the development of the education sessions? Were they able to contribute to the content based on their perceived needs? Were they involved in determining the best time for the training and who should provide it? (In many companies, the speaker is interviewed by a safety team or task force to ensure that the presentation style will be compatible with the employees' learning styles.)
- *Flexibility:* Do the employees feel that they can ask questions and bring up issues related to back care during the sessions? Is there time to discuss personal injury prevention issues with the speaker after the session or during breaks? If it becomes apparent that a

particular training class isn't helpful, is it possible to determine what the problems are and to remedy the situation before training continues? This demonstrates that the training is more than just something the company wants to offer; it is something that should make a difference.

- *Accountability:* Are there clear expectations about what is supposed to happen now that the training is complete? What does the company expect the employees to do differently now that they have been trained? What are the expectations of management and supervisors to keep the information fresh? Who is evaluating the effectiveness of the training and whether people need additional training?
- *Respect:* Are the sessions scheduled in a way that is respectful of the employee population? Are classes scheduled when the employees are fresh and awake or when the shift is over and everyone is tired? Does the length of the class or scheduled breaks take into account the attention span that most people have for this kind of training? Does the training respect the employees' intelligence, or is it condescending and presented in an impractical way? Are the employees surveyed early in the process to evaluate whether the training meets their needs, and if not, what changes might be helpful?
- *Fun:* Is the training presented in a way that conveys the seriousness of the information but allows people to enjoy themselves during the learning process?
- *Recognition:* As much as possible, equate the information that is presented to the audience members and their specific needs. Also, be willing to recognize the limitations of a 1-hour class. Inform the audience at the beginning that they are not expected to change their behaviors simply because they attended a 1-hour class. True change takes more time. This recognition seems to help the audience relax a bit more because they realize that they are not being expected to become experts as a result of this one class.
- *Creativity:* Be willing to do a series of 15-minute meetings once a month at the employees' workstations if this works best for the company. Do not assume that the way information has been conveyed to employees in the past is the best way. It is the way we have become accustomed to doing it.

Ergonomics

Good ergonomic design is important for efficient and comfortable work performance. However, ergonomic redesign may not be possible for some jobs, nor may it be the panacea to all workplace injuries. For example, what can be done about employees who don't use the equipment properly or fail to use it because they are resistant to change?

Numerous companies have implemented one or two ergonomic changes. Fewer have established a comprehensive process that mirrors the systems that have been created for productivity and quality. To ensure positive results in an ergonomics process, apply the 10 elements to the process. One of the best ways to incorporate ergonomics into an injury prevention process is to look at a situation and determine why the job is leading to increased risk of injury. In most cases, it will be the result of workstation design, employee workstyle, or a combination of both. If workstation design is determined to be a cause, an evaluation of the job will help identify the risk factors associated with the task. Once these have been identified, the organization can begin exploring options for eliminating or reducing the risks. This can be accomplished through engineering redesign and administrative changes (reduce the time a person spends on the task, rotate individuals, etc.) (see Chapter 14). It is important to keep in mind that an effective evaluation of the workplace and implementation of effective physical changes in the workplace dictate close attention to the 10 essential variables.

- *Commitment:* Has the company demonstrated a willingness to follow through on projects? This is not determined as much by the amount of money that is spent as it is by the length of time the process continues.

- *Consistency:* Are ergonomics projects just as important when the company is busy as they are when the company is slow? Do the employees perceive that safety is less important than productivity and quality? By maintaining a consistent level of activity relative to the ergonomics process, a pattern of consistency can be developed.
- *Communication:* Does the company have a formal method for communicating within the ergonomics process? All too often, good ideas are lost because of a lack of communication, and people become discouraged because recommendations they made regarding an ergonomic issue were not followed through with or addressed. Communication does not mean that every idea must be acted on and ultimately lead to change. It means that every communication from an employee or supervisor leads to a response that informs them of the status of their ideas.
- *Flexibility:* Does the process allow for steps such as beta sites or prototypes when determining the best job design or process format? The ability to modify a process as new information is gathered is as important to ergonomics as it is to quality and productivity.
- *Accountability:* Who is responsible for the ergonomics process? In fact, everyone is responsible, but if there are not individuals who have specific responsibilities and accountabilities, projects will fall through the cracks. Everyone at any time during the ergonomics process needs to know the right person to talk to in order to get something done and whom to talk to if something does not get done.
- *Inclusion:* The best ideas come from those who perform the jobs. In many instances, the employees may not have the engineering background to solve the problem, but they certainly have the ability to identify the problem. Allowing the people who do the job to participate in problem solving will always lead to greater acceptance of whatever changes are made.
- *Respect:* Volvo builds its cars with the cars tipped on their sides. This allows workers better access to the car and keeps the employees in less-demanding positions while they are working. There is no such thing as a bad idea in an ergonomics program. Even the most outrageous ideas may have merit at some basic level, and every idea should be treated with respect. If people feel that their ideas are not respected, the ideas will stop coming, not only from those who feel rejected, but from their peers who do not want to experience the same thing.
- *Fun:* If a company is trying to get volunteers for the ergonomics committee, the task will be much easier if the potential members perceive the position as fun to hold.
- *Creativity:* Ergonomics leaves a great deal of room for creativity. One of the best ergonomics exercises is to announce to a room full of employees that a particular job can be redesigned and money is no object. Then go to a flip chart and let them shout out new designs that would make the job easier. Many of them will be outrageous and impractical (and the employees will recognize this), but many of the ideas will contain value that can be built on for actual changes.
- *Recognition:* Recognition takes on two meanings in ergonomics. The first is to recognize that the company may be changing something that an employee has become accustomed to over the past 25 years. The company needs to understand that it can be very difficult for an employee to embrace this change. That is why the employee needs to be included in the process from the very beginning. It is also important to recognize an employee's efforts in the ergonomics process. For example, one company followed through on an employee recommendation to raise a piece of equipment. The management team purchased a small plaque, put

the employee's name on it along with his recommendation, made a small statement regarding the value this idea had to the company, and then welded the plaque right to the machine. Needless to say, the employee began each day polishing the symbol that (for decades to come) acknowledges his value.

Stretching and Warming Up

A great deal of conflicting information exists about stretching—most of which is anecdotal (see Chapter 14). In the programs that have proven successful for me (resulting in a reduction in injuries), the stretching was actually one part of a comprehensive program. Stretching is not a way to eliminate the demands of an ill-designed workstation. However, is it an appropriate tool in an environment that challenges the muscles on an ongoing basis? In my 15 years of experience, stretching programs, when combined with a comprehensive safety process, can play a major role in the reduction of work injuries. Stretching and warm-up is one small piece of the injury prevention process. Why can stretching contribute to an injury prevention process?

- Is it because warm muscles are stronger and at less risk of a strain or sprain?
- Is it that taking the time to stretch reminds employees to be careful and makes them focus on the task at hand?
- Is it because the employees appreciate management's commitment to safety, and as a result they are more careful about how they perform their tasks?
- Is it because a periodic stretch performed throughout the day reduces muscle fatigue and helps the employees remain fresh and functioning at full capacity?

The answer to all these questions is "Probably." The fact is these are *all* reasons why stretching is important. Since no study states unequivocally the value of stretching in the workplace, care needs to be taken in how a stretching program is set up, how it is started, how it is maintained, and how its effectiveness is measured. The value of stretching is difficult to identify because it is difficult to isolate and measure. For example, it is assumed that warming up and stretching help to keep baseball pitchers healthy. However, baseball pitchers are usually in good shape, have coaches to teach the best technique, have athletic trainers to ice their muscles at the end of a game, and do not pitch if they are tired. It is difficult to separate stretching from any one of these health-maintaining behaviors. The same holds true in the workplace. Again, the 10 elements are critical in its implementation.

- *Commitment:* Stretching programs often take time and energy, not only to develop and implement them, but also to maintain them. Companies need to recognize that fluctuations in participation are not unusual. Commitment is demonstrated by meeting these challenges and finding ways to effectively deal with them on an ongoing basis. It is significantly easier to develop ways to keep the program alive than it is to restart it.
- *Consistency:* In many companies the stretching program will be put on hold because of productivity issues. However, if a stretching program truly interferes with productivity, it is not a good program. A stretching program that is set up appropriately will improve productivity and quality, not adversely affect them. Companies will benefit from beginning with a basic stretching program and maintaining it for a length of time to demonstrate that it can be implemented without compromising productivity or quality. Once it is demonstrated that it is not a time-consuming factor, the program can be expanded.
- *Communication:* Particularly in the beginning of a stretching program, the reminder to stretch needs to be communicated on a daily basis. Often the company assumes that *"If we teach them, they will stretch."* Companies must realize that incorporating stretching into one's daily routine, particularly if one has never exercised before, is a major behavior change that needs support. Communication can take

place in a variety of ways, including formal stretching times, encouragement over an intercom system, small work groups who encourage each other, or supervisors who invite participation on a daily basis. There isn't a right or wrong way to communicate the message as long as it is communicated regularly.

- *Flexibility:* The company needs to be willing and able to modify the stretching program as new information and employee feedback become available. The company may find that it makes more sense to all involved to stretch in the middle of the day rather than at the beginning or that there are stretches that are more appropriate for one department than another. It is the ability to react to these situations in a timely manner that lets the employee population know that this is something that is important to the company, and something they are willing to maintain and grow over time.
- *Inclusion:* It is always easier to invite people to stretch than it is to force them to stretch. Stretching by invitation means that the implementation of a stretching program involves gathering employee feedback early in the process and addressing the pros and cons and concerns before the program is implemented. It is not uncommon to have many people expressing an interest in a stretching program, only to have participation decrease after the program is implemented. Much of this decrease can be offset by actively seeking participation in the formation of the program, so that representatives of the employee population can have an influence on the events taking place in their environment. This can make the introduction of a stretching program much less threatening to employees and reduce resistance to the program.
- *Accountability:* Accountability in a stretching program can be difficult. Some may like to think that all people believe taking care of one's body is the individual's responsibility. However, if that were true, people would do this without the policies and procedures that require the use of hard hats, safety glasses, and steel-toed shoes. People need encouragement and training in the right way to care for their bodies at work if they are not accustomed to doing so. Therefore, if a company wants to implement a stretching program, the company has to be willing to help the employees make the change. Creating an environment that invites, rather than discourages, stretching throughout the day helps this endeavor. If the environment encourages stretching, and that is what everyone is doing, that is what everyone does. On the other hand, there are few things in the typical work environment that invite stretching. That is why at the beginning of the program the messages and invitations to stretch need to be strong. Employees, over time, can begin to look at their workplace as an environment in which stretching is a normal part of the workday.
- *Respect:* It is important that a company recognize that stretching and warming up at work are new and sometimes threatening activities for some employees. The reasons can include embarrassment, concerns about wasted time, or previous injuries that an employee does not want to aggravate. The company can demonstrate respect toward the employees by acknowledging these issues and addressing them as valid concerns.
- *Fun:* Stretching is one of the activities in the workplace that provides an opportunity for employees to have some fun. It should not be disruptive or silly, but something that is relaxed and enjoyable. Many companies have developed ways to make their stretching programs more fun by incorporating music, enlisting energetic leaders, or providing participants with T-shirts that say "I survived the stretching program!"
- *Creativity:* Stretching programs have much room for creativity. I have clients who stretch

to music and others who use egg-timers to signal the times for the stretch that most complements the work they are performing. The point is to be creative enough to establish a stretching program that looks less like a ritual and more like the normal course of business.

- *Recognition:* Companies must recognize that many of the people being asked to stretch have not done a great deal of stretching in their lives, and certainly are not accustomed to doing so in front of their co-workers. Stretching programs are often best implemented in the later stages of an injury prevention process, once the employees are convinced that management is committed. One client started the program by having the employees perform a bit of a warm-up and a single stretch at the end of the daily shift meeting. After a week or so another stretch was added, and within a couple of months a respectable warm-up and stretch program had been implemented. The point is that the company recognized the employees' need to ease into something that was different from what they were accustomed to.

Measuring the Efficacy of Programs

Companies measure success of injury prevention programs by reductions in incidents, lost time from injuries, lower expenses incurred by injuries, increases in production, improvements in quality, reductions in rework or waste, and improvement in morale. These can be measured formally with employee surveys or informally through supervisor and employee interactions (see Chapter 17 for a complete discussion on outcome assessment).

ONE COMPANY'S APPROACH TO IMPLEMENTING A STRETCHING AND WARM-UP PROGRAM

Background

The department had 30 employees whose job responsibilities included a variety of material-handling activities. Before implementation of the program, the department reported an average of eight recordable injuries per year, most related to strains or sprains of the back, neck, and shoulders.

Program Development and Implementation

Task Force Organization and Orientation

A task force of motivated and interested employees from the department was organized. It was their responsibility to work closely with me, promote the program within the department, and monitor the feedback of their co-workers.

The program began with a task force orientation to provide the task force with an introduction to the program, including the rationale and proposed methods. The orientation offered the task force members an opportunity to ask questions and discuss options that might improve the acceptance and effectiveness of the program.

During the orientation, a question was raised as to whether or not the program should be mandatory. There was concern that there would be resistance to a mandatory program and lack of participation in a voluntary program. It was determined that the program would be voluntary but would be presented to the employees as a job function. To date (nearly 4 years into the program), no one has refused to participate.

Employee Orientation

This meeting, like that for the task force, was to orient the employees to the program and provide them with the rationale and methodology for putting the program into place.

Prior to my involvement with the company, a survey had been distributed to all the employees. A cover sheet provided them with background information on the need for a stretching program. The survey asked them questions regarding their interest in a program, discomfort experienced during the day, and other general information. I was given access to the survey results and was therefore better able to address the employees' specific concerns during the orientation. The orientation addressed the following.

- The areas of basic anatomy and biomechanics
- How certain movements affect the body
- The effects of work
- The need for compensating for work demands throughout the day

Each of the stretches was demonstrated with the employees at the end of the orientation. After the orientation, the official starting date of the program was chosen. The stretching program was introduced as a two-part program: warming up first thing in the morning to prepare the body for work, and stretching periodically throughout the day to allow the body to remain fresh.

The morning portion was formally organized, and the periodic stretches were to be performed at the employees' discretion. Because early in the development of the program it was determined that this program should be fun and upbeat, an employee suggested that a cassette player be brought in. Employees were encouraged to bring in music they would like to listen to while stretching. Employees could then choose to talk among themselves while stretching or just listen to the music.

It was agreed that a volunteer leader would time the stretches. The leader was expected only to tell the employees when to perform a different stretch, not how to do it. This was seen as less threatening than having a leader feel compelled to demonstrate a stretch or answer questions about the stretches.

Employee Survey

During the orientation, I worked hard to generate enthusiasm for the program and to ensure that I addressed all of the employees' ideas and concerns. I also informed the employees that this was not their last opportunity to offer feedback, and that I would survey them after the stretching program had begun. If the majority of the surveys come back negative, I would inform management that it was not a good idea to proceed. If they came back primarily positive, however, we would move on and get more established. I have yet to see a stretching program really be successful if the employees weren't happy with it.

Evaluating the Worksite

The next step was a worksite evaluation. The purpose was twofold: to introduce myself to the employees, and to gather the relevant information to customize the stretching program. During the evaluation, jobs were closely examined to determine the movements and muscle groups used. In addition, photographs (slides) were taken to customize the employee orientation program. I also talked with the employees about their jobs and solicited their input on the stretching program.

After the worksite evaluation was completed, I wrote a report that outlined the job demands and the stretches that would be most appropriate. The results of the worksite evaluation were then formally presented to the stretching task force for their review.

Getting Started

For the first 3 minutes of the program, the employees would warm up their bodies by marching in place, swinging their arms, and getting their blood circulating. The warm-up portion was readily accepted, and many employees described it as the stimulus they needed to start their day. Many of the participants were athletes (softball) and understood the need to warm up before they started stretching.

All of the stretches in the program were performed in the standing position. These stretches included low-back extension, low-back flexion, calf stretch, hamstring stretch, rotation stretch, shoulder stretch, side stretch, overhead stretch, and neck stretch.

On any given day, six of the preceding nine exercises were performed. The group chose the six stretches they felt were most appropriate for that day. The only rule was that the stretches address all the primary muscle groups. In other words, the group could not choose to do only neck stretches or only back stretches. They had to include stretches for the neck, shoulders, back, and legs.

I was present on two days during the first and second weeks and then 1 day per week for the next 2 weeks to ensure that the stretches were being performed properly and to answer any questions. Modifications or alternative stretches were provided to those who experienced undue discomfort or who had existing disorders that precluded a specific stretch.

Program Maintenance

To ensure the longevity of the program, meetings with the task force were held on a monthly basis for the first few months to discuss follow-up activities. The consultant would come to talk and stretch with the employees one or two mornings per month. This gave the consultant the opportunity to observe techniques and address any questions.

Ongoing Commitment

After a few months, several of the employees approached their manager with the request for a stretching program for home use. As a result of this request, a program was developed that allowed the interested employees to be evaluated on-site by a physical therapist for development of this program.

The assessment took place in the nurse's office in the plant, and each assessment lasted approximately 30 minutes. The evaluation was to determine if there were any conditions that would preclude the performance of specific stretches. The employees were told that all the information from their assessment would remain confidential and would not be shared with their employer.

As a result of the assessments, a few employees were found to have conditions that warranted treatment. In these cases, management encouraged them to seek treatment, and they were switched to exercise programs that dealt specifically with their conditions.

Every employee in the department volunteered for the assessment, and management considers this preventive care approach a cost-effective way to address problems before they become more serious. Many report that they continue to do at least some of their home program exercises.

I also conducted quarterly education programs, which included 1-hour discussions on general health and safety concerns. The first program focused on upper extremity care and the second on fitness facts and fallacies. A list of topics was provided to the employees, and they could choose the subjects that interested them most.

One issue that arose was the staggered start times for many employees. In this case, there were employees who did not have the group leader to take them through the stretches. The task force recommended that a tape be made that walked the participant through the routine. The employees chose the music, and the instructions and timing of the stretches were dubbed onto the tape. The program also encouraged the employees to perform the stretches briefly throughout the day. Stretching posters were placed throughout the facility to remind the employees and task force members to stretch periodically. The goal was for these activities to become routine work behaviors.

Results

Before the program was implemented, the department typically experienced eight recordable injuries related to strains and sprains. Total days of restricted duty averaged approximately 100 days per year. Since the inception of the program nearly 5 years ago, the department has averaged zero recordable injuries and no days lost.

As stated earlier, there are a number of factors present that can be attributed to this reduction in injuries. Although the stretching program certainly can be considered as one of these factors, management and employee involvement, good communication, high visibility, and ongoing commitment are all factors that contributed to these results.

START AT THE END AND WORK BACKWARD

What does this mean? It means that if you want to help a company reduce its injuries, you need to start with the end result (i.e.,What behaviors do you want to see? What changes in the environment do you want to see?) and work backward. What happens is that we all get caught up in the logistics of the activities but we lose sight of the goal. Often, getting through the employee training or getting the new piece of equipment in place becomes the goal, and once the goal is met, everyone relaxes, assumes that the goals have been met, and considers the program over. A consultant needs to develop a long-term vision for a company's injury prevention process. If the end result is that six months from now, a year from now, and five years from now the company wants to see ongoing ergonomics changes, employees performing warm-up and stretching activities that are specific to their jobs, and supervisors who are consistently reinforcing safe techniques with their employees, sequential short- and long-term goals will be needed for the company to arrive at the final goal. This way of setting goals means that there has to be an independently functioning process in place that is self-sustaining and is considered by everyone in the company as an integral part of the business model.

In effect, a consultant is helping the company create an injury prevention framework or culture. Over the years a consultant will work into this framework new methods for training employees and supervisors, new ergonomics strategies, and new ways to implement successful stretching and warming up. A company that has a strong framework need only add these new strategies into the existing framework and build on a process that is already working for them. When it is done well, an injury prevention process is barely visible to the untrained eye.

A DAY IN THE LIFE OF AN INJURY PREVENTION PROCESS

Employees enter the building at the beginning of their day and proceed to warm up and perform some simple stretches. A supervisor comes by to conduct the Monday morning shift meeting, and at the end, she adds in a quick injury prevention message. The ergonomics committee is having their monthly meeting at 10:00, and they are reviewing the latest recommendations that have been received from employees and determining which recent changes need to be reviewed again to ensure that the changes are working for the employees.

An employee is performing a job and stops for a minute to grab an assistive device. A supervisor observes this behavior and walks over and thanks the individual for taking the time to do it right. Later that day a therapist does a brief walk-through of the facility to answer employee questions and meet with the safety committee or ergonomics committee. He stops in a couple of departments to lead their weekly 15-minute shift meeting. At lunchtime, a supervisor brings a stack of pizzas into the department as a surprise for her staff because they have gone 6 months without a recordable injury. She thanks them for their efforts, they enjoy the pizza, and they go back to work. Down the street, a clinic is performing some preplacement assessments on a group of new hires, and in the same clinic, a therapist is going to the workplace with a discharged client to review the safe performance of the job right at the worksite. As you can see, none of these things are events. They are normal day-to-day occurrences that coexist in harmony with productivity and quality. Consultants need to work closely with companies to create a workplace that treats safety as a normal part of that process.

RESOURCES

Canfield, J., Hansen, M.V., Rogerson, M., Rutte, M., & Clauss, T. (2001). *Chicken soup for the soul at work: 101 stories of courage, compassion and creativity in the workplace.* Deerfield Beach, FL: Health Communications Inc.

Canfield, J., & Miller, J. (1996). *Heart at work.* New York: McGraw-Hill.

Geller, E. S. (1998). *Working safe: How to help people actively care for health and safety*. Boca Raton, FL: CRC Press.

Manning, M. V. (1998). *Safety is a people business: A practical guide to the human side of safety*. Knoxville, TN: Abs Group Inc.

APPENDIX 16-1

Developing a Proposal

January 26, 1999
Frank A. xxxxxxx
Senior Safety/Environmental Engineer
xxx Telecommunications
P.O. Box xxxx
Minneapolis, MN 55440-1101
Dear Frank:
Attached is an outline of proposed activities for the LaSeur facility. Please send as many copies as necessary to the plant for their review. Once you have all had a chance to take a look at this, we can talk again, and I can address any questions the group has. I would be happy to schedule a time to sit with your safety team and discuss the proposal in more detail if you think that will be beneficial to the group and help them in the decision-making process. As I mentioned in the meeting, the goal is to establish an ongoing, consistent injury prevention process that gradually becomes the "normal course of business" for the company.

I enjoyed the recent visit to the plant and look forward to the possibility of providing injury prevention services for your company in LaSeur. Please thank everyone involved for taking the time to meet with me on Friday and for showing me around. I will talk with you soon.
Sincerely,
Michael S. Melnik, MS, OTR

Proposed Injury Prevention Services for xxx Telecommunications
Submitted by: Prevention Plus, Inc.
Date: 1/24/1999

Proposed Activities

1. Meeting with Management/Safety Committee: The purpose of this meeting is to introduce the process to the management team and enlist their support. A meeting with the safety committee is also recommended. This group will be instrumental in maintaining and growing the process.
2. Supervisor Orientation: The purpose of this meeting is to introduce the supervisors to the prevention process. Their involvement and support are essential for process success, so it is important to offer them a forum to voice questions, concerns, and ideas.
3. Worksite Evaluation: The purpose of the worksite evaluation is to familiarize myself with the work environment, provide the employees with an opportunity to meet me before the training sessions, and allow me to customize the training sessions for your organization.

4. Employee Training Sessions: These sessions are designed to accomplish two things.
   a. Provide the employees with the information they need to know to work safely.
   b. Serve as a motivational session to encourage employees to get involved in the process.

   The session focuses on identifying risk factors, developing problem-solving methods for reducing these demands, and establishing some initial action items to get the process started.
5. Supervisor Training Sessions: These sessions provide the supervisors with some of the initial tools to help them actively supervise the process in their work areas. Of primary concern is the supervisors' ability to effectively communicate injury prevention with their employees and to reinforce safe behaviors.
6. Ongoing Injury Prevention Activities: The key to the injury prevention process is the continuation of activities once the initial activities (1-5) are completed. These activities include the following.
   a. Ongoing safety committee meetings
   b. Ongoing communication with employees
   c. Ergonomics activities/physical changes in the facility
   d. Ongoing evaluation of the injury prevention process

   It is also important that the facility establish a more formal method for identifying symptomatic employees as well as a system for a consistent return-to-work process. Prevention Plus can work with you and your local health providers on this effort.

Investment

1. Meeting with management: $xxx.00 (1-hour session)
   Meeting with safety committee: $xxx.00 (1-hour session)
2. Supervisor orientation: $xxx.00 (1-hour session)
3. Worksite evaluation: $xxx.00/hr (approx. 3 hours)
4. Employee education sessions: $xxx.00/class (1 hour each). Approx. 25 employees per class.
5. Supervisor education sessions: $xxx.00/class (1 hour)
6. Ongoing activities: Consulting billed at $xxx.00/hr; Classes billed at $xxx.00/hr; Travel billed at $xx.00/hr

Approximate investment: Meetings with management/safety committee: $xxx.00
   Supervisor orientation: $xxx.00
   Worksite evaluation: $xxx.00
   Employee training: 18 sessions @ $xxx.00/per: $xxx.00
   Supervisor training: 2 Sessions @ $xxx.00/per: $xxx.00
   Ongoing activities: Approximately $xxx.00 for first quarter of process
   Travel: Approximately $xxx.00 for first quarter of process

Approximate investment for first quarter of process: $xxx.00

CHAPTER 17

Outcome Assessment of Prevention Programs

Richard K. Schwartz

A PRAGMATIC APPROACH TO PROGRAM EVALUATION

Outcome assessment is an evaluative process. It is most simply described as a process used to determine the extent to which organizational or program goals have been met. Possible outcomes range from finding that goals have *not* been met to finding that goals have been exceeded. Discrepancies between goals and outcomes can suggest where changes in programs are warranted. Outcomes that fail to meet goals may require greater investment of resources or alterations in intervention strategies. Outcomes that exceed goals not only identify the elements of intervention and prevention programs that work well, but also suggest where resources may be cut back, freeing them for activities that may have a higher return-on-investment.

The utility of program evaluation depends on the selection of appropriate outcome variables and the reliability and validity of outcome measurements. There are no formulas, checklists, or methodologies that mandate clearly those prevention options most suitable for particular groups, industries, job categories, or regions. It is imperative that those who undertake musculoskeletal disorder (MSD) prevention programs document a given program's effectiveness, lack of effectiveness, or, ideally, relative effectiveness compared to other options. Both quantitative and qualitative evaluations are necessary.

Those responsible for MSD prevention programs are unlikely to have formal training in outcome evaluation research. As a result, outcome assessment is rarely conducted. When it is done, evaluation of prevention programs is often simplistic and biased. When starting a new program, consider including a part-time consultant with expertise in outcome evaluation as a member of the program team.

This chapter describes the importance and complexity of outcome evaluation studies. Some very powerful outcome analysis tools are presented in this chapter, but procedural instruction in statistical techniques is avoided. Those interested in developing such skills independently would benefit from consulting Borich and Jemelka (1982) on the evaluation of programs and systems, Cascio (1991) on determining costs related to human behaviors in organizations, and Hayes (1997) on how one can extrapolate the immediate data from a sample and make inferences about larger systems and organizations. Although not as detailed as some of the preceding sources, Milstein, Wetterhall, Christenson, Dennis-Flagler, and Harris, (1999) provide an excellent guide to program evaluation related to public health that can be obtained from the Center for Disease Control and Prevention (CDC).

The outcome evaluation process requires an organization to clearly define the goals of the prevention programs being evaluated. It is essential to delineate indicators of successful programs prior to program implementation. This generally occurs in two stages. The first stage involves assessment of the needs of the organization and establishment of measurable prevention program goals. The second stage requires that a commitment be made to measure and record data needed to determine whether or not the program goals have been met.

The first stage requires that baseline or historical measures be compiled to document the problems that the program is to address. This documentation should give a picture of human activity and costs at the beginning of the program. These measurements permit trend and projection analyses to be conducted so that the benefits of a program for any given year are measured not only in comparison to the previous year but also in comparison to the prediction of the costs of injuries if no intervention was ever conducted. This stage of the outcome evaluation process should also include qualitative assessments of factors such as job satisfaction, employee stress, morale, and attitudes of employees toward supervisors, managers, and the employer.

The second stage entails the compilation and maintenance of an accurate MSD injuries and losses database. This means not only incorporating data that will describe human behaviors (e.g., types of injuries, lost time, trends over time), but also developing information that allows the organization to evaluate productivity and dollar costs associated with injuries. Experienced evaluators know that MSD incidence rates often *increase rather than decrease* during the first several years of a successful MSD prevention program. This increase in the number of cases (such as number of workers' compensation claims or number of "OSHA Recordable" injuries) does not necessarily mean that the program does not work. By documenting that the severity of accidents and injuries declines and that total dollars lost diminishes even with increasing numbers (incidence), it is possible to show that workers' awareness has been enhanced by the program. Effective prevention programs encourage workers to report signs and symptoms of cumulative trauma earlier than they did prior to the program. With earlier detection and intervention, early symptoms of MSDs can be effectively treated with conservative measures, reducing severity, lost time, and medical expenses.

Outcome assessment is not a hard science. It is more than the collection of statistical and informational techniques used to measure performance. It requires both qualitative and quantitative evaluation. Properly conducted outcome assessment always indicates the congruence between what is valued by an organization and how the organization actually behaves. It answers the question, "Are we really doing the things we should be doing to meet our goals and fulfill the mission of the organization?"

COMPILING AN MSD INFORMATION SYSTEM

The starting point of any approach to risk reduction is an injury information system containing all relevant data that the company has about each injury and each injured employee. Such data are compiled from Occupational Safety and Health Administration (OSHA) 300 logs, from illness and injury reports, and from occupational health records. The creation and maintenance of such an electronic database make it possible to pinpoint specific categories of employees, specific types of injuries, and even specific locations where interventions are most needed. Table 17-1 shows data from such a database and shows how information that is readily available can be formatted for storage, retrieval, and statistical analyses. Although only part of a page of this database is shown here, the actual database records more than 400 injuries reported over a 5-year period and is updated annually.

The database has two important epidemiologic features. First, it permits a given workforce to be compared with state and national data in terms of incidence, severity, and risk factors for specific injuries. Second, it permits both descriptive and inferential statistical analysis of the company's

Table 17-1
Sample Data from Injury and Illness Tracking Database

Name	Year	Total Incurred	Total Paid	Line	Supervisor	Cause	Days Lost	Injury Date	Body Part	Job
Brent	2001	$276	$276	VC	JLD	Other		1/11/01	LE	Prod oper
Sam	2001	$458	$459	LM	EG	Cumulative trauma	12	2/21/01	UE	Prod oper
Edith	2001	$96	$96	TEC	CI	Other	0	8/1/01	UE	Prod oper
Arnold	2001	$29,632	$22,530	AT	JM	Slip, trip, fall	0	3/5/01	LE	Prod oper
Rose	2001	$0	$0	PH	K Barger	Cumulative trauma	0	11/20/01	UE	Prod oper
Becky	2001	$8948	$8750	TEC	CI	Slip, trip, fall	0	3/7/01	UE	Prod oper
Sid	2001	$654	$654	VC	JLD	Cumulative trauma	0	3/2/01	UE	Prod oper
Mark	2001	$4822	$175	AT	BA	Other	0	10/17/01	Back	Prod oper
Jesus	2001	$0	$0	HA	KB	Manual handling	0	3/1/01	UE	Prod oper
Andy	2001	$0	$0	VC	JLD	Manual handling	0	1/20/01	UE	Prod oper
Sara	2001	$0	$0	MK	MM		0	5/10/01	UE	Eng
Mary	2001	$0	$0	QA	KM	Cumulative trauma	0	12/8/01	LE	Eng
Paul	2001	$0	$0	TEC	CI	Manual handling	0	4/24/01	UE	Prod oper
Dick	2001	$0	$0	TEC	CI	Cumulative trauma	0	5/8/01	UE	Prod oper
Gayle	2001	$101	$101	VC	JLD	Other	0	4/9/01	UE	Prod oper
Sue	2001	$0	$0	Ship	CC	Other	0	7/10/01	LE	Stock hand
Ramon	2001	$0	$0	QA	CC	Other	.	2/6/01	UE	QC
Arturo	2001	$15	$15	VC	JLD	Manual handling	0	8/8/01	Back	Prod oper
Jessie	2001	$0	$0	VC	JLD	Cumulative trauma	0	6/14/01	UE	Prod oper
Frank	2001	$0	$0	VC	JLD	Other	0	5/3/01	UE	Prod oper

LE; Lower extremity; *UE*; upper extremity.

injuries over time. Both types of information are quite useful in targeting the most important problems for intervention and in assessing the impact of all interventions over time by comparing preintervention data with postintervention data.

Data related to work-related illnesses and injuries are readily available through the United States Bureau of Labor Statistics (BLS) web site *http://www.bls.gov/iif/home.htm#data*. Such information permits comparison of a particular employer's injury and illness records to national data gathered by the U.S. Department of Labor by year, industry group, type of injury, lost days incidence, restricted days incidence, gender, and other significant variables.

The injury and illness database allows the evaluator to study the significant causal and outcome variables over specified time periods to determine if there are trends or patterns. Run charts, one of the most useful means of determining how an outcome or performance measure has changed over time, can easily be generated from these databases. As shown in Figure 17-1, a run chart is simply a graphic display of data with time plotted on the x-axis

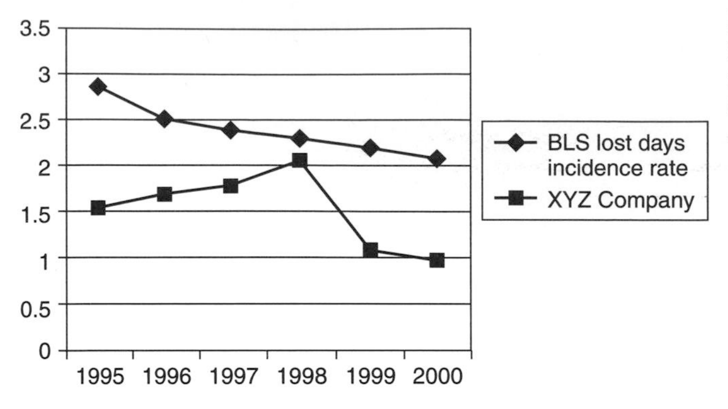

Figure 17-1 Comparison of XYZ's lost day injury and illness rates to those for all manufacturers, 1995–2000. From Bureau of Labor Statistics, US Department of Labor, 2002. *Note:* All incidence rates are expressed as rates per 100 workers per year (or 200,000 hours worked).

and an outcome or performance variable plotted on the y-axis (Brassard & Ritter, 1994). Figure 17-1 shows the lost days injury and illness incidence rate for the years 1995 through 2000 for manufacturers in the United States in comparison with the lost days injury and illness incidence rates for Company XYZ for the same period that were calculated using the company's injury and illness database.

Figure 17-2 is another example of a simple run chart showing how days lost to cumulative trauma injuries have varied for one particular company over the past 4 years. The program marker indicates the point at which a "Job Specific Fitness for Duty Testing Program" was implemented. The information shown here is one indicator that this program has been a success over the past three years.

Although information from an injury and illness database can be useful, it can also be misleading if considered in isolation. For example, if one finds consistent gender differences in injury rates, lost time, or type of injury, it could be misleading to attribute such differences simply to gender. An equally plausible explanation might be that height, strength, or weight differences are determinants of injury rates, lost time, and type of injury, and that gender differences only show up because there are significant differences in physical traits between the genders. If employees must lift parts from a shelf 72 inches above the ground, and the shortest workers are therefore most likely to sprain their shoulders or wrists while reaching overhead, it might appear that being female is a predisposing factor for injury. This fact that the shortest males are also at an increased risk for injury could be obscured by the fact that the majority of the shortest workers happen to be women. It is important to remember that statistical associations should not be confused with causal relationships.

DETERMINING COMPANY LOSSES

A database recording financial and other losses associated with occupational illnesses and injuries can enhance the value of the injury and illness database by revealing the effects of prevention programs on important resources of the organization. Although the injury database is a *sine qua non* of effective outcome assessment, it would be misleading to equate injuries and accidents with losses. This is especially true when evaluating the prevention of MSDs because the very best programs are those that seek to detect the signs and symptoms of problems long before there are medical costs, lost time, or other losses. Likewise, initial injuries to a given employee are almost always both less severe and less expensive than subsequent injuries to the same employee. A single surgical case for a ruptured intervertebral disc can cost over $100,000 in compensation, medical costs, administrative costs, and disability settlement. In contrast, 20 back sprains, if treated conservatively

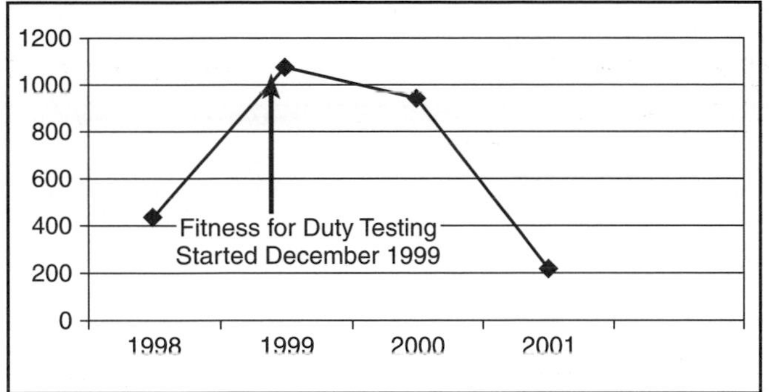

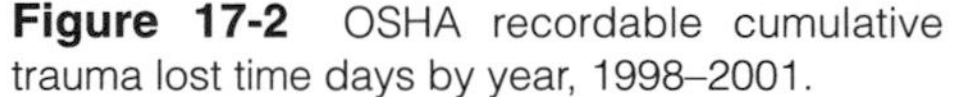

Figure 17-2 OSHA recordable cumulative trauma lost time days by year, 1998–2001.

on-site by an occupational health service—thus avoiding any visits to the doctor—may cost an average of less than $50 per case, with a total cost of no more than $1000 to treat all 20 employees with back sprains.

The adverse impact of injuries on an organization cannot always be measured solely in direct injury costs. For example, consider the case of a lead technician on a project who is out of work for several weeks at a cost of $1000 to $2000 in medical and lost-time expenses. If this worker's absence delays the launch of a new product and causes the company to default on a major contract, actual losses in present and future business from that account could be astronomical.

Assessment of losses requires that additional data concerning productivity, medical, and administrative costs of occupational injuries and illnesses be integrated into the assessment database for later analysis and interpretation. This risk-management data system integrates direct and indirect costs of prevention with other outcome measures to permit comprehensive statistical analysis of program activities and outcomes. Table 17-2 shows some of the data required in addition to the injury data provided in Table 17-1.

Risk-Management and Loss-Control Information Systems

The concept of risk management defies a single definition. In some contexts, the risks to be managed are those related to natural disasters such as tornadoes, floods, and drought, whereas in other contexts, risks are related to uncertainties about the demand for goods and services, to delays in production schedules, or to unanticipated taxation or governmental regulation. A risk-management program designed to reduce the adverse impact of workers' compensation claims, injuries, and lost time must be driven by risks related to employee health and safety. Organizations are faced with decisions concerning two categories of risk: pure risk and speculative risk (Mehr, 1983). *Pure risks* are risks that lead to losses without opportunity for any net gain. Included among these are losses from injuries, illnesses, lost time, and litigation brought against an employer on behalf of an employee. *Speculative risks* offer the opportunity for both losses and gains and include the hiring of new employees, decisions to offer a new product or service, and investment of organizational resources. Although pure and speculative risks may appear to be independent, persons responsible for loss-prevention programs, including those responsible for MSD prevention, appreciate relationships between the two that affect management decisions. For instance, a wellness program requiring a fitness center and trained staff is a speculative risk. If it decreases a single year's incidence rate for workers' compensation injuries without lowering workers' compensation insurance premiums, it may be said to reduce pure risk yet still be a net financial

Table 17-2
Sample Data from Loss Control Database

Name	Year	Total Incurred	Total Paid	Line	Cause	Days Lost	Claims Admin.	Temporary Emp. Costs	Production Shortfall Replacement Cost
Brent	2001	$276	$276	VC	Other	0	$44	$0	$0
Sam	2001	$458	$459	LM	Cumulative trauma	12	$71	$1262	$5160
Edith	2001	$96	$96	TEC	Other	0	$32	$0	$0
Arnold	2001	$29,632	$22,530	AT	Slip, trip, fall	0	$128	$0	$7102
Rose	2001	$0	$0	PH	Cumulative trauma	0	$22	$0	$0
Becky	2001	$8948	$8750	TEC	Slip, trip, fall	0	$93	$0	$4224
Sid	2001	$654	$654	VC	Cum trauma	0	$47	$0	$388
Mark	2001	$4822	$175	AT	Other	0	$33	$0	$166
Jesus	2001	$0	$0	HA	Manual handling	0	$22	$0	$0
Andy	2001	$0	$0	VC	Manual handling	0	$22	$0	$0
Sara	2001	$0	$0	MK		0	$22	$0	$0
Mary	2001	$0	$0	QA	Cumulative trauma	0	$22	$0	$0
Paul	2001	$0	$0	TEC	Manual handling	0	$22	$0	$0
Dick	2001	$0	$0	TEC	Cumulative trauma	0	$22	$0	$0
Gayle	2001	$101	$101	VC	Other	0	$26	$0	$0
Sue	2001	$0	$0	Ship	Other	0	$22	$0	$0
Ramon	2001	$0	$0	QA	Other	0	$22	$0	$0
Arturo	2001	$15	$15	VC	Manual handling	0	$23	$0	$0
Jessie	2001	$0	$0	VC	Cumulative trauma	0	$22	$0	$0

loss. However, if both occupation-related and non-occupation-related injuries and illness are reduced to a significant extent by such a program, premiums for both workers' compensation and health insurance may be decreased, and assets beyond those required by the fitness center may be conserved, resulting in a net "profit" to the cash flow of the organization.

Risk management has often been identified closely with the transference of risks from one party to another through the purchase of insurance. For many organizations, the risk manager is little more than an insurance manager. At its best, risk management is a process whereby certain risks that cannot be controlled are transferred (insured) and those that can be controlled are retained with programs undertaken to reduce or eliminate the behaviors and events that lead to losses.

For some organizations, the notion that risks should be assumed and not transferred is novel and unacceptable. Yet, risks need not be transferred to be managed effectively. Indeed, on the contrary, the transference of risks via insurance has led to the concept of acceptable risks and acceptable losses, even when the dollars to effect such transfer of risk represent a huge opportunity cost. This is especially true in cases in which losses are unnecessary, being attributable to human behaviors that can be modified, and in cases in which the causes and patterns of losses are known in advance. Risks may be managed proactively through the decision to assume responsibility for the prevention of undesirable events that lead to losses. Regardless of the type of risk or whether a prevention program does or does not depend on transferred risks (insurance) or retained risks (management programs), two classes of losses—direct and indirect—must be measured and accounted for to assess prevention program outcomes.

Direct Injury Costs: Indemnity

Organizations that carry workers' compensation insurance or use insurance products to cover losses from MSDs are charged a premium in advance of each covered time period to indemnify or reimburse such losses, either in whole or up to some prestated limit or cap. This premium usually covers (1) usual and customary medical expenses incurred in the treatment of occupation-related illness and injury; (2) compensation expenses, including the payment of a significant portion of wages that the worker otherwise would lose if unable to work; (3) administrative costs of documentation; (4) reserves that must be deposited in an account and remain available for future payments as the claim develops over time; and (5) actuarial adjustments, including experience modifiers (i.e., multiples of a standard premium for a group at risk that are used to pass along unexpected losses to future policy premiums). The amounts paid for medical services and wage replacement, large as they may be, are only a fraction of the actual premium cost. Profit for the insurance company, commissions for the agents, and state insurance taxes are also included in the premium.

This challenging and potentially confusing description of insurance issues is necessary to show that the true cost of illnesses and injuries is both complex and difficult to document. Because not all those who develop and offer MSD prevention programs are necessarily knowledgeable about cost accounting, tax laws, and insurance, a caveat is in order; determining the actual costs of a program requires special expertise. Simple approaches will most likely be inappropriate. A financial analyst, accountant, chief financial officer, or attorney is an important expert to consult when developing the measures to be used in prevention program outcome assessment.

Sources of data required to calculate direct costs of programs and losses are the risk manager, chief financial officer, accountant, and insurance provider. Loss runs from the insurance company will detail medical indemnity, amounts paid to date, amounts reserved for future claim development, and what remains encumbered at any given point in time after an occupational illness or injury. Unfortunately, there are often constraints that hinder access to the data needed to fully document losses. In some cases, businesses that operate from multiple locations pool their insurance costs and cannot accurately break out the costs for any one location. In other cases, loss information is considered "sensitive" and is not released for use in program evaluation.

Indirect Injury Costs

The true costs to companies of injuries and accidents go far beyond the obvious medical, rehabilitative, and even compensation costs. For each day an employee is unable to work, there is lost productivity, disruption in the work schedules of others who must temporarily replace the injured worker, and documentation costs for the company that eventually may include costs of determining liability and other legal services. If the employee cannot return to work, there are the costs of hiring and training a replacement and then a productivity differential in the output or work capacity of the new employee that seldom equals that of the injured person being replaced.

Incremental increases in cost per unit of goods or services produced and the cost of compensatory overtime or replacement of workers are significant costs that can and must be determined to evaluate an MSD prevention effort. Settlements with injured workers and short-term and long-term disability status must also be considered. In addition, there may be tax-supported state, local, and even federal disability benefit costs financed by taxpayers in each jurisdiction. There will be lost tax revenues such as unpaid Social Security contributions, Federal Insurance Contribution Act (FICA) funds, state and federal income taxes, and sales tax revenues that would have been generated by a healthy worker and returned to society to meet our common needs. Clearly, it is not possible to document all indirect costs of work-related injuries and illnesses. Costs that will actually be included in the formal outcome assessment of the prevention program must usually be acknowledged to be an underestimate of actual losses. If possible, those costs that cannot be measured should be identified.

Other Costs

Not all costs can be converted directly to simple indicators such as dollars. One of the most insidious costs of MSDs is that these injuries affect the morale and attitudes of subpopulations of workers, often within small work groups. The stress of working short-handed, having to adjust to the absence of a valued employee, and placing demands for attention on immediate supervisors may be significant. Such stress can lead to increased errors, quality deterioration, interpersonal tensions, and decreased productivity. These effects are often described by managers and supervisors but nonetheless prove difficult to measure.

THE GOAL-SETTING PROCESS: FOUNDATION OF OUTCOME EVALUATION

Outcome evaluation is most effective when built into a prevention program at its inception. Adding an unplanned outcome assessment to a program will limit its usefulness. Outcome assessment should begin during the earliest stages of program planning and continue throughout the lifetime of the program. It is my experience that organizations more often conceptualize evaluations as activities to be performed only at periodic intervals, and most often these organizations prefer that such evaluation periods be as brief and infrequent as possible. However, outcome assessment is linked inextricably to the goals of the program being assessed. Therefore, the first step in outcome assessment is to define the goals of a particular prevention program. This is also the first step in program development.

Clearly, if they are to be measured, program goals must be measurable. The essential question that is repeatedly asked is, "To what extent has our prevention program fallen short, hit the mark, or exceeded our expectations?" An approach to defining and prioritizing program goals that is worthy of consideration is formally known as *needs-discrepancy analysis*. It is based on the work of Borich (1990) at the University of Texas at Austin. This approach has proved especially useful in large organizations in which a committee or group has been charged with the task of developing a comprehensive prevention program. A particular advantage of this approach is that it develops the consensus of a large group (12 to 30 people at a time) without permitting excessive discussion, argumentation, or turf battles among the participating stakeholders. *Stakeholders* are those who have a direct interest in the prevention program—its administration, funding, or outcomes. Ideally, a stakeholders' group will include representatives of all major organizational constituencies from upper management to direct labor and support staff. A minimum of 10 participants is required to minimize systematic bias within the planning group.

Needs-discrepancy analysis is predicated on the belief that goals are established to organize activities that will change the behavior of an organization. If there existed no discrepancy between the present and the desired state of affairs within the organization, there would be no need for a prevention program.

The group leader or facilitator for these sessions begins by asking all stakeholders to take a seat in a circle facing one another. The leader then instructs participants that the first meeting is to be a brainstorming session. This process will generate an exhaustive list of both currently existing and desirable but undeveloped activities designed to realize the organization's injury and illness prevention and occupational health mission. The leader should summarize the ground rules as follows: Each participant will speak in turn. No participant is allowed to comment on or react to what any other participant says. The leader will call on each person in turn, proceeding around the circle, asking each to identify and describe the single most important problem related to MSDs (or any similar problem) faced by the organization. Each person's comments are recorded. Then, after everyone has had a turn to speak, the leader proceeds around the circle, once again asking the same question. This continues until there are no new responses. The leader then repeats the process, this time asking participants to identify and describe any activities that they believe are essential to an injury and illness prevention program. At the end of this second round of brainstorming, the meeting is adjourned *without discussion* among participants.

This process encourages all stakeholders to listen to one another and prevents any participant from intimidating, questioning, or negating the perceptions of any other participant. The facilitator or leader uses the transcripts to develop a *needs-analysis survey,* a comprehensive list of perceived needs in the form of a dual-rating scale (Figure 17-3).

The second stakeholders' meeting requires participants to rate on two scales each item developed on the needs analysis survey. The first of these scales, which appears in the left-hand column of Figure 17-3, assesses the extent to which the activity currently is being performed. The second scale, which appears in the right-hand column of Figure 17-3, assesses the extent to which the activity is valued. After all stakeholders have completed the formal survey (which should take 40 minutes to 1 hour), the leader explains the entire process to participants.

Between the second and third meetings, the surveys are analyzed statistically and presented graphically to represent the group's assessment of needs (Figure 17-4, *A*). A schematic representation of the four data quadrants (Figure 17-4, *B*) indicates which goals are (1) high need and high priority (highly valued), (2) high need and low priority (less valued), (3) low need and low priority, and (4) low need and no priority (not valued).

These results are then used to prepare a prioritized list of all project goals (Box 17-1), which will serve as a road map for program-planning activities.

Note that the goal with the highest perceived need and lowest perceived attainment becomes the highest priority goal. All other goals with high perceived importance are similarly rated in order of the magnitude of discrepancy between perceived need and perceived attainment. Goals that are perceived to have low need but high attainment suggest areas where resources are invested that do not serve current needs and may represent opportunities to cut back on budgets that support these activities. Finally, goals that are neither valued nor achieved are to be ignored. Following the prioritization of goals based on stakeholders' data, a final session with the stakeholders is usually devoted to creating a list of task-oriented objectives and a timetable to serve as an action plan for this project. Regardless of the methodology used to determine goals, the ability to evaluate outcomes depends on the ability to appropriately define how goal achievement will be measured. These measures include both objective and subjective indicators of program accomplishments, as will be discussed.

CONDUCTING OUTCOME EVALUATIONS

Issues in Outcome Evaluation

The outcome of any musculoskeletal treatment or prevention program can only be assessed in

This is a sample page of an actual Needs-Discrepancy Analysis questionnaire as filled out by a participant in the process.

Richard K. Schwartz, MS, OTR
Consulting Services
San Antonio, TX. 78217

This is a listing of the issues as seen by the stakeholders group.	To What Extent Does ________ Currently Do the Following?					To What Extent Should ________ Be Doing the Following?				
	Check one					Check one				
	To a great extent	To some extent	Very little	Not at all	Don't know	To a great extent	To some extent	Very little	Not at all	Don't know
1. Provide Job Safety Analyses for each position to identify potential risks/hazards?				✓		✓				
2. Provide training on how to prevent repetitive motion problems?			✓			✓				
3. Provide adequate breaks or rest periods to minimize fatigue?			✓			✓				
4. Provide appropriate chairs for those who work primarily in the seated position?			✓			✓				
5. Provide opportunities for changing positions while working?		✓				✓				
6. Offer accommodations to employees returning to work after injuries/illnesses?			✓			✓				
7. Respond to concerns raised by the Ergonomics Committee?			✓			✓				
8. Analyze accidents/injuries and illnesses to determine if there are underlying patterns?				✓		✓				
9. Enforce existing safety and health policies.		✓				✓				
10. Provide an administrative environment responsive to the needs and concerns of employees?			✓			✓				
11. Provide appropriate tools and equipment to perform work assignments?			✓			✓				
12. Provide adequate space to work?				✓		✓				
13. Train employees for the tasks they are assigned?			✓			✓				
14. Provide for rotation of duties or tasks assigned to a given employee?		✓				✓				

Figure 17-3 Stakeholders' ratings of perceived goal status and perceived goal need.

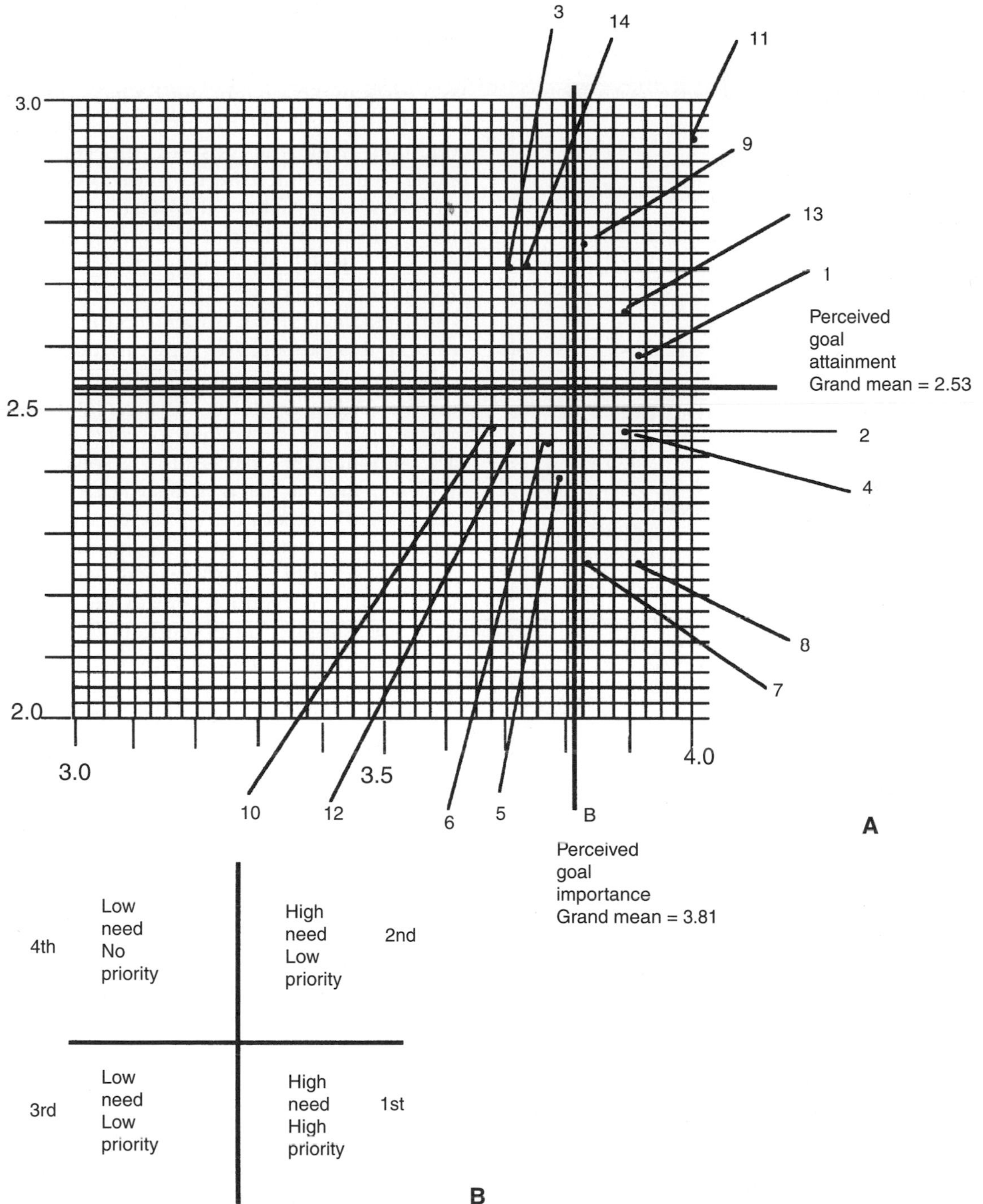

Figure 17-4 Needs assessment.

BOX 17-1
Prioritized Program Goals Based on Needs-Discrepancy Analysis

High Priorities (in order of importance): Lower Right Quadrant

- Analyze accidents and injuries to determine if underlying patterns exist.
- Respond to concerns raised by Ergonomics Committee.
- Provide training on how to prevent repetitive motion injuries.
- Provide appropriate chairs for those who work primarily in the seated position.

Low Priorities (in order of importance): Upper Right Quadrant

- Provide job safety analyses for each position to identify potential risks and hazards.
- Provide opportunities for changing positions while working.
- Offer accommodations to employees returning to work after injuries and illnesses.
- Provide administrative environment responsive to needs and concerns of employees.

Conserve Resources: Upper Left Quadrant

- Provide appropriate tools and equipment to perform work assignments.
- Enforce existing safety and health policies.

No Need Exists: Lower Left Quadrant

- Provide adequate breaks or rest periods to minimize fatigue.
- Provide for rotation of duties or tasks assigned to a given employee.

comparison to defined standards. Imagine two friends on a camping trip. Sound asleep in the middle of the night they are awakened by a bear outside their tent. One friend wakes the other says, "There's a bear outside. We're going to have to run for our lives!" As the second friend arises, the first starts for the entrance of the tent, ready to run. The second friend, however, awakes, sits up, and starts putting on his running shoes. Confused, the first friend says, "Why are you putting those on? You know you can't outrun a bear!" And the second friend calmly replies, "I don't have to outrun the bear. I just have to outrun *you*."

Outcome evaluation only has meaning in relation to organizational goals. For example, a prevention program that reduces the number of MSD cases by 80% might not be judged unsuccessful if the cost of the prevention program combined with the cost of the remaining injuries remains unchanged. On the other hand, a prevention program that leads to a 50% increase in the number of MSD cases might be very successful if the cost of the prevention program combined with the cost of all injuries is 30% less than the cost of injuries the previous year. Can this happen? Not only can it happen, it is the expected or predicted outcome because effective MSD prevention usually requires employers to encourage workers to report problems early. Although this may lead to a spike in the incidence rate of MSDs, it also leads to early correction of ergonomics problems, early intervention and treatment of symptoms, and decreased severity of work-related illnesses and injuries. Such interventions greatly decrease the need for surgical intervention, leading to dramatic savings in medical expenses, lost time, and workers' compensation payments.

Defining "successful outcomes" in relation to program goals is a necessary first step in program evaluation. The second step is to ensure that both the data and methods to measure outcome goals are available. It is an inescapable principle that outcomes must be predefined, in terms of measurable objectives, in one or more of the following ways.

- *In relation to prior outcomes:* requires analysis of differences over time within samples and populations. For example, the costs of losses for an entire organization, a department, or a work group could be compared from one year to the next.
- *In relation to normative data from a comparison population:* requires the identification of a criterion for success (benchmarking). For example, if the MSD incidence rates and standard distribution are known for those organizations within a specific Standard Industrial Code group, then the organization's

incidence rate for any period can be compared to the industry as a whole.

- *In relation to cost-benefit and return-on-investment:* for example, determining the ratio of net dollars saved in comparison with total dollars invested in a program or activity.
- *In relation to the judgment of putative experts:* that is, those responsible for conducting the program.

Whereas the first three of these methods of assessment require objective quantifiable results from data that must be as free as possible from evaluator bias, the fourth and final type of assessment must rely on judgment data that are both subjective and biased. In some cases, such outcome assessment will intentionally represent the biases of a single expert. This expert could be the owner of the business, its chief financial officer or director of human resources, or an outside consultant with no stake in the outcome of the evaluation. A panel of experts including both stakeholders and outside consultants could also provide expert judgment.

Competent program evaluators understand that subjective assessment is bound by the same rules of evaluation, statistical analysis, and causal inference as is objective outcome assessment. The major difference between these types of evaluation is not the procedural rigor or the need for reliable and valid measurement but simply the nature of the data itself.

Qualitative Measures of Outcome

Organizational behavior and the behavior of individuals in organizations are not always rational. The opinions, needs, beliefs, perceptions, and desires of people are often called into play in organizational decision-making processes. Despite their qualitative or subjective nature, these factors can be described and used to interpret programmatic outcomes. It may be extremely useful to know, for example, that the vast majority of supervisors on production lines that have few injuries believe that workers' input is very important, whereas supervisors on production lines with numerous injuries believe that workers' input is unimportant. Being able to quantify, rank, describe, and correlate such subjective information can provide reliable and valid predictors of organizational or employee behavior even when such behaviors are not rational. Examples of the types of data that may be collected before, during, or after prevention program activities include the following narrative records, case studies, interviews, focus groups, and checklists and attitude rating scales.

Narrative Records

One of the simplest methods of outcome evaluation is a journalistic or narrative record of prevention program activities. For example, a log of the ways that specific work-related complaints of symptoms or discomforts are addressed over time, including both the pre- and postintervention periods, can be used to identify changes in the number and quality of complaints. An interviewing technique called "Think Aloud Protocols" is especially good at eliciting such information. Several types of think aloud protocols exist. One type is the "Task Responding" protocol. This technique asks the worker to be talking only during the execution of certain predetermined tasks or task elements, such as only while using a particular tool or only when work is being inspected. A second type is the "Problem Protocol." This is used only when the employee is having difficulty or encounters a problem related to the work being performed. To use these as evaluation tools, workers in high-risk positions or workstations are videotaped after being instructed to speak continuously as they work. A transcript of their "thinking aloud" is produced and can be analyzed for numbers of complaints, comments about symptoms, percentage of comments that are task-related versus non-task-related. Following programmatic interventions, the same employees are again videotaped "thinking aloud" as they perform the same work and changes in the content and frequency of their thoughts are noted and compared to preintervention data.

Case Studies

Case studies have the advantage of providing in-depth accounts of how specific problems are addressed by the prevention program. The major strength of case studies is that they can provide a longitudinal description that is both interesting and informative. The major weakness, however, is that they can be biased and select only certain kinds of information to report and systematically ignore other information.

Interviews

Interviews are the single best method for establishing a program context and perspective that is independent of the inherent limitations of a particular study design. The potential sophistication of this approach generally is not well appreciated. For example, interviews may be structured (fixed-format questions addressed to each respondent) or unstructured using open-ended questions such as "Tell me what you like and dislike about this job." Interviews may be given to individuals, entire groups, or representatives of groups. Interviews may be overt or covert, in that the interviewer can reveal the purpose and nature of the interview or can keep the interviewee from knowing that the actual interview is taking place. Interview data can be recorded in journal format, on audiotape, on videotape, at fixed intervals, or randomly, using what is termed a *systematic time sampling strategy* (Borich, 1990).

Focus Groups

A simple, direct assessment of outcomes can be obtained by forming a small group of experts in the prevention of MSDs and charging them with the responsibility of performing on-site, direct observation analysis of a group or organization. The group should be independent experts or evaluators rather than individuals known to one another. The first step in using a focus group for assessment requires that the program goals and objectives be shared with the focus group. The group then develops a list of natural-language questions concerning the program that will guide the group's observations. Examples of the kinds of questions focus groups might address that are not likely to be answered by objective data include the following.

- Who seems to benefit most from the program? The least?
- Do employees really seem to have a better understanding of MSD risk factors after training than they had before training?
- After training, do employees show any noticeable changes in work postures or body mechanics?
- Will those supervisors who initially are resistant support the program to make it work for their employees or undermine the program to show their opposition?

The second step in the focus group evaluation process requires that the group spend one to two days talking with workers while gathering information and observing activities that the group members deem relevant. At the end of their visit, the group members will meet and provide verbal feedback, which should be followed by a written report of recommendations for changes and improvements in the program. Such a group may meet at fixed intervals, such as semiannually or annually, or before and after the program implementation in a pre- and posttest comparison design. It is useful to assign at least one key management person in the organization to be available to the group to clarify impressions, answer questions, and provide access to whatever information the group requires. A special strength of this approach is that the experts often ask questions that were not initially anticipated, whereas a distinct weakness is that the limited observation periods may give a biased rather than a representative sample of employee behaviors.

Checklists and Attitude Rating Scales

Although data gathered from checklists and attitude scales are subjective, the format often permits statistical analysis across a representative sample of employees or, in some cases, from an entire group or organization.

The clear advantage of such an approach is that it provides a common set of issues and reactions from individuals, permitting comparison of attitudes, values, and beliefs across demographic groupings or actual work groups or with other settings. Such checklists and scales can be completed either by trained observers or by individual program participants. A weakness of the approach is that comparisons can be made only between groups on any single item. Comparison of one item to another is problematic because there is no way of knowing which items are more important or more highly valued.

Employee Interviews and Surveys

It must be recognized that many corporate decisions are not made solely on the basis of financial considerations. In U.S. industry today there are very powerful moral and humanitarian considerations that support prevention concepts for other than economic reasons. It should not be assumed that an adversarial relationship always exists between managers and workers. Likewise, it should not be assumed that only economic costs and benefits of prevention must be studied.

A survey form was distributed to more than 900 employees of a government agency to determine the effects of an office ergonomics and MSD prevention program. A parallel version of this survey was administered simultaneously to 140 supervisory and management personnel in the same settings, and the perceptions of these groups were compared. Significant differences by role and by location were noted when respondents were asked to describe the aches, pains, and discomforts experienced at work. It was found that supervisors had significantly fewer complaints on average than either their employees or their own supervisors (i.e., chiefs). This was valuable information in assessing the role of supervisors in the prevention program, since supervisors (because they rarely complained) were viewed favorably by their chiefs and unfavorably by employees, who believed that supervisors were insensitive to employee complaints (perhaps because these supervisors did not experience the same stressors as their employees).

The role of qualitative outcome assessment in general, and the effects of prevention programs on morale specifically were described earlier. Evaluation of such outcome measures provides insight into psychosocial and group dynamics that are influenced, both for better and worse, by MSD prevention programs.

Quantitative Measures of Outcome

Many excellent texts can be consulted for those who wish to learn the models, methodologies, and step-by-step techniques for performing program analysis using objective data. Anderson et al. (1989) provide an excellent perspective for business data, whereas Borg and Gall (1983) present clear direction for the analysis of educational and behavioral data. Because these and other texts treat this subject in great deal and with more expertise than can be offered here, the focus of this section is on methods of looking at objective variables that are especially useful in the assessment of MSD-prevention programs.

Equally important is consideration of the vast array of computational tools available to analyze data and develop statistical inferences. Should one use simple two-variable models or multivariate analysis? Should one rely on strong associations or correlations or require more rigorous causal analysis? What type of experimental design is appropriate: randomized clinical trials, crossover design, blocking? Hayes (1997) provides an excellent starting point for those with some background in statistics. However, for most readers, such issues are too technical and esoteric. More important than being competent to conduct these analyses is to be aware of the tools and options available. Consultation with a research methodologist, statistician, or evaluation consultant may save much time and energy and avoid pitfalls that could fatally flaw an outcome evaluation.

Many obvious outcome measures warrant little or no comment. Among these are injury and illness incidence rates (i.e., per 200,000 hours worked), program costs (discussed later), lost workdays, medical and indemnity costs, employee turnover rates, absenteeism, numbers of nursing or other medical visits, complaints, near-misses, injuries, nonsurgical cases, and surgical cases. Other measures, such as the cost of specific or aggregated employee-related losses per unit of production or services, are illustrated in the case studies at the end of this chapter.

Some independent outcome measures, such as time from onset of injury until return to work, may not reveal much about a program, but when combined with demographic and behavioral data such as age, gender, ethnicity, employment tenure, number of previous jobs, educational level, smoking history, and prescription drug use, the possibilities for more meaningful analysis expand greatly. One of the most useful methodologies for combining outcome measures with demographic and behavioral data is *trait-treatment interaction* (Berliner & Cahen, 1973). For example, we would assume the success of a program if the average time between injury and return to full duty after unilateral carpal tunnel surgery to the preferred hand declined from 4 months before the implementation of an early-return-to-work accommodated-duty program to 1 month after the implementation of such a program. Yet, secondary analysis that evaluates the influences of gender, age, tenure, or smoking history on such an outcome might reveal that smokers still averaged 4 months per case but that nonsmokers averaged only 3 lost workdays per case for surgery. In such an instance, the secondary analysis is more helpful in evaluating and revising the program than was the primary analysis.

Pareto charts offer a simple means for identifying and prioritizing problems. The simplicity of this technique makes it readily accessible to even untrained evaluators. The appeal of this technique is that it enables the evaluator to focus on the most serious problems at any given point in time. Essentially, a Pareto chart is just a bar graph of some problem or problem dimension presented in descending order of frequency (importance) from left to right. A simple (single time point) Pareto chart can be used to target interventions designed to reduce exposure to cumulative trauma and reduce intervention costs by only addressing MSD issues in those departments, plants, or areas where losses are abnormally large. Implementing an ergonomics and safety training program throughout a large manufacturing facility can be very costly. Using a Pareto chart of Average Cost of Workers' Compensation Claims per Employee, where each production line or area is represented separately, may suggest a limited intervention that could address a significant proportion of the problem. Figure 17-5 is a Pareto chart showing the number of workers per line and average workers' compensation cost per worker for that line.

Using this Pareto chart, a decision was made to include only those workers who were employed on lines 5, 7, and 1 in an ergonomics education and prevention training program. This meant that only 185 (65 + 49 + 71) of the total 465 production workers were targeted for inclusion in the intervention, whereas the other 280 workers were intentionally not included.

Statistical analysis of the relationship(s) between and among variables is one of the more powerful quantitative analysis tools. Many excellent statistical software packages are available, usually requiring only a basic course background in statistics to use appropriately. Figure 17-6 shows the results of an analysis to determine whether or not lost days are related to the type of injury. This analysis shows that the average number of days for manual handling injuries for the population and period studied was over 25 days per injury or illness, whereas the average number of days for cumulative trauma injuries for the population and period studied was just under 16 days per injury or illness. Note that the P-value for these findings is

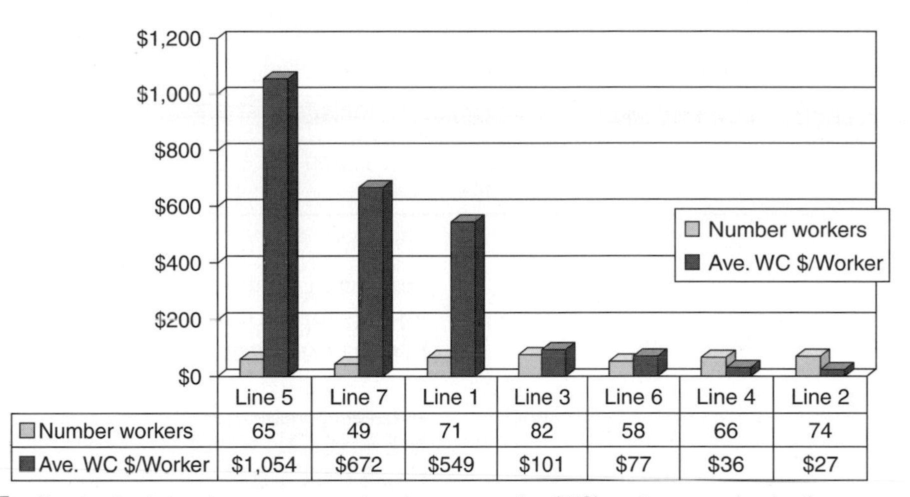

	Line 5	Line 7	Line 1	Line 3	Line 6	Line 4	Line 2
Number workers	65	49	71	82	58	66	74
Ave. WC $/Worker	$1,054	$672	$549	$101	$77	$36	$27

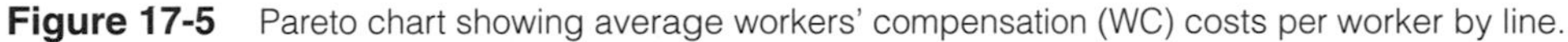

Figure 17-5 Pareto chart showing average workers' compensation (WC) costs per worker by line.

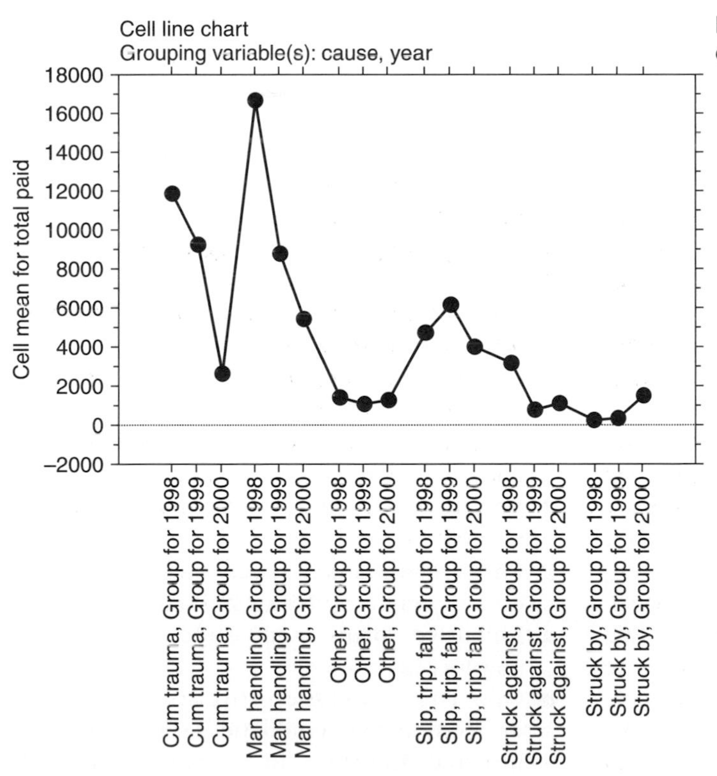

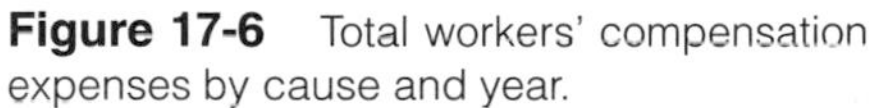

Figure 17-6 Total workers' compensation expenses by cause and year.

Table 17-3
Analysis of Variance Showing Relationship of Lost Days to Cause of Injury: ANOVA Table for Lost Days

	DF	Sum of Squares	Mean Squares	F-Value	P-Value	Lambda	Power
Cause	5	15516.228	3103.246	2.929	0.0140	14.646	0.852
Residual	219	232018.154	1059.444				

Table 17-4
Analysis of Variance Showing Relationship of Lost Days to Cause of Injury: Means Table for Lost Days Effect: Cause

	Count	Mean	Std. Dev.	Std. Err.
Cumulative trauma	51	15.922	36.348	5.090
Manual handling	58	25.086	45.027	5.912
Other	56	4.214	13.940	1.863
Slip, trip, fall	34	13.471	30.909	5.301
Struck against	13	7.462	26.015	7.215
Struck by	13	0.692	2.213	0.614

0.0140, meaning that the likelihood of finding a distribution of results this great being due to chance alone is very small (Tables 17-3 and 17-4). Although this statistic reassures the evaluator that it is highly likely that a significant relationship exists between type of injuries and lost days, what is most important is that the magnitude of this difference showing an average of nine more lost days per manual handling injury compared to cumulative trauma injury is one indicator that manual handling problems are a greater problem in this setting than cumulative trauma.

Statistical analysis can be useful in determining the impact of an MSD prevention program over time. Figure 17-6 and Table 17-5 show the impact on total dollars paid medical and leave for workers' compensation for the period January 1, 1998, to December 31, 2000. In December 1998, an MSD prevention and training program that targeted manual handling and cumulative trauma injuries was initiated. The data in Table 17-5 show that the average total paid workers' compensation cost per case declined for both cumulative trauma (MSD) and manual handling injuries for each of the two years following the intervention program.

METHODS FOR DETERMINING COST-EFFECTIVENESS

Quantitative outcome analysis is also an essential tool for determining the cost-effectiveness of achieving a particular outcome. Businesses and organizations recognize that dollars must be invested wisely.

The benefits of prevention include the following.

- Decreased lost time related not only to injuries but also to a wide range of health problems
- Decreased medical and workers' compensation costs
- Reductions in reserves or insurance costs
- Decreased employee turnover
- Increased productivity

The costs of prevention programs may include the following.

- Management costs to design and implement prevention programs
- Consultancy and fee-for-service agreements for professional services
- Clerical and data-processing services to document and evaluate programs
- Release time during which employees will be trained
- Physical resources, space, and materials to conduct safety activities and training
- Incentive plans and direct payouts to employees
- Opportunity and alternative investment costs or income that could be earned by funds invested in prevention programs if such

Table 17-5
Total Paid Workers' Compensation Expenses by Cause by Year

Group, Year	Count	Mean	Standard Deviation	Standard Error
Cumulative trauma, 1998	21	11,923	14,648	3197
Cumulative trauma, 1999	16	9405	13,106	3277
Cumulative trauma, 2000	14	2675	5353	1431
Manual handling, 1998	17	16,751	30,159	7315
Manual handling, 1999	19	8825	15,448	3544
Manual handling, 2000	22	5532	6945	1481
Other, 1998	17	1485	2619	635
Other, 1999	21	1171	2898	632
Other, 2000	18	1349	3742	882
Slip, trip, fall, 1998	16	4795	8355	2089
Slip, trip, fall, 1999	6	6238	10,758	4392
Slip, trip, fall, 2000	12	4041	10,500	3031
Struck against, 1998	3	3194	4345	2508
Struck against, 1999	1	801	—	—
Struck against, 2000	9	1098	1926	642
Struck by, 1998	4	302	209	105
Struck by, 1999	3	418	421	243
Struck by, 2000	6	1538	2350	959

funds were invested in other activities of the company

Not every alternative approach to injury prevention and risk management is equally cost-effective, and some may actually be cost-ineffective. Are those programs most cost-effective that target workers with the highest risk of injury? How often must training, safety inspections, and other prevention activities be conducted to maximize the return on dollars invested in prevention? Beyond the benefits of prevention programs to individual employers, what are the economic benefits of such programs to society at large?

Economic data and evidence of cost-effectiveness of prevention programs are needed for two reasons. First, such information provides an excellent decision-making support tool to assist management in allocating prevention dollars. Second, it serves as a powerful marketing tool to drive home the need for such programs.

Cost Accounting and Return-on-Investment Analysis

Although often thought of as a methodology, prevention is, first and foremost, a way of conceptualizing work processes, environments, tools, equipment, and labor that emphasizes the appreciation and consideration of human beings as valuable biomechanical and biocomputational tools with which to accomplish corporate or organizational objectives. Prevention of MSDs is not only a safety or risk-management or human factors activity, but is also a comprehensive approach to organizational problems that can and must permeate every activity within the system (Schwartz, 1995).

A key question that an organization with an MSD prevention program must ask is, "What is the opportunity cost in present and future dollars of *not* providing such programs?" An MSD prevention program should pose alternative solutions to problems and permit the attribution of costs and benefits to the various alternatives. This means that even when assumptions must be made and information is not complete, there is a methodology for accurate estimation of return on investment (ROI) from each alternative. As a decision-making tool, outcome assessment provides a framework within which engineering and procedural activities can be translated into a cost-accounting model and evaluated technically and from a bottom-line and investment-risk perspective. Information such as anticipated payback periods for capital investments (how long it will be until the benefits realized from a particular activity equal the additional cost of the activity); effects of changes in human behaviors on cycle time, errors, and labor costs; and analyses of value added to a product or service by a particular improvement in the methods used to produce that commodity or service are essential to the evaluation of specific outcomes anticipated from MSD prevention programs.

Those seeking to implement a responsible prevention program must be prepared to compete for the dollars required for the implementation. These dollars must be justified with respect to the desirability of the projected outcomes, and they must be justified as a better investment of resources than competing alternative activities that desire to use these same scarce resources. Often, a worst-case analysis should be conducted to minimize the risk of the prevention program itself becoming a deficit operation. In those instances in which the certainty of outcomes is difficult to predict, small pilot studies are a more responsible and less risky alternative than full-scale program implementation. Pilot programs can cap losses and permit the development and refinement of both prevention program activities and evaluation activities that will be used to assess program outcomes. The case studies at the end of this chapter illustrate both cost accounting and ROI analysis.

Injury Cost Trend Analysis

A risk-management and ergonomics program designed to reduce the adverse impact of workers' compensation claims, injuries, and lost time must be assessed in relation to historical trends, not simply in terms of the absolute value of dollars spent or saved from one year to the next. Figure 17-7 shows that for one company, actual losses from worker's compensation claims resulting from MSDs were \$473,764 in 1998. To assess the value of the prevention program established in December 1998, a cost-benefit analysis was done, based on a model comparing losses in each of the two subsequent years to the losses in 1998. The actual losses in 1999 declined by nearly \$300,000 to \$173,907. Actual losses in 2000 declined an additional \$47,425 to \$126,482. However, these savings from one year to the next do not accurately reflect the true value of the prevention program to the organization. The actual *value* of saving \$299,857 in the first year of the program must be reduced by the cost of the program—that is, \$37,598. Actual

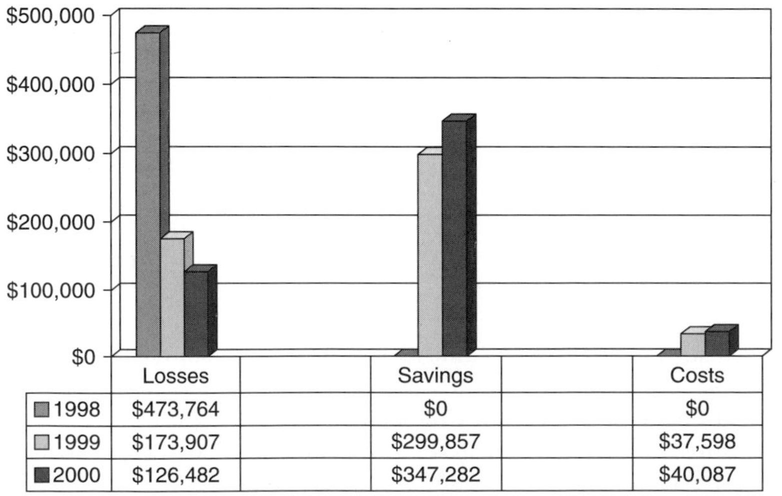

	Losses	Savings	Costs
1998	$473,764	$0	$0
1999	$173,907	$299,857	$37,598
2000	$126,482	$347,282	$40,087

Figure 17-7 Impact of prevention program on losses from 1998 to 2000.

savings is therefore $262,259. Between the first and second years of the program, actual losses were reduced another $47,425 minus the $40,087 in program costs for an actual additional savings of only $7,338. Even though the 2-year difference by this analysis seems to be $269,597 (the sum of $262,259 and $7,338), this is an underestimate of the actual savings of the program. Taking into account the fact that losses in 1998 had increased almost linearly for the four years from 1995, when losses were $344,233, to 1998 when losses peaked at $473,364, expected losses for 1999 should be equal to or greater than the losses of 1998.

Thus, in the analysis provided in Figure 17-7, a decision was made to use the losses in 1998 as a baseline and measure future losses against this baseline year.

Productivity and Labor Costs Analysis

Even in profitable organizations in which there is insignificant risk of injury and minimal repetitive motion, prevention of MSDs is important. In fact, it could be argued that the more successful a company or group is in reducing losses from MSDs, the more prevention and ergonomic approaches are the *only* ways to increase the ROI of capital and labor. Ergonomic interventions designed to reduce the physical and psychologic demands on workers result in energy conservation, work simplification, stress reduction, and time and motion reduction, thereby allowing workers to be more efficient and effective. Ergonomics is an important tool in quality enhancement, cycle time reduction, and optimization of the marginal value of labor dollars invested in production or services (Schwartz, 1994).

The literature on multiphasic health screening has failed to find that comprehensive screening and testing of all employees is a cost-effective means of controlling risk. However, there is reason to believe that screening for certain specific health limitations may be an additional tool in a total risk-management strategy. One example of a screening tool that may lower total risks is preemployment screening for illegal drug use. Such screening is undertaken not to eliminate from consideration for hire those individuals with significant health problems but rather to discourage the application of persons who abuse drugs. Drug screening also sends a strong message that the company will not condone the abuse of scheduled drugs and the attendant health risks.

Another screening tool is physical capacities testing to determine a minimal skill level, such as the ability to lift a 50-pound load from 12 to 48 inches off the ground. Such screening may identify those persons who are unable to meet strenuous job demands. If these tests are job specific and are conducted as post-offer, preplacement tests, they are both appropriate and legal under the Americans with Disabilities Act (Equal Employment Opportunity Commission, 1993) (see Chapter 15 for further discussion).

Simulation of alternative duties that are being considered for an employee may reveal which duty can be best tolerated with the highest levels of productivity. Direct analysis of labor costs per unit of production or unit of service provides a powerful indicator of improved efficiency in worker performance as a result of a prevention program.

Reduced employee turnover, with its associated reduction in hiring and replacement costs, is another example of a labor cost that can be used as an outcome indicator in evaluating a prevention program. In one 2800-employee firm in which the author has worked for more than 4 years to establish a comprehensive loss-control and risk-management program based on prevention principles, the savings for the first two years of the program exceeded $1,400,000. In the third year of the program, actual losses were less than $300,000, and there appeared to be no way to equal the savings of the previous years. However, an astonishing trend began to emerge. Whereas turnover of employees had averaged more than 19% annually for many years, it suddenly dropped in the third year to less than 10% per year, and the savings attributable to reduced hiring, replacement, and training costs were approximately $1300 per position; multiplied by 260 fewer-than-expected employee turnovers, the estimated savings totaled $338,000. The employees perceived that the same work that had been done in the past now was easier to accomplish because of ergonomic interventions and training and was safer because of the prevention program activities, and this perception was a major factor in retaining employees who were otherwise at high risk for leaving the company.

AN EXPLANATORY NOTE

A search of the literature on injury and illness prevention programs, outcome analysis, and MSDs and ergonomics is unlikely to uncover instruction related to outcome evaluation of prevention programs. The reader may wonder whether anyone else has attempted such evaluation or whether it is merely an esoteric and academic exercise of little or no use to actual organizations.

Most organizations are extremely reluctant to allow outsiders access to information that is a business asset. The great value of such evaluations to employers, the costs of bringing in outside consultants, and the competitive advantage of using information to improve the organization all mitigate against sharing these studies. An honest picture of organizational behaviors, organizational losses, waste, and harm done to humans is vital to comprehensive outcome evaluation. Outcome evaluations are typically conducted using data that are restricted, confidential, and potentially damaging to the organizations profiled by such data. These data also are potentially "discoverable"—that is, they could be subpoenaed as evidence in litigation and used against those who had the courage and foresight to conduct an honest self-appraisal. No organization wants to air its dirty laundry in public. One *can* find in the literature the successes of prevention programs, but these often are published long after the programs have been in place and only after they have been scrutinized, and often sanitized, by attorneys and executive officers.

The figures cited earlier in this chapter and those in the case study that follows are actual data from the author's clients that have been merged and disguised. Evaluation is both art and science. Knowledge of spreadsheets, databases, statistics, and accounting is insufficient to conduct useful outcome assessments. There will always be those who use such information tools in a procrustean manner, avoiding the issue of appropriateness of approach and the need to assess continually and to refine the techniques. Those looking for quick-and-dirty, turnkey systems for outcome evaluation are bound to be disappointed, since these do not exist currently, and it is unlikely that they ever will.

CASE 1

A consulting firm for a large Midwestern manufacturer had been providing both an ergonomics injury prevention and early return-to-work program for almost five years, when there was a management change at the company that led to the appointment of a new plant manager from outside the firm. This person immediately fired the middle managers responsible for the Human Resources, Environmental Health and Safety, and Employee Training departments. Of course, these were the very people with whom the outside ergonomics consultants had worked closely on a day-to-day basis. When the time came to renew the consulting agreement, the new manager asked for a proposal and set up a 15-minute meeting for an oral presentation by the consultants.

Knowing that their contract was on the line, what could the consultants do to convince the new management to continue the programs that the consultants had established and operated for the previous 5 years? Since the consultants would be meeting the new plant manager for the first time, and since there was so little time to explain what they did or how successful it had been, a decision was made to sell the programs on their bottom-line dollar value to the company.

Using the accident and injury database and risk management databases, the consultants decided to provide an overall summary of program costs, which were $60,741 for the period,

Table 17-6

Cost-Benefit Analysis of Ergonomics and RTW Prevention Programs 1998–2002

ANALYSIS OF IMPACT OF GSF CONSULTING SERVICES, INC. ON REDUCTION OF WORKERS' COMPENSATION CLAIM LIABILITY AT MIDWEST MANUFACTURING CO. FOR PERIOD 1/1/98 TO 9/30/02

		Savings Resulting from Services	Consultant Costs	Losses Not Prevented	Benefits (Net Savings)
Ergonomics Workstation Evaluations					
Intervention services (438 evaluations)			($47,360)		
Number of WC claims completely prevented	305				
Average cost per WC claim prevented	$6718				
Savings on claims from intervention services		$2,048,990			
Number of WC claims following intervention services	66				
Cost of claims not prevented				($368,458)	
Net savings from intervention services.					$1,633,172
RTW Evaluations					
RTW Evaluations	106		($13,382)		
Number of RTW evaluations without added WC claim	96				
Number of RTW WC claims prevented	76				
Savings on claims from RTW evaluations		$499,714			
Number of WC claims not prevented by RTW evaluations	10				
Cost of claims not prevented				($74,677)	
Net savings resulting from RTW evaluations					$425,037
Totals		**$2,548,704**	($60,741)	($443,135)	**$2,044,828**
Cost/Benefit Ratio		**$60,741/$2,044,828 equals 1/33**			

RTW, Return to work; *WC,* workers' compensation.

and the overall program benefits, which were savings of $2,044,828 (Table 17-6). It should also be noted that losses from injuries and illnesses are especially burdensome because they are paid for at the time they occur and therefore directly reduce gross revenues from sales and services. Each dollar paid in losses (or each dollar saved if there is no loss) would otherwise be a dollar of profit to the organization.

Using these figures, they calculated the overall cost/benefit ratio for their work to be an impressive 1/33. Table 17-6 was presented at the meeting, and the presentation concluded with the consultants noting, "We have saved you $33 for every $1 you have invested in our services. If you can get a better return by taking the money from our contract and investing it elsewhere, we will understand. If you do not have such an alternative, we would appreciate continuing our partnership with you." To the credit of these consultants, the new management team renewed the contract.

These consultants had carefully documented and quantified program outcomes related to their work. Because they were able to demonstrate both the reduction of occupational injuries and illnesses and the actual savings directly attributable to the interventions they conducted, it was relatively simple to compute program costs and determine the cost/benefit ratio for their work. If the same efforts had been made without planning for and conducting systematic and routine outcome evaluations, it would have been difficult for these outside consultants to prove their value to the client.

REFERENCES

Anderson, D. R., Sweeney, D. J., & Williams, T. A. (1989). *Quantitative methods for Business* (4th ed.). St. Paul: West Publishing.

Berliner, D., & Cahen, L. (1973). Trait-treatment interaction and learning. In F. Kerlinger (Ed.), *Review of research in education*. Itasca, IL: Peacock.

Borg, W. R., & Gall, M. D. (1983). *Educational research: An introduction* (4th ed.). New York: Longman.

Borich, G. D. (1990). *Review notes for evaluation models and techniques*. Austin: The University of Texas.

Borich, G. D., & Jemelka, R. P. (1982). *Programs and systems: An evaluation perspective*. New York: Academic Press.

Brassard, M., & Ritter, D. (1994) *The memory jogger II*. Methuen: GOAL/QPC.

Cascio, W. F. (1991). *Costing human resources: The financial impact of behavior in organizations.* Boston: PWS-Kent Publishing.

Equal Opportunity Employment Commission (1993). 29 CFR, Chapter 14, part 1630: *The regulations to implement the Equal Employment Provisions of the Americans with Disabilities Act* and, from the Appendix to Part 1630: *Interpretive guidance on title I of the Americans with Disabilities Act.* 391–424. Washington, DC: U.S. Government Printing Office.

Hayes, W. L. (1997). *Statistics* (5th ed.). New York: Holt, Rinehart & Winston.

Mehr, R. I. (1983). Risk management and risk analysis. In *Fundamentals of insurance*. Homewood, IL: Richard D. Irwin.

Milstein, R. L., Wetterhall, S. F., et. al. (1999). Framework for program evaluation in public health. *Morbidity and Mortality Weekly Report, 48*(RR11), 1–40. Atlanta, Center for Disease Control and Prevention.

Schwartz, R. K. (1994). Why ergonomics is good economics. In T. Harkins (Ed.), *Workers compensation update 1994*. Walnut Creek, CA: Council for Education in Management.

Schwartz, R. K. (1995). OSHA's pending ergonomic rules. In M. Fox (Ed.), *Personnel law update.* Walnut Creek, CA: Council on Education in Management.

PART FIVE

Managing MSDs in Home and Leisure Environments

CHAPTER 18

Ergonomics in the Home

Martha J. Sanders
Robyn Stricoff

HOME-WORK CONTINUUM IN THE DEVELOPMENT OF MUSCULOSKELETAL DISORDERS

For those who work for pay outside the home, at least 30% to 40% percent of each weekday is spent in home-related activities (based on an 8-hour workday and 7 to 8 hours of sleep per night). This percentage increases for those who do not work for pay or volunteer outside the home. Although we associate the development of musculoskeletal disorders (MSDs) with biomechanical exposures in the workplace, the home environment is not without ergonomic exposures that may exacerbate or initiate the development of MSDs. Since MSDs are caused by cumulative exposure to risk factors throughout the day, the clinician must consider the sum of all exposures at home and at work in the treatment and prevention of MSDs.

A Case for Addressing Ergonomics in the Home

Ergonomic applications relative to the prevention of MSDs have focused on primarily industrial and office settings. Such applications have sought not only to decrease the risk of injury but also to maximize efficiency, eliminate waste, and improve productivity and comfort. Ergonomics has not traditionally addressed home and leisure activities, possibly because there are few direct business incentives or monies driving such interventions. However, many reasons exist why the home environment is an area ripe for ergonomic intervention. First, business and industry may inadvertently be subsuming the costs for home-related injuries, since, according to the criteria for an OSHA recordable injury, a work-related injury includes any illness that is exacerbated by a work-related activity, including an injury that may have been precipitated by activities at home (see Chapter 4 for a thorough discussion). Second, whether workers' compensation or healthcare insurance pays for the medical treatment, home-related injuries contribute to the overall cost of health care. Third, healthy employees may be more productive and enjoy better quality of life. Fourth, the performance of domestic work is still one of the world's primary occupations, with a significant number of accidents occurring inside the home as compared to outside (Grandjean, 1973).

Risk Factors in Home Activities

The same types of biomechanical risk factors exist in the performance of home-related activities as in the performance of workplace tasks (e.g., excessive force, awkward or static posture, repetition, vibration, acceleration, mechanical compression), although these risk factors are *not usually* considered to occur with the same intensity or duration as they occur at work (see Chapter 10 for a complete discussion). However, when individuals become involved with intrinsically motivating activities such as crafts, gardening, or sports, or activities in which the outcome is highly valued (such as finishing a present for the holidays, raking the leaves before snow, or repairing the family car), individuals may spend a prolonged duration of time in such an activity. Csikszentmihalyi (1990) describes the optimal "flow" experience in which individuals enter a state of focused concentration and effortless control when engaged in a particularly meaningful and challenging activity. In such a state, a sense of time and perhaps musculoskeletal discomfort may be overridden by the exhilaration of the task. To that end, some exposures in home-related activities may, in fact, reach or surpass the intensity of those at work.

This chapter discusses the application of ergonomic principles to activities in the home. The existing principles for optimal use of the body (not typically described in ergonomic terms) are presented. Ergonomic risk factors and recommendations to improve the safe and effective performance of common home maintenance activities of cooking, cleaning, and laundering are presented. Finally, the current issues in ergonomics for children are addressed.

USING THE BODY FOR OPTIMAL FUNCTIONING: A REPRESENTATION OF ERGONOMIC IDEOLOGIES

Health care professionals who treat clients with disabilities have addressed safe and effective use of the body in home environments for decades (Trombly, 1997). Although not conceptualized as ergonomic principles, joint protection, body mechanics, and energy conservation techniques all deal with efficient use of the body during activity. *Joint protection principles* were originated to promote function in clients with rheumatoid arthritis (Cordery, 1965); *body mechanics* have focused on back safety in industry (Saunders, 1993); and *energy conservation techniques* have been implemented to conserve energy in those with limited endurances, such as multiple sclerosis or pulmonary disease (Trombly, 1997). In reality, these principles are based on sound biomechanical guidelines that encourage efficient use of the body for all populations. As worker populations age, these measures will become increasingly important in preventing injury and promoting function in both work and home environments. These principles are listed in Box 18-1. The reader is referred to the appropriate references for a complete discussion of each.

Protecting One's Joints

Joint protection principles have been an integral component of client education for rheumatologic diseases, primarily rheumatoid arthritis

BOX 18-1
Principles for Optimal Use of the Body

Protecting the Joints

1. Distribute the load over as many joints as possible
2. Use larger and stronger joints to accomplish the task
3. Use each joint in its most stable position to reduce pressure on the joint
4. Ensure correct patterns of movement
5. Avoid deforming positions and stresses that contribute to deformity
6. Avoid staying in one position for long periods of time
7. Balance between moving a joint and resting a joint

Conserving Energy

8. Pace activities throughout the day and week
9. Alternate heavy and light tasks throughout the day and week
10. Balance rest and activity: take rest breaks during prolonged activity
11. Organize one's environment for optimum efficiency
12. Use correct working positions: sit versus stand when able

Protecting the Back

13. Keep the load close to the body
14. Move with the feet first
15. Avoid forward bending and twisting
16. Use a wide base of support and staggered stance

(RA), for over three decades. More recently, joint protection principles have been applied to osteoarthritis (OA), which is relevant to an aging population. Joint protection principles are based on the theory that forces generated in everyday use of the joints may contribute to structural damage and subsequent deformity for involved joints, particularly in the hand (Cordery, 1965; Cordery & Rocchi, 1998). Intervention principles focus on reducing internal and external mechanical loading on joints (which will subsequently reduce microtrauma to the articular cartilage and subchondral bone) and promoting muscular support to absorb the loads around a joint (Cordery & Rocchi, 1998; McCloy, 1982). The ultimate goal is to maintain functional use of the extremity. Box 18-1 outlines the most widely accepted joint protection principles (Cordery, 1965; Cordery & Rocchi, 1998; Hammond, 1994; Stamm et al., 2002).

The application of joint protection principles to everyday activities consists of techniques to decrease loads on joints through using the body in biomechanically advantageous positions and by using adaptive equipment. A classic application of the principles is carrying a heavy pot by placing one hand (palm-up) under the pot base and steadying the pot with the other hand on the handle. This technique both distributes the weight of the pot over several joints (thus minimizing the external torque at any one joint) and uses the stronger biceps muscles rather than the hand intrinsic musculature to sustain the load.

Another example is removing water from a sponge by pressing it with an open palm rather than grasping it and wringing it out. The process of wringing a washcloth forces the metacarpophalangeal (MCP) joints into flexion and ulnar deviation, which can be potentially deforming. In general, the more resistive the activity or grasp demands, the greater the deforming forces (Cordery & Rocchi, 1998). Recommendations suggest that individuals should strive to maintain full range of motion of the joints in order to adequately distribute the loads over the largest area, thereby reducing the load on each joint. Adapted tools and devices are designed to encourage a more neutral position of the wrist and hands and decrease forces necessary for tool use. For example, the pistol grip eliminates ulnar deviation of the wrist by placing the handle 90 degrees to the blade or working piece. A pistol grip can be applied to knives, saws, gardening tools (see Chapter 20), and paintbrushes, to name a few. Other adapted tools now mainstreamed for everyday use are screwdrivers with a large ball to grasp as a handle and extended handles on doors or faucets. (Refer to Cordery and Rocchi (1998) for a complete discussion of joint protection principles and adaptive equipment.) The principle of avoiding deforming hand forces during tool use has also been suggested by Tichauer (1966) relative to use of tools in industry and has been integrated into ergonomic tool design (see Chapter 11 for a full discussion).

Although joint protection principals have been recommended based on biomechanical theory, the efficacy of joint protection intervention for OA has only recently been addressed. Stamm et al. (2002) examined the effect of joint protection and home exercises on hand function of clients with hand OA in a randomized control trial of 40 clients with OA. Clients were assigned to two groups: One group received joint protection and hand exercises (JPE), and the control group received information on OA. Outcomes measures were grip strength, visual analogue scales (VAS) for pain and hand function, and the Health Assessment Questionnaire (HAQ). After 3 months of intervention, researchers found a significant gain in hand function in the JPE group as compared to the control group. Grip strength in the JPE group improved by 25% ($p < 0.0001$ right hand; $p < 0.0005$ left hand). Self-perceived hand function was improved in 65% of the JPE group as compared to 20% in the control group ($p < 0.05$). No differences were found in health assessment questionnaires between JPE and control groups.

Most individuals over the age of 65 show evidence of articular damage with 60% to 70%

of all those over 65 seeking medical attention for this condition (Kraus, 1997). Since mechanical stress is an important facilitator of the degenerative process, joint protection techniques would appear to be prudent prevention techniques for all individuals performing work- or home-related activities. The principles *should* be considered universal design for all ages. The Joint Protection Behavior Assessment is a tool that measures a person's use of joint protection principles (Hammond, 1994; Klompenhouwer, Lysack, Dijkers, & Hammond, 2000). This assessment requires observing a client performing 20 subtasks, then assigning a score to the performance of each task according to whether joint protection principles were used to complete the task.

Protecting One's Back

Body mechanics is a term that has been equated with proper use of the body, primarily the back, to prevent injuries associated with lifting or weighted activities (Saunders, 1992). Lifting injuries can be classified into three groups: accidental, caused by overexertion, and cumulative (Pheasant, 1991). Tasks performed in the home environment certainly lend themselves to all three groups. Years of subclinical damage to joints, ligaments, disc, and other tissue from cumulative performance of seemingly innocuous activities of daily living may result in soft tissue damage far greater than one may expect.

Intervertebral disc pressure (IVDP) is the criterion used to assess risk of low-back injury in the workplace (Kroemer & Grandjean, 2001). NIOSH estimates that 770 pounds of disc compressive force will be stressful for some members of the workforce and 1430 pounds will be stressful to most members of the workforce. IVDP is lowest with lying supine, next highest with standing and highest with sitting. The greater the kyphosis to the lumbar spine, the greater the IVDP.

Proper body mechanics techniques are taught to minimize the effects of a posturally induced strain or a load-induced strain to the low back. An example of an everyday activity performed at least two times per day and placing stress on the low back is brushing one's teeth. As one leans over the sink, the head is displaced in front of the body, far away from the center of mass, causing both increased IVDP and high internal muscle forces to sustain that position. Trunk angle for people brushing teeth may vary; however, most assume a posture of kyphosis to the lumbar spine. The farther one bends over, the greater the IVDP, and the greater the load of the head and upper body on the back. The weight of the entire upper body is being supported entirely by back musculature and ligaments. Disc compressive force could be estimated at approximately 400 pounds in this head-forward posture (see calculations in Appendix 18-1). By supporting upper body weight on the counter with the nondominant hand and staggering one's stance, a decrease in disc compressive forces of about 30% is possible, and internal muscle forces required to maintain this position are decreased. Since back injury at home tends to occur more so from the cumulative trauma just described than overexertion, it is important that body mechanic principles become integral in the correct means of performing common household tasks.

Conserving Energy

Managing fatigue has been an important aspect of managing the disease for many individuals with chronic illnesses such as rheumatoid arthritis, multiple sclerosis, postpolio syndrome, and chronic fatigue syndrome (Cordery & Rocchi, 1998; Trombly, 1997). Fatigue, in this case, refers to a generalized exhaustion of the entire body related to central nervous system function rather than localized muscle fatigue, as discussed in Chapter 9. As our overall energy level becomes subjectively less as we age, energy conservation techniques may help us to continue to perform those activities that are important to us.

The two main concepts of energy conservation or energy management are preserving energy (by using good body mechanics, organizing the workplace, delegating tasks) and budgeting energy (through prioritizing the activities on which to spend the energy). A critical feature of energy conservation is finding a balance between rest and activity (Cordery & Rocchi, 1998). Melvin (1989) suggests that the most effective means to increase functional endurance is to take a 5- to 10-minute rest before becoming tired or exhausted. In a prospective, randomized study of energy conservation and joint protection techniques, this principle was found to be effective for individuals with RA who completed a 6-week energy conservation program. At a 3-month follow-up, 50% of those who took a 10-minute rest break after performing prolonged activity were more physically active throughout the day as compared to 11% in a control group that received traditional instruction about the disease process (Gerber et al., 1987). Although results did not reach significance, authors suggest that this preliminary data may draw an important relationship between energy conservation techniques and increased overall physical activity. Such principles may be useful for an aging population in the home.

ERGONOMIC CONSIDERATIONS FOR HOME MAINTENANCE ACTIVITIES

Considerations for ergonomics in the home include design features for specific workspaces, ergonomic tools, task modification, and optimal use of the body as discussed previously. Home workspaces may be created for optimal performance by incorporating principles of work design: work flow, work layout, anthropometrics, optimal tool use, work physiology, and biomechanics into the architectural layout. The term *gerotechnology* has been used to describe ergonomic interventions for older adults with age-related impairments (Pinto et al., 2000). Pheasant (1996) provides a complete discussion on these topics. Ergonomics approaches for specific home-related tasks are discussed following and in Tables 18-1 through 18-4.

Cooking

Kitchen Layout and Storage

A myriad of specific tasks are incorporated into the entire cooking process, many of which expose individuals to biomechanical risk factors including prolonged standing, awkward postures of the hand and wrist, and static and forceful grasps. Table 18-1 provides an outline of such factors. Basic principles of *workplace layout* can be applied to overall kitchen design and storage of utensils in order to maximize efficient use. Relative to the general location of components, these principles suggest that the most important and frequently used items should be placed in convenient locations. Relative to the specific arrangement of components, items with similar functions should be located together, and items that are commonly used in a sequence should be laid out in the same sequence (Sanders & McCormick, 1993). (These principles are also aspects of energy conservation techniques.)

Two basic philosophies of kitchen design exemplify the general location principles for the three work surfaces that constitute the "work triangle" of the kitchen: the sink, the stove, and the refrigerator.

1. The path from the stove to sink is the most frequently used route. These appliances should be located in close proximity to each other.
2. For a right-handed person, the sequence of activity proceeds from left to right—that is, from the sink to the main work surface to the stove to the accessory work surface (Pheasant, 1996).

These principles become especially important when transporting pots, pans, or dishes from one surface to another.

When specifically arranging items, the most accessible storage space is the countertop. How-

Table 18-1
Modifying Cooking Tasks

Task	Ergonomic Risk Factor	Recommendations
Overall cooking process	Prolonged standing Upper extremity force and repetition Static grasps	Use a good kitchen layout to minimize distances between frequently used components Purchase ergonomic mats Build a foot bar into work areas Use a stool to elevate legs Wear insoles Vary standing and sitting Use utensils with a soft, oval shape and larger-diameter handles Stretch frequently
Cutting	Awkward wrist position Repetition Static grasp on knives	Use ergonomic knives with pistol grip Learn proper technique (professional) Use a food processor when possible
Stirring	Repetition Awkward wrist position Static grasp on spoon handle	Use utensils with a soft, oval shape and larger-diameter handles Use a power grasp with the thumb up Move entire arm Use an electric mixer
Transporting pots, pans, and dishes	Excessive forces Awkward postures when lifting dishes to and from cupboards	Place dishes on a pushcart Organize kitchen so that heavy and frequently used items are at waist height Use two hands to carry heavy pots

ever, the countertop can potentially become cluttered, which clearly defeats its ergonomic purpose. (Pheasant [1996] refers to this as "ergonomic decay.") Therefore, functional groupings and frequency of use should guide placement. For example, heavy and frequently used items such as pots and pans should be located between knee and shoulder heights, preferably under countertops. Food storage should be arranged to minimize reaching, bending and lifting: a bag of potatoes should be stored between knee and shoulder height; the dishwasher and the cupboard for plates and glasses should be located close to each other to minimize reach distances when putting away plates; a lazy Susan can minimize awkward reaches to the back of cabinets; cooking utensils should be located close to the stovetop; and frequently used spices and condiments can be purchased in bulk, with smaller amounts stored on the countertop.

Kitchen Utensils

Kitchen utensils, similar to industrial tools, are undergoing revolutionary design changes in response to users with special needs and aged consumers. Ergonomic design for kitchen utensils is important both in opening food products and in using them in the cooking process.

Opening products such as jars with vacuum-sealed lids and sealed plastic containers presents a major problem for many consumers (Kelsheimer & Hawkins, 2000; Voorbij & Steenbekkers, 2002). Kelsheimer & Hawkins (2000) found that 85% of an elderly population reported some type of difficulty in performing kitchen tasks. The most difficult tools to use effectively were reportedly a jar opener, paring knife, kitchen scissors, and a can opener.

When Voorbij and Steenbekkers (2002) examined the methods and forces used to open jars in an elderly population, they found that 50% of elderly users had difficulty opening a jar

Table 18-2
Modifying Cleaning Tasks

Task	Ergonomic Risk Factors	Recommendations
Cleaning toilet	Static and awkward position of wrist and entire body while kneeling and rotating brush	Use long-handled toilet scrubber Wear knee pads for prolonged kneeling Build a bridge to support upper body by grasping a grab bar while cleaning toilet
Cleaning shower	Static finger flexion while holding sponge Awkward body posture Excessive reach to top of shower	Use an open palm on sponge Use overnight cleaner Use lightweight mop with extended handle
Mopping floor	Excessive load to the low back while lifting bucket full of water Twisting motion of the trunk while moving mop	Use a bucket on wheels Fill bucket using a hose from sink Empty bucket by tilting Use a mop with longer handle and two points of grasp Follow good body mechanics; move feet first
Vacuuming	Push-pull forces to the low back and shoulder Carrying vacuum up and down stairs	Use self-propelled vacuum Design home with central vacuum connections Have car vacuums available in upstairs rooms Have a vacuum for upstairs and downstairs Follow good body mechanics; move feet first
Dusting	Repetitive use of upper extremity Excessive reaches Static grasp on cloth	Use spray to most efficiently gather dust Use long handles for out-of-reach locations Use an open palm to move cloth rather than a static grasp
Emptying garbage	Carrying heavy loads held away from the body	Use smaller garbage cans and transfer to large can Place large garbage can on wheels Place liner in garbage cans or tip garbage can to empty

with or without tools. Elderly men used 5.7 Nm of force to open a jar, and women used 3.9 Nm. All subjects used two hands to open the jar, one for stabilizing and the other for turning. Rahman, Thomas, and Rice (2002) did not find a strong relationship between the participants' maximum grip strengths and the amount of force used to open containers. However, researchers found that elderly populations used a greater percentage of their maximum grip strengths than younger participants to access containers. The maximum forces measured by force-sensing resistor for opening containers ranged from 8 lb to 20 lb (on a large bottle), well above the minimum required to open a container. Researchers recommend that manufacturers should strive for an opening torque of 2 Nm for jars so that the greater majority of individuals over age 50 would be able to open jars independently. Kitchen accessories and appliances such as rubber gripping pads and manual and electric can openers are clearly necessary to meet such everyday problems for consumers. Consumers should try to use their hands in the most efficient and least resistive manner possible.

Ergonomic design changes for utensils commonly address the position of the wrist during use, the anatomy of the MCP joints during grasp, the texture of the handle, and the overall weight of the utensil. *Pistol grips* on knives (see preceding discussion) require a more neutral wrist position during use as compared to an ulnarly deviated position of the wrist while using a traditional straight-blade knife. *Bent blades* for cake decorating enable elevating the hand above frosting rather than awkwardly abducting and internally rotating the shoulder. *Oval or curved handle* designs with a larger diameter follow the transverse arch of the MCP joints, thus allowing for a more efficient gross grasp and efficient use of the flexor tendons (Figure 18-1). *Soft, nonslip handle textures* provide optimal grasping conditions even when wet. Ergonomic utensils utilizing the design criteria just discussed have been introduced by such companies as OXO Good Grips and Smith and Nephew Rehabilitation (see resources at end of chapter). Such utensils increased the ease of task performance in an elderly population (Kelsheimer & Hawkins, 2000).

The use of small appliances, such as can openers, food processors, and electric mixers, can also greatly decrease the workload of the upper extremities. Newer appliances further combine and minimize functions to decrease upper-extremity strain. For example, OXO Good Grips offers a teapot that automatically opens once it is lifted, thereby minimizing strain on the hands, a liquid measuring cup with angled measuring lines to facilitate reading measurements from above, and a jar opener with an extended handle and "teeth" to secure the jar lid (Figures 18-1 and 18-2). Readers are referred to Trombly (1997) for further discussions related to consumers with disabilities.

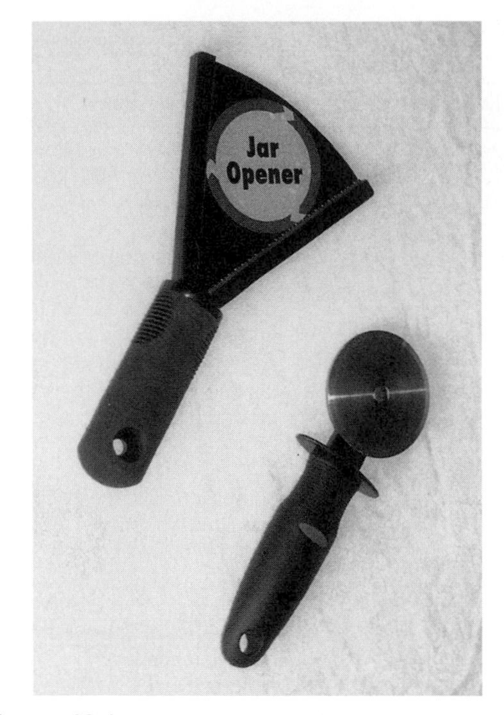

Figure 18-1 The OXO Good Grips Y Pizza Cutter features a soft, oval-shaped grip that follows the arches of the hand; the Jar Opener minimizes deviation of the wrist and the need for high hand forces to open a jar.

Cleaning

The tasks involved in cleaning the home expose individuals to the biomechanical risk factors of awkward and static postures at the shoulder, back, and hands while cleaning toilets and showers; excessive forces to the low back and hands while emptying garbage, lifting a vacuum cleaner, and scrubbing tile; and repetition primarily to the upper extremity during all motions (see Table 18-2 for specifics). In 1973, Grandjean (1973) noted that performing housework was particularly stressful to the low back, especially when stooping, lifting, and carrying loads with poor posture. He suggested five rules that closely approximate the principles of body mechanics discussed previously.

Overall, design modifications for cleaning involve extending handles on tools to clean surfaces out of one's reach (such as a shower stall), placing wheels on water buckets and garbage cans to decrease the loads carried, and using the most efficient housework equipment. For example, a well-maintained, self-propelling vacuum cleaner will take less energy to use than a standard one. Practicing good preventive maintenance by using daily shower cleaning products and keeping vacuum cleaner bags empty further increases task efficiency and minimizes ergonomic exposures.

When cleaning bathrooms, a number of ergonomic design issues increase efficiency and ease. Bathrooms may be designed with ample

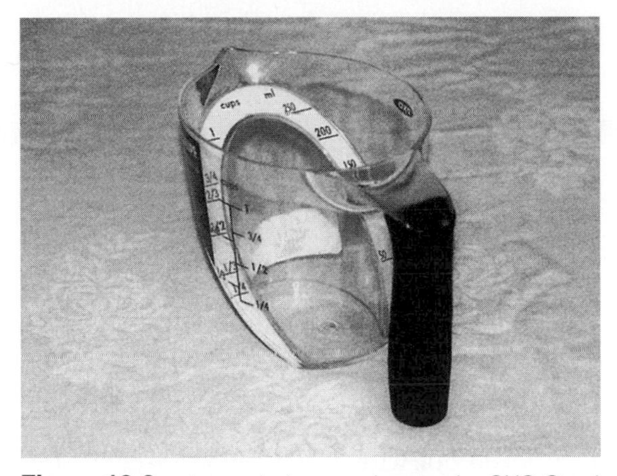

Figure 18-2 An angled measuring cup by OXO Good Grips eliminates awkwardly positioning the neck to measure liquids.

room around toilets to allow better access for cleaning, thus eliminating awkward postures from working in a cramped workspace. Installation of grab bars may allow one to support upper body weight while bending over to scrub a toilet. Use of a flexible shower head nozzle allows one to rinse off the entire area of the shower without bending and reaching. Knee pads minimize the contact stress from kneeling on hard surfaces. Sized gloves and effective cleansing agents help to reduce grip forces used. Finally, individuals should be reminded to alternate hands and arms for repetitive cleaning, such as showers and mirrors.

Laundry

Laundering has certainly evolved from the days when washboards were used to manually scrub and wring clothes before hanging them out to dry. The postures associated with using the washboard were so stressful that early doctors called the cluster of symptoms that arose from laundering "Washerwoman's Strain" (Armstrong, 1992). Although the washing machine reduced the time involved in laundering and eliminated the risk of injury from repetition and awkward hand postures, other risks were created, an all-too-common occurrence in the design process. This section examines these risk factors and how to minimize them in the home environment.

Exposure to risk factors associated with doing the laundry varies from home to home, depending on the volume of laundry and the time allotted to complete the task. For a single person, laundry may be a small job; for individuals with back strain or with a large family (many families do more than six loads per week), the task becomes monumental. If the task of doing the laundry falls on one person who has limited time during the week, that person may find himself or herself doing 7 days' worth of laundry in a condensed weekend period. In this case, the person should consider energy conservation principles such as pacing work throughout the week and job sharing with other members of the household.

Ergonomic Risks to the Low Back from Laundering

Exposure to low-back risk factors occurs as one reaches into the washing machine to pull out the wet clothes and then put wet clothes into the dryer. The design of the washer contributes to this exposure. For a top-loading washer, the top of a washer is typically 36 inches off the floor, and the depth inside the drum is 24 inches. To reach to the bottom of a washing machine drum, one must forward flex the trunk 45 to 80 degrees, depending on one's stature. After flexing the trunk and pulling out a heavy load, one is inclined to flex, twist, and reach into the dryer, lowering the load to approximately 13 inches off the floor. Since the door on some dryers extends 15 inches in front of the dryer when open, one would have to step back 15 inches while holding the wet clothing and step to the side to position himself or herself directly in front of the dryer to avoid up to 90 degrees of spine twist. Disc compressive forces for a 150-pound person could be as much as 578 pounds under these conditions.

When disc compressive estimates are applied to reaching above the washing machine to access a large container of liquid detergent placed on a shelf, a disc compressive estimate of 453 pounds results. According to NIOSH, 770 pounds of disc compressive force is stressful for some members of the workforce, and 1430 pounds is stressful to most members of the workforce. Although these activities fall below the NIOSH limit, it is understandable how a person working as a material handler and recovering from a work-related low-back injury could reinjure himself or herself or prolong recovery by doing the family laundry.

Ergonomic Risk to the Shoulders from Laundering

Although back strain is the greatest risk in performing laundry, strain to the shoulder musculature can occur by reaching to grab a large container of liquid laundry detergent. The moments (loads) at the shoulder caused by the total weight of the arm, load in the hands, the distance of the load to the shoulder joint, and the angles of the elbow and shoulder joints can be analyzed (Bloswick, 2001). Shoulder moment is expressed as a ratio. Ratios above 1 are representative of tasks likely to cause shoulder injury, and ratios below 0.5 are deemed safe unless there is a high degree of repetition. Under normal circumstances, reaching to obtain a full container of laundry detergent yields a shoulder ratio of 1, indicating shoulder injury is likely. By placing the detergent on top of the dryer and sliding it toward the washer, shoulder moment is reduced to a ratio of 0.1 (please see reference for a complete discussion).

Ergonomic Recommendations for Laundering

Table 18-3 provides practical solutions to reduce risks to the body while laundering. By addressing home layout, work organization, design issues, and body mechanics, risk of injury through laundering can be minimized. A home space that is laid out with the washing machine area upstairs will eliminate carrying loads up and down stairs. Use of front-loading washers can help minimize spine twist while transferring clothes if a person kneels and laterally transfers clothes from the washer to the dryer. A dryer that is oriented so that the door opens on the opposite side of the washer will eliminate stepping around the dryer door to deposit clothes. If the work area is organized so that the laundry detergent is stored on the same level as the washer (on top of the dryer) it can be slid into position and tilted for pouring, thus eliminating awkward trunk postures and reach, which may also contribute to low-back pain. Disc compressive force and strain to the

Table 18-3

Minimizing Risks Factors and Twisting while Doing Laundry

Task	Ergonomic Risk Factors	Recommendations
Placing laundry in washer	Lifting laundry basket from floor to washer	Place laundry basket at waist height
	Reaching to access laundry detergent	Place laundry soap at waist height or store on top of dryer
Transferring clothes from washer to dryer	Strain to low back when pulling heavy, wet clothes from washer	Loosen tangled items before pulling out of washer Remove only a few items at a time
	Trunk flexion to reach into washer	Use golfer's lift or brace knees to decrease trunk flexion
	Twisting motions to spine when loading dryer	Move feet first to face dryer straight on Kneel in front of dryer to load clothes
Folding and distributing	Static postures to neck to look down Carrying loads of laundry Repetition to fold	Place folded laundry directly in baskets according to family member; this saves added time for distribution

supportive muscles and ligaments for pouring laundry detergent could be lessened using these work organization techniques.

Proper body mechanics for removing wet clothes from the washer include staggering one's stance to lower center of gravity, bracing one's knee on the front of the washer or extending one leg as in the golfer's lift (Saunders, 1993) to disperse the forces acting on the low back, using one hand to support the weight of the upper body, and grabbing only one handful of wet laundry at a time. These practices could reduce disc compressive forces from approximately 578 to 305 pounds for a 150-pound person. See Appendix 18-1 for specific calculations.

ERGONOMIC CONSIDERATIONS FOR CHILDREN

As ergonomic applications expand into the home and leisure activities, it becomes apparent that little recognition has been given to the ergonomics involved in children's activities and workspaces. Children are increasingly experiencing low-back pain from carrying heavy loads and developing musculoskeletal conditions from playing with video and computer games. Further, they sit long hours at school on furniture that is not designed for their needs (Jacobs et al., 2002). Fortunately, children's normal play of sports and recreation seems to have protective value for such musculoskeletal conditions (Grimmer & Williams, 2000). The following section addresses three areas relative to youth and ergonomics: backpacks, video games, and handwriting. Chapter 24 discusses the ergonomics of children and computer use.

Backpack Use in Children and Adolescents

Backpacks have become an integral aspect of the dress code for youth of all ages, grades, and nationalities. In the United States an estimated 40 million students carry backpacks to school daily (Pascoe & Pascoe, 1999). In Italy 34.8% of Italian schoolchildren were found to carry backpacks weighing at least 30% of their body weights at least one time per week (Negrini, Carabalone, & Sibilla, 1999). In Australia over 20% of students ages 12 to 18 had low-back pain relative to backpack use (Grimmer & Williams, 2000). The U.S. Consumer Product Safety Commission reports that over 7000 emergency room visits in 2001 were related to students wearing backpacks and handling books (U.S. Consumer Product Safety Commission, 2001). With these statistics in mind, researchers have recently begun to investigate the variables involved with children, backpacks, posture, and low-back pain.

Grimmer, Williams, and Gill (1999) and Grimmer and Williams (2000) examined changes in spinal posture of 985 Australian adolescents ages 12 to 18 who carried backpacks at school. Researchers found significant differences in the students' craniovertebral angle (CVA) or forward head angle when they wore loaded backpacks as compared to wearing empty backpacks. This forward head posture was apparent even when backpacks were positioned over both shoulders. The largest differences were seen in younger students, suggesting that as the spine matures youths develop different postural responses and adaptations to the loads. In a separate study, Chansirinukor, Wilson, Grimmer, and Dansie (2001) also found that craniovertebral angle increased for students ages 13 to 16 who carried backpacks (1) for at least a 5-minute duration and (2) that weighed 15% of their body weight.

The relationships between reported low-back pain and environmental variables in students were further investigated. Low-back pain in students was related to carrying heavier loads relative to their body weights, sitting for longer periods after school, and carrying backpacks for longer amounts of time. Regular participation in organized sports was protective of low-back pain for most students. Grimmer and Williams (2000) found that younger students, ages 12 to 14 who carried backpacks greater than 6% of their body weight were at the greatest risk for low-back pain.

Organizations such as the American Occupational Therapy Association (AOTA, 2003), American Physical Therapy Association (APTA,

2003), and American Chiropractic Association (ACA, 2003) have focused prevention efforts on educating parents, youths, and school administrators about this issue. Although public health efforts globally endorse decreasing the present weights of students' backpacks, recommendations as to the percentage of body weight differ among organizations. The AOTA and the APTA recommend wearing backpacks no more than 15% of a student's body weight as this is a feasible yet prudent goal. The ACA suggests wearing backpacks no more than 5% to 10% of a child's body weight secondary to the danger of excessive loads placed in maturing spines. Table 18-4 provides suggestions for choosing the best design, wearing the backpacks properly, and initiating administrative solutions that may decrease the need for transporting books daily. Although transporting bookbags on wheels seems to be an obvious solution, experts caution that they can be dangerous to transport up and down stairs and can easily tip and fall if not designed properly, causing torque injury to the wrist. Further, they rarely fit in lockers (ACA, 2003; Hamilton, 2001). Other creative administrative solutions to carrying fewer books include managing students' notebooks as part of the daily curriculum (transferring daily papers to a smaller notebook) and altering heavy homework days among classes (Hamilton, 2001). Most important, students need to develop an awareness of these issues in order to monitor their own practices.

Gaming

Video games often entice youths to spend hours engaged in front of a television. Although this practice may increase concentration skills, typically children sit in unsupported postures performing repetitive thumb motions. Thumb injuries related to overuse of video games became so common in the 1990s that doctors coined the term "Nintendo Thumb" to describe a tendinitis of the dominant thumb extensor tendons caused by overuse of the thumb while playing video games. In fact, as Figures 18-3, *A*, and 18-3, *B*, demonstrate, many children's games require sustained, repetitive, and forceful exertions of the thumbs in order to operate triggers and push buttons. Overall, the major risk factors during gaming are prolonged durations in an awkward posture and exposure of the thumbs to a repetitive activity. Table 18-4 summarizes means to decrease such exposures by changing positions, taking breaks, and using any programmable features of the game that can

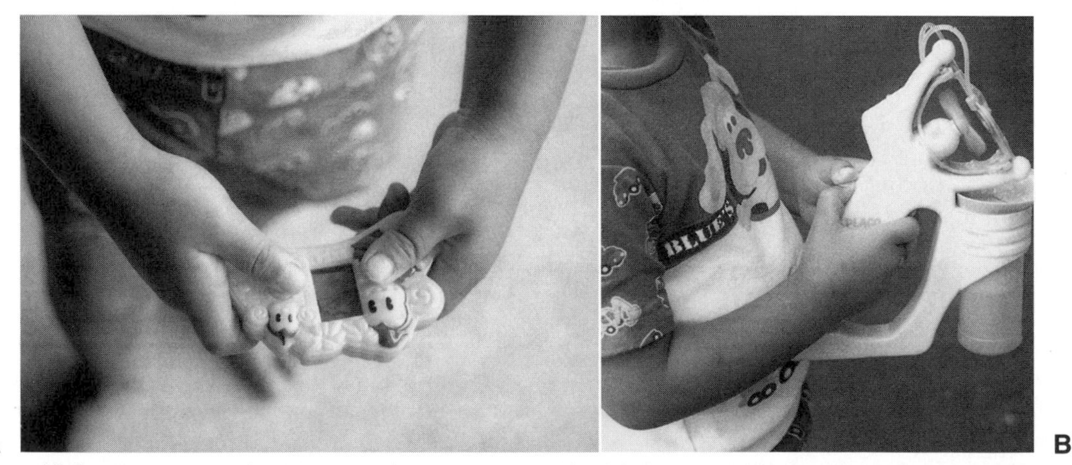

Figure 18-3 The thumbs of children may be prone to repetitive injuries caused by handheld electronic games and other toys with resistive trigger devices.

decrease the repetitive motions by grouping common functions or key sequences together (Healthycomputing.com, 2003).

As with computing, youths should sit with proper back support, keep the wrists straight while holding the controllers, position the television so as not to bend or rotate the neck, and minimize glare. They should press the gaming controller buttons lightly and hold the game controller with a relaxed hand. Finally, youths should change methods for inputting such as using the controller pad instead of the control stick (Xbox Game Review, 2003). Finally, parents may consider limiting the time spent playing video games, particularly if children are performing other activities using the same musculature such as computing or a TV remote control.

Handwriting

Handwriting is a daily task in the occupational role of a student. Although countless hours are spent in learning, practicing, and using handwriting skills, this task can be difficult for many children. Handwriting involves a myriad of complex skills including coordinating the fingers, gripping the pencil, forming letters, and adjusting one's body to the task (AOTA, 2003). Problems with handwriting may stem from ergonomic issues as well as from developmental

Table 18-4

Modifying Youth Activities to Minimize Ergonomic Risks

Task	Ergonomic Risk Factors	Recommendations
Carrying backpacks	Low-back pain Neck and shoulder pain Forward head posture	*Choose a good design* Wide, padded, adjustable straps Padded back Multiple compartments to distribute loads Waist or hip belts Consider bookbag on wheels cautiously *Wear the backpack correctly* Make sure backpacks weigh no more than 10% to 15% of body weight Wear both straps on shoulders Adjust backpack so that bottom is just above the low back Pack heavy items close to back *Healthy alternatives* Keep one set of books at home Carry only books that are needed Use a locker, if available
Gaming	Low back pain Neck and shoulder pain Thumb pain "Nintendo thumb" Neck pain	Take frequent breaks! Change positions Grasp the joystick lightly Use any "programmable" features that minimize repetitive actions For forced-feedback game pads, eliminate vibration component or take breaks more frequently
Handwriting	Difficulty writing Prolonged time in poor posture	Provide a workstation that encourages good posture Provide breaks every 20 to 30 minutes Perform warm-up stretches before writing activities Perform relaxation techniques Increase hand strength and coordination with activities such as jacks, marbles, and painting

issues. Therefore, parents and teachers are advised to thoroughly investigate the root cause of the problem before making changes in the child's environment. Occupational therapists suggest that parents and teachers help students assume a proper posture for writing by providing support to the arms and hands. Students should take regular breaks every 20 to 30 minutes, position the paper and document relative to the body, and perform warm-up activities and relaxation techniques (AOTA, 2003; Jacobs et al., 2002; Tseng & Cermack, 1993). These techniques can relax the child and enhance the proximal stability necessary for distal control.

SUMMARY

Ergonomic risks are inherent in the daily maintenance activities we perform at home. Although ergonomic principles have been applied to tasks for individuals with special needs, only recently have consumers universally realized the benefits of using well-designed equipment and good body mechanics for increased comfort and productivity at home. This chapter addresses the historic uses of joint protection, body mechanics, and energy conservation techniques, suggesting these principles are prudent for all those performing activities. Ergonomics applications are presented for common household tasks with the goal of providing practical solutions to decrease ergonomic exposures. Finally, children should grow up with these principles as part of their everyday knowledge base.

REFERENCES

American Chiropractice Association (ACA). (2003). Health tips. Retrieved on January 5. 2003 at *http://www.acatoday.com/media/tips/backpacks.html*.

American Occupational Therapy Association (AOTA). (2003). Backpack facts: What's all the flap about? Retrieved on January 6, 2003 at *www.aota.org/backpack/index.asp*.

American Physical Therapy Association (APTA). (2003). Backpack talking points. Retrieved on August 10, 2003 at *http://www.apta.org/news/featurereleases/backpack/backpackpoints*.

Armstrong, T. J. (1992). Cumulative trauma disorders of the upper limb and identification of work-related factors. In L. H. Millender, D. S. Louis, & B. P. Simmons (Eds.) *Occupational disorders of the upper extremity.* Churchill Livingstone: New York.

Bloswick, D. (2001) *Ergonomics and the workplace workshop.* Chicago, IL: Ergoweb, October 11-13.

Chansirinukor, W., Wilson, D., Grimmer, K., & Dansie, B. (2001). Effects of backpacks on students: Measurement of cervical and shoulder posture. *Australian Journal of Physiotherapy, 47*(2), 110-116.

Cordery, J. (1965). Joint protection: A responsibility of the occupational therapist. *American Journal of Occupational Therapy, 19*(5), 285-294.

Cordery, J., & Rocchi, M. (1998). Joint protection and fatigue management. In J. Melvin & G. Jensen (Eds.), *Rheumatologic rehabilitation series.* Vol 1. Bethesda, MD: American Occupational Therapy Association.

Csikszentmihalyi, M. (1990) *Flow: The psychology of optimal experience.* New York: Harper Perennial.

Gerber, L. H., Furst, G. P., Smith, C., Shulman, B., Liang, M., Cullen, K., et al. (1987). Patient education program to teach energy conservation behaviors to patients with rheumatoid arthritis: A pilot study. *Archives of Physical Medicine and Rehabilitation, 68*(7), 422-445.

Grandjean, E. (1973). *Ergonomics of the home.* New York: John Wiley & Sons.

Grimmer, K. A., Williams, M. T., & Gill, T. K. (1999). The associations between adolescent head-on-neck posture, backpack weight, and anthropometric features. *Spine, 24*(21), 2262-2267.

Grimmer, K. A., & Williams, M. T. (2000). Gender-age environmental associates of adolescent low back pain. *Applied Ergonomics, 31*(4), 343-360.

Hamilton, A. (2001). Sounding board: Prevention of injuries from improper backpack use in children. *Work, 16*(2), 177-179.

Hammond, A. (1994). Joint protection behaviors in patients with rheumatoid arthritis following and education program: A pilot study. *Arthritis Care and Research, 7*(1), 5-9.

HealthyComputing.com (2003). Backpacks. Retrieved on 1/5/03 at *www.healthycomputing.com/kids/backpacks/html*.

Jacobs, K., Bhasin, G., Bustamante, L., Buxgton, J.C., Chiang, H-Y., Greene, D. et al. (2002). Everything you should know about ergonomics and youths, but were afraid to ask. *OT Practice, 7*(10), 11-19.

Kelsheimer, H. L., & Hawkins, S.T. (2000). Older women find food preparation easier with specialized kitchen tools. *Journal of the American Dietetic Association, 100*(8), 950-959.

Klompenhouwer, P. J., Lysack, C., Dijkers, M., & Hammond, A. (2000). The joint protection behavior assessment: A reliability study. *American Journal of Occupational Therapy, 54*(5), 516–524.

Kroemer, K. H. E. & Grandjean, E. (2001). *Fitting the task to the human* (5th Ed.). London: Taylor & Francis.

Kraus, V. B. (1997). Pathogenesis and treatment of osteoarthritis. *Medical Clinics of North America, 81*(1), 85–112.

McCloy, L. (1982). The biomechanical basis for joint protection in osteoarthritis. *Canadian Journal of Occupational Therapy, 49*(3), 85-87.

Melvin, J. (1989). *Rheumatic disease in the and child: Occupational therapy and rehabilitation* (3rd. ed). Philadelphia: F. A. Davis.

Negrini, S., Carabalone, R., & Sibilla, P. (1999). Backpack as a daily load for schoolchildren. *Lancet, 354*(9194), 1974.

Pascoe, D. D., & Pascoe, D. E. (1999). Book bags help to shoulder the burdens of school work. *Teaching Elementary Physical Health,* March 18–22.

Pheasant, S. (1991). *Ergonomics, work and health*. Aspen Publishers: Gaithersburg: MD.

Pheasant, S. (1996). *Bodyspace: Anthropometry, ergonomics and the design of work* (2nd ed.). London: Taylor & Francis.

Pinto, M. R., De Medici, S., Van Sant, C., Bianchi, A., Zlotnicki, A., & Napoli, C. (2000). Ergonomics, gerotechnology, and design for the home-environment. *Applied Ergonomics, 31,* 317–322.

Rahman, N., Thomas, J. J. & Rice, M. S. (2002). The relationship between hand strength and the forces used to access containers by well elderly persons. *American Journal of Occupational Therapy, 56*(1), 78–85.

Sanders, M. S., & McCormick, E. J. (1993). *Human factors in engineering and design* (7th ed.). New York: McGraw-Hill.

Stamm, T. A., Machold, K. P., Smolen, J. S., Fischer, S., Redlich, K., Graninger, W. et al. (2002). Joint protection and home hand exercises improve hand function in patients with hand osteoarthritis: A randomized controlled trial. *Arthritis Care & Research, 47*(1), 44–49.

Saunders, D. (1993). *For your back*. Chaska, MN: Saunders Group, Inc.

Tichauer, E. (1966). Some aspects of stress on forearm and hand in industry. *Journal of Occupational Medicine, 8*(2), 63–71.

Tseng, M. H., & Cermack, S. A. (1993). The influence of ergonomic factors and perceptual-motor abilities on handwriting performance. *American Journal of Occupational Therapy, 47*(10), 919–925.

Trombly, C. A. (Ed.). (1997). *Occupational therapy for physical dysfunction* (4th ed.). Philadelphia: Lippincott Williams & Wilkins.

U.S. Consumer Product Safety Commission National Electronic Injury Surveillance System (NEISS) database, 2001.

Voorbij, A. I. M., & Steenbekkers, L. P. A. (2002). The twisting force of aged consumers when opening a jar. *Applied Ergonomics, 33*(1), 105–109.

Xbox Game Review (2003). *Xbox Healthy gaming guide*. Retrieved on January 26, 2003 at *http://www.xboxgamereview.net/www/gamingguide.htm*.

RESOURCES

Good Grips™
OXO International
75 Ninth Avenue, 5th Floor
New York, NY 10011 USA

Smith and Nephew Rehabilitation
One quality Drive, P.O. Box 1005
Germantown, WI 53022-8205

AliMed Ergonomics
297 High Street
Dedham, MA 02026
www.alimed.com

APPENDIX 18-1

Calculations for Disc Compressive Force Estimate Using Good and Poor Mechanics during Laundering

Calculating Disc Compressive Force Estimate

In order to calculate an estimate of disc compressive force, measure the following.

1. Body weight (BW)
2. Load in hands (L)
3. Horizontal distance from hands to low back (HB)
4. Torso angle (cos theta)

These numbers will be applied the following general formula:

A + B + C = Back compressive force

A = Effect of upper body weight on compressive force

B = Back muscle force reacting to distance of the load from the spine

C = Upper body weight and load contribution to compressive force

Specific weightings are given as follows:

A = 3(BW)cos(theta) =

B = 0.5(L × HB) =

C = 0.8(BW/2 + L) =

Estimations for A depend on the torso flexion angle.

Torso angle (COS THETA)

Vertical torso use cos(theta)	= 0
Torso bent ¼ use cos(theta)	= 0.38
Torso bent ½ use cos(theta)	= 0.71
Torso bent ¾ use cos(theta)	= 0.92
Torso horizontal use cos(theta)	= 1

Disc Compressive Force Estimates Applied to Laundering

Application of preceding to removing wet towels without proper body mechanics.

Where:

A = 3(BW)cos(theta) = 3(150) × (0.71) = 320

B = 0.5(L × HB) = 0.5(10 × 38) = 190

C = 0.8(BW/2 + L) =0.8(150/2 + 10) = 68

Disc compressive force ESTIMATE 578 pounds

Application of preceding to removing wet towels with proper body mechanics.

Where:

A = 3(BW)cos(theta) = 3(150) × (.38) = 171

B = 0.5(L × HB) = 0.5(5 × 28) = 70

C = 0.8(BW/2 + L) = 0.8(150/2 + 5) = 64

Disc compressive force ESTIMATE 305 pounds

CHAPTER 19

Ergonomics of Child Care

Martha J. Sanders

Ergonomics has assisted industry in decreasing workers' compensation costs, increasing productivity, and improving efficiency and comfort in workers through optimizing the worker–workplace interactions (Pheasant, 1991). Although caring for young children is the occupation of millions of parents and over 1.2 million child care workers and 423,000 preschool teachers, it has been largely ignored from an ergonomics perspective (Bureau of Labor Statistics, 2002a; Calabro et al., 2000). Qualitative narratives describe parents' physical and emotional strains arising from the routine tasks of lifting, carrying, bending, and caring for young children (Griffin & Price, 2000; Hochschild, 1989). Descriptive surveys find that 11% to 47% of all child care workers complain of low-back pain related to lifting and handling children (Calabro et al., 2000; Child Care Employee Project, 1983; Gratz & Claffey, 1996). The Bureau of Labor Statistics (BLS) reports that close to 5000 child care workers, family care providers, and preschool teachers suffered an illness or injury in the year 2000 (BLS, 2000). Unfortunately, fewer studies have provided information about the frequency of musculoskeletal complaints in parents, as if parents are predestined to suffer from musculoskeletal pain. The implications for preventing musculoskeletal pain exist not only for the improved health of adults but also for enhanced quality of care in fulfilling the child care provider and parental roles.

This chapter reviews the research on the musculoskeletal symptoms and ergonomic risks related to caring for children in child care providers, preschool teachers, and parents. It discusses the job tasks and physical demands related to caring for children and provides recommendations designed to minimize the risk of developing musculoskeletal pain. As in most industrial situations, the exposures can be effectively minimized but rarely eradicated.

MUSCULOSKELETAL SYMPTOMS AND PSYCHOSOCIAL STRAIN IN CHILD CARE WORKERS AND PRESCHOOL TEACHERS

A paucity of literature exists relative to the biomechanical and psychosocial strain involved in adults caring for children in child care centers or preschool. Researchers first began to address the work-related tasks of child care providers within the context of improving the work environment for adult child care workers in order to maximize their quality of work with children. Most studies focused on the infectious disease, burnout, and environmental concerns in child care work (Bright & Calabro, 1999; Pickering & Reeves, 1990). However, the Child Care Employee Project (CCEP) noted ergonomics as an important concern for child care providers across the United States. Results of a child care employee newsletter survey indicated that 48%

of child care workers had experienced back strain from lifting children, 69% reported moving heavy furniture, and only 25% of the centers had adult-size furniture available for the workers (CCEP, 1983).

When epidemiologic studies began to address the musculoskeletal health of adult child care workers, wide discrepancies in the frequency of musculoskeletal discomfort were reported. Brown and Gerberich (1993) examined the worker injuries in 440 child care workers in Minnesota and found that 1.94 per 100 workers were injured from 1985 to 1990. Injuries involving the low back accounted for 34% of the injuries, followed by injuries to the lower extremity (20%), upper extremity (12%), and multiple sites (13%). Over 50% of all injuries were sprains, the majority caused by overexertion (44%); 48% of all back injuries were associated with lifting children.

Gratz and Claffey (1996) addressed the overall health status and health behaviors in 446 early childhood workers in both day care centers and in-home day care settings. Workers indicated high frequencies of both musculoskeletal complaints and psychosocial stress since working in child care. Seventeen percent to 18% of all child care workers and directors noted back pain, 30% to 35% noted headaches, and 23% to 36% noted fatigue on a weekly basis. Child care workers reported that these symptoms had dramatically increased in frequency since working in child care. Twenty-nine percent to 35% of the child care workers and in-home providers rated the jobs as stressful to very stressful. Calabro et al. (2000) surveyed 240 child care workers in 34 day care centers and found that 11.5% of child care workers suffered low-back pain; 21.5% suffered falls or trips related to the job.

Finally, Manlove (1993) specifically addressed the psychosocial strain in day care work through assessing the organizational and personal issues related to burnout in 188 day care workers. Manlove found that higher levels of neuroticism, work role conflict, and role ambiguity were positively associated with higher levels of burnout. Those who demonstrated greater organizational commitment, better relationships with supervisors, and a sense of work autonomy reported less depersonalization and emotional fatigue at work. Although these self-report surveys were conducted on nonrandom samples and thus must be interpreted cautiously, collectively the outcomes indicate that both musculoskeletal and psychosocial health are valid concerns that must be further addressed.

The BLS contends that child care is a relatively "safe" industry, with an illness and injury rate of only 2.6 per 100 full-time workers in 1999 (BLS, 2002b). However, the true incidence of musculoskeletal injuries in teachers and child care workers may be significantly underreported for a number of reasons, including the following.

1. Many child care workers are employed by businesses with fewer than 11 employees and therefore do not need to report OSHA statistics.
2. Many data sources include only lost-time injuries involving 3 days or more.
3. These types of injuries are difficult to attribute to the workplace and thus may not be reported (Bright & Calabro, 1999; Brown & Gerberich, 1993; Morse, Dillon, Warren, Levenstein, & Warren, 1998).

Calabro et al. (2000) further propose that child care work is an at-risk safety culture, since workers do not perceive the risks in child care work as great. Workers perceive a favorable health and safety climate in spite of reporting high frequencies of injuries, illnesses, and turnover.

MUSCULOSKELETAL SYMPTOMS AND PSYCHOSOCIAL STRAIN IN PARENTS AND FAMILY PROVIDERS

The studies related to adult health while caring for children have been conducted within the context of promoting workplace health and safety. Without this framework, concern for parents' health has not been addressed in a coordinated approach. Russell, Andersson, Taub, O'Dowd, and Reynolds (1993) and Breen, Ransil, Groves, and Oriol (1994) expressed concern about the frequently reported low-back pain in new mothers as related to use of epidural anesthesia during delivery. In a sample of 1015 women who delivered their first child, Russell et al. (1993) found that 30% had backache lasting 6 months or longer after childbirth. Fifteen percent of the women had no previous problems with their backs; 18% of those receiving an epidural developed new onset back pain as compared to 12% in those who did not have an epidural. Back pain was reportedly exacerbated by lifting and carrying children.

Conversely, Breen et al. (1994) found no difference in the prevalence of low-back pain reported by those using epidural anesthesia. Forty-four percent of 1042 women in their sample suffered postpartum low-back pain when interviewed 2 months after delivery. Breen et al. (1994) found that low-back pain was related to a history of low-back pain, younger age, greater weight, and shorter stature in mothers.

Sanders (2002) examined the frequency of musculoskeletal pain as related to child care practices in a sample of 130 parents with at least one child under the age of 4 years old. Sixty-six percent of the sample noted the presence of musculoskeletal pain in at least one part of the body. Low-back pain was most commonly reported (48%), followed by neck (17%), upper back (16%), shoulder (11.5%), knee (10%), fingers and thumb (8%), and wrist pain (7%). The presence of musculoskeletal pain was positively related to performing high-risk child care practices ($p = 0.001$; CI = 59% to 95%) and the parents' perception that caring for children was a highly demanding job ($p = 0.005$; CI = 65% to 83%) (see Chapter 8 for a complete discussion of significance (p value) and confidence intervals (CI). Thus, both physical and psychosocial issues appeared to contribute to musculoskeletal pain in this sample.

Griffin and Price (2000) more qualitatively examined mothers' perspectives on performing the child care tasks that involved lifting. This study addressed the methods mothers used to lift and handle children and their decision-making processes in choosing these methods. Mothers indicated that they used primarily the "stoop lift" method of lifting (bending at the waist with knees straight). Their decisions to use certain lifting and carrying methods were based on contextual factors such as time constraints, equipment options available, number of children, duration and frequency of the task, and ways to conserve energy. Overall, mothers used the quickest, safest, and most efficient methods to accomplish the task based on concern for the children's needs rather than their own posture. Mothers' reasons for using incorrect lifting methods included lack of time, overall fatigue, laziness, habit, and simply not thinking about it.

Finally, Hochschild (1989) examined the sociologic issues relative to child rearing in the 1980s as increasing numbers of women reentered the workforce. Hochschild documented the fatigue, emotional stress, and individual coping strategies resulting from the "double shifts" that women undertake to manage careers and families. Dyck (1992) discussed the social constraints and complex social network women use to negotiate their childrearing tasks.

Overall, high frequencies of musculoskeletal pain and emotional strain have been reported in both child care workers and parents. A closer examination of child care tasks will better elucidate the origins of these health problems. The following job analysis and related discussion on ergonomic risk factors will help to focus prevention efforts.

JOB ANALYSIS OF CHILD CARE WORK

Child care workers are responsible for meeting the basic needs of children (feeding, hygiene, physical and emotional comfort, stimulation) in addition to providing activities that stimulate the children's physical, emotional, intellectual, and social growth (BLS, 2002a). According to the

Bureau of Labor Statistics (BLS), many categories of employment exist related to caring for children. *Child care workers* nurture children outside the home in child care centers, nursery school, preschools, community centers, and public schools; *family child care providers* care for children in the providers' own homes; *private household workers* or *nannies* care for children in the homes of their employers; and *preschool teachers* teach basic physical, mental, and development skills in public or private schools. Child care workers may work full- or part-time (BLS, 2002a).

The tasks involved in the jobs of child care workers vary according to the ages of the children under their care. However, the major tasks of these providers involve greeting parents and children, playing with children (including singing and assisting with developmentally appropriate games and crafts), teaching basic social and gross motor skills, feeding children, diapering and dressing and undressing children, putting them to bed, writing notes, cleaning equipment, moving furniture or cots, transporting laundry or garbage, and conversing with colleagues and parents. In general, those working with younger children tend to perform more lifting, holding, and carrying of children than those working with older children. Additionally, child care workers are expected to display positive attitudes and be constantly vigilant in monitoring children for disruptive or unsafe behavior. Teachers in supervisory positions and directors spend part of their time in scheduling, administrative duties, and program development (BLS, 2002a,b).

The physical demands of the child care worker's job may include frequent lifting and carrying of children, sitting on the floor, sitting on low furniture, squatting, kneeling, reaching to various heights, moving furniture, carrying, prolonged standing, pushing children on toys and swings, and writing (BLS 2002b; King, Gratz, Scheuer, & Claffey, 1995).

Work sampling studies on a group of 22 child care workers indicated that teachers spent 63% of their time with the children, 8.4% talking to another teacher, 14.3% taking notes, and 14.3% cleaning or setting up for an activity. Postural observations indicated that on an average, 25% of teachers' time was spent squatting, kneeling, or sitting on the floor when working with children. For those working with younger children, the frequency was higher at 31%. Teachers spent an additional 26% of their time sitting on small, child-sized furniture when helping children with an activity. Eighteen percent of teachers' activities involved flexing at the trunk greater than 20 degrees. Again, these frequencies were higher for those working with young children (Grant, Habes, & Tepper, 1995).

Work-related postures in kindergarten and nursery school teachers in Japan have been addressed in relation to strain to the low back and shoulders (Kumagai et al., 1998; Nagira, Suzuki, Oze, Ohara, & Aoyama, 1981). In a sample of 1059 nursery school teachers, 36% of their time was spent in hands-on activities with children, 17% holding or carrying objects, and 9% of the time holding or moving children. No short breaks were observed other than lunchtime. Postures involving bending, squatting, or kneeling were assumed for 30% of their workday. Similarly, in a group of 12 kindergarten teachers, 36% of their time was spent standing bent forward, squatting, or kneeling. The frequency of lifting one's trunk from a severe forward flexion (45 degrees) was 95 times per hour. Although the frequency of lifting and carrying kindergartners is generally thought to be less than infants, researchers found that these teachers spent considerable time in postures that placed significant load on their backs.

No job analysis or work sampling studies have been performed on parents of young children. However, parents must perform all the child care tasks mentioned in addition to bathing, transporting, putting children to bed and waking them, and participating in family recreational activities. In a grander scope, parents must further orchestrate the functioning of a household within the demands of jobs and community activities. Therefore, parents find themselves multitasking to take care of children while performing household chores, laundry, answering the phone, or writing shopping lists, to name a few (Hochschild, 1989; Pirie & Herman, 1995). Although child care providers perform child care tasks with greater frequency in an 8-hour day (or less), workers usually receive short breaks or relief from a coworker. Such breaks are often nonexistent in a parent's day (Hochschild, 1989). Many parents describe the emotional strain of taking care of children as fatiguing as the physical stresses, particularly after a long day for both parents and children (Hochschild, 1989; Sanders, 2002).

BOX 19-1
Ten Child Care Practices Rated as the Most Physically Stressful for Child Care Workers

Lifting child from the floor
Lifting child up to a changing table
Lifting child into and out of a pushcart
Lifting child into and out of a crib
Bending to help wash hands
Lifting child onto a toilet
Bending to help with feeding and playing
Stacking and unstacking cots and toys
Holding and carrying children
Bending to clean the room and equipment

Note: Practices were rated on a scale of 0 to 9, with 0 being no physical stress and 9 being extremely stressful.

ERGONOMIC RISK FACTORS

The job analyses demonstrate that child care workers spend substantial portions of their days in postures that stress the back and lower extremities. King et al. (1996) and Owen (1994) examined the specific tasks and ergonomic risk factors in 125 child care workers in a large metropolitan child care center. For those workers who cared for younger children (ages 6 weeks to 2.5 years), lifting was the primary ergonomic concern. Children were lifted in and out of cribs, high chairs, strollers, diaper changing tables, and up from the floor using awkward postures. Those staff working with children older than 2.5 years reported the demand for physical endurance to be a major concern along with the need to be "vigilant and continuously responsive" to these very active and mobile children. Lifting children this age was even more stressful because of the weight of the children. For all groups, sitting on small-sized furniture, unsupported sitting, and awkward lifting were problematic.

Owen (1994) examined issues related to low-back pain in 27 child care workers in five Midwestern day care centers. Owen identified the 10 tasks perceived to be the most physically stressful for this sample of child care workers (Box 19-1). These tasks involved primarily lifting, bending, and stooping. Small furniture designed for children's use demanded that adults frequently bend or stoop to assist the children. Observations of child care workers further indicated that workers used poor lifting technique, lifting children from a kneeling position, at one's side, or away from the worker's body.

Sanders (2002) similarly asked parents to rate child care tasks according to their perceived levels of physical stress. Parents indicated that the most stressful tasks involved prolonged carrying in awkward positions and assuming awkward postures of the upper trunk, as well as tasks involving lifting, bending, and squatting. Box 19-2 summarizes the top 10 practices that parents considered to be the most stressful. When the NIOSH Lifting Formula was applied to lifting a child from a crib or from the floor to a standing position, results indicate that child care workers or parents may be required to lift greater loads than would be recommended (Grant et al., 1995). For example, when lifting a child weighing 20 to 30 pounds over the rails of a crib into a caregiver's upright position, the recommended weight limit would be approximately 15 pounds. Because many babies weigh more than this, this act may increase the risk of low-back injury (Grant et al., 1995).

Overall, the major risk factors for child care workers are frequent and improper methods of lifting and lowering children and supplies,

BOX 19-2
Ten Child Care Practices Rated as the Most Physically Stressful for Parents

Carrying a child in a car seat (while doing errands)
Breast and bottle feeding in awkward positions
Carrying a child while bending down
Carrying a child on hip while doing chores
Prolonged squatting
Pushing child on low toy
Lifting child from floor
Placing child in car seat
Bathing child (lifting, kneeling to wash)
Bending to walk child

Note: Practices were rated on a scale of 0 to 9, with 0 being no physical stress and 9 being extremely stressful.

sitting on inadequately sized furniture, sitting on the floor unsupported, bending down to the floor, and excessive reaching above shoulder heights. The risk factors for parents focus more on prolonged carrying of children in awkward positions while multitasking and awkward upper-extremity postures in addition to frequent lifting, bending, and squatting. Mundt et al. (1993) substantiate that lifting children, especially over 25 pounds, is a risk factor for herniated lumbar intervertebral disc. Russell et al. (1993) suggests "as posture would seem to be an important factor in the development of long-term backache, there should be greater efforts to make mothers more aware of their posture."

ERGONOMIC RECOMMENDATIONS TO MINIMIZE PHYSICAL STRESSES

Although many ergonomic risks exist in the occupations of parents and child care workers, many of these risks can be substantially minimized by improving one's body mechanics during the performance of child care tasks and by improving the design of child care equipment. Whitebrook, Belm, Nattinger, and Pemberton (1989), as part of the CCEP, recognized that child care workers should follow basic principles in order to minimize stresses to backs. However, no publications have specifically discussed body mechanics for child care tasks, with one notable exception: Pirie and Herman's *How to Raise Children without Breaking Your Back.* These authors offer numerous suggestions for caring for children as safely as possible and for regaining musculoskeletal strength and flexibility following childbirth.

The next section describes basic body mechanics principles and then discusses specific recommendations and tips for performing the most common (and stressful) child care tasks. Table 19-1 identifies common child care equipment, the ergonomic design problems, and recommendations to enhance parents' or child care workers' body mechanics while using the equipment.

Principles for Good Body Mechanics

The reader is referred to many books and journals that describe in more detail the theory and biomechanics behind proper use of the body (Chaffin & Andersson, 1984; Pirie & Herman, 1995; Pope, Andersson, Frymoyer, & Chaffin, 1991; Saunders, 1992) (also see Chapter 18). Overall, the basic tenet is to keep the body in neutral so that the muscles are balanced and in the proper alignment while performing the task, thereby utilizing the least of amount of energy necessary to complete the task. Once a body segment is out of alignment, the moment or torque placed on that joint increases (LeVeau, 1992; Pope et al., 1991).

A neutral position of the body is one in which both sides of the body are symmetrical; the head is aligned with the trunk; the shoulders, ribs, and hips are level; and the feet are not rotated inward or outward. From a lateral view, the ears should be aligned with the midpoint of the shoulders, hips, knees, and ankles; the cervical, thoracic, and lumbar curves should not be exaggerated. Individuals are reminded to move carefully and deliberately while lifting, lowering, and carrying equipment in order to use proper body mechanics.

Table 19-1

Commonly Used Child Care Equipment, the Ergonomic Design Problems, and Suggestions for Use Based on Proper Body Mechanics

Child Care Equipment	Ergonomic Design Problem	Recommendations for Use
Inside swing	Low height of swing necessitates bending at waist to place child; the frame prevents caregiver from getting close to swing.	Kneel to place or remove baby from swing, or slide the baby in swing from behind.
Bouncy seat	Wide rims and hanging straps prevent caregiver from getting close to seat.	Kneel next to swing; hold the baby at the waist, leaning forward over caregiver's arms; place baby's feet in first and then place baby upright.
Round exercise saucer	Wide rims prevent caregiver from getting close to seat.	Straddle the walker and squat slightly to lower or lift child.
Child gates	Awkward height creates an awkward leg lift and may stress low back.	Open gates; do not step over.
Walker	Wide rims prevent caregiver from getting close to seat.	Straddle the walker and squat slightly to lower or lift child.
Backpack	Extra weight of child may cause upper or lower back discomfort.	Start using backpack for short periods and then build up duration; request assistance for putting on back or place on a high (safe) surface; adjust waist strap and torso straps to fit firmly on hips and close to body.
Frontpack	Extra weight of child may cause neck, shoulder, and back pain.	Adjust carefully; the infant's body should be at the level of the chest; back straps should be snug and symmetrical.
Stroller	Low height of stroller causes forward bending at waist to place child.	Squat or kneel with one leg to the side of the stroller and then slide baby in.
Baby jogger	Constant grasp on jogger can cause wrist or arm pain.	Periodically stretch fingers and rotate wrists. Avoid excessively tight grip (always use safety strap).

The following are the basic principles of body mechanics. These principles should be integrated into the performance of all child care tasks.

- Keep the load close to the body. If squatting, place the load between the legs.
- Lift with the back straight, bending at hips and knees simultaneously.
- Do not twist or rotate the back or trunk. Move the body starting with the feet first.
- Position the feet shoulder distance apart or more for support.
- Push a load rather than pull.
- Raise one foot on a low stool while standing to support low back.
- Use the stronger muscles to perform a task; use a whole-hand grasp instead of a pincer grasp.

Lifting and Lowering Children

A lift that is performed 12 inches from the ground is much less stressful on back structures than a lift performed at ground level (Pirie & Herman, 1995). Therefore, if the child is able to stand or bear weight, parents or child care workers should place the child upright prior to lifting and then lower the child to a standing position. This practice eliminates the need to squat or bend completely to the floor.

Alternately, older children can be lifted or lowered to a stool, sturdy surface, or short stepladder from which they can climb down independently (Pirie & Herman, 1995). Figure 19-1, *A-D* demonstrates a sequence of lifting a baby from the floor using the body mechanics principles just listed. It is important to remember the following when lifting or lowering a child.

- Always keep the baby as close as possible to you while lifting and lowering. Try sliding the baby down your body instead of holding the baby away from your body.

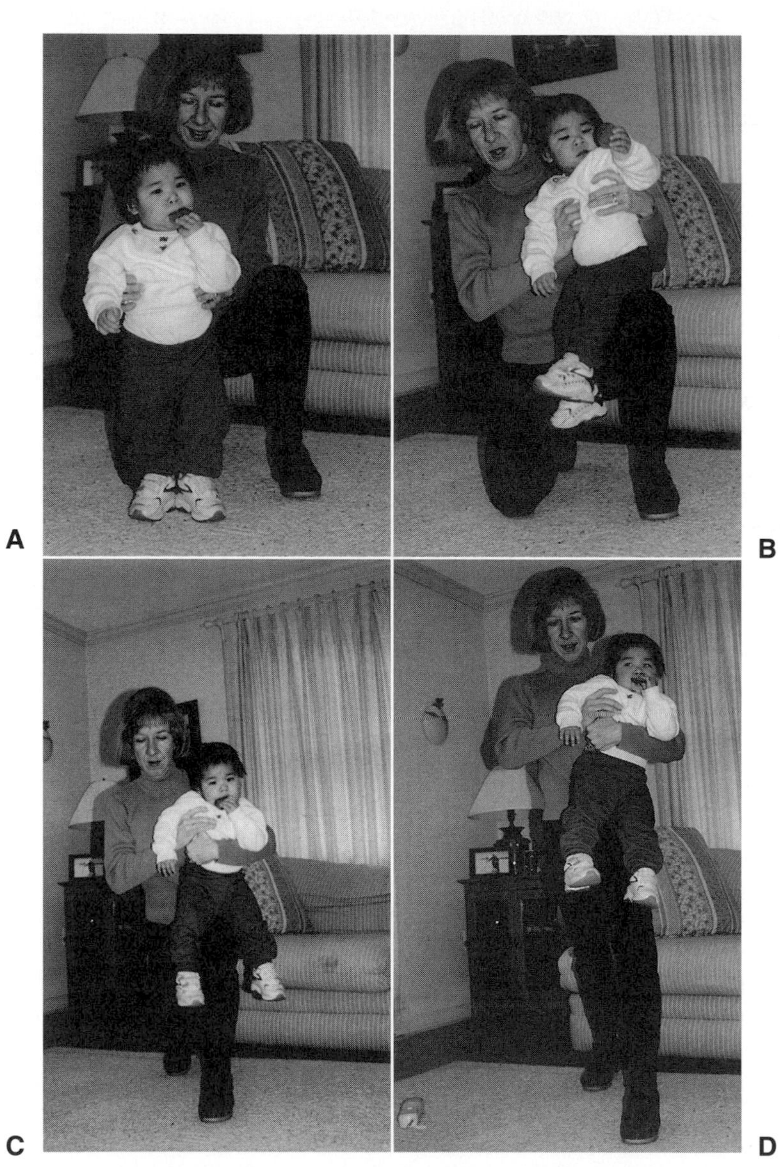

Figure 19-1 Sequence of lifting a child from the floor. **A,** Bring the child to a standing position. **B,** Place the child on one knee. **C** and **D,** Support the child close to the body while coming to a stand.

- When lifting a child from the floor, use a *partial squat* if the child is able to stand (also called a *power lift*). Maintain the head up, back arched, and one foot slightly ahead. If lifting from the floor, place one knee on the floor and keep one knee bent. Bring the baby close to you, place the baby on the bent knee, and gradually come to a stand, keeping the baby close to your body (also called the *tripod lift*). If squatting, make sure the child is between your legs (adapted from Saunders, 1992).
- Keep your feet at least shoulder length apart for good balance.

Carrying Children

An unlimited number of options exist for carrying children. Pirie and Herman (1995) describe four types of carries commonly used. The *hip carry* involves the caregiver supporting the child on one hip. Although convenient, leaving one hand free, this carry tends to exaggerate lateral flexion of the spine and hip in order to support the child. The *front carry* (holding a child in front of the body with both arms) keeps the baby's weight as close as possible to the caregiver's center of gravity. However, one must be careful to maintain the shoulders in a retracted position to prevent a round-shouldered posture. The *football carry,* holding the child across one's body with the head in one arm and pelvic girdle in the other, allows for some distribution of the child's weight between two arms. However, the uneven distribution becomes fatiguing in the shoulder and arms. The *shoulder carry* is comfortable carrying for infants. However, when used for older children, the shoulder carry shifts the center of gravity backward and places strain on the back. Table 19-1 outlines other equipment such as front-packs and backpacks that offer other options for prolonged carrying. Whichever methods parents or child care workers choose, they should remember the following points.

- Vary the type of carry used. Consider the use of backpacks and frontpacks for longer durations of carrying.
- Alternate the sides on which the child is carried.
- Avoid carrying the child while bending down since this increases strain on the back.
- Be conscious of maintaining an upright, erect posture while carrying children.

Transporting Children

Placing a Child in a Car Seat

Car seats are crucial to child safety. However, placing a child in the car seat can put strain on the low back or shoulders when performed incorrectly. If the car seat is placed next to the door, the parent can lift the child outside of the car so that the child's body is parallel to the car seat and supported by the parent's flexed elbows. The parent can then move close to the car and lift the child into the car seat, keeping the weight as close to the body as possible. If the car seat is placed in the center of the back seat, the parent can sit on the seat with the child on his or her lap, move close to the car seat, and then rotate toward the car seat to lift and place the child.

Carrying a Child in a Portable Car Seat

Car seats can be practical for transporting sleeping children. However, when carrying portable car seats, the size and shape of child carriers demand that they are held away from the body, thus placing much increased torque on the upper back, trunk, and shoulders to accommodate this weight (Figure 19-2, A). The most prudent method of transporting a child seat is to carry the child in one arm and the car seat in the other. However, if the child must be carried in a car seat, a parent may carry the car seat sideways in front of the body, with arms supporting either side or carry the car seat in one arm with the handle placed on the proximal forearm and the elbow flexed (Pirie & Herman, 1995) (Figure 19-2, *B*). In the latter option, the car seat can be carried in front of the body with the opposite hand providing added support at the handle. The following information is important to remember.

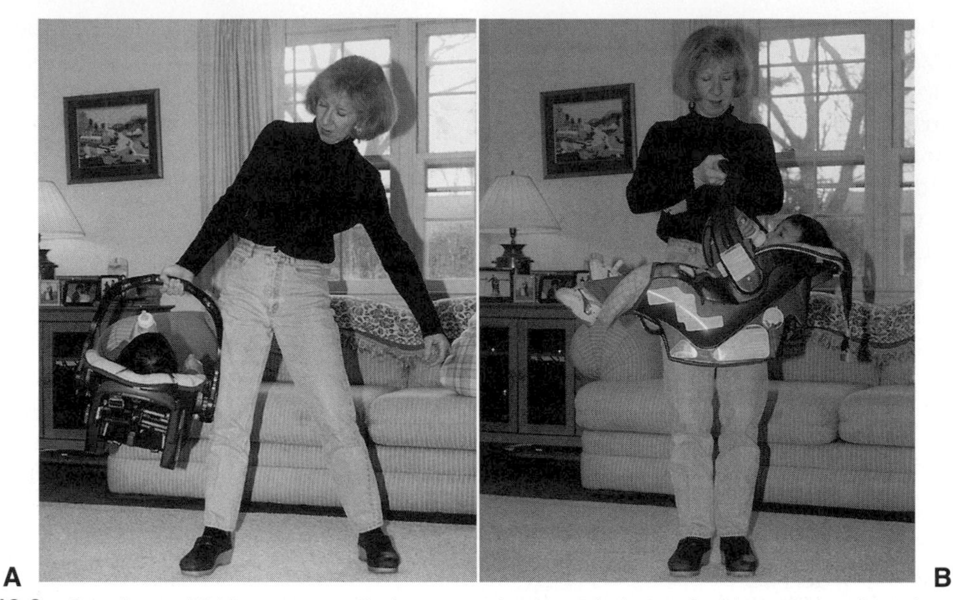

Figure 19-2 Carrying a child in a car seat. **A,** A car seat that is carried at one's side creates awkward postures and excessive torques at the trunk and shoulder. **B,** A car seat that is carried in front of the body allows for a symmetrical upright posture.

- When *placing* a child in a car seat, get as close to the car seat as possible.
- Lift the child first, then place the child in the car seat. Avoid scooping and twisting.
- If *carrying* a child in a car seat, carry the car seat close to the body (either in front with two arms or to the side with a flexed elbow) and alternate arms.
- Try to limit the distances the child is carried in the car seat. Other options for transporting a child include transferring the car seat to a stroller or using a frontpack or backpack to carry the child.

Feeding: Breastfeeding, Bottle Feeding, and Baby Food

Proper intake of food is clearly important to a child's growth. However, parents often sacrifice their own musculoskeletal comfort for their children's ease of eating. A caregiver's typical position for breast or bottle feeding involves neck flexion and rotation, shoulder protraction, elbow flexion, and possibly wrist flexion. Such a posture may strain the neck, shoulder, and thoracic region over a period of time (Chaffin & Andersson, 1984). Elevating the baby's position will help decrease this muscle strain (Pirie & Herman, 1995). Those who consistently extend the thumb to position the breast for the baby may develop pain in the first dorsal compartment of the thumb extensor musculature. Such a thumb position may develop into deQuervain's disease over a period of time (Kirkpatrick & Lisser, 1995).

The following tips will help the caregiver achieve an upright and neutral upper body position during feeding:

- If using a cradling position, place a pillow on your lap under the baby's head to elevate the baby, or use a Boppy pillow (half-moon-shaped pillow) around your waist to achieve the same effect.
- Try bottle feeding the baby in a seated position. Seat the baby on one or both legs with the baby facing away from you. Put your arm under the baby's arm, and place

the bottle in the baby's mouth. The baby is securely held against you, and the wrist is in a straight (neutral) position.

- Use a cupped hand rather than a flat hand with an extended thumb for positioning the breast.
- Alternate sides of the body and positions for breast and bottle feeding. Rotate your neck periodically, or perform gentle neck stretching exercises on a regular basis (Pirie & Herman, 1995).
- Place a pillow behind your low back for support when sitting to breast or bottle feed a baby.
- When feeding the baby solid food from a jar, remove food from the jar into a bowl for feeding. This will eliminate repetitively flexing your wrist into the small jar.
- Use an electric jar opener to remove tops of jars and cans.

Dressing and Changing

The height of a changing table impacts the back position while changing a baby. A changing table that is too low may strain the mid and lower back while bending over; one that is too high may strain the upper back and shoulders because the baby must be lifted over the lip of the table. A waist-height table is optimum for most people (Pirie & Herman, 1995). Those who change diapers on a bed should either kneel by the bed if low enough or sit sideways on the edge of the bed with one foot on the floor and one leg flexed toward the trunk. Keep the back straight, and use an arm as support as needed. It is important to remember the following.

- Change the child on a changing table or surface at waist height whenever possible.
- Avoid lifting and twisting motion simultaneously. Lift the child first and then turn your trunk toward the table. Alternately, use a small stool for older children to climb up to in order to avoid lifting from the floor.
- Distract the child by singing or making animal sounds to calm her while dressing. A calmer baby is much easier to dress!

Bathing the Child

Bathing can be a source of great pleasure for both parents and children. However, the presence of water and soap puts safety issues at the forefront during this activity. In order to avoid falls and strains, keep in mind the following tips.

- Make sure the floor is dry and nonslip strips are placed in the tub floor.
- When washing the child, kneel next to the tub on a small foam mat and support your elbows on the tub rail. Alternately, use a kneel chair with an angled seat and thick knee and elbow supports to wash the child.
- To remove a child from the tub, get close to the tub, place one knee on the tub rail, wrap a towel around the child (to more easily hold the child), position the child close to you, and remove the child. If a waist-height surface is close by, seat the child on the surface to dry.
- Wash infants in the sink, using a small foam pad or reclined surface. The sink height is usually ideal for washing and removing the baby.

Bedtime and Napping

Traditional cribs are typically designed with adjustments for the surface of the mattress and height of the rails. Portable cribs, although convenient, subject a caregiver's body to awkward positions in order to place and remove a baby. The following information is useful to keep in mind when using a crib.

- When using a traditional crib, be sure to lower the crib rails before putting the baby in or removing the baby from the crib. Move the baby closest to the side rail, and place the child in a sitting position if possible. Turn the child so that the back is closest to your body (Grant et al., 1995) (Figure 19-3, *A* and *B*).
- When lifting a child from a portable crib, roll the baby close to the side of the crib, bring your feet as far under the crib as possible, bring the child to a sitting position, and bend your knees and hips to lift the child.

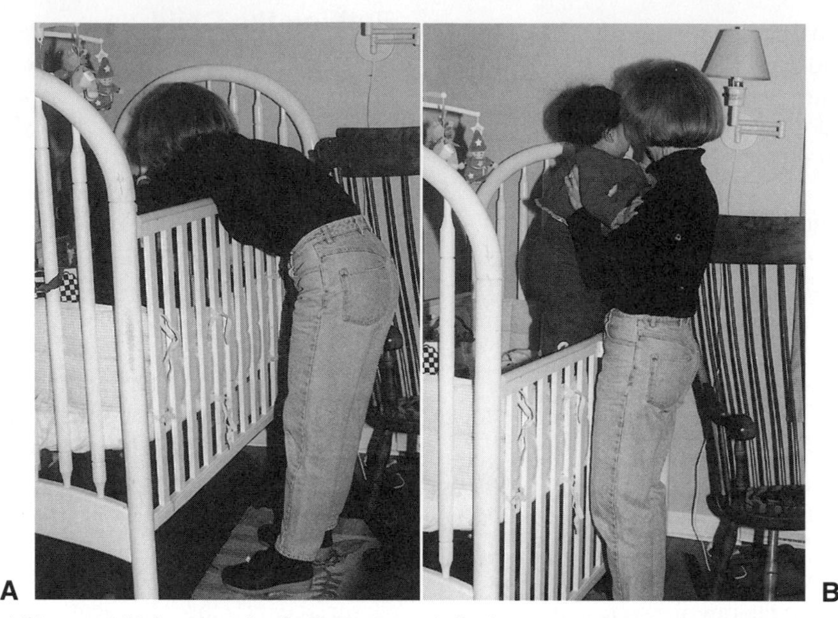

Figure 19-3 Lifting a child from a crib. **A,** Extreme trunk flexion posture results from high crib rails and a child positioned at the opposite side of the crib. **B,** Roll the child to one's side and lower crib rails for a more upright posture.

- When reading bedtime stories, support the back and arms with a pillow.

Play Time and Family Recreation

Children's play is the vehicle for a child's intellectual, physical, and emotional development (Case-Smith, 1997). Play is crucial to a child's development and should be a positive aspect of both the child's and the parent's day. The following suggestions may help parents and caregivers prevent stress to the low-back, shoulder, and neck areas when playing with children.

- Purchase a toy scooter or bike with an extended handle (push bar) to push the child at waist height (Figure 19-4 *A* and *B).*
- When placing child in a swing, kneel with one leg close to the swing.
- When playing on the floor, place a pillow behind your back and sit against a wall or furniture for support.
- Backpacks and frontpacks: See Table 19-1 for suggestions for use.

Performing Chores

Housework and chores are necessary for maintaining a household or child care business. Although multitasking with children afoot may appear efficient, it may compromise the successful accomplishment of both tasks.

Try to limit prolonged carrying of the child on one hip. Consider sitting down, placing the child in a backpack (for vacuuming or laundry), or placing the child in a seat or swing next to you while you complete your task. To pick items off the floor, put the baby down before retrieving the item. The baby's weight can place a great strain on your back in this position. Finally, make sure to carry loads of laundry, diapers, or garbage at waist height.

SUMMARY

The roles of parents and child care workers encompass numerous tasks that nurture children's emotional, intellectual, physical, and social growth. These tasks involve awkward postures,

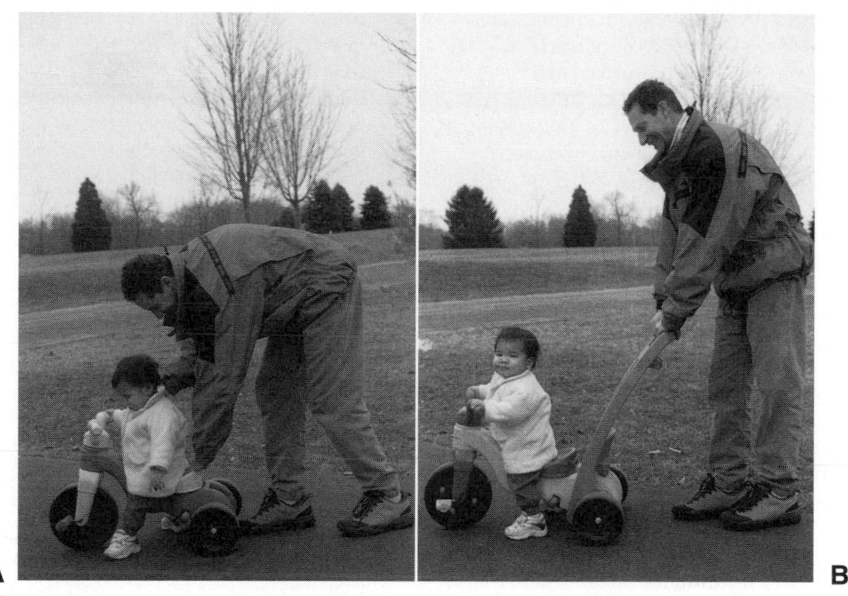

Figure 19-4 Recreational options. **A,** Pushing a child on a low push toy causes extreme trunk flexion. **B,** An extended handle on a push toy allows for a more upright posture.

frequent lifting, bending, carrying, and holding the children. Most parents and child care workers maintain a focus on the child rather than on their bodies during the performance of these tasks. In fact, over 66% of all parents and 11% to 44% of all child care workers have complained of musculoskeletal discomfort that may interfere with the performance of these tasks. This chapter addresses the ergonomic risks and offers suggestions to minimize risks based on body mechanics principles.

REFERENCES

Breen, T.W., Ransil, B. J., Groves, P. A., & Oriol, N. E. (1994). Factors associated with back pain after childbirth, *Anesthesiology, 81*(1), 29-34.

Bright, K. A., & Calabro, K. (1999). Child care workers and workplace hazards in the United States: Overview of research and implications for occupational health professionals. *Occupational Medicine, 49*(7), 427-437.

Brown, M. Z., & Gerberich, S. G. (1993). Disabling injuries to childcare workers in Minnesota, 1985-1990. *Journal of Occupational Medicine, 35*(12), 1236-1243.

Bureau of Labor Statistics (BLS). (2000). Number of nonfatal occupational injuries and illnesses involving days away from work by occupation and selected body parts affected by injury or illness, 2000. Available at http://www.bls.gov/iif/oshwc/osh/case/ostb1043.txt.

Bureau of Labor Statistics (BLS). U.S. Department of Labor. (2002a). Occupational outlook handbook 2002-2003 Edition: Child care workers. Available at http://www.bls.gov/oco/ocos/170.htm.

Bureau of Labor Statistics (BLS). U.S. Department of Labor. (2002b). Career guide to industries 2002-2003 Edition: Child care services. Available at http://www.bls.gov/oco/cg/cgs032.htm.

Calabro, K. S., Bright, K. A., Cole, F. L., Mackey, T., Lindenberg, J., & Grimm, A. (2000). Child care work: Organizational culture and health and safety. *American Association of Occupational Health Nurses Journal, 48*(10), 480-486.

Case-Smith, J. (1997). *Pediatric occupational therapy and early intervention* (2nd ed.). Stoneham, MA: Butterworth-Heinemann.

Chaffin, T., & Andersson, G. (1984). *Occupational low back pain.* New York: John Wiley & Sons.

Child Care Employee Project (1983, Spring). Warning: Child care may be hazardous to your health. *Child Care Employee News, 1,* 1-2.

Dyck, I. (1992). The daily routines of mothers with young children: Using a socio-political model in research, *Occupational Therapy Journal of Research, 12*(1), 16-35.

Grant, K. A., Habes, D. J., & Tepper, A. (1995). Work activities and musculoskeletal complaints among preschool workers. *Applied Ergonomics, 26*(6), 405-410.

Gratz, R., & Claffey, A. (1996). Adult health in child care: Health status, behaviors, and concerns of teachers, directors, and family child care providers. *Early Childhood Research Quarterly, 11,* 243-267.

Griffin, S. D., & Price, V. J. (2000). Living with lifting: Mothers' perceptions of lifting and back strain in child care. *Occupational Therapy International, 7*(1), 1-20.

Hochschild, A. (1989). *The second shift: Working parents and the revolution at home.* New York: Viking Press.

King, P. M., Gratz, R., Scheuer, G., & Claffey, A. (1996). The ergonomics of child care: Conducting worksite analyses. *Work, 6,* 25-32.

Kirkpatrick, W. H., & Lisser, S. (1995). Soft-tissue conditions: Trigger fingers and deQuervain's disease. In J. M. Hunter, E. J. Mackin, & A. D. Callahan (Eds.), *Rehabilitation of the hand: Surgery and therapy* (4th ed.). St. Louis: Mosby.

Kumagai, S., Tabuchi, T., Tainaka, H., Miyajima, K., Matsunaga, I., Kosaka, H. et al. (1998). Load on the low back of teachers in kindergartens. *Sangyo Eiseigaku Zasshi, 40*(5), 204-211.

LeVeau, B. F. (1992). *Williams and Lissner's Biomechanics of human motion* (3rd ed.). Philadelphia: W.B. Saunders.

Manlove, E. E. (1993). Multiple correlates of burnout in child care workers. *Early Childhood Research Quarterly, 8,* 499-518.

Morse, T., Dillon, C., Warren, N., Levenstein, C., & Warren, A. (1998). The economic and social consequences of work-related musculoskeletal disorders: The Connecticut upper-extremity surveillance project (CUSP). *International Journal of Occupational and Environmental Health, 4*(4), 209-216.

Mundt, D. J., Kelsey, J. L., Golden, A. L., Pastides, H., Berg, A. T., Sklar, J. et al. (1993). An epidemiologic study of non-occupational lifting as a risk factor for herniated lumbar intervertebral disc. *SPINE, 18*(5), 595-602.

Nagira, T., Suzuki, J., Oze, Y., Ohara, H., & Aoyama, H. (1981). Cervicobrachial and low-back disorders among school lunch workers and nursery-school teachers in comparison with cash-register operator. *Journal of Human Ergology, 10,* 117-124.

Owen, B. D. (1994). Intervention for musculoskeletal disorders among child-care workers. *Pediatrics, 94*(6 Pt 2), 1077-1079.

Pheasant, S. (1991). *Ergonomics, work, and health.* New York: Aspen Publishers.

Pickering, L. K., & Reeves, R. R. (1990). Occupational risks for child-care providers and teachers, *Journal of the American Medical Association, 263*(15), 2096-2097.

Pirie, A., & Herman, H. (1995). *How to raise children without breaking your back.* Somerville, MA: IBIS Publications.

Pope, M. H., Andersson, G., Frymoyer, J., & Chaffin, D. (1991). *Occupational low back pain: Assessment, treatment and prevention.* St. Louis: Mosby.

Russell, R., Groves, P., Taub, N., O'Dowd, J., & Reynolds, F. (1993). Assessing long term backache after childbirth. *British Medical Journal, 306*(6888), 1299-1303.

Sanders, M. (2002). The ergonomics of caring for children, National American Occupational Therapy Association conference, May 6, 2002, Miami, FL.

Saunders, D. (1992). *Self-help manual for your back.* Chaska, MN: The Saunders Group.

Whitebrook, M., Belm, D., Nattinger, P., & Pemberton, C. (1989). *Staying Healthy. Unit II Working for quality child care.* Oakland, CA: The Child Care Employee Project.

CHAPTER 20

Ergonomics of Leisure Activities

Cheryl Atwood

The importance of maintaining recreational and leisure activities throughout an individual's ever-changing life span cannot be underestimated. The experience of developing one's creative potential, which includes involvement in hobbies, is essential to a joyful life and emotional well-being (Cameron, 1992). Participation in a variety of leisure activities has also been associated with active participation and productivity in the workplace (Karasek & Theorell, 1990). Thus, continued involvement in leisure activities may be beneficial both to the individual and society at large.

Physical and emotional changes can occur throughout one's life that threaten the ability to perform leisure activities. Although leisure activities directly impact our life satisfaction, few studies have applied ergonomic principles to our nonoccupational endeavors. Ergonomic principles can be applied to leisure activities in order to achieve and maintain a meaningful leisure activity schedule in absence of injuries that may interfere with leisure or work-related tasks. Individuals' capabilities and limitations relative to specific components of each leisure activity are also key factors to consider. This chapter discusses the application of general ergonomic design principles to leisure activities, with specific focus on the leisure activities of gardening, quilting, and knitting. Within each section, the biomechanical risks inherent within each leisure activity are briefly addressed, as well as ergonomic designs and modifications for special populations (notwithstanding that everyone benefits from good ergonomic design).

GENERAL CONSIDERATIONS

Although a leisure activity may be ultimately pleasurable and not "work for pay," the potential still exists for stressing the body. In fact, it is possible to spend more continuous time involved in a leisure activity than a work activity because of the anticipated outcome and pleasure gained from the process. As a result, one may become so interested in the activity that the mind may override the body's perception of pain. Individuals should therefore consider the biomechanics of leisure activities with the same importance as that given to work activities.

Prior to starting an activity, a few general questions can help determine whether ergonomic modification will be necessary to ensure a safe and stress-free leisure environment.

- Is the work surface the proper height? Is the work surface too low, causing trunk flexion, or too high, causing increased shoulder flexion and hyperextension of the back?
- Does the activity require heavy lifting?
- Does the activity require working in awkward positions for extended periods of time?
- When lifting is required, what steps can be taken to minimize the loads?
- Are the necessary tools located close to the work area?

- Can the necessary tools be adapted to reduce strain on the body and minimize the forces used?
- Does the activity require continuous repetitive motions?
- Does the activity require staying in the same position for a continuous period of time (Kroemer & Grandjean, 2001)?

Once the risks are determined, broad recommendations for all activities as well as specific recommendations for certain hobbies can be defined. In general, regardless of the task, it is important to take frequent rest periods from the leisure activity. Hobbyists should alternate work and break periods such that they avoid becoming fatigued. Depending on the activity, it may be beneficial to exercise, stretch, or move during break periods. Exercise may include taking a walk for overall cardiovascular health and circulation or stretching specific muscle groups, such as hands and fingers.

ERGONOMICS OF GARDENING

The motivations for gardening are as varied as gardeners themselves. Gardening offers endless opportunities for problem solving and developing a sense of pride and accomplishment. Growing and cultivating plants can be aesthetically pleasing to the senses and challenges our creativity and imagination. However, gardening may result in sore and aching muscles, back and joint pain, insect bites, and overexposure to environmental elements.

Task Components and Risks Associated with Gardening

The typical components of gardening include the following.

- *Digging:* Most often using a shovel or spade, digging is required to excavate and prepare the soil for planting by turning over and breaking up the soil. This task is performed either prior to or at the beginning of the gardening season, usually in early spring. The end of the growing season also requires digging to remove dead plants and to prepare the soil for the next growing season.
- *Raking:* Raking is performed to clear the ground of loose debris and smooth the planting surface. Most raking occurs during the spring and fall.
- *Hoeing:* The hoe is a multiple-use tool that aids the gardener in creating rows for planting seeds at a variety of soil depths and in removing weeds throughout the growing season.
- *Seeding:* Adding seeds to a prepared garden bed can be performed by hand or with the aid of a tool.
- *Watering:* Supplying water to gardens with a hose, under- or above-ground sprinkler, or watering can is necessary for plant growth in dry conditions.
- *Weeding:* Management of unwanted plants in the garden can be done by pulling out weeds by hand or by using a hoe or other tool that digs out the weeds' root system. Weeding is performed throughout the growing season as needed.
- *Harvesting:* Gathering and reaping the rewards of one's labor is usually done by hand. Flowers, herbs, vegetables, and fruits can be picked and collected in a variety of containers or simply in the hand. Plants mature at different rates and will therefore be harvested at different times of the season.

Each of these tasks potentially involves biomechanical risk factors that may contribute to or aggravate a musculoskeletal disorder (MSD). (For a complete discussion of biomechanical risk factors, see Chapter 10.) Table 20-1 outlines the risk factors and potential solutions for the gardening tasks described. When gardening at ground level, most aspects of gardening involve some degree of dynamic trunk and low-back flexion, kneeling, and repetitive grasping of tools or plants. When these postures are assumed for an extended period, strain on the knees, hips and ankles, back, and hands may develop. Raking and soil tilling are both strenuous activities that require substantial upper-body and back strength, as well as good

Table 20-1
Ergonomic Risks Associated with Gardening and Potential Solutions

Tasks	Biomechanical Risk Factors	Solutions
Digging	Prolonged trunk flexion posture Forceful grasping Force applied to feet	Use extended-handle tools Dig using feet against shovel instead of using hands Wear heavy shoes if digging using foot
Raking	Repetitive flexion and extension of the shoulder Trunk flexion	Take frequent breaks (every 20 minutes) Use proper size and type of rake
Hoeing	Prolonged kneeling and trunk flexion while assuming awkward positions or overreaching to maintain plants Awkward and forceful hand positions	Use a kneeling mat as cushioning for knees. Take stretch breaks every 20 minutes Use ergonomic tools to permit a neutral wrist position and greater leverage
Seeding	Prolonged kneeling and trunk flexion Static posturing	Use a kneeling mat for cushioning Stretch in extended position every 20 minutes
Watering	Heavy load on shoulder and back musculature	Use a sprinkler Carry smaller quantities of water Carry watering can (close to your body) on arm with elbow bent Water in the early morning or at dusk to maximize water absorption into soil Choose plants according to tolerance for sun and location to be planted
Weeding	Prolonged kneeling and trunk flexion Forceful hand grasping	Use a kneeling mat for cushioning and small bench for rests Use gloves with rubber palms for efficient grasping
Harvesting	Prolonged trunk and low back flexion	Take frequent breaks

balance to support and use these tools properly. The process of weeding involves high-grip forces in addition to a typically stooped (flexed low back, trunk, and knee) posture.

Although tools enable gardeners to work more efficiently with less force, gardening tools can be heavy and cumbersome for even the most physically fit gardeners when used repetitively. The handles of many hand trowels forks, rakes, and weeders are made of smooth wood with small diameters that can be slippery, necessitating increased force in the hand, wrist, and arms for effective use (see Chapter 11 for a complete discussion of tools). The following discussion provides an overview of the common designs that have been implemented by horticultural and gardening organizations to enable more and more individuals to enjoy the fruits of gardening.

Ergonomic Designs for Gardening

Strain to the back or neck and knees typically occurs while maintaining awkward postures or while overreaching to maintain plants. In order to keep plants within a comfortable reach, a garden bed should be no wider than 2 feet if it is accessible from only one side, and no more than 4 feet wide if accessible on both sides (Relf, 1995). Many options are available to eliminate or reduce this strain by using raised bed gardens, container gardening, or vertical growing.

Raised Beds

Raised bed gardening offers many options for gardeners who want to prevent low-back pain or increase access to beds because of limited mobility. Raised beds can be constructed at any height. Beds at 6 to 12 inches above ground level can greatly reduce the amount of trunk flexion necessary to complete tasks; a raised bed of 36 inches will nearly eliminate low-back flexion for most adults. Some options for raising the height of beds are frames made from cedar boards, chimney flue tiles, stacked cinderblocks, or old washtubs.

Plants that are grown in raised platforms and containers require more frequent watering than ground-level gardens. Therefore, the location of the water source should be taken into consideration before deciding where to place the garden bed. If a water source is not close by, extension hoses can be used to transport the water. A nozzle attachment with an on-off switch should be on the end of the hose.

If a raised bed is to be used by a gardener in a wheelchair, a paved surface surrounding the garden will be necessary. Paved paths leading to the garden will also be required. Although the width of wheelchairs can vary greatly, a paved path of at least 36 inches is wide enough for most wheelchairs to fit comfortably. However, a path of this width does not allow for turning a wheelchair or allow for an accompanying person to walk at the gardener's side. A path at least 48 inches wide is recommended for two people to be able to walk side by side or when one person is using a wheelchair. A path that is at least 6 feet wide (72 inches) allows enough turning radius for a wheelchair (Adil, 1994). The same dimensions would apply for use with a power scooter. A paved surface also reduces the risk of falling and tripping for gardeners who use walkers or canes.

Gardeners who are constructing garden beds that will become permanent structures should consider the following questions prior to construction.

- Are the tools conveniently located for easy access?
- Is the water supply easily available?
- Is the ground surface smooth enough for intended use?

Professional assistance may initially be required in the construction of the raised bed.

Containers

The goal of gardening with containers is to increase accessibility of gardens by limiting overextension of the trunk. The availability of containers is endless. Clay and terra-cotta pots are obvious choices, but wagons, paint cans, plastic buckets, watering cans, toy dump trucks, sand pails, and even old boots are possibilities. Containers can be raised higher to decrease reach distances by placing them on the steps of an old stepladder. A simple plant stand can be made by stacking two sets of clay or terra-cotta pots, upside-down, one on top of the other, to a height of about 24 inches. By placing either a 2 × 10 in board or a preassembled window box across the top of the pots (Figure 20-1), individually potted plants can be set across the board or into the window box.

Regardless of the containment system, it is important to consider the needs of the plants that will grow in them before deciding on the placement of the containers. The sun exposure must be considered as well as the proximity to the home or garden shed.

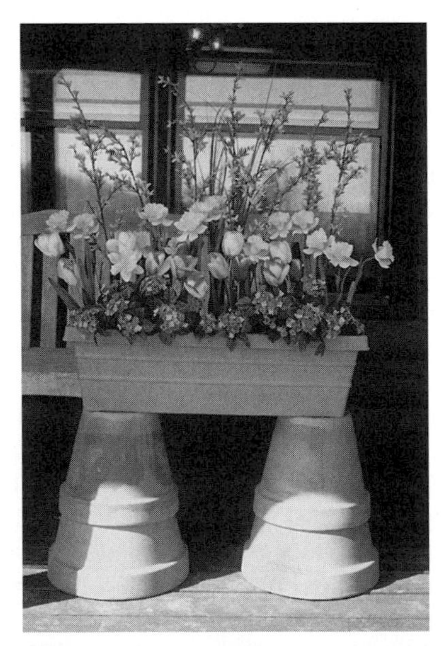

Figure 20-1 14-in and 10-in terra-cotta pots placed on top of each other form a raised plant stand.

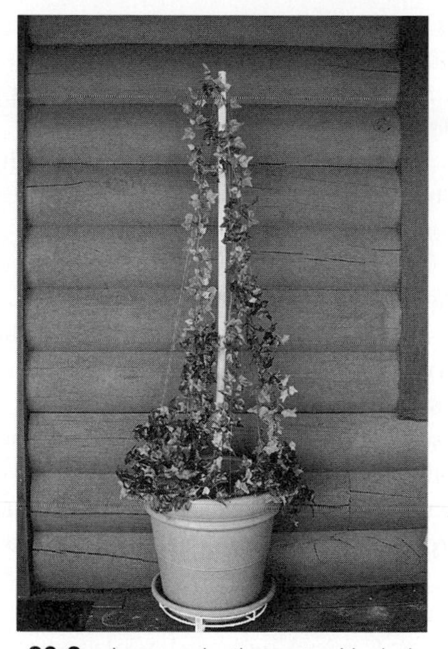

Figure 20-2 Large plastic pot with holes drilled around top. String is tied from drilled holes of the planter to the top of the pole inserted in the middle of the pot to support growing plants.

Vertical Growing

Growing plants vertically can also reduce the amount of trunk and low-back flexion. Trellises of all sizes can be added to increase vertical growing space in a ground-level bed or in containers. A trellis can be created by drilling a series of holes along the top edge of a large plastic planting container. Place a 5-ft-high pole in the center of the pot filled with soil and attach wire or string from each drilled hole to the top of the pole (Figure 20-2). Pole beans, cucumbers, tomatoes, squash, and eggplant grow well this way. Such containers can be used indoors or outdoors.

Gardening Tools

In selecting proper garden tools, it is important to consider the weight and length of the tool, the design of the handle, and the wrist position with which the tool is used. As the user grips the handle of the tool, the wrist should remain in a neutral position, which will allow for the greatest amount of grip strength (see Chapter 11). Ergonomic weeders, trowels, and fork tools are now designed with a pistol grip to maintain the wrist in a neutral position (Figure 20-3). The handle surface should be a comfortable, textured grip. Arm support cuffs can be further added to the tool to provide greater leverage and stability (see the Resource list at the end of this chapter). These tools weigh only about half a pound.

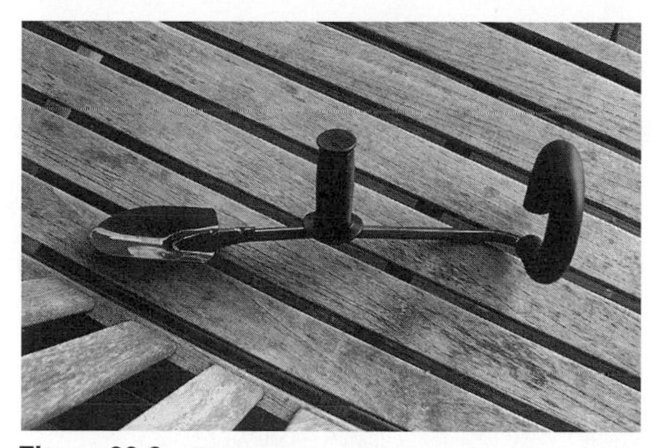

Figure 20-3 Pistol grip trowel with arm support.

Keeping the body in a neutral position while sitting or standing is of utmost importance in reducing proximal loads on the back and shoulders while using hand tools. A gardener should therefore make sure the handle is long enough to limit excessive reaching or bending. Many tools are now available with extension handles (trowel, hoe, rake), measuring from 31 to 35 inches (Figure 20-4). These long-reach garden tools safely increase reaching potential without increasing strain on the back. To further increase stability, it is advisable to add arm support attachments to these long-reach tools. Alternating between sitting and standing will also help reduce muscle fatigue.

When selecting ergonomically designed tools and products, one should be certain that the items provide the benefits described by the manufacturer. Many items are sold as ergonomically designed products with little evidence that substantiates the claim. At this time there is no standard that manufacturers must meet in order to label their products as ergonomically designed.

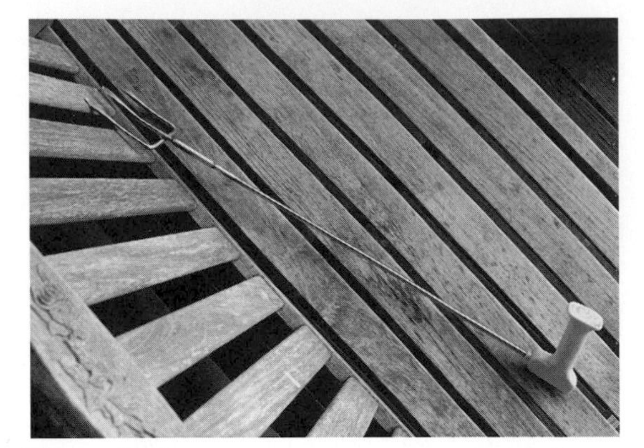

Figure 20-4 Long-reach fork measures 32 inches to increase reach without strain.

Gardening Products

In addition to implementing good ergonomic design, gardening products are available that can potentially minimize the overall work required in gardening. For example, as an alternative to using backyard soil for containers and raised beds, a soil product can be purchased that is lighter than dirt and reduces the risk of introducing soil-borne diseases, insects, and weeds to the garden plants. These products contain potting soil and a mixture of vermiculite, peat moss, or perlite. Application of this product can reduce the work required to maintain such garden beds. If these products cannot be found in a commercially prepared mixture, most garden centers carry the products individually packaged and they can be easily combined.

When planning a garden, one should consider using both perennials and annuals. However, perennials have the benefit of requiring less work, since the life cycle of a perennial plant is longer than one season. Most perennials will last for many years, dying at the end of the growing season only to return in full growth the following spring.

Using fertilizers in the garden may not reduce the workload required to maintain the garden but will increase the harvest quality and perhaps the quantity. The key to successful use of fertilizers is knowing the soil's requirements. Soil pH kits to determine a soil's acidity are available at most garden centers. Once the pH has been determined, a suitable fertilizer can be applied. A wide range of fertilizers is available, from chemically processed to organic. Individual needs must be taken into account to determine what fertilizer works for a particular individual.

Modifications for Special Users

Gardening is ideally suited for those with limited mobility. When constructing a garden, an individual's current and future needs must be addressed including the gardener's current use of a walking aid such as a cane or walker or the eventual use of a wheelchair. Most wheelchairs that are made for adult use measure approximately $28\frac{1}{2}$ inches from the ground to the top of the armrests and approximately 24 inches to the thighs. A raised bed garden platform can be built out of two sets of "A" frame posts that suspend a rectangular garden bed or by using an old picnic table (Figure 20-5). This garden bed has enough space under it to allow the wheelchair to get close to the bed. A wheelchair that is equipped with desktop armrests or removable arms will allow the user greater access to the garden bed.

The length of the bed can vary according to the space available, although consideration should be given to the weight of the raised platform bed. As the length of the bed increases, extra support is needed under the bed. It would be advisable to keep the bed short enough so additional support is not needed and so the accessibility of the wheelchair is not hindered.

Finally, when gardening, it is imperative to keep the body hydrated. Taking frequent breaks from the activity and gently stretching at this time along with drinking plenty of water will help to ensure a safe and rewarding day in the garden.

ERGONOMICS OF QUILTING

As long as fabric pieces are available, either old or new, someone will have an amazing ability to produce quilts. Quilting presents a myriad of

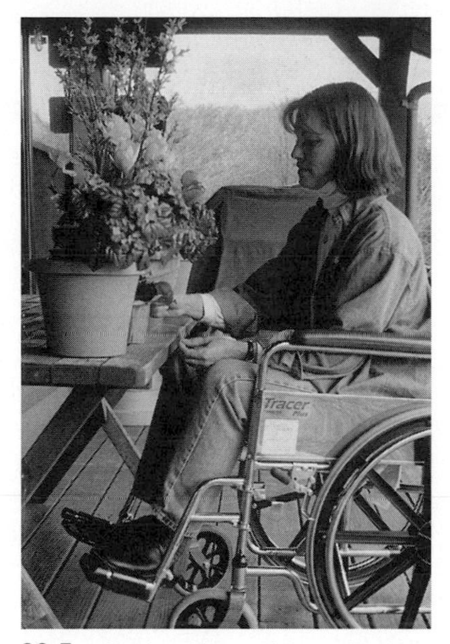

Figure 20-5 Picnic table used as a raised garden bed is high enough for a wheelchair to get close to it from all sides.

opportunities to be creative with an endless array of quilting patterns and fabric color choices available. One can reap the rewards of quilting after spending hours planning, visualizing, and constructing a glorious quilt.

Task Components and Ergonomic Risks Associated with Quilting

Quilting does not come without challenges. To produce a quilt, either big or small, a variety of steps must take place. Fabric and pattern selection is usually the starting point. This requires attention to color variations in value and intensity. The ability to differentiate between colors can be a difficult procedure if an individual is visually impaired or color blind. Once the fabric selection has been completed, the cutting begins.

Cutting is usually done with rotary cutters that come in a variety of shapes. Risks associated with cutting stem from both excessive force while cutting and awkward positions of the wrist, neck, and shoulders (Watts, 1996). Excess muscle force may be generated in the finger flexors and hand intrinsics from statically gripping the cutter handle. Additionally, the shoulder flexor and extensor muscles generate force while swiping with the cutter.

Once the cutting has been completed, the assembly of the quilt top takes place. This is referred to as *piecing*. Piecing may be done either by machine (machine piecing) or sewing by hand (hand piecing). *Quilting* refers to the process of sewing all of the layers of the quilt together, either by hand or by machine. Some of the challenges associated with piecing and quilting depend partly on whether an individual will stitch by hand or by machine. When stitching by machine, the process can move along rapidly if done by chain piecing. *Chain piecing,* sometimes referred to as fast feeding, is a process that involves sewing fabric patches in a consecutive line without cutting the thread in between the patches. By working in this manner, the piecing is done in a fast and efficient method, therefore reducing the repetitive and finite motions otherwise required by hand stitching. The primary concerns in machine stitching are the height of the sewing machine, which influences the individual's posture, and the static position of the individual.

Hand stitching requires keeping the hand in a prolonged static position with the fingers in a precision grip, repeating a tiny rocking motion with the sewing needle. Hand quilting needles are very thin and approximately $1\frac{1}{8}$ inches long. Appliqué needles can be longer than hand quilting needles, but they also tend to be thinner, which can increase the need for gripping tightly. When hand quilting, one hand remains under the layers of the quilt and the sewing hand remains on top. At this time the body remains in a very static position that can strain the back if proper posture is not maintained.

Ergonomic Design for Quilting

Workspace

When designing the workspace for quilting, a few things should be considered. Cutting and sewing should be performed at different-height tables to maintain proper posture. The table height for using a rotary cutter while standing will vary, depending on the height of the person. To determine an appropriate table height for the user, stand and measure the distance between the floor and the elbow flexed to 90 degrees. Subtract about 3 inches from this measurement, and adjust the table to this height. A folding conference table available at most office supply and discount stores works well for this. Lengths of $1\frac{1}{4}$-inch PVC pipe (Figure 20-6) can be cut to fit onto the legs of the table, thereby raising it to the proper height (Hargrave & Craig, 2000).

Although not always practical, it is recommended that the sewing machine be enclosed in a sewing cabinet (Johnson-Srebro, 1998). This ensures that the sewing table surface is level with the top of the machine sewing surface. Many quilters do not have a sewing cabinet, so the sewing machine is usually placed on top of a table. The sewing surface of a cabinet is about 30 inches from the floor, whereas most conference tables measure about 28 to 29 inches from the floor. By placing a portable sewing machine on top of the table, the sewing surface is raised another 3 to 4 inches to a total surface height of 31 to 33 inches. This height may be acceptable for a very tall person, but it may cause others arm or back strain.

While sitting at the table, the knees, hips, and elbows should be flexed to about 90 degrees. The elbow should be about the same height as the table. Adjustable office chairs work well for quilting. If using a conference table that is too high, the table height can be altered by measuring the height of the elbow from the floor and shortening the legs on the table to match the elbow height (Hargrave & Craig, 2000).

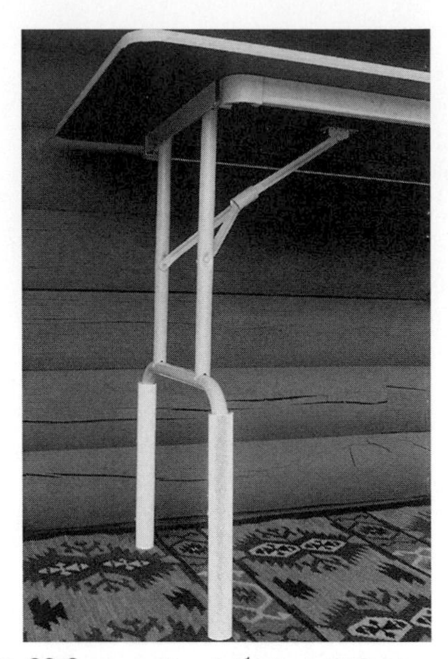

Figure 20-6 Lengths of $1\frac{1}{4}$-inch PVC pipe used to raise a conference table to proper height for cutting.

Lighting

Lighting not only affects our vision, it can also affect how we interpret color values and intensity. How we see and differentiate between colors depends greatly on the lighting provided. Sunlight contains every wavelength of visible light. As the light travels to the earth, most of the long wavelengths—the oranges and reds of the spectrum—are absorbed into the atmosphere. Standard lightbulbs contain full-spectrum light, too, but most of the light comes from the longer wavelengths of oranges and reds. As a result, if a workspace is lighted only with the use of standard bulbs, the workspace and fabric selections may appear to have a yellow or red tint. Fluorescent bulbs contain a higher degree of short wavelengths, or violets and blues. This type of lighting gives a brighter appearance to fabrics and surroundings.

Lights that are placed close to the working area to enhance the lighting of a particular area are called task lights. In general, it is important to keep the work area very well lit so the eyes do not become strained during any stage of the quilting process. Choose lightbulbs that do not increase the glare on the working surface. Translucent bulbs offer good lighting while reducing glare (Hargrave & Craig, 2000). Full-spectrum bulbs offer lighting that most closely resembles natural sunlight. Fabric colors and interior surroundings will appear vibrant and true with the use of these bulbs. Some brand names of full-spectrum bulbs and lighting products are Ott-lites (www.ott-lite.com), Chromalux incandescent, and Lumichrome fluorescent (www.blanksfab.com) (see Resource list at end of chapter).

Tools for Quilting

Rotary cutters come in a variety of shapes and sizes. A style that keeps the wrist in a neutral position and with a large gripping surface will put the least strain on the muscles and tendons of the hand, wrist, and lower arm and increase the user's grasping strength (Figure 20-7). Cutting blades should always be sharp to ensure ease of cutting. Rotary cutting mats are needed when using a rotary cutter. These mats are made of heavy-duty plastic and are unharmed by the razor edge of rotary cutting blades.

When using a rotary cutter, ruler, and mat, place a rubber needle puller on top of the fabric so that it rests between the fabric and the ruler. Needle pullers are small, flat, round rubber disks traditionally used for pulling needles through thick fabric. This will keep the ruler from slipping on the fabric and reduce the amount of pressure needed to hold the ruler in place while cutting. When using the rotary cutter, one should use the following technique to minimize discomfort and muscle strain when cutting.

- Hold the rotary cutter so that the thumb is on top of the cutter. Place the ruler on the fabric with the noncutting hand holding the ruler firmly, with even pressure, and with the thumb at the bottom of the ruler and the fingers comfortably spread apart.
- Hold the cutting hand at a 45-degree angle from the table top, and cut away from the body until the blade is even with the noncutting fingertips (Johnson-Srebro, 1998).

When using rotary cutters, be certain to close the rotary cutter immediately after use for safety purposes.

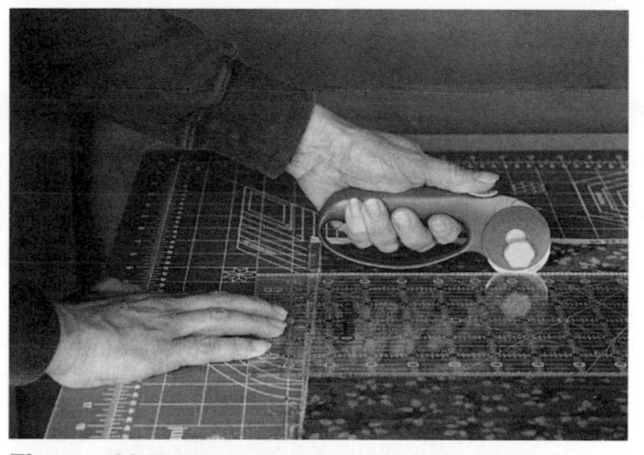

Figure 20-7 Rotary cutters come in a variety of shapes.

Suggested Stretches

As with any activity, it is critical to take frequent rests in order to prevent cumulative strain of tendons and soft tissue structures (Kroemer & Grandjean, 2001). Experts suggest that removing oneself completely from the activity and taking a 10-minute break every hour will increase productivity and ease tension buildup from the quilting. If a repetitive strain injury already exists, it is recommended that two 10-minute breaks be taken every hour (Delany-Mech, 2000).

Stretches for quilting should address the upper trunk and low back as well as the hands. Stretches for the upper back and trunk include stretching from side to side while sitting in the sewing chair or while standing. This stretch is performed as follows: While sitting straight, extend the right hand straight above the head and place the left hand at the hip. Stretch the extended hand to the left without leaning forward or back and briefly hold the stretch (Figure 20-8). Repeat to the other side. Alternate this stretch several times for maximum benefit.

To stretch the muscles of the back and side, a variation of the Hatha yoga simple twist is beneficial. Slide to the front of the chair and place the right hand on the outside of the left knee. Reach the left hand behind as far as possible without straining, and hold the back of

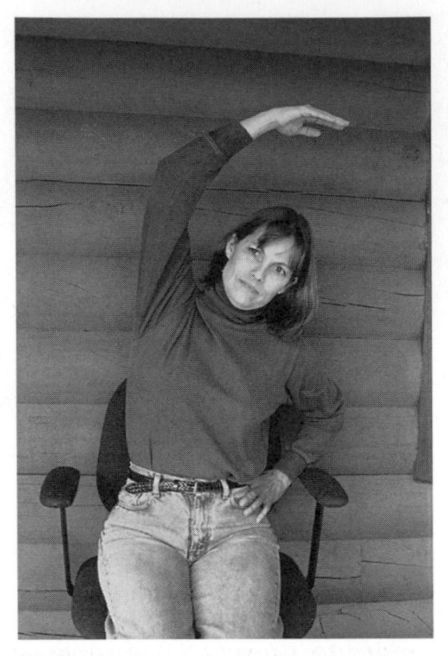

Figure 20-8 Stretches for the back can be performed sitting or standing, alternating each side.

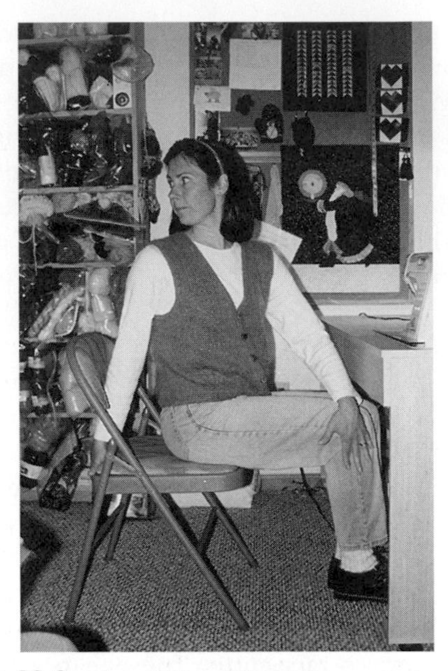

Figure 20-9 A variation of the Hatha yoga simple twist is beneficial for the muscles of the back and sides.

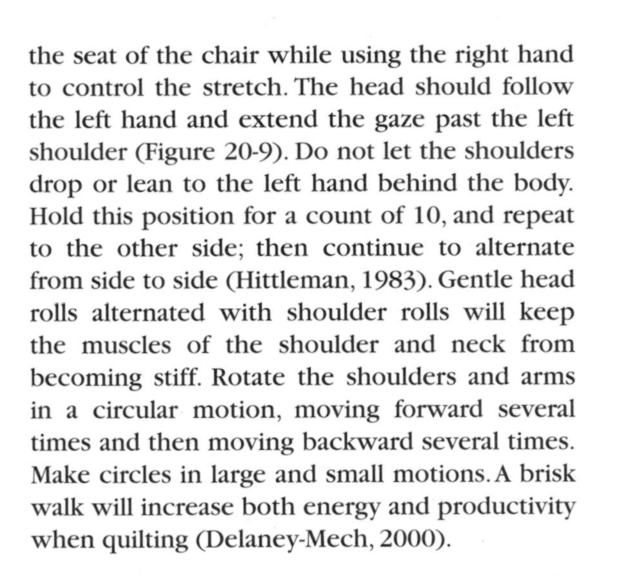

the seat of the chair while using the right hand to control the stretch. The head should follow the left hand and extend the gaze past the left shoulder (Figure 20-9). Do not let the shoulders drop or lean to the left hand behind the body. Hold this position for a count of 10, and repeat to the other side; then continue to alternate from side to side (Hittleman, 1983). Gentle head rolls alternated with shoulder rolls will keep the muscles of the shoulder and neck from becoming stiff. Rotate the shoulders and arms in a circular motion, moving forward several times and then moving backward several times. Make circles in large and small motions. A brisk walk will increase both energy and productivity when quilting (Delaney-Mech, 2000).

ERGONOMICS OF KNITTING

For centuries, people young and old have been diligently knitting items to wear. Bathing suits, diapers, silk stockings, lace shawls, sweaters, pants, mittens, hats, gloves, vests, and blankets were knitted out of necessity and more recently for pleasure. The opportunity to sit and knit among friends of various ages renews and calms one's hurried spirit of our present times. Knitting guilds and less formal knitting groups continue to form as the popularity of knitting continues to increase. Elizabeth Zimmerman (1989) captures the sense of joy obtained when knitting: "Really, hand knitting is a dreamy activity, built into many people's thumbs and fingers by genes already there, itching to display their skills and achievement possibilities."

Task Components and Ergonomic Risks Associated with Knitting

The process of knitting involves the preparation of yarn that may or may not need winding into a ball or skein form, either by hand or with the use of a ball winder. In order to select knitting needles, one should knit a gauge sample to determine if the recommended needles will produce the required finished measurements. After selecting the proper needles, the project may begin. The project may be simple and completed in a short time on large needles using heavy yarn, or it may be very time consuming using very fine needles and thin yarn. The stitch pattern affects the amount of work. Once the main body of the project has been completed, the pieces need to be attached together, as in sweater construction. Trimming, accessorizing, and embellishing are the final steps in the knitting process, along with weaving in the loose ends of yarn where skeins of yarn began and ended.

The biomechanical processes of knitting involve maintaining a static tripod grasp on the knitting needles, tightly gripping the working yarn and needles with flexed fourth and fifth fingers, and repetitively flexing and extending the fingers to complete the stitches. The position of the wrist while knitting a straight knit or purl is relatively neutral. However, when knitting a pattern, the wrists tend to be positioned in flexion as the hand manipulates the stitches in a more complex manner. Significantly more concentration and attention to details are required. Thus, a protruded and flexed posture of the neck may typically occur for long periods, causing increased loading and overstretching of cervical ligaments. New and inexperienced knitters may easily fatigue in the fingers and hands after only a short period of time, since their muscles are not conditioned to this fine and repetitive work. Although general soreness that is alleviated by rest may not be problematic, the knitter should be aware of bodily signs that signal further concern: pain at the base of the neck, frequent headaches or headaches spreading from this area, a burning sensation across the shoulders, pain in the elbows or wrists, and tingling in the fingers (Stove, 1995).

Ergonomic Design for Knitters

Knitting is less conducive to ergonomic design changes than many other activities. However, precautions can be taken to prevent injury or further aggravate any current conditions. As with any activity, the individual's current and future needs should be addressed.

Workspace

The workspace for knitting requires very little in terms of equipment. A supportive chair and adequate lighting are the basic requirements. As with any activity, maintaining proper alignment of the spine is of utmost importance, not only to reduce stress but also to prevent injury.

Tools

The tools required for knitting include, but are not limited to, knitting needles, tapestry needles, rubber point protectors, cable needles, stitch markers, stitch holders, and scissors. Needles come in a variety of sizes and styles. The lower the size number, the smaller the diameter of the needle. The smaller the diameter of the needle, the more stress created as the work continues. Needles can be made of metal, wood, bamboo, and plastics. Straight needles are nonflexible and come in lengths of 10 inches and 14 inches. Circular needles have a shorter working needle surface, connected together either by a metal or plastic cable. The length is measured from needle point to needle point and comes in lengths of 11, 16, 24, 36, and 40 inches. Seamless knitting may be accomplished with circular needles, or they may be used in place of traditional straight needles. Some straight needles have points at both ends. Double-pointed needles are available in sets of four or five needles. They may be used in the same manner as circular needles for seamless knitting and are mostly used on smaller projects such as mittens, gloves, and socks. They are available in 7-, 10-, and 12-inch lengths. Double-pointed needles can also be found in 16-inch lengths but not in many sizes—usually U.S. sizes 1 through 6. These are designed to be used with a knitting belt.

A knitting belt is a small leather pouch with many holes in it attached to a belt strap. The belt is worn around the waist with the pouch in front. The end of one 16-inch double-pointed needle is inserted into one of the holes of the belt (Figure 20-10). Knitting belts were traditionally used to increase the speed at which one could knit because the hands no longer needed to support the knitting needle, so the knitter could wrap the working yarn and pass stitches from one needle to the other more quickly. Knitting belts still prove to be of value today. Not only can they increase knitting speed, if that is the individual's goal, but more important, they simultaneously reduce the strain and tension of the knitter's hands, wrists, and arms.

Another method for reducing finger strain when knitting is to use wood or bamboo needles. These needles are much lighter than metal needles. Circular needles have even greater benefits over straight needles. Because of the circular shape of the needle, the knitted fabric being created rests on the individual's lap as he or she knits instead of in the hands. Straight, single-point needles are supported only by the hands and wrists. Any fabric created by knitting is therefore supported in the same manner. By switching to a knitting belt or a circular needle, much tension in the hands and wrists can be reduced.

Needle size should also be considered. Many knitters enjoy using very small needles, such as U.S. sizes 0 to 4. These needles are used often with lace, fingering, and sport-weight yarn and can produce very delicate knitted articles. As stated previously, the finer the needle, the greater the strain on the muscles and tendons. The tiny stitches are more difficult to see, require a greater tension on the working yarn, and require more stitches per inch to create fabric than do heavier yarn and larger needles. Larger needles—U.S. sizes 8 and higher—worsted weight or bulky yarn may be all that is needed to reduce the tension in the hands, arms, and neck while knitting. The type of yarn used can also be a factor to consider.

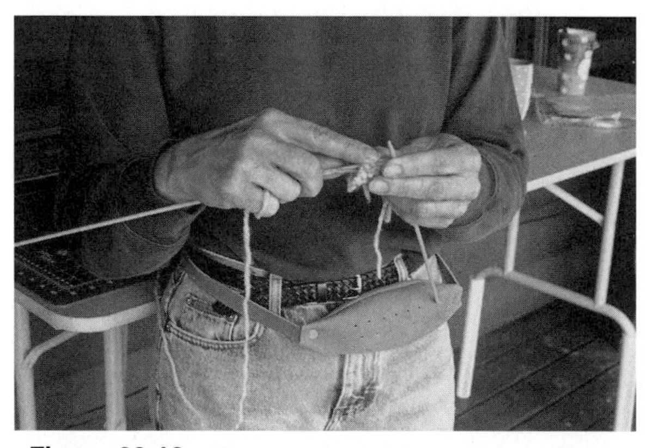

Figure 20-10 The use of a knitting belt reduces the strain on hands, arms, and shoulders because the hands are not required to support the weight of the knitting needles.

For those who prefer the finer work and would not consider larger needles and yarn as an alternative, the use of a freestanding or necklace style magnifying lens may be helpful to reduce eye strain (Figure 20-11). More frequent rest periods may also be required to allow the muscles and tendons to adequately recover from the repetitive strain of the activity.

Knitting Products: Knitting Materials, Gloves, Glasses

As previously mentioned, yarn comes in a variety of weights, known as fingering, sport, double knitting, worsted, bulky, and chunky weight. Yarn can also be made of various materials such as lambswool, cotton, alpaca, llama, Angora rabbit, Angora goat, camel, synthetics, and more. Cotton is more difficult to work with than wool or synthetic yarns because it has no elasticity to it and requires a tighter hold on the working yarn to keep the stitch size consistent. Support gloves are available and do offer comfort and support when working with any yarn (Figure 20-12). When working with cotton and some very fine yarns, a simple glove can be worn to increase tension on the working yarn without increasing gripping tension. Rubber gloves made for cleaning and general purpose can be used. Cut off the tips of the glove fingers about halfway on the finger length. This allows the tips of the fingers to be exposed, yet keeps the hand covered where the working yarn is held. The rubber itself provides the needed increased tension, giving the muscles and

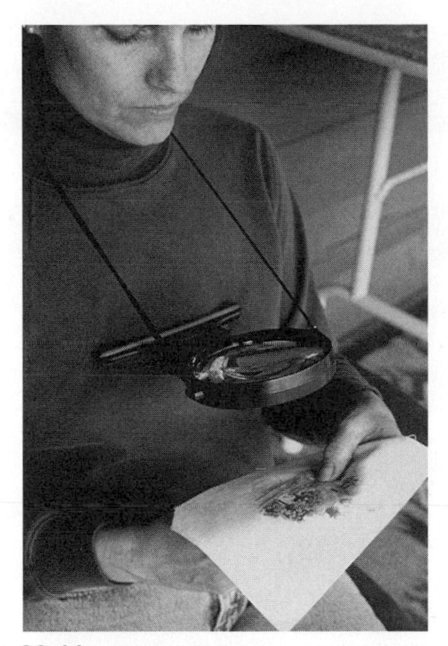

Figure 20-11 A magnifying lamp provides increased visibility when needed.

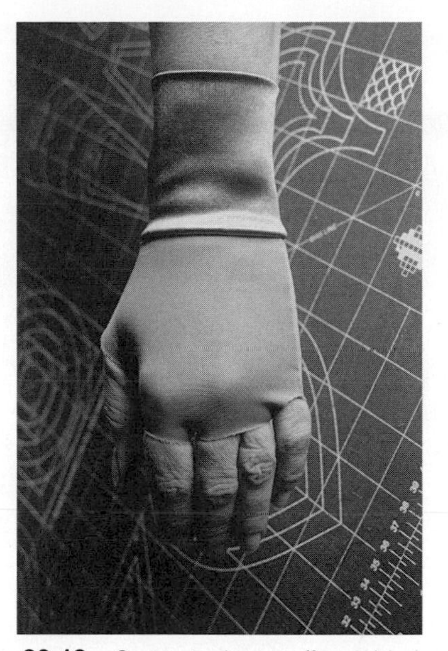

Figure 20-12 Support gloves offer added comfort and support.

tendons a chance to relax. Both support gloves and rubber gloves should be used only for support and reduced tension and not as an excuse to begin marathon knitting sessions.

Under all circumstances, frequent rest periods that include exercises for the fingers, wrists, and arms should be incorporated into any knitting program right from the start. A 10- to 15-minute rest period every hour, along with a series of stretching exercises, will help to condition muscles and tendons. In my experience, it appears that knitters, both experienced and novice, do not currently incorporate exercises into their knitting routine. Even with a known repetitive strain injury most knitters still do not incorporate any exercises into their knitting schedule.

Suggested Stretches

Prior to beginning knitting, it is advisable to soak the hands and wrists in comfortably hot water for a few minutes to warm stiff muscles. Once the hands are warmed up, a series of exercises should follow and be repeated every hour. Because knitting requires repeated gripping of the hands and fingers, performing exercises that require the opposite movements are beneficial and refreshing. With palms facing the lap and the arms reaching out in front, extend the fingers as wide as possible. Rotate the hands so the palms are up, and then turn them down (Figure 20-13). Repeat the same exercise with the arms extended out to the sides at shoulder level. Repeat 10 to 20 times in each direction. To stretch the fingers, place hands together so just the fingertips are touching each other. Stretch the fingers out as far as possible, gently pushing the hands against each other, then bring all fingers and thumbs closely together. Repeat this rhythmic motion 20 times while breathing deeply and slowly (Figure 20-14). As with quilting, gently rotating the neck in circles in both directions will help to keep the shoulders and neck from becoming tense (Larson Line & Loving Tubesing, 2000). As with any exercise or activity, it is critical to stop if any discomfort is experienced. The benefits of including

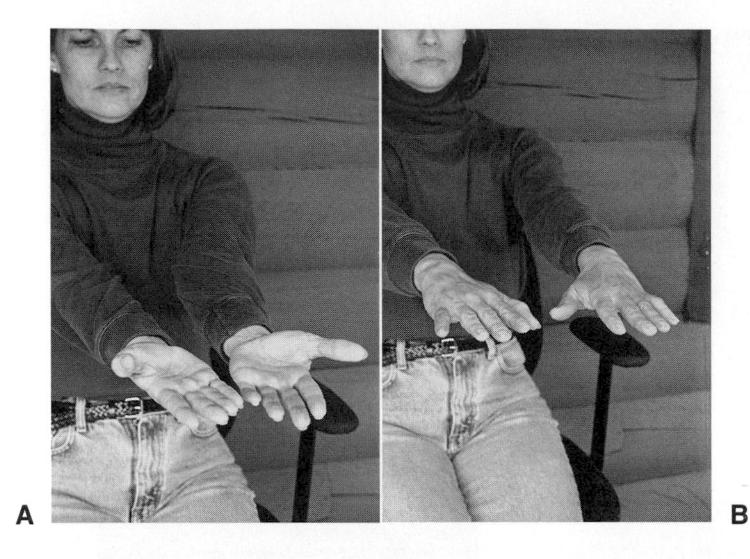

Figure 20-13 **A** and **B,** Rotating extended arms and fingers helps stretch finger flexors and muscles of the shoulders.

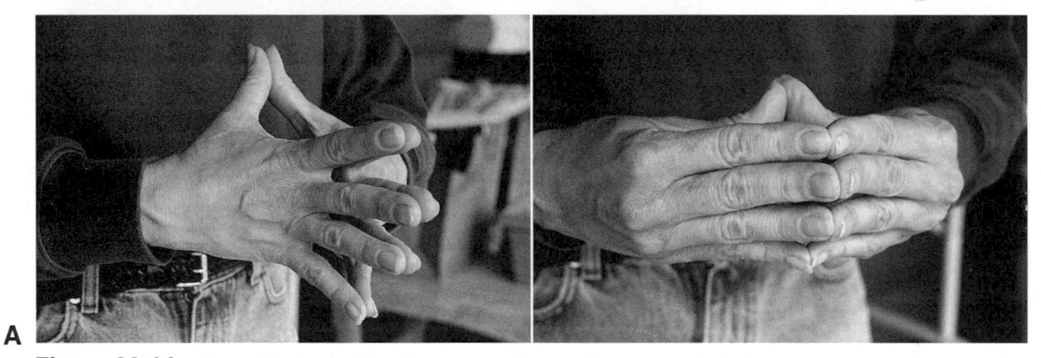

Figure 20-14 **A** and **B,** Performing finger stretches reduces muscle fatigue.

these and other exercises into a knitting routine cannot be underestimated. Careful attention to reducing strain and allowing adequate time for muscles to recover are key factors in enjoying our leisure activities.

Finally, when knitting, be sure to sit in a supportive chair, with feet on the floor. Keep the knees, hips, and elbows bent at a 90- to 100-degree angle. During at least two rest periods, it is advisable to completely remove oneself from the activity. Taking a brisk walk outdoors will not only clear the mind, but also increase energy and heighten the senses.

Adaptive tools are not readily available for the average knitter to use to prevent injury or to use once an injury has occurred. Preventing an injury by taking precautions through exercise, rest, and listening to the body is always of utmost importance. With a few simple steps any activity program can safely be maintained, and new activities can be started.

REFERENCES

Adil, J. R. (1994). *Accessible gardening for people with physical disabilities, a guide to methods, tools and plants.* Bethesda: Woodbine House.

Cameron, J. (1992). *The artists way, a spiritual path to higher creativity.* New York: Penguin Putnam.

Delaney-Mech, S. (2000). *Rx for quilters: Stitcher-friendly advice for everybody.* Lafayette: C&T Publishing.

Hargrave, H., & Craig, S. (2000). *The art of classic quiltmaking.* Lafayette: C&T Publishing.

Hittleman, R. (1983). *Richard Hittleman's yoga, 28 day exercise plan* (Reissue edition). New York: Bantam Books.

Johnson-Srebro, N. (1998). *Rotary magic, easy techniques to instantly improve every quilt you make.* Emmaus, PA: Rodale Inc.

Karasek, R., & Theorell, T. (1990). *Health work: Stress, productivity and the reconstruction of working life.* New York: Basic Books.

Kroemer, K. H. E., & Grandjean, E. (2001). *Fitting the task to the human* (5th ed.) Philadelphia: Taylor & Francis.

Larson Line, J., Loving Tubesing, N. (2000). *Quilts from the quiltmaker's gift.* Duluth: Pfeifer-Hamilton.

Relf, D. (1995) Gardening in raised beds and containers for older gardeners and individuals with physical disabilities. Virginia Polytechnic Institute & State University, 426-020. Retrieved at www.hort.vt.edu/human/pub426020d.html.

Stove, M. (1995). *Creating original hand-knitted lace.* London: Robert Hale.

Watts, C. (1996). *The hidden hazards of quilting.* Saskatchewan, Canada: Physio-Diversity.

Zimmerman, E. (1989). *Knitting around.* Pittsville, WI: Schoolhouse Press.

RESOURCES

Leisure for Special Needs
www.arthritis.org
www.aota.org
www.thewright-stuff.com

Gardening Supplies
www.earthbudeze.com
www.gardeners.com (Gardeners Supply Company)

Ergonomic Gardening Tools
www.gardenscapetools.com
www.gardentalk.com (Walt Nicke Company)
www.hort.vt.edu
www.lifewithease.com (Long reach tools, arm support attachments)
www.dynamic-living.com
www.plowhearth.com
www.earthbudeze.com

Lighting and Quilting
www.ott-lite.com
www.clotilde.com
www.blanksfab.com
www.dynamic-living.com
Jo-Ann Fabrics
www.thewright-stuff.com

Knitting
www.fiber-images.com
Schoolhouse Press (800-968-5648)

PART SIX

Specific Programs for High-Risk Populations

CHAPTER 21

The Older Worker

Robert O. Hansson
James H. Killian
Brendan C. Lynch

INTRODUCTION

In the year 2000, the median age of the American labor force was 39.3 years. More than 67% of men and 51% of women aged 55 to 64, and 17% of men and 9% of women aged 65 to 74 remained at work (Fullerton & Toossi, 2001). Middle-aged and older employees thus comprise a large and important component of the workforce. However, they also account for substantial numbers of occupational injuries and disorders.

For purposes of this chapter, we define the term *older worker* to include persons aged 40 and older. By age 40, observable age-related changes will have already occurred for many persons, and this is the age at which one becomes eligible for protection by federal law from age discrimination in employment. Within this vast age-range, however, there is much variability, and for most people age-related changes are not likely to become problematic until the 50s and 60s. In addition, there is great diversity across individuals with respect to the experience and consequences of aging. Nevertheless, available research provides considerable insight into the implications of the aging process for the management of health in the work setting.

In 1999, workers aged 45 or older accounted for 28% of all reported occupational injuries and illnesses. Within this population, however, days lost from work for a case of occupational injury or illness increased with age, with persons aged 45 to 54 missing eight days, those aged 55 to 64 missing 10 days, and those aged 65 and older missing 11 days per incident (Bureau of Labor Statistics, 2001a). Table 21-1 further illustrates the incidence for 1999 in the United States of (a) traumatic occupational injuries and disorders, and (b) systemic occupational diseases and disorders among these three age groups (Bureau of Labor Statistics, 2001b). Systemic occupational diseases and disorders in this analysis include diseases of the blood, inflammatory diseases of the central nervous system, disorders of the peripheral nervous system (such as carpal tunnel syndrome and neuropathy), hypertensive disease, tendinitis, dermatitis, and so on.

AGE-RELATED CHANGES IN HEALTH AND DISABILITY AS A CONTEXT FOR EXPERIENCE OF MSDs

It is important to consider musculoskeletal disorders (MSDs) in the context of an older person's broader health picture. In modern industrialized countries, the healthy life span has substantially lengthened in recent decades, allowing many persons to continue to work into later life.

Table 21-1
Incidence in 1999 of Traumatic Occupational Injuries and Disorders and Systemic Occupational Diseases and Disorders

	Traumatic Occupational Injuries and Disorders		Systemic Occupational Diseases and Disorders	
Age Category	Number	Percentage	Number	Percentage
45-54	278,287	17.9%	25,251	23.2%
55-64	124,322	8.0%	10,985	10.1%
65 and older	20,655	1.3%	1,462	1.3%

Source: Bureau of Labor Statistics, 2001b.
Percentage is of all accupational injuries.

Issues of health and disability, however, do arise at some point for most older working adults. Normal aging involves a progressive deterioration of physiologic functioning of the immune response, cardiovascular, skeletal, endocrine, and sensory systems, central and peripheral nervous systems, aerobic capacity, and so on (Hayflick, 1994). In addition, advancing age is often accompanied by an accumulation of chronic disorders and conditions, including heart disease, arthritis, diabetes, impaired vision, hearing, and sense of balance. Such changes can result in reduced strength and endurance, metabolic function, lung function, tolerance for pain, resistance to disease, reduced adaptive reserves, and capacity for physiologic self-repair (Rowe, 1985). Chronic disease, then, is a major obstacle to rehabilitation and recovery (Lichtenberg & MacNeill, 2000), and some 23% of persons aged 45 to 64 report limitations of their activities because of their chronic conditions. As might be expected, among employees aged 45 to 64, those with such chronic conditions are also more likely to miss work and to prematurely drop out of the workforce (Summer, 2000).

As we age, injuries are also more likely to result from internal causes (rather than environmental factors). For example, with increasing age the causes of falls in the workplace increasingly involve such factors as postural instability, diminished mobility, multiple medications, cardiac status, deteriorated vestibular or proprioceptive feedback, impaired vision, or perceptual capacity (Ketcham & Stelmach, 2001; Ochs, Newberry, Lenhardt, & Harkins, 1985).

It is relevant, also, that many of an older person's other chronic conditions have the potential to exacerbate or be exacerbated by a newly acquired MSD. Arthritis and orthopedic impairments would be expected to be primary candidates for such interactions (see Chapter 7 for a complete discussion). However, a variety of more subtle complications exists as well. For example, diminished kidney functioning may limit one's ability to take antiinflammatory or pain medications. Any medications given to treat an MSD may subsequently create issues of multiple medication interactions, which commonly become a problem with middle-aged and older adults.

Similarly, diabetes can be a concern. Diabetes among older adults is in many ways a condition that accelerates aging and its consequences (Morley, 2000). The disease is progressive, it becomes harder to manage over time, and it increases vulnerability to other forms of disorder or dysfunction. It is a risk factor for falls, impaired wound healing, diminished nerve function and blood flow to extremities, blindness, and hyperglycemia. Diabetes could become an issue, then, if the pain associated with an MSD in later life were to inhibit rigorous physical exercise, making glucose levels more difficult to control and increasing the likelihood of neuropathy, which could in turn mask or complicate the symptoms of an MSD. Even the physical and psychologic stress likely to be associated with MSD-related symptoms may increase glucose levels.

In late life, the probability also increases that an MSD will play a role in the broader process of disablement, in which chronic disease or injury contribute to the impairment of major organ or body systems, in turn affecting functioning in work and life roles. For example, an MSD may mandate inactivity or immobility, in time reducing the muscle and cardiopulmonary conditioning required for safe, productive work and for independent living (Jette, 1996).

These examples, then, illustrate the problem of multiple chronic conditions in later life. More than 60% of adults aged 55 years and older report having more than one chronic condition, and the additive and interactive effects of such conditions tend to increase risk for poor health and disability. In this connection, a secondary concern for older workers experiencing an MSD, impairment, chronic pain, or functional limitations involves how the situation is interpreted by the individual or others. In many cases, chronic pain and a difficult prognosis may be interpreted by the individual as that point at which they progressed from "not being old" to "being old" (Kemp, 1985). It could also lead employers to prematurely conclude that an older person is becoming less fit for employment. Such beliefs can encourage premature decline and dependency (Jette, 1996).

However, injury and disease do not always lead to disablement among older adults. Older employees are a heterogeneous population. Each person brings to the workplace a different mix of experiences, dispositions, physical and cognitive abilities, vulnerabilities, and coping resources. Older workers also vary considerably in their ability to recover from or manage the consequences of injury (including MSDs), trauma, medication, and surgical intervention (Rowe, 1985).

IMPACT OF CHANGES ON WORK

Many age-related changes in capacity have implications for work safety and performance (Charness & Bosman, 1990; Fisk & Rogers, 1997; Hoyer, Rybash, & Roodin, 1999; Simoneau & Leibowitz, 1996; Spirduso & MacRae, 1990; Whitbourne, 1999). For example, there are important changes in body structure, particularly over the age of 50 years. Standing height tends to decrease because of bone loss, compression of the spine, and diminished joint function. There is also a reduction of muscle size, strength, endurance, and tone. Bones become more vulnerable to physical pressure and fracture. Range of motion and speed of movement are reduced, with consequences for posture, cramping, gait, mobility, and vulnerability to work-related accidents.

With age, there are also important changes in many of the body's vital functions, with substantial decreases in cardiac reserve, respiratory capacity, and immune function. These can impact capacity for the safe and continued performance of strenuous work in an industrial environment.

The degradation of neural tissue with age impacts sensory and higher-integrative processes of the brain, with implications for many psychomotor functions such as reaction time, eye-hand coordination, balance, and postural control, as well as for vision and hearing. Vision changes include lower quality of image (especially under poor lighting) and decreased capacity to adjust focus and adapt to glare or darkness. There are also declines in depth perception, color perception, peripheral vision, and perception of moving objects or of rapidly changing objects. Hearing changes include diminished sensitivity to high frequencies and impaired speech perception. There is also a general slowing of motor and cognitive behavior and a need for increased time to process information. Sensitivity to temperature changes is diminished, incurring risk for hypothermia or frostbite. Pain thresholds are heightened and can mask injury or illness. Kinesthetic abilities are impaired, reducing one's ability to sense location of limbs and increasing the risk of falls. Age-related changes in the sense of balance may reflect an interaction of factors, such as an impaired vestibular system (which may result in dizziness or vertigo), disturbances of vision, reduced ability to function with degraded sensory information and to notice or compensate for the onset of a fall, and so on.

Age-related physiologic problems and MSDs tend to co-occur. Declines in muscular strength, flexibility, and endurance after the 20s and 30s increase the risk for developing a musculoskeletal disease (Spirduso & MacRae, 1990). As a consequence, older people often experience limitations that can negatively affect job performance. They are especially vulnerable to identified risk factors for the development of chronic musculoskeletal pain (Headley, 1997). For example, the diminished capacity of muscles caused by injuries or other age-related physical declines may compromise dynamic posture and proper form in performing many job-related tasks. Postural problems, in turn, may undermine lower body strength, increasing the risk of strain—a concern for many older people (Kovar & LaCroix, 1987). Also, poor work design (e.g., lifting an overload, working on a task at an improper height or without support for one's arms) may cause wear, tear, and fatigue (Kroemer, 1997). Decreased muscle elasticity and flexibility among older persons should also increase susceptibility to tendon or muscle deformations and muscle tears.

Many older workers also complain about sedentary work as well. For example, among working men and women aged 60 to 64, 10% report having difficulty sitting for periods of longer than 2 hours because of muscle stiffness; 6% report being unable to do so (Kovar & LaCroix, 1987). Acute injuries or chronic MSDs are also more serious among older workers because recovery time increases with age. Additionally, older workers are more likely to develop chronic conditions as a result of an acute injury that can seriously impede their ability to either perform job duties or return to them in a timely fashion.

ADAPTIVE STRATEGIES FOR OLDER WORKERS

The good news, however, is that older working adults can often successfully cope with or adapt to age-related declines in health and physical function. They do benefit from employers' accommodative efforts in the areas of accident prevention and rehabilitation and from workplace interventions involving training and job redesign. They also benefit disproportionately from access to higher-quality tools at work (Hansson, Robson, & Limas, 2001). Unfortunately, less than one half of older workers who have experienced a job-threatening health incident are likely to receive special accommodation by employers. It is also an issue that older workers who have been disabled appear to have less access to occupational rehabilitation services. They tend to receive less encouragement from employers to attempt full rehabilitation, and they are less likely than their younger counterparts to ever return to work (Thomas, Browning, & Greenwood, 1994). Such patterns should be a concern among employers and among those involved in the formulation of employment and health policy.

The older worker, however, must also assume an active role in coping with age-related vulnerabilities. There is much evidence, for example, regarding the role of physical exercise and fitness in deferring (and in some instances, reversing) many of the age-related declines just described. A growing body of epidemiologic and intervention studies among older persons has shown that exercise and physical fitness tend to be associated with a slower rate of decline in speed of behavior, in changes of muscle structure and endurance, in bone strength, and joint flexibility. Similarly, physical activity is associated with increased heart volume and output, lower blood pressure, and reduced risk for heart disease. It is a factor in controlling glucose levels and the complications of diabetes. Maintenance of physical fitness and health is central to maintenance of cognitive function and general well-being (Hoyer et al., 1999; Keysor & Jette, 2001; McAuley & Katula, 1999; Spirduso & MacRae, 1990; Vercruyssen, 1997). It is consistent, then, that among occupations such as police officer or firefighter, in which all employees are routinely required to demonstrate a continued level of physical fitness for the job, the usual age disadvantage with respect to accidents and disability is reduced (Landy, 1996).

In addition, many older workers have been in their job or occupation for many years, and will have acquired broad experience and expertise in that job that may help them in finding ways to adapt to or compensate for declines in function. They may also have considerable job seniority and organizational status, which makes it more likely that organizational support resources will be made available to them during any periods of adjustment or rehabilitation (Park, 1994). Of particular interest is that in the process of adapting to a loss in function, many older persons will be able to develop alternate (and unforeseen) functional skills or strategies for dealing with the loss.

It is clear, however, that at some point for each individual, age-related concerns will emerge with respect to diminishing work capacity and increased vulnerability to the consequences of stress, disease, and injuries (including MSDs). At this point, demands to adapt to a stressful or physically difficult job are likely to surpass the limits of the older worker's available coping reserves. The psychologic literature suggests two important themes associated with continued ability to function under such circumstances. These have to do with emotion regulation in later life and strategies for successful aging.

Emotion Regulation

Reactions to pain and loss of function associated with serious injury often involve an emotional component. It is especially interesting, therefore, given the age-related increase in risk for pain, injury, and disability, that reports of psychologic well-being actually increase in later life. This may reflect a dampening of emotional responsiveness on the part of older adults (Lawton, Kleban, Rajagopal, & Dean, 1992). They appear to react to fewer worries, but they are also less likely to report strongly positive emotional experiences (such patterns have been confirmed using physiologic measures). These findings may reflect a growing sense of resignation to the negative consequences of age for health and functioning. They may also reflect the process of emotion regulation (Aldwin, Sutton, Chiara, & Siro, 1996).

Older adults also appear to adopt specific cognitive strategies for the regulation of emotional reactions to stressful life events. They often become more realistic in their coping efforts, setting achievable goals. They may begin to compare themselves with age-peers only and are likely to reappraise the implications of an age-related problem in search of a balance between related costs and gains. Because older workers are also likely to be coping with different kinds of stressors (e.g., chronic pain or health conditions, or age discrimination), they are more likely to appraise the problem as less changeable or controllable. It is consistent, then, that older persons tend to reduce their emphasis on problem-focused coping and adopt an emotion-focused coping style that places greater emphasis on managing their emotional reactions to the inevitable consequences of age-related loss or injury (Aldwin et al., 1996).

Additional cognitive mechanisms may also play an increasing role in emotional reactions in later life. Of particular relevance are the effects of age-related experience, learning, and maturity. For example, older workers are likely to have acquired much experience with stressful life and health events that is useful to them in coping with newly emerging problems. Having faced and coped with similar events in the past, older persons will likely have learned the limits of their potential exposure to negative consequences, the nature of those consequences, and the relative utility of available coping strategies.

Strategies for Successful Aging

We have learned much from those older persons who have aged more successfully than most with respect to health, well-being, and occupational outcomes. Of primary importance is the need in later life to continue to assert control over lifestyle factors that influence functional decline: nutrition, exercise, and continued social and intellectual engagement (Rowe & Kahn, 1997). It is also important that older workers take personal initiative to develop strategies for preventing or deferring deterioration of job skills, find ways to compensate for irreversible loss or disability, and find ways to enhance their functioning and value to their employer, perhaps by developing alternative skills and abilities. They need to manage their own careers, assertively seek training and employer resources designed to accommodate age-related changes, and make career choices carefully and in such a way as to try to turn potential setbacks to their strategic advantage (Sterns & Gray, 1999).

When significant declines are experienced, however, an adaptive response is that of Selective Optimization with Compensation (SOC) (Baltes & Baltes, 1990). The first step in the SOC model recognizes the need for specialization, identifying those most critical skills and areas of performance in one's job and setting priorities (selection). The second step involves focusing increased efforts (e.g., training, practice, rehabilitation) exclusively on those most critical domains of the job (optimization). Finally, it is necessary to find ways to compensate for irreversibly diminished or lost skills or abilities that could impact job performance (compensation). This last step may involve the introduction of orthotic devices, machinery, or computers, but it could also involve redesigning the workplace to redistribute workloads.

Implementation of these adaptive strategies, however, can be constrained by a variety of factors. In the work setting, for example, the ability to become more selective in one's activities and responsibilities may be constrained among older employees who lack organizational status, power, or job discretion (Abraham & Hansson, 1995). Similarly, among older persons with MSDs, some kinds of activities (e.g., personal care or mobility) may be too important for selection to be a coping option. For other activities, it may be less feasible or practical to emphasize optimization efforts (e.g., costly training or rehabilitation programs) or compensatory strategies (e.g., too personal a need to ask others for assistance or too expensive to redesign the physical environment). It is consistent, then, that older persons with MSDs have been found to engage in adaptive behaviors reflecting selection, optimization, and compensation to manage their disability. However, they do so with varying frequency across different domains of life activity, reflecting the kinds of constraints noted previously (Gignac, Cott, & Badley, 2000).

ERGONOMIC ISSUES AND THE OLDER WORKER

Problems associated with auditory and visual acuity, muscle sprains and strains, posture, psychomotor performance, endurance, and general muscle strength become more likely with age (Paneck, 1997). Corporations should then find it useful to be proactive in addressing older employees' ergonomic needs. Fundamental to this effort is some regular form of assessment to identify individual needs for workplace modification. Ergonomic assessment and intervention efforts to improve the person-environment fit for older workers can be highly relevant in several areas.

For example, human factors engineers have proposed guidelines for designing favorable visual and auditory environments in which older persons operate. There are available recommendations regarding enhanced levels of illumination for various home and work environments (Illuminating Engineering Society, 1981a,b), although it appears important to involve the older workers themselves in evaluating the appropriateness of illumination levels to the task demands of a particular environment or to give older workers control over illumination levels. It is especially important as well to control glare through the use of nonreflecting materials on interior surfaces, placement of light fixtures and windows, and so forth. Guidelines also focus on simplifying the visual field, providing contextual, textural, and linear-perspective cues to reduce problems of depth perception and risk of falling, reducing task requirements for frequent changes between near and distant focus, and using change of size or color to set off important visual cues or warning signals (Charness & Bosman, 1990; Kline & Scialfa, 1997).

To enhance the auditory environment for older persons, it is important to minimize distracting background noise. This might be accomplished through the use of sound-absorbing construction materials. Important signals or messages should be designed to enhance clarity, slowing their pace of presentation to increase distinctiveness, increasing volume, and avoiding high frequencies. Performance may also be enhanced by varying pitch, providing concurrent visual signals as a backup for auditory signals, and reducing the number of competing auditory stimuli (Charness & Bosman, 1990; Kline & Scialfa, 1997).

In addition, tools might be redesigned to altered specifications that account for older adults' increased vulnerability to the consequences of repetitive bending or deviating the wrist and the need to place less stress on joints, ligaments, tendons, and muscles (Spirduso & MacRae, 1990). Work stations might be redesigned to accommodate older workers' declining ability to reach switches and controls with ease, use forceful exertions, or to stand or sit over long periods of time. Similarly, moveable workstations that allow some standing and some sitting could help to minimize symptoms associated with poor circulation, arthritis, and general stiffness. Physical work environments could be designed to allow greater use of lifting equipment, more frequent breaks, and collaboration with others on strenuous work tasks. Greater care could be taken to prevent falls. Ensuring that slippery surfaces are well marked, that handrails are provided along inclined walking areas, and that walkways are free of obstacles could be particularly effective steps in reducing falls among older employees. These are simple and cost-effective accommodations for many employers (Perrell et al., 2001).

ISSUES IN ASSESSMENT OF OLDER WORKERS

A variety of issues cloud the assessment of older persons. The experience of illness or disorder tends to change with aging. For example, older persons' health problems are more likely to reflect internal and nonspecific causes and the interactive deterioration of multiple body functions or systems. So health problems may be less attributable to any single cause. Diagnoses can therefore become more complicated, reflecting a need to rule out potentially confounding variables such as cardiac dysfunction, infection, medications, and arthritis. They are also more likely to be chronic in nature, progressive, and more likely to lead to increased physiologic vulnerabilities rather than enhanced protective resistance (Rowe, 1985).

Among older persons, presenting symptoms of a disease or disorder may also be less predictable, and the relationship between a given diagnosis and its functional consequences tends to become more variable. Some older persons will have long since adopted more effective health behaviors and coping strategies. Others may ignore or underreport symptoms because they assume them to be associated with normal aging, or they fear what they may discover if they submit to further testing (Rowe, 1985).

Because the illness experience in later life tends to be more chronic and progressive in nature, and because with age we lose adaptive and restorative capacity, assessments need to go beyond simple diagnosis. Practitioners should also try to estimate ability to function in the work environment to which the client must return. This will, of course, require a more comprehensive assessment of the demands and supports characteristic of such environments, an endeavor that transcends usual practice.

The chronic and progressive nature of health problems in later life also suggests a role for at least minimal psychologic assessments. Chronic pain, physical stress, or diminished functional ability often co-occur with the psychologic experience of stress or with depressive symptoms, both of which can undermine problem solving, adaptive health behavior, and motivation to rehabilitate. Brief screening measures for stress and depressive symptoms are widely available as a complement to physical assessment of older adults (Kane & Kane, 2000).

The assessment of pain, numbness, and diminished physical function associated with MSDs can also become more complex among older persons. Older persons may already be experiencing such symptoms because of arthritis, osteoporosis, cardiovascular conditions, diabetic neuropathy, or old injuries (Parmelee, 1994). Pain is in great part also a subjective experience, and the anatomical and subjective experiences of pain do not always correlate. One can feel pain in the absence of a physical cause, and the sensory experience can vary in both intensity and quality—for example, throbbing, burning, or piercing (Parmelee, 1994). It may reflect actual tissue damage or vary with one's fearful expectations. Thresholds at which we report pain may also reflect changing adaptation levels, functional status of the nervous system, masking effects of other sources of pain, cognitive impairment, or emotional response sets (e.g., fearful anticipation, assumptions that it is just age-related arthritis acting up, or depression). Researchers have made considerable progress in assessing the experience of pain. To date, however, there is little agreement regarding how best to deal with the added complexity of physical and psychologic assessment in an older population (Kane & Kane, 2000; Parmelee, 1994).

CASE STUDY

The case of a 60-year-old professional employee illustrates how a variety of age-related problems can mask the symptoms of MSDs among middle-aged and older employees. This employee works up to 3 hours per day at a computer work station. For several years he had noticed minor stiffness and pain in his right wrist after working on his computer. However, 2 years ago he had also been diagnosed with diabetes. Coincidentally, he had also begun to experience arthritis-related pain and stiffness in the metacarpophalangeal joints of his right hand. It is understandable, then, that the symptoms of what could be an emerging MSD in that hand could be confused with those of diabetes-related neuropathy, poor circulation that can cause numbness, the arthritis, accumulated old injuries, or simply the employee's expectations regarding normal aging. In this case, such confusion resulted in a lengthy delay in self-referral for assessment of numbness along the top of the hand and diminished treatment options. His physician recommended that he take occasional breaks from the computer and that he frequently massage his hand and arm to try to restore some nerve function.

PSYCHOLOGIC ISSUES IN TREATMENT AND MANAGEMENT OF MSDs IN OLDER ADULTS

We have described how a serious loss of function or a disability among older persons is more likely to have nonreversible consequences. In such cases, it may be necessary to establish more flexible goals for treatment or rehabilitation and to focus more on management of symptoms and maintenance of function rather than on recovery (APA Working Group on the Older Adult, 1998). This frustrating circumstance, understandably, is often associated with increased risks for emotional distress (perhaps depression), which can further complicate efforts to manage an MSD or participate in rehabilitation (Kraaij, Arensman, & Spinhoven, 2002). Older workers can experience most of the psychologic problems that occur among younger workers, but here, too, assessment and understanding of symptoms may be more complex. This suggests that any psychologic interventions be coordinated with providers of medical and rehabilitation treatment, pain control, any environmental modifications of the workplace, and so on.

Many existing psychologic interventions appear beneficial, regardless of a worker's age. A goal of Cognitive Behavioral Therapy, for example, might be to help clients to recognize any thoughts of hopelessness or helplessness that may be affecting mood. Discussions with the older MSD client might also focus on expected links between physical distress, functional limitation, and emotional reactions. In this connection, clients may be asked to list all of the obstacles they encounter in the home or work environment to completing routine tasks and to list the times and places when they feel most depressed. Such efforts are often helpful in identifying for discussion interactive patterns of physical pain, loss of function, inconvenience, and onset of psychologic distress.

Providing therapeutic information in an educational format, then, appears useful in helping clients to understand and cope with likely psychologic complications of physical disorder and loss of function. However, intervention protocols may need to be adjusted to compensate for slower learning or problem-solving processes in older employees. Therapy itself should also be conducted in a format that is conducive to the older worker's abilities, conducting therapy in a well-lit room, and ensuring that the older worker has any needed hearing or visual aids. In addition, it may be important to recognize any relevant generational differences with regard to a worker's views or feelings about mental health treatment. Older workers' perceptions of mental health care likely have been shaped by historical experiences in which mental illness was much more stigmatized than today. So embarrassment about receiving mental health services may need to be addressed more frequently among older adults. Older adults may thus require more education with regard to the rationale, structure, and goals of psychologic interventions. Therapies that include an educational aspect as well as clear, definable goals have been shown to be effective in conducting therapy with older adults (APA Working Group on the Older Adult, 1998).

CONCLUSIONS

A number of points from the preceding discussion deserve emphasis. Older workers experiencing an MSD usually do so in the context of greater baseline frailty. They are likely to require more intensive and comprehensive attention and intervention. Yet, assessment and diagnosis are likely to be more difficult in later life, reflecting issues of multiple causation, multiplicity of conditions, increased population heterogeneity with regard to vulnerabilities, and coping resources and styles. Assessment and intervention should also reflect an appreciation of the progressive nature of disease and disorder in later life and an increased interrelatedness between physical, cognitive, and emotional symptoms. On the other hand, many older persons exhibit considerable potential for coping and rehabilitation, and a variety of preventive and therapeutic interventions appear to be effective with older persons, as they are with younger persons. Exploiting such interventions, however, will likely require the collaborative efforts of many disciplines from the fields of medicine, health, psychology, and human engineering, in addition to those of employers.

REFERENCES

Abraham, J. D., & Hansson, R. O. (1995). Successful aging at work: An applied study of selection, optimization, and compensation through impression management. *Journal of Gerontology: Psychological Sciences, 50B*, P94–P103.

Aldwin, C. M., Sutton, K. J., Chiara, G., & Siro III, A. (1996). Age differences in stress, coping, and appraisal: Findings from the normative aging study. *Journal of Gerontology: Psychological Sciences, 51B*, P179–P188.

APA Working Group on the Older Adult. (1998). What practitioners should know about working with older adults. *Professional Psychology, 29*, 413–427.

Baltes, P. B., & Baltes, M. M. (1990). Psychological perspectives on successful aging: The model of selective optimization with compensation. In P. B. Baltes & M. M. Baltes (Eds.),

Successful aging: Perspectives from the behavioral sciences. Cambridge: Cambridge University Press.

Bureau of Labor Statistics (BLS). (2001a). *News, USDL 01-71.*

Bureau of Labor Statistics (BLS). (2001b). *Injuries, illnesses, and fatalities. Case and demographic characteristics for workplace injuries and illnesses involving days away from work—1999. Table R45: Number of nonfatal occupational injuries and illnesses involving days away from work by nature of injury or illness and age of worker, 1999.* Http://stats.bls.gov/iif/oshcd99.htm.

Charness, N., & Bosman, E. A. (1990). Human factors and design for older adults. In J. E. Birren & K. W. Schaie (Eds.), *Handbook of the psychology of aging* (3rd ed.). San Diego: Academic Press.

Fisk, A. D., & Rogers, W. A. (1997). *Handbook of human factors and the older adult.* San Diego: Academic Press.

Fullerton, H. N., & Toossi, M. (2001). Labor force projections to 2010: Steady growth and changing composition. *Monthly Labor Review,* November, 21-38.

Gignac, M. A., Cott, C., & Badley, E. M. (2000). Adaptation to chronic illness and disability and its relationship to perceptions of independence and dependence. *Journal of Gerontology: Psychological Sciences, 55B,* P362-P372.

Hansson, R. O., Robson, S. M., & Limas, M. J. (2001). Stress and coping among older workers. *Work, 17*(3), 247-256.

Hayflick, L. (1994). *How and why we age.* New York: Ballantine Books.

Headley, B. J. (1997). Physiologic risk factors. In M. J. Sanders (Ed.), *Management of cumulative trauma disorders.* Boston: Butterworth-Heinemann.

Hoyer, W. J., Rybash, J. M., & Roodin, P.A. (1999). *Adult development and aging* (4th ed.). Boston: McGraw-Hill.

Illuminating Engineering Society. (1981a). *IES lighting handbook: Application volume.* New York: Waverly.

Illuminating Engineering Society. (1981b). *IES lighting handbook: Reference volume.* New York: Waverly.

Jette, A. M. (1996). Disability trends and transitions. In R. H. Binstock & L. K. George (Eds.), *Handbook of aging and the social sciences* (4th ed.). San Diego: Academic Press.

Kane, R. L., & Kane, R. A. (2000). *Assessing older persons.* Oxford: Oxford University Press.

Kemp, B. (1985). Rehabilitation and the older adult. In J. E. Birren & K. W. Schaie (Eds.), *Handbook of the psychology of aging* (2nd ed.). New York: Van Nostrand Reinhold.

Ketcham, C. J., & Stelmach, G. E. (2001). Age-related declines in motor control. In J. E. Birren & K. W. Schaie (Eds.), *Handbook of psychology of aging* (5th ed.). San Diego: Academic Press.

Keysor, J. J., & Jette, A. M. (2001). Have we oversold the benefit of late-life exercise? *Journal of Gerontology: Medical Sciences, 56A,* M412-M423.

Kline, D. W., & Scialfa, C. T. (1997). Sensory and perceptual functioning: Basic research and human factors implications. In A. D. Fisk & W. A. Rogers (Eds.), *Handbook of human factors and the older adult.* San Diego: Academic Press.

Kovar, M. G., & LaCroix, A. Z. (1987). Aging in the eighties, ability to perform work-related activities. *National Center for Health Statistics Advance Data, 136,* 1-12.

Kraaij, V., Arensman, E., & Spinhoven, P. (2002). Negative life events and depression in elderly persons: A meta-analysis. *Journal of gerontology: Psychological Sciences, 57B,* P87-P94.

Kroemer, K. H. E. (1997). Anthropometry and biomechanics. In A. D. Fisk & W. A. Rogers (Eds.), *Handbook of human factors and the older adult.* San Diego: Academic Press.

Landy, F. J. (1996, March). Mandatory retirement and chronological age in public safety workers. Testimony before the United States Senate Committee on Labor and Human Resources. Washington, DC: American Psychological Association.

Lawton, M. P., Kleban, M. H., Rajagopal, D., & Dean, J. (1992). Dimensions of affective experience in three age groups. *Psychology and Aging, 7*(2), 171-184.

Lichtenberg, P. A., & MacNeill, S. E. (2000). Geriatric issues. In R. G. Frank & T. R. Elliott (Eds.), *Handbook of rehabilitation psychology.* Washington, DC: American Psychological Association.

McAuley, E., & Katula, J. (1999). Physical activity interventions in the elderly: Influence on physical health and psychological function. *Annual Review of Gerontology and Geriatrics, 18,* 111-154.

Morley, J. E. (2000). Diabetes mellitus: A major disease of older persons. *Journal of Gerontology: Medical Sciences, 55A,* M255-M256.

Ochs, A. L., Newberry, J., Lenhardt, M., & Harkins, S. W. (1985). Neural and vestibular aging associated with falls. In J. E. Birren & K. W. Schaie (Eds.), *Handbook of the psychology of aging* (2nd ed.). New York: Van Nostrand Reinhold.

Paneck, P. E. (1997). The older worker. In A. D. Fisk & W. A. Rogers (Eds.), *Handbook of human factors and the older adult.* San Diego: Academic Press.

Park, D. C. (1994). Aging, cognition, and work. *Human Performance, 7,* 181-205.

Parmelee, P. A. (1994). Assessment of pain in the elderly. *Annual review of gerontology and geriatrics, 14,* 281-301.

Perrell, K. L., Nelson, A., Goldman, R. L., Luther, S. L., Prieto-Lewis, N., & Rubenstein, L. Z. (2001). Fall risk assessment measures: An analytic review. *Journal of Gerontology: Biological Sciences, 56A,* M761-M766

Rowe, J. W. (1985). Health care of the elderly. *New England Journal of Medicine, 312*(13), 827-835.

Rowe, J. W., & Kahn, R. L. (1997). Successful aging. *Gerontologist,* 37(4), 433-440.

Simoneau, G. G., & Leibowitz, H. W. (1996). Posture, gait, and falls. In J. E. Birren & K. W. Schaie (Eds.), *Handbook of the psychology of aging* (4th ed.). San Diego: Academic Press.

Spirduso, W. W., & MacRae, P. G. (1990). Performance and aging. In J. E. Birren & K. W. Schaie (Eds.), *Handbook of the psychology of aging* (3rd ed.). San Diego: Academic Press.

Sterns, H. L., & Gray, J. H. (1999). Work, leisure, and retirement. In J. C. Cavanaugh & S. K. Whitbourne (Eds.), *Gerontology: An interdisciplinary perspective.* Oxford: Oxford University Press.

Summer, L. (August, 2000). *Workers and chronic conditions.* Washington, DC: National Academy on an Aging Society.

Thomas, S. A., Browning, C. H., & Greenwood, K. M. (1994). Rehabilitation of older injured workers. *Disability and Rehabilitation, 16*(3), 162–170.

Vercruyssen, M. (1997). Movement control and speed of behavior. In A. D. Fisk & W. A. Rogers (Eds.), *Handbook of human factors and the older adult.* San Diego: Academic Press.

Whitbourne, S. K. (1999). Physical changes. In J. C. Cavanaugh & S. K. Whitbourne (Eds.), *Gerontology: An interdisciplinary perspective.* Oxford: Oxford University Press.

CHAPTER 22

Preventing Work-Related MSDs in Dental Hygienists

Martha J. Sanders
Claudia Michalak-Turcotte

Musculoskeletal disorders (MSDs) have become a significant occupational hazard for the dental hygiene profession (Akesson, Johnsson, Rylander, Moritz, & Skerfving, 1999; MacDonald, Robertson, & Erickson, 1988; Murphy, 1998). Studies indicate that 6.4% to 11% of all dental hygienists are diagnosed with carpal tunnel syndrome (CTS), and up to 56% of all dental hygienists complain of carpal tunnel-like symptoms (Lalumandier & McPhee, 2001; MacDonald et al., 1988; Osborn, Newell, Rudney, & Stoltenberg, 1990). The prevalence of general musculoskeletal pain in dental hygienists is much higher, with studies reporting 63% to 95% for combined low-back, neck, shoulder, arm, and hand pain (Akesson et al., 1999; Atwood & Michalak, 1992; Osborn et al., 1990; Shenkar, Mann, Shevach, Ever-Hadani, & Weiss, 1998). A 5-year prospective study illustrates the breadth of the problem. Ninety-six percent of all dental hygienists developed symptoms in at least one body part over a 5-year period. Ninety-five percent reported physical findings consistent with MSDs, and 57% were diagnosed with an MSD (Akesson et al., 1999). Not surprisingly, research suggests that MSDs represent a significant cause of attrition from the dental hygiene field (Akesson et al., 1999; Lalumandier & McPhee, 2001; Ylippa, Bengt, & Preber, 1999).

Although dental hygienists acknowledge that MSDs interfere with their comfort and quality of work, quality of life also seems to suffer. Dental hygiene professionals report difficulty performing hobbies, household chores, functional activities, and social recreation (Atwood & Michalak, 1992; Shenkar et al., 1998). Overall, 88% of all workers in the 5-year longitudinal study described functional disturbances both at work and at home (Akesson et al., 1999).

Although many dental hygienists are now aware of the risk factors inherent in their profession because of large-scale efforts at addressing this issue in dental hygiene journals (Michalak-Turcotte, 2000; Michalak-Turcotte & Atwood-Sanders, 2000), the majority are not trained to specifically recognize and improve ergonomic hazards. Basic ergonomic information has only recently been introduced into dental hygiene educational curricula. In most programs, this information is limited to client positioning and instrumentation; body mechanics and preventive exercise are rarely addressed (Beach & DeBiase, 1998).

Although health care professionals are well suited to provide prevention services to dental hygienists, they must truly understand the biomechanics and job-related issues of dental hygienists in order to provide services that are effective. This chapter addresses the risk factors inherent in the dental hygiene profession, current research related to these risk factors and specific MSDs common to dental hygiene professionals. It then presents a case study that illustrates recommendations for minimizing the risk of developing an MSD.

PROFESSIONAL BACKGROUND AND ROLES

The profession of dental hygiene was first introduced in the United Stated in 1917, in response to the need for dental auxiliary personnel to deliver preventive oral health care services. Since then, the role of dental hygiene has emerged gradually under the general auspices of dentistry. Most states require dental hygienists to complete a 2-year professional program and pass a national registry examination as well as a clinical examination in order to obtain a license to work. The practice of dental hygiene is overseen by three governing bodies in most states with clearly delineated functions: Dentists provide work guidelines, the American Dental Hygiene Association provides professional standards, and state and federal regulators (e.g., the Occupational Safety and Health Administration) provide mandates regarding occupational health and safety in the workplace.

JOB ANALYSIS

The most common role of a dental hygienist is to provide preventive oral health care. However, dental hygienists may also participate in other roles, such as scheduling clients, maintaining equipment, assisting dentists, and planning treatment within their daily work roles. Dental hygienists work in a variety of traditional and nontraditional settings that influence both the role of the dental hygienist and the biomechanics of the task. The settings have expanded from primarily private offices to wellness clinics, school systems, and insurance offices. Branches of dentistry in which a hygienist may be employed include family practice, school dental care, geriatrics, orthodontics, periodontics (gum and bone), and pediatric dental care (Shenkar et al., 1998; Wilkins, 1994).

Scheduling

Dental hygienists typically treat 8 to 14 patients per 8-hour day, averaging 50 minutes per appointment, although variation exists (Atwood & Michalak, 1992). Pediatric and elementary school dental hygienists provide dental hygiene services within a 30-minute session; periodontal practice hygienists provide services within a 45- to 60-minute session; and family practice hygienists provide services within a 30- to 60-minute session.

Job Tasks in a Typical Treatment Session

A typical dental treatment session proceeds as follows: The dental hygienist first updates the medical history prior to performing dental hygiene services. The hygienist then inspects the extraoral tissues (face and neck regions), intraoral (within the mouth) tissues, bone levels around teeth, gingival (gum) tissues, and the teeth of the client. The dental hygienist then removes the deposits of calculus and stain and smooths the roots of the teeth to deter further calculus deposits from adhering to the teeth. After cleaning the teeth, the dental hygienist may polish the teeth to remove any remaining stains or may simply floss and brush the teeth. Last, the dental hygienist reviews client education and records the treatment session in the medical chart. Radiographs may be exposed and processed at the beginning or middle of an appointment session. The proportion of time spent in each task of the treatment session is estimated at 50% spent in scaling, 10% in probing, 25% in polishing, and 15% in flossing (Bramson, Smith, & Romangnoli, 1998).

Dental Instruments

Hand and mechanically driven instruments are the primary tools dental hygienists use during treatment sessions (Pattison & Pattison, 1992; Shenkar et al., 1998). For examination procedures, dental hygienists most commonly utilize hand instruments called explorers and probes; for tooth cleaning or deposit removal, scalers or curettes are employed. These hand instruments are thin, cylindrical tools with handle diameters ranging from 1/4 inches to 5/8 inches.

The instruments have a sharp, angled tip at one or both ends for examining or removing debris. The instrument ends tend to be mirror images to be used in different areas of the oral cavity. The handle surfaces are usually textured with serrated, longitudinal, knurled, crosscut, or ribbed patterns. Typically, handles are composed of stainless steel ("Karl Shumacher," "Sci-Dent"), chrome-plated brass ("Sci-Dent"), carbon stainless steel (G. Harzell and Son, "Sci-Dent"), or a combination of high carbon and chromium steel alloy (Immunity Steel, Hu-Friedy). Some handle designs include a rubber synthetic applied to the handle to increase the diameter, but there is also an increase in weight. Resin handles are lighter in weight and can tolerate repeated sterilization (American Eagle, Hu-Friedy).

Dental hygienists also use mechanically driven instruments, including slow-speed hand pieces for polishing and ultrasonic scalers for removing calculus and stains. Both ultrasonic scalers and polishing devices use high-vibration frequencies ranging from 25,000 Hz to 30,000 Hz for ultrasonic scalers and from 500 Hz to 600 Hz for polishing instruments (Cherniak, 1998). The ultrasonic scaler has a rapidly vibrating tip that is cooled with water being released. The water bubbles are released from the tip and burst, actually breaking down the hard deposits and disturbing bacteria formation. The dental hygiene profession recommends that practitioners use ultrasonic scalers rather than hand-scaling to remove heavy calculus deposits, since a light grasp and activation stroke is required to operate the ultrasonic scaler. Researchers estimate that dental hygienists may be exposed to high-frequency vibration for up to 50% of their treatment session, depending on their ultrasonic use (Bramson et al., 1998). A gross power grasp is used for pulling cords, suctioning, and grasping the overhead light (Pattison & Pattison, 1992).

Proper Instrumentation Techniques

The primary grasp used for instrumentation is called the "modified pen grasp" (Figure 22-1).

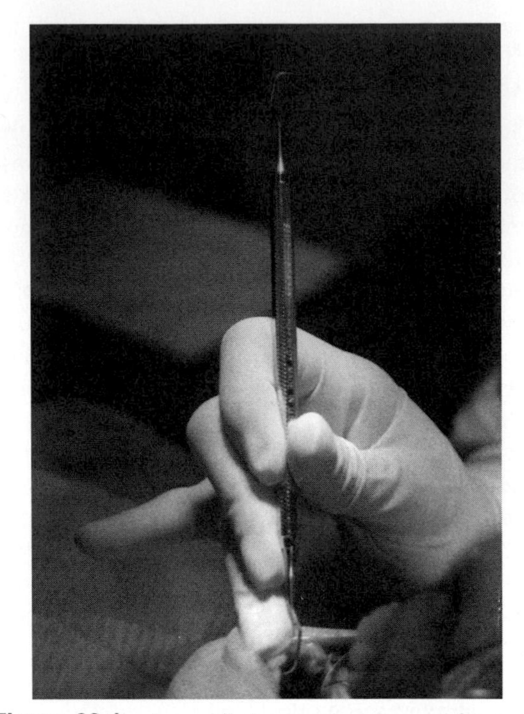

Figure 22-1 A modified pen grasp is used for most dental hygiene instrumentation.

Traditionally, the instrument is held between the thumb and radial aspects of the index and middle fingers, while the fourth finger is positioned in extension on an adjacent tooth or a hard, stable tissue. This fourth finger acts as a fulcrum to stabilize the hand and leverage both hand and forearm forces (Pattison & Pattison, 1992). Hygienists may also use an extraoral fulcrum when working on the maxillary posterior region.

In proper technique, the fingers gently guide the instrument to "sense" the amount of pressure needed while the stronger wrist and forearm motions direct and power each stroke. Instrument procedures should be performed with minimal finger movements and the thumb flexed at both joints. Excessive use of finger motions places high load demands on the small finger musculature and increases repetitive use of flexor tendons (Meador, 1993; Pattison & Pattison, 1992). When properly executed, the wrist constantly moves from 5 degrees of flexion to 35 degrees of extension as the forearm rotates from pronation to supination, as shown in Figure 22-2 (Nunn, 1998).

Dental hygienists are taught to use *indirect vision*, a technique in which a small mirror is used to view teeth that are not in direct line of sight. This practice allows dental hygienists to maintain an upright position during instrumentation rather than flexing their trunks or laterally bending their necks to view teeth (Nunn, 1998; Pattison & Pattison, 1992; Wilkins, 1994).

Posture and Mode of Delivery

In the early years of practice, dentists and dental hygienists worked standing up, with the client seated in an upright position. This position probably contributed to the first reported MSD in dentistry: low-back pain. Over the years, dentistry and dental hygiene have moved to a sit-down delivery system, with the client in a semireclined supine position. Most dental hygienists maintain a static, seated posture for the majority of the treatment session. Back pain is still noted to be a problem for dental professionals in addition to upper-extremity complaints resulting from static loads on the neck and shoulders (Ratzon, Yaros, Mizlik, & Kanner, 2000).

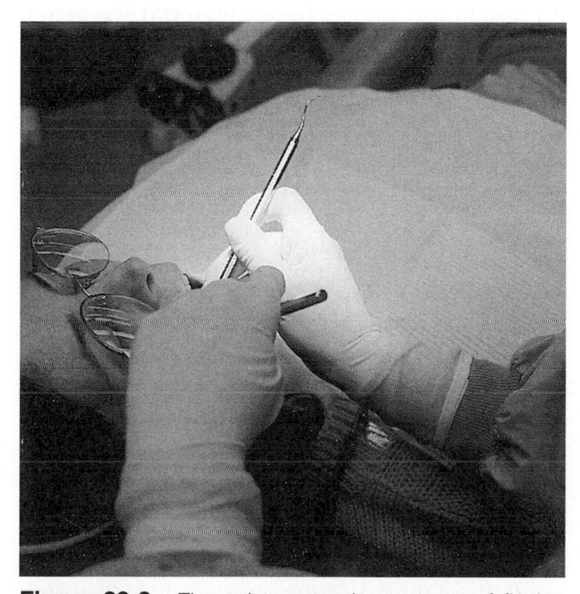

Figure 22-2 The wrist moves in extremes of flexion and extension during root planing and scaling procedures.

Dental hygienists' mode of delivery corresponds to hands on a clock as they orient themselves from the head of the client. With the client's head at 12:00, the right-handed clinician moves from the 7:00 to the 1:00 position around the client. The left-handed clinician moves from the 11:00 to the 5:00 position.

The delivery system (instrument table) is located close by the clinician within arm's reach. It is preferable that the delivery system be moved with the dental hygienist to avoid torso twisting or overreaching (Nunn, 1998; Wilkins, 1994).

The ideal sitting posture for the dental hygienist is assumed by sitting himself or herself correctly in the chair and adjusting the client's chair so that the client's mouth is slightly below the height of the clinician's elbow. The dental hygienist should strive for "neutral position" in which the trunk and neck are erect; the neck flexed to no more than 15 degrees, with no side bending or rotation; the shoulders relaxed at the side (not abducted); the elbows flexed to about 90 degrees; the hips flexed to about 90 degrees or greater with slight abduction and external rotation; and the back supported in lumbar lordosis with the feet flat on the floor (Murphy, 1998).

RISK FACTORS FOR MSDs IN DENTAL HYGIENISTS

The job analysis describes the work of dental hygienists as static, yet precise and exacting, using a firm, repetitive grasp on small-diameter instruments for the majority of tasks. These factors, among others, place dental hygienists at risk for developing some type of MSD when combined with less-than-ergonomic workstations, instruments, and high standards for care. The following discussion highlights specific risk factors in the job tasks just discussed that may predispose dental hygienists to an MSD. The risk factors are organized into work task, work organization, and worker-related factors for ease of discussion notwithstanding that categories overlap (see Chapter 8 for a complete discussion of these categories). Table 22-1 provides an outline of work task–related risk factors.

Work Task Factors

Table 22-1 presents the work task risk factors that are believed to contribute to MSDs in dental hygienists. This category of risk factors refers to performance of the actual job task. These biomechanical risk factors have been related to MSDs in industry and are reviewed here in terms of specific dental hygiene tasks.

Table 22-1

Work Task–Related Risk Factors for Developing an MSD

Risk Factor	Job Task or Movements
Repetition	Instrumentation procedures: wrist flexion, extension, forearm rotation, and finger movements at >30 exertions per minute; writing progress notes, exposing radiographs, cleaning instruments
Force	Firm grasp on instruments during root planing and scaling; firm grasp on ultrasonics, mirror, and writing utensils
Awkward posture	Neck flexion >30 degrees; lumbar and thoracic flexion; shoulders protracted, internally rotated; shoulders flexed or abducted >30 degrees; elbows flexed >90 degrees; wrists flexed or deviated while grasping; thumbs hyperextended at IP joint
Static posture	Similar position maintained for more than 20 minutes
Vibration	Cumulative use of nondampened vibrating instruments (ultrasonic scaler, polishing instrument, slow-speed handpiece)
Contact stresses	Pressure from instrument edges on fingers; tight gloves constrict wrist and fingers
Equipment	Thin-diameter hand-scaling instruments

IP, Interphalangeal joint.

Repetition

High-repetition jobs have been defined as those that involve greater than 30 movements per minute or those involving the same motions for more than 50% of the cycle time (Moore & Garg, 1995; Silverstein, Fine, & Armstrong, 1987). Dental hygienists' instrumentation tasks of scaling and root planing have been measured at 50 to 60 strokes per minute in ergonomic analyses and would therefore considered to be highly repetitive (Bramson et al., 1998; Sanders & Turcotte, 2002). Repetitive use of similar muscle groups is apparent not only during instrumentation but also in the other tasks that dental hygienists perform throughout the day. These tasks include writing the client's progress notes, filing charts, and exposing radiographs (MacDonald, 1987).

Force

Dental hygienists use varying amounts of grip and prehension forces during instrumentation. Although few studies have measured the actual muscle forces generated during instrumentation, Bramson et al. (1998) attempted to measure forearm and grip forces by applying surface EMGs to the bellies of the extrinsic flexor and extensor muscles of the wrist during simulated root planing procedures. In this study, dental hygienists generated from 9.22 to 16.79 pounds of flexor and extensor muscle force in the dominant hand. These forces represented between 15% and 22% of dental hygienists' maximum voluntary contraction (MVC), using the Jamar dynamometer to measure maximum grip strength.

When researchers estimated the prehension forces (considered to be 15% to 20% of the grip forces), the values ranged from 1.34 to 2.8 pounds, representing 12.45% to 16.3% of the MVC. Some pinch forces were measured as high as 20.2% of the MVC (Bramson et al., 1998). Both grip and prehension forces would be considered high, given that forces exerted during tasks should not exceed 8% to 10% MVC in order to sustain work for several hours a day without fatigue.

Overall, dental hygiene studies need to further examine the total accumulation of prehension forces developed during the day. Studies need to more closely examine the clinical variables that affect prehension forces such as the increased forces required to remove heavy calculus, increased muscle tension when working with an anxious client, and the need for more grip force when pulling cords on ultrasonic equipment during use. Finally, prehension forces need to be directly evaluated rather than estimated based on predictive models. When all these factors are accounted for, excess force is considered to be a greater risk factor than repetition in developing an MSD in dental hygienists (Strong & Lennartz, 1992).

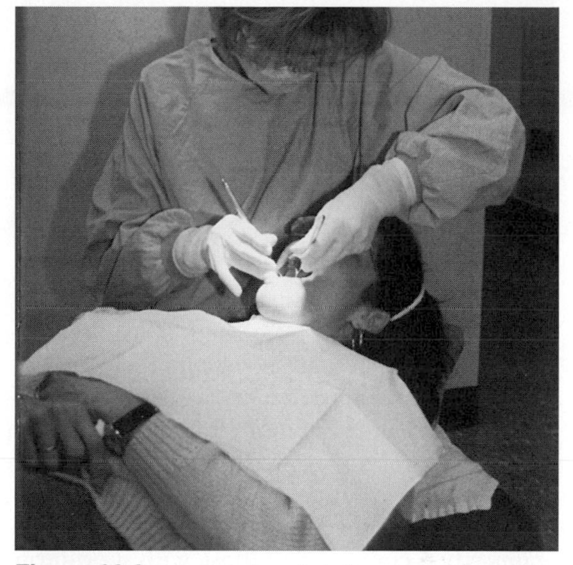

Figure 22-3 Awkward and static neck and shoulder posture contribute to dental hygienists' discomfort at work.

Awkward Postures

Although dental hygienists are taught to work in an upright position with the shoulder at the side (refer to the preceding job analysis), actual observations of dental hygienists typically reveal the following awkward postures: neck flexion greater than 30 degrees, with side bending or rotating to the right or left; shoulder abduction greater than 45 degrees; wrist flexion or extension greater than 30 degrees; and thoracic and low-back flexion (Oberg, 1993; Sanders & Turcotte, 2002) (Figure 22-3).

Research indicates that such postures cause heavy loads and increased intramuscular pressure on the cervical, shoulder, and wrist musculature. Chaffin and Andersson (1984) propose that a posture of 30 degrees of cervical flexion creates a load on cervical muscles equivalent to 13% of one's MVC. Such a load will cause significant muscular fatigue within 4 to 5 hours of work, even with a 10-minute rest break every hour.

Werner, Armstrong, Birkus, and Aylard (1997) verify that the intracarpal canal pressures (ICCP) are greatly increased with the wrist positioned in extreme flexion or extension (>40). These pressures continue to increase when the hand is grasping (increases 200%) or supinating (increases 250%) when extending (see Chapter 10 for a complete discussion). Such wrist postures are common during instrumentation.

Branson, Williams, Bray, McIlnay, and Dickey (2002) have developed the Posture Assessment Instrument (PAI), an instrument that guides the assessment of dental hygienists' posture using a semiquantitative approach.

Static Posture

The awkward postures discussed previously are often maintained as static postures for extended periods of time as dental hygienists stabilize their trunks and shoulders in order to perform precision work with their hands. Oberg et al. (1995) found high static loads and significant localized muscular fatigue in the trapezius muscle of dental hygienists after performing intensive tasks such as scaling. Research has documented that even low-level static loads at 10% to 15% of one's MVC maintained for a long duration create excessive loads on the neck and shoulder musculature that contribute to muscle strain and fatigue over time (Akesson, Hansson, Balough, Moritz, & Skerfving, 1997). This fatigue may be caused by disturbed microcirculation, increased intramuscular pressure, and inefficient removal of lactic acid from the area (Sjogaard, Savard, & Juel, 1988). Oberg (1993) suggests that this static posture is related to acute and chronic neck and shoulder pain in dental hygienists.

Vibration

Several studies have examined dental professionals' changes in sensory perception related to high-frequency vibration exposure. Ekenvall, Nilsson, and Falconer (1990) found that dentists with long-term exposures to vibration had a higher frequency of neurological symptoms and larger vibration threshold differences on vibrograms when compared to those with short-term exposures. Yoshida, Nagata, Mirbod, Iwata, and Inaba (1991) found a positive correlation between the prevalence of numbness and cold sensation in the fingers and the daily usage time of high-frequency machines in dental technicians. Conrad, Conrad, and Osborn (1991) found that 12% of all dental hygienists participating in a study tested positive for mild median nerve dysfunction using digital vibrometry.

Although researchers have continued to find higher percentages of neuropathies and impairments of vibrotactile sensibility in samples of practicing dental hygienists exposed to high-frequency vibration, the mechanism is still unclear (Akesson et al., 1999; Cherniak, 1998; Stentz, Riley, Stanton, Sposato, Stockstill, & Harn, 1994). Researchers still query whether the changes are due to the vibrational frequency or the biomechanical aspects of grasping the instruments. Dental hygiene educators still advocate the ultrasonic scalers to remove calculus and stain deposits rather than using hand instruments that require heavy prehension forces (Wilkins, 1994).

Mechanical Stresses

Contact stresses from instrument edges are potential sources of trauma to the neurovascular bundles lateral to each finger (Johnson, 1990). Instrument handles with longitudinal ridges may cause discomfort over a period of time. Tight gloves and wristwatches that place direct pressure at the wrist may also contribute to symptoms associated with CTS.

Instruments

As discussed in the job analysis, dental hand instruments have very small diameter shafts for grasping and manipulating the tool. Biomechanical models explain that high finger forces are needed to operate instruments with small diameter handles because the extrinsic finger flexors are contracting from an already shortened position. The intrinsic hand musculature must therefore overcompensate for the finger flexor muscles, particularly when the wrist is positioned in flexion. Further, added stress is placed on the first carpometacarpal ligament when using small diameter instruments (Johnson, 1990).

Other aspects of instrumentation that may contribute to higher hand forces are the use of dull or unbalanced instruments. Dull instruments require higher hand forces to remove calculus. Unbalanced instruments (instruments whose center of mass is not in the center of the instrument because of poor manufacturing, dropping, or frequent use) may require increased prehension forces to maintain the position in the hygienist's hand.

Recovery Time

Recovery time greatly influences the ability of the muscle to heal from strenuous exertions or repetitive use. When Oberg, Karzina, Sandsjo, and Kadefors (1995) evaluated the static load and occurrence of muscular fatigue in the trapezius muscle of dental hygienists, recordings from myoelectric signals indicated significant localized fatigue after rigorous instrumentation procedures. The recovery period for this muscle fatigue exceeded 2 hours. When the use of rest pauses was investigated, it was found that hygienists took many short pauses during the day but none for longer than 5 seconds. Complete recovery of muscle fatigue could therefore not occur.

When microbreaks were examined in jobs with less exertion, such as computing, evidence exists that microbreaks had a positive effect in reducing discomfort in the neck, shoulder, wrist, and back when taken at 20-minute intervals (McLean, Tingley, Scott, & Rickards, 2001). Lack of breaks for recovery time even with low loads has also been suggested as a causative factor in work-related muscle pain (Akesson et al., 1999; Chaffin & Andersson, 1984; Oberg et al., 1995).

When all work task risk factors are considered, epidemiologic studies indicate that the overall biomechanical risk factors for neck and shoulder problems in dental hygienists include prolonged static cervical flexion, shoulder flexion or abduction greater than 60 degrees, forceful exertions, lack of upper-extremity support, and inadequate rest breaks (Murphy, 1998; Bernard, 1997; Ylippa et al., 1999). Predictors for developing a disorder of the hand or wrist include awkward wrist posture with repetitive use, extended duration of work, the trunk rotated relative to the upper body during instrumentation, and treatment of clients with heavy calculus.

Workplace Organization Factors

Workplace organization factors refer to how the job is organized toward the ultimate product or service. It involves the organizational structure of the workplace or lines of authority and policies, the job content and productivity demands, degree of worker control, and daily operations, including maintenance schedules, scheduling, and ordering supplies for the workstation setup. Specific aspects of these have been related to the development of MSDs (see Chapter 8).

Job Content

Organizational issues that influence both dental hygienists' satisfaction at work and the development of MSDs have recently been addressed. The size of the dental practice has been related to job content and organizational issues. Swedish dental hygienists who worked in large practices (more than nine hygienists) experienced increased pressures related to business finances, role anxiety (conflicts in work tasks and lack of support from dentists), and increased job demands as compared to those who worked in smaller practices. Dental hygienists in smaller practices reported more opportunity to develop new skills, control their work, and engage in positive relationships among workers. Job content issues identified as predictors of MSDs were dental hygienists' lack of control over job functions, physical exposure from clinical job tasks, lack of work breaks, and anxiety over role competition with dentists (Ylippa et al., 1999). Rolander and Bellner (2001) found a high correlation between the physical demands of work and intensity of pain in the neck and shoulders ($r = 0.73$ and $r = 0.67$, respectively, $p < 0.05$).

Further studies that examine dental hygienists' satisfaction with their jobs find that even though dental hygienists are generally satisfied with their jobs, they cite physical exposures, low salary, no advancement, and little control over job functions as reasons to consider leaving the profession (Ylippa, Bengt, Preber, & Sandelin, 1996). Researchers concluded that decidedly more job control and role clarity were needed to improve dental hygienists' working conditions along with opportunities for professional development and supportive relationships with dentists (Ylippa et al., 1996; Ylippa et al., 1999).

Scheduling

Dental hygienists may or may not schedule clients themselves. Therefore, the number and type of clients that dental hygienists treat on a daily basis may not be within their control. Studies indicate that dental hygienists who treat more than 11 clients per day or work more than 34 hours per week are at higher risk for developing an MSD than those who treat fewer clients or work fewer hours (Atwood & Michalak, 1992; Shenkar et al., 1998). Further, those dental hygienists who treat many clients with heavy calculus consecutively are also more likely to develop an MSD (MacDonald et al., 1988; Shenkar et al., 1998). Clients should be scheduled for an amount of time that is required to complete dental hygiene services while keeping the client comfortable.

Organizational Policies

Dental hygiene practices need to philosophically decide whether to polish their client's teeth after cleaning. *Polishing* refers to buffing the teeth after debridement in order to remove any remaining extrinsic stains from teeth. Polishing is most often completed using a power-driven polisher. Although clients enjoy the feeling of polished teeth and often view polishing as the "reward" at the end of a visit, polishing may be harmful to the client by removing microns of tooth enamel and to the dental hygienist by exposure to vibration. Dental professionals recommend *selective polishing,* which refers to polishing only those areas of the teeth that are stained. Flossing removes any abrasive particles from polishing and any soft deposits remaining between the teeth.

Instrument Maintenance

Sharp instruments require less time, force, and repetition of the dental clinician to remove deposits. Dental hygienists are trained to sharpen instruments as needed; however, studies indicate that most hygienists do not sharpen instruments regularly (Atwood & Michalak, 1992; Strong & Lennartz, 1992). Hygienists should check instrument sharpness prior to use to determine if sharpening is needed.

Workstation Setup

The workstation for a dental hygienist includes the client and operator chairs, the delivery system (instrument tray), and the cleaning and charting area. As a general rule, the dental hygienist should be positioned as close to the client as possible (see Figure 22-3) and move both the chair and the delivery station around the client according to the part of the mouth (as discussed in the job analysis). Frequently, overreaching occurs, which places stress on the low back. The hygienist's chair should be adjustable and have lumbar, thoracic, and arm supports. Electromyography studies indicate that the use of lumbar supports significantly reduces muscle loads on the upper and lower back during dentistry procedures (Hardage, Gildersleeve, & Rugh, 1983). Informal observations indicate that many dental hygienists sit forward on the edge of the chair and therefore do not use the lumbar support available.

Problems arise when the height of the operator's chair (the dental hygienist's chair) does not match that of the client's chair. If the operator's chair is too high, the dental hygienist must increase neck flexion and lumbar flexion to reach the client. Most likely, the feet will not be flat on the floor. If the chair is too low, the dental hygienist must elevate the arms during instrumentation, thereby increasing static loads on the shoulders (Meador, 1993; Pattison & Pattison, 1992).

Environmental Factors

Factors such as lighting, ventilation, and a comfortable temperature are usually adequate in dental offices. However, these factors, along with the social and organizational factors (e.g., the relationship between the dentist and the dental hygienist), incentive plans, and workers' compensation issues should be addressed.

Worker Risk Factors

The impact of personal factors on dental hygienists' work cannot be underestimated. The profession consists primarily of women, whose profession demands perfection and who may be balancing several roles outside of work. Health care practitioners treating dental hygienists need to understand their clients' job-home stress and other role obligations. Health care practitioners need to examine a client's entire day with the understanding that hobbies or chores that involve a repetitive or static grasp (e.g., gardening, quilting, latch hook, carpentry, or constantly picking up a child) may also contribute to MSD symptoms (see Chapters 19 and 20 for further discussion). Further, client anxiety may have an impact on a dental hygienist's anxiety because the hygienist tenses his or her muscles in efforts to avoid inflicting pain on the client.

Hygienist Size

The hygienist's physical size may be an issue for those who are appreciably larger or smaller than population norms. The adjustable range on chairs must be specifically addressed. Instruments and gloves may be ordered to accommodate the appropriate hand size.

Work Style

Work style refers to the individual variation in dental hygienists' instrumentation performance. Current research suggests that the manner in which individuals perform their jobs may increase the susceptibility to MSDs by creating higher intensity of exertions, muscle tension, and fewer rest breaks than the job demands. Balogh, Hansson, Ohlsson, Stromberg, and Skerving (1999) found great individual variation in the EMG results and muscular load of the shoulder among workers performing the same task. Feurerstein (1996) suggests that employees who work despite the pain, employees who report the need to achieve, and those who perform perfectly at work every day may be predisposed to developing an MSD when exposed to other ergonomic factors.

MUSCULOSKELETAL DISORDERS COMMON TO DENTAL HYGIENISTS

Prior to 1985 low-back pain was the most commonly reported source of musculoskeletal pain in dental hygienists. In the late 1980s CTS emerged as the greatest musculoskeletal concern once results of a large-scale survey indicated that 6% of all dental hygienists in California had been diagnosed as having CTS and 32% demonstrated one or more symptoms associated with CTS (McDonald et al., 1988).

A later Minnesota study expanded investigations to document the overall musculoskeletal pain in dental hygienists. Osborn et al. (1990) found that 63% had experienced back, neck, shoulder, or arm pain in the previous year. A Connecticut study found even greater prevalence of musculoskeletal pain, with 8% of the sample diagnosed with CTS and an overwhelming 93% of the sample experiencing some type of musculoskeletal pain (Atwood & Michalak, 1992). Most recently, a 5-year prospective study showed that 95% of the sample reported physical findings consistent with MSDs, 57% were diagnosed with a MSD, and 96% of all dental hygienists in the study developed symptoms in at least one body part over a 5-year period (Akesson et al., 1999).

Although wrist and hand pain was assumed to be the most common site of pain, the shoulder and neck (71%) are documented as the most common site for musculoskeletal pain, followed by the low back (56%), hand and wrist (65%), and forearm and elbow (27%) (Atwood & Michalak, 1992). Internationally, these results compare with researchers from Sweden, who report similar frequencies of shoulder and neck pain (82%), wrist pain (46%), and elbow pain (18%) (Akesson et al., 1999).

Even though CTS may be the most costly and feared condition of dental hygienists, neck and shoulder pain may interfere equally if not more so with dental hygienists' quality of work, job satisfaction, and energy level (Atwood & Michalak, 1992). Health care practitioners must be vigilant in examining the entire upper extremity for clinical symptoms and muscle tenderness, since research indicates that neck and shoulder pain may be related directly to a diagnosis of CTS. Table 22-2 outlines the common musculoskeletal conditions found in dental

Table 22-2
Common MSDs of the Upper Extremity in Dental Hygienists

Body Part	Musculoskeletal Problem	Contributing Factors	Recommendation
Neck	Tension neck syndrome	Neck flexion posture	Decrease neck flexion
	Trapezius myalgia		Wear magnifying glasses
	Thoracic outlet syndrome	Client positioned too low	Reposition client's chair higher
		Frequent reaching backward	Position instruments close by
Shoulder	Supraspinatus tendinitis	Abducting shoulders >30 degrees	Reposition client's chair lower
	Bicipital tendinitis		Keep shoulders at side
	Scapular myalgias	Static abducted position	Stretch shoulder girdle frequently
			Take longer breaks after intense scaling
Elbow	Lateral epicondylitis	Static or forceful grasp on instruments	Use light grasp on instruments
	Radial tunnel syndrome		Stretch wrist extensor muscle groups regularly
	Pronator teres syndrome	Repetitive forearm rotation	
	Cubital tunnel	Excess elbow flexion	Position elbow in less than 90 degrees
Wrist	Carpal tunnel syndrome	Extremes of wrist flexion and extension	Minimize extremes of motion
	Wrist tendinitis		
		Forceful and repetitive use of instruments	Minimize force on instruments
			Take stretch breaks
		Pressure on carpal canal	Use ergonomic instruments
			Avoid constriction at wrist
Finger	deQuervain's disease	Frequent thumb abduction	Minimize finger movements during instrumentation
	Finger flexor tenosynovitis	Repetitive finger flexion	
	Heberden's nodules	Overuse of joints	Allow for soft tissue recovery

hygienists along with the contributing biomechanical sources of the problem.

Neck

Tension neck syndrome along with trapezius myalgia, levator scapula myalgia, and thoracic outlet syndrome have been documented as frequent problems (Akesson et al., 1999). This is not surprising, since dental hygienists frequently assume a static forward head posture that causes tightness and spasms of the upper trapezius and scalene muscles (see Figure 22-3). Researchers suggest that neck symptoms relate to the degree of neck flexion assumed during work. Thoracic outlet syndrome may be related to tight neck muscles combined with frequently reaching backward to procure instruments. Neck pain has been associated with static neck flexion of over 20 degrees or static muscle work that exceeds 5% to 6% of the MVC (Luopajärvi, 1990).

Shoulder

Shoulder pain is not uncommon in dental hygienists. In a typical posture, the shoulders are elevated, protracted, and internally rotated while working (see Figure 22-3). Over a prolonged period, this posture may contribute to shortened pectoral muscles and the potential for developing supraspinatus tendinitis or bicipital tendinitis. This potential is exacerbated by high static loads when the shoulders are abducted or flexed more than 30 degrees (Palermud, Forsman, Sporrong, Herberts, & Kadefors, 2000). In a recent 5-year study, dental personnel demonstrated a significantly higher number of shoulder symptoms in the last 12 months as compared to a referent group (Akesson et al., 1999).

Elbow and Forearm

Pain at the elbow arises from repetitive forearm rotation, particularly when combined with static

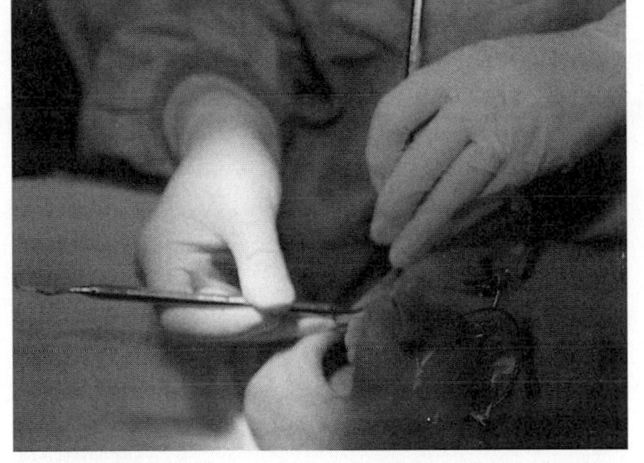

Figure 22-4 Elbow pain may develop from isometric contractions of the extensor musculature while grasping the instrument.

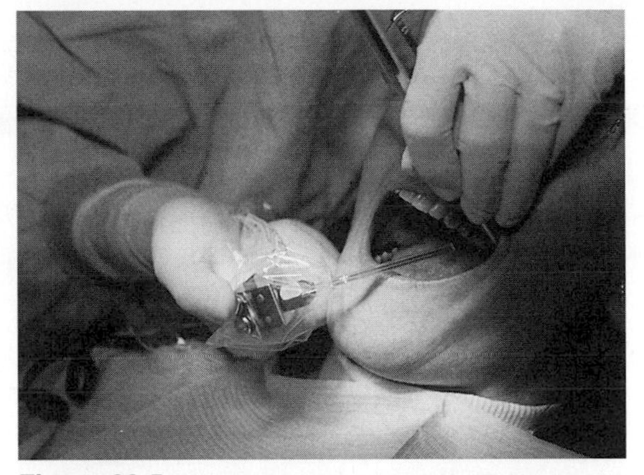

Figure 22-5 Tasks such as spraying or irrigating the mouth also demand a static forceful grasp.

grasping, wrist deviation, and excessive elbow flexion (Figure 22-4). Dental hygienists may develop lateral epicondylitis because the wrist extensor musculature statically contracts during instrumentation and writing. The condition is aggravated by forceful manual periodontal debridement with forearm supination or pronation. Health care practitioners should rule out radial tunnel syndrome for lateral epicondylitis (see Chapters 5 and 6 for further discussion). Nerve entrapment syndromes, such as cubital tunnel syndrome, or pronator teres syndrome, may occur in hygienists who work with the elbow flexed more than 90 degrees or who rotate the forearm repetitively.

Wrist and Fingers

Tasks such as irrigating or spraying the mouth with water, processing radiographs, and writing progress notes in addition to instrumentation contribute to wrist and finger conditions (Figure 22-5). CTS is the most recognized of all MSDs that affect dental hygienists, although not necessarily the most prevalent. In a recent prospective study, 46% of all dental hygienists complained of pain in the hands and wrists, and 50% noted symptoms over the last 7 days (64% over the last year). Although 62% noted findings consistent with an MSD, only 5% were diagnosed with an MSD of the hand or wrist (Akkeson et al., 1999).

CTS may develop from compression of the median nerve during extremes of wrist flexion or extension or from pressure placed on the median nerve when finger or thumb flexor tendons become inflamed. Conditions such as tenosynovitis often are misdiagnosed as CTS because of the common complaint of pain. Finger flexor tenosynovitis should be ruled out for CTS.

Heberden's nodules and a positive selective muscle flexor digitorum superficialis test (which is related to the diagnosis of pronator teres syndrome) have also been documented in dental hygienists (Akesson et al., 1999). Ganglion cysts, trigger fingers, and cubital tunnel syndrome are other less common conditions that may develop from overuse of the finger flexor tendons and pressure placed on the ulnar side of the hand.

Thumb

Thumb pain is a common complaint that has yet to be fully analyzed. Dental hygienists who use excessive thumb extension, abduction, and radial-ulnar deviation of the wrist may be sus-

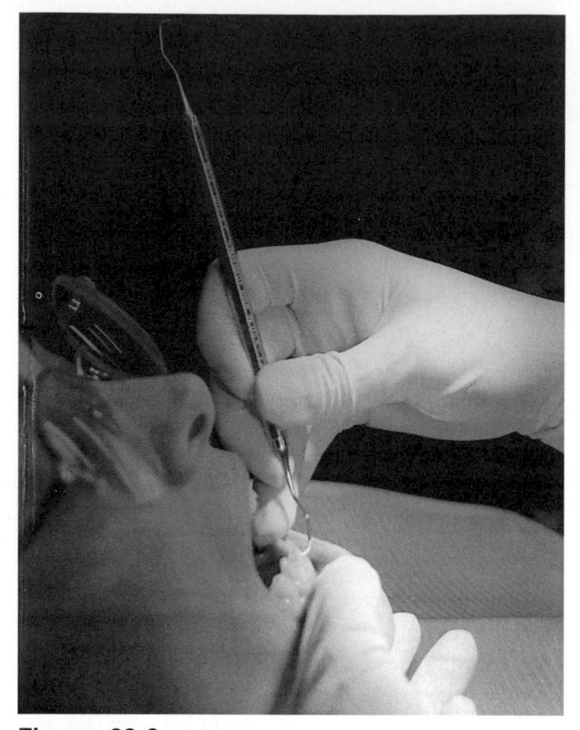

Figure 22-6 Hyperextension of the thumb interphalangeal joint places excess pressure on the collateral ligaments of the thumb metacarpal joint.

ceptible to deQuervain's disease. Many dental hygienists also hyperextend their thumb metacarpophalangeal (MP) or interphalangeal (IP) joints during instrumentation, thereby placing increased stresses on thumb musculature (Figure 22-6). Dental hygienists who hyperextend the MP joint and simultaneously hyperflex the IP joint require excessive use of the flexor pollicis longus. Overuse of the thumb flexor muscles may cause a trigger finger. Dental hygienists who hyperflex the MP joint of the thumb and extend the IP joint place additional stresses on the collateral ligaments, particularly the radial collateral ligament of the thumb.

RECOMMENDATIONS TO REDUCE THE RISK OF DEVELOPING AN MSD

Recommendations to reduce the risk of developing an MSD are listed in Table 22-3. Although these strategies are based on sound theory and current research, no outcome studies have yet documented the effectiveness of the strategies on the overall prevention of MSDs in dental hygienists. The recommendations are organized to reflect the current strategy that OSHA uses to control risks: engineering controls (relating to the design of the task), administrative controls (relating to the work organization), work practice controls (relating to a worker's protection of himself or herself at work) and worker controls (lifestyle changes a worker can make) (see Chapter 14 for a complete discussion of the controls).

Engineering Controls

Engineering controls address changes in design of the equipment so that everyone who uses the equipment benefits. This discussion briefly highlights ergonomic design for dental equipment. Ergonomic instruments have been available for over a decade. Dental hygiene schools have only recently begun to train dental hygienists with ergonomic instruments so that they will be inclined to routinely order such equipment as clinicians. Although the designs of ergonomic instruments are based on material properties and biomechanics of the hand, no studies have proven that ergonomic handles prevent injuries or minimize fatigue. Comfort appears to be the subjective seller for the instruments thus far. The issue for many smaller dental clinics is one of costs and benefits. If the benefits are not proven, the costs of ergonomic equipment must be reasonable.

The ergonomic design of operator chairs is also continually being modified and improved. Whereas lumbar supports were initially introduced into chair designs, arm supports have been found to minimize fatigue to the upper trapezius of some dental hygienists. Operator chairs are now available with arm supports, trunk support bars, and adjustable lumbar pads to support the dental hygienist as he or she moves. Finally, adjustable and moveable delivery systems are increasingly important as several dental hygienists may now be using the same workstation. Moveable delivery stations can be

Table 22-3
Recommendations to Decrease the Risks of Developing an MSD

Controls	Recommendations
Engineering	**Use ergonomic instruments and equipment**
	Larger-diameter, hollow handles, balanced, lightweight
	Silicone-coated handles or waffle-iron serrations
	Dampen vibration components of mechanical instruments
	Use straight cord handpieces with swivels
	Purchase sized gloves for the right or left hand
	Choose an adjustable operator chair with arm supports, lumbar support, and trunk bar
Administrative	**Scheduling**
	Allot adequate time for each client
	Alternate scheduling for clients with heavy and light calculus
	Schedule no more than 10 clients in one full day
	Policies and procedures
	Take periodic breaks throughout the day with a longer break at lunch
	Recall clients according to individual health needs
	Perform selective polishing
	Training
	Gradually increase work tolerance from part-time to full-time
	Train dental hygienists in new instrumentation techniques
	Provide opportunities for professional development
	Maintenance
	Sharpen instruments regularly
	Maintain equipment
	Workstation setup
	Organize workstation to minimize reach distances
	Use moveable delivery systems
	Authority relationships
	Clarify roles of dentist, dental hygienist, and dental assistant
	Discuss productivity standards
Work practice	**Use proper instrumentation techniques**
	Avoid thumb hyperextension
	Keep wrist in neutral during forearm rotation
	Minimize extreme wrist motions
	Use indirect vision
	Use ultrasonic scaler and slimlines to remove heavy calculus
	Alternate work positions and move delivery systems as needed
	Maintain upright posture when possible
	Stretch between procedures and between clients
	Use peer and self-monitoring: videotaping
Worker	**Work style**
	Use least amount of force necessary
	Try not to tense other parts of body during instrumentation
	Monitor work-related stress

adjusted to right- or left-handed practitioners of varying heights.

Administrative Controls

Administrative controls attempt to minimize exposure to risk factors according to how the job may be organized. Policies on scheduling, recalling clients, and selective polishing are an area that may impact exposures to high hand forces throughout the day. Increasingly, dental hygienists have the independence to determine the amount of time needed for clients. Traditionally, clients were recalled every 6 months for a 1-hour examination and cleaning, regardless of whether the client developed heavy calculus more rapidly. Today, more and more dental hygienists schedule clients for visits according to their particular oral health needs. This practice helps to prevent periodontal disease and minimize the forces needed for dental hygienists to remove calculus. Unfortunately, insurance companies typically pay for only two preventive visits per year, regardless of whether the client needs more frequent visits to prevent problems. Dental hygienists therefore have the burden of convincing high-risk clients to visit more frequently even if insurers won't pay for the treatments. The policy of *selective polishing,* as discussed earlier, is a beneficial control for both client and hygienist. However, implementation requires educating the client as to the benefits of polishing selectively and replacing that procedure with brushing or flossing.

Training dental hygienists in proper ergonomic instrumentation and workstation setup is valuable for both the present and the future. New techniques in instrumentation can minimize the stressors to the hand (e.g., changing extraoral fulcrums). Many options exist in educating clients with computerized programs to allow time for the dental hygienist to stretch or take microbreaks.

Work Practice Controls

Although ergonomic evaluations provide suggestions for optimal workstation setups, the responsibility for maintaining an optimal posture lies with the dental hygienist. The task of improving posture can be especially daunting for those who have worked in awkward postures for many years. In such cases peers can offer powerful support in reminding each other of the correct methods.

Stretching activities are designed to interrupt the static positions and promote blood flow in body areas used. Stretches can be performed at lunch, integrated into setup routines (such as reaching for supplies and files), or can be performed while a client is watching a client-education video. Stretches are demonstrated and reviewed in Figures 22-7 to 22-9. Additional stretches recommended are wrist flexion with the elbow extended, wrist rotation, and thumb extension. We recommend performing these stretches after every client (at least one time per hour), holding the stretches for at least 7 seconds, and integrating the stretches into the office routine. For example, dental hygienists can stretch the fingers between placing and retrieving instruments (Figure 22-10).

The following case study illustrates ergonomic recommendations for the dental hygienist with proximal musculoskeletal discomfort.

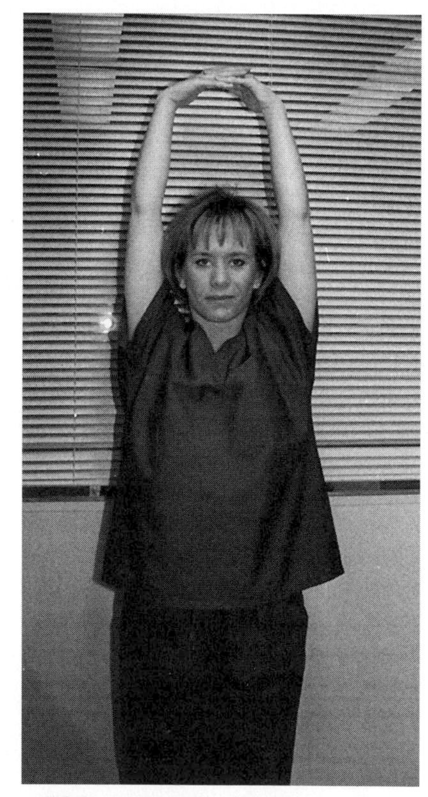

Figure 22-7 Extending the arms overhead stretches the shoulder and elbow musculature while reinforcing good posture.

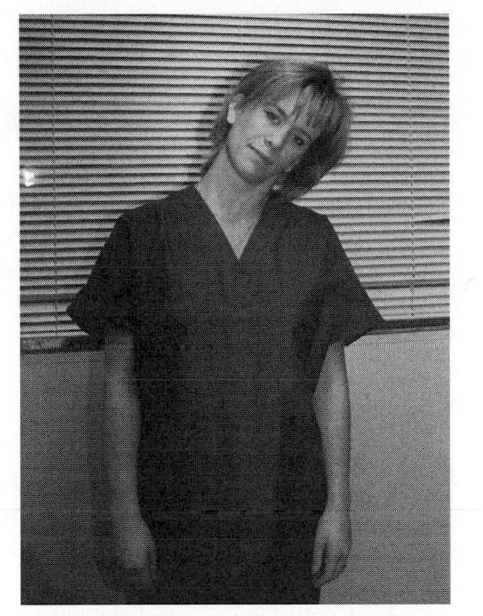

Figure 22-8 Gentle neck circles stretch trapezius, scalene, and sternocleidomastoid muscles.

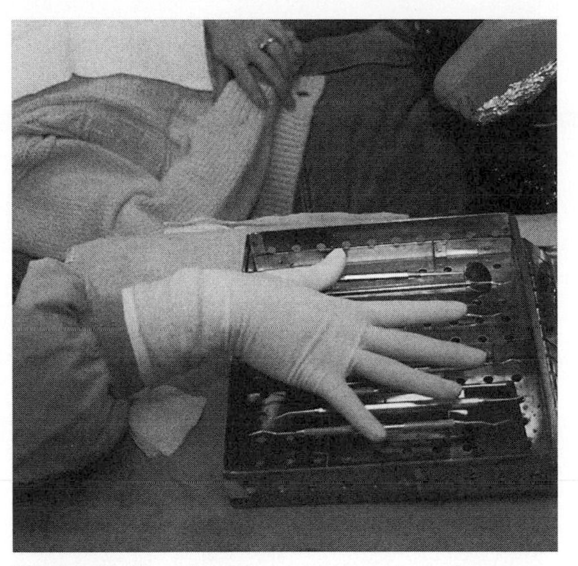

Figure 22-10 Extending the fingers during instrument retrieval helps relieve tight thumb and finger flexor musculature.

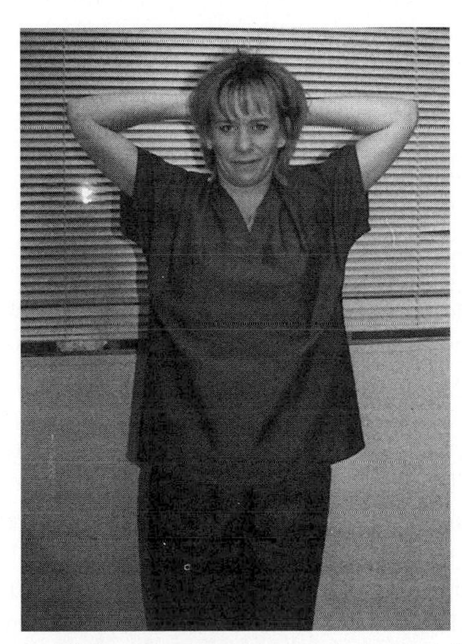

Figure 22-9 Clasping the hands behind the neck gently stretches pectoral muscles.

CASE STUDY

Deidre is a 35-year-old female who has worked as a private practice dental hygienist for 12 years. In November of last year, Deidre noted increased discomfort in her left scapula, low back, and neck that appeared to coincide with recent changes in the setup of her work environment. Deidre has had recurrent back problems and pain in her upper thoracic and cervical spines since her L5S1 laminectomy at age 19. An ergonomic job hazard analysis and body map were performed on Deidre, with the goal of enhancing her comfort and productivity at work.

Ergonomic Job Analysis

Deidre is a single mother of an 8-year-old boy. She works 3½ days per week in a family practice for 6 to 9 hours per day. Deidre provides dental hygiene services to an average of 13 clients per 9-hour day for 30 to 60 minutes per client, depending on the procedures. She is paid on commission, which is a percentage of client charges that she renders. Therefore, her motivation to provide dental hygiene services to as many clients per day as possible is high. Most clients that Deidre treats show significant amounts of calculus and periodontal (bone loss) disease. Deidre begins her day with a short staff meeting and works continuously through the day, taking breaks only between procedures or when clients are late for an appointment.

Work Tasks: Instrumentation

Deidre is right-handed and uses ⅜-inch handled instruments with a cross-cut pattern on the handle. She performs hand scaling for lighter calculus removal and states she uses the ultrasonic scaler to remove heavy calculus. She applies significant hand forces during instrumentation (estimated at 10% to 30% of her maximum strength) but does not appear to tense other parts of the body. She performs similar hand and finger movements for greater than 50% of her work cycles and performs 50 to 60 exertions or hand motions per minute within a typical scaling session. She wears one-sized latex gloves, designed with the thumbs in extension (rather than abduction) and a tight band at the wrist.

Postures

Deidre works in a seated position for most of her day. Her low back assumes a kyphotic posture and she uses no lumbar support. She moves from the 9:00 position to the 12:00 position during the treatment session. Her neck and trunk are sidebent to the right (to view the mouth), and her neck is flexed to at least 30 degrees and rotated to the left. Her left shoulder is abducted to 70 degrees to retract (hold) the mirror. Deidre's right arm is adducted, and her elbows are flexed to 100 degrees. Her forearms move from midposition to full pronation during instrumentation; the right wrist moves from 15 degrees flexion to 35 degrees extension with the fingers statically flexed on the instrument and thumb hyperflexed at the MP joint and hyperextended at the IP joint. The left fingers statically grasp the smooth handle of the mirror.

Workplace Organization

Deidre works in a well-lit office with a stationary but adjustable client chair in the middle of the room and ample space around the client. The delivery system is stationary and nonadjustable, placed behind and to the right of Deidre. Deidre enjoys her work schedule because it allows free time during the week. However, after several 9-hour days, the pain intensity in her left scapula increases.

Worker

Deidre adores gardening but confides that it aggravates her neck and back pain. She used to regularly perform T'ai Chi for relaxation and back pain control but has not participated lately. She has a supportive boyfriend who is interested in fitness and who has introduced her to the gym for strengthening and stretching.

Body Map

The body map revealed areas of pain in the left scapula (rhomboids) (3/5), bilateral low back (2/5), and occasionally the neck (2/5). Palpation of the left scapula revealed multiple chronic active trigger points. She stated that the pain traveled toward her neck periodically. Overall, the pain level was 2 at the lowest and 4 at the highest on a scale of 5.

Summary

Results of the ergonomic job analysis and body map reveal the primary risk factors related to Deidre's symptoms to be awkward and static postures in the neck and shoulder. Specific postures that appear directly related to her scapular trigger points and neck and low-back pain are neck flexion and sidebending to the right, neck rotation to the left, trunk bending to the right, prolonged left shoulder abduction, scapular protraction, and unsupported sitting. These positions result from assuming the same position relative to the client for the entire treatment session. A poor workstation setup causes her to frequently twist her body backward to the right to procure instruments and reach forward to position the overhead light. The operator chair is too high, causing her to lean forward during instrumentation; the operator chair is not adjusted to provide lumbar support.

Her schedule of four consecutive 6- to 9-hour days, with no scheduled breaks, also leaves little time for muscle recovery. Although she has control over her work schedule, she does not schedule her clients according to calculus levels or intensity of service needed. Finally, her personal risk factors include little involvement in a regular exercise and stretching program and a hobby that contributes to her discomfort.

Although Deidre does not have distal soft tissue symptoms, she uses small diameter instruments that create the potential for increased finger forces. Her work demands high prehension forces and repetition during instrumentation with mechanical stresses placed on the fingers.

Recommendations

Recommendations focus on decreasing Deidre's neck, shoulder, and back discomfort at work and minimizing her risk of developing further problems. Recommendations are summarized in Table 22-4.

Work Task–Related Concerns

Awkward postures were addressed through examining Deidre's positioning around the client during the treatment session and educating her as to the importance of striving for a "neutral" position when working. Because Deidre sits in the same position for the majority of the treatment, she assumes awkward trunk and shoulder postures in order to access posterior portions of the mouth. Such extreme positions may be avoided by positioning herself as close as possible to the client and moving herself to different positions around the client to better access specific locations.

The use of magnifying glasses further minimizes neck flexion and thus facilitates a neutral posture. Even though the ideal distance between the client and the hygienist is 14 to 16 inches, many hygienists work much closer to the client for better visibility. A variety of magnifying lenses are available, including those that are stationary, mounted on a headband, or those similar to reading glasses. As with any vision product, issues such as degree of magnification required, depth of field, convergence angle, and working distance must be properly assessed and individually prescribed. Magnifying glasses are routinely used by dentists and are slowly gaining popularity with hygienists.

Prolonged static posturing can be effectively addressed by stretching the neck, shoulder, low back, and upper extremity regularly throughout the day. Deidre was given a series of stretches to perform between clients. Deidre should obtain arm supports to minimize the static loading on shoulders while working with her hands or utilize a trunk support bar. These supports are attached to the sides of the operator chair so that a hygienist may rest his or her forearm while using the hand, thus decreasing the load on the shoulders.

Instrumentation can be improved to prevent further problems caused by her job. Deidre was encouraged to continue use of the ultrasonic scaler, use the least amount of force necessary to remove calculus, and instruct clients in techniques to minimize calculus buildup. It was suggested that she order larger-diameter ergonomic instruments with at least $^5/_8$-inch diameter and a hollow shaft to minimize the loads to her fingers. Finally, she was encouraged to learn updated instrumentation techniques to vary her use of hand musculature.

Workplace-Related Concerns

Work organization issues such as Deidre's work schedule, break times, and client scheduling need to be addressed. Deidre should consider changing her schedule to Monday, Wednesday, Friday, and alternate Saturdays in order to allow for soft tissue recovery time between days and between clients. Further, since Deidre does have control over her scheduling, she should schedule clients according to intensity of treatment, alternating between difficult and less difficult

Table 22-4
Risk Factors, Description of Related Activity, and Recommendations for Case Study

Risk Factor	Description	Recommendation
Work Task–Related		
Awkward posture	Neck and thoracic flexion >30 degrees	Increase height of client chair Use magnifying lens
	Neck sidebending to the right and rotation to the left	Turn client's head toward hygienist to view mouth
	Shoulder abduction >70 degrees Unsupported sitting	Lower left arm by repositioning self around client
	Dynamic reaching behind and in front	Move delivery system closer to avoid twisting
	Thumb MP hyperextension	Flex MP and IP joints of thumbs
Static posture	Maintains same posture for >20 minutes: neck and thoracic flexion, scapular abduction	Stretch neck, shoulders, back between clients Use arm supports on chair to minimize static loading on shoulders
	Finger flexion on instruments	Take breaks to allow for recovery Stretch hands and arms between tasks
High repetition	Repetitive wrist flexion and extension and forearm rotation during instrumentation and writing	Take breaks in morning and afternoon
High force (effort)	Firm grasp on instruments during scaling of heavier deposits	Use ultrasonic scaler to remove gross calculus Sharpen instruments after each client Alternate heavy- and light-calculus clients Educate client as to preventive measures
Extended duration of exertion with limited recovery time	Greater than 50% of time spent in tasks requiring hand-intensive exertions	Educate clients about flossing, tartar control, brushing techniques to decrease buildup of tartar Schedule frequent appointments to avoid long sessions Take breaks to allow for recovery
Mechanical stresses	Edges of instruments press on digital neurovascular structures	Select round instrument handles with rubber coating or cross-cut patterns
	Tight gloves constrict wrist and thumb	Wear sized gloves that roll past wrist
Instruments	Small-diameter instruments	Use largest and lightest handles possible
	Dull instruments	Sharpen instruments regularly Learn updated techniques for fulcrum use
Workplace-Related		
Workstation setup	Operator chair too high	Adjust chair so that elbows are at client's mouth height
	No lumbar support on chair	Use chair with adjustable lumbar support
	Nonchanging delivery system	Move delivery system as needed
	Hygienist works in stationary position	Gain better access to client by moving around client
Work organization	Three 9-hour days with no break	Working more days with fewer hours per day
	Scheduling clients with heavy calculus consecutively	Alternate between heavy- and light-calculus clients
Worker-Related		
Life style	No involvement in exercise or stretching	Begin a stretching and strengthening program
Hobby	Hobby that contributes to neck and low-back pain	Return to T'ai Chi Gain assistance with stressful gardening chores; pace duration of gardening

IP, Interphalangeal; *MP*, metacarpophalangeal.

clients throughout the day. Finally, Deidre should schedule a 1-hour lunch break and take mini "pause" breaks whenever possible. She should try to allow slightly longer breaks. In terms of *workstation set-up,* Deidre needs to adjust the height of the clinician's chair so that her elbows are level with the client's mouth. Deidre should also establish the practice of moving the delivery system (instrument tray) around the client as she changes position. This practice will eliminate her frequent twisting of the body. Finally, she needs to use the lumbar support of her chair by positioning herself farther back on the seat and adjusting the lumbar support along with arm supports.

Worker-Related Concerns

Personal factors to improve Deidre's comfort were to begin a stretching and strengthening program at home once she has received treatment for her trigger points. Scapular and back strengthening exercises were provided in conjunction with therapy. She was encouraged to return to T'ai Chi for movement and postural control.

Follow-Up

One week later, Deidre was revisited at her workplace to observe and problem-solve any difficulties in implementing ergonomic changes. She had begun stretching between clients, changing positions during instrumentation, and adjusting her workstation heights. These changes had improved her posture significantly. Notably, she was using less apparent effort to remove calculus deposits, and her wrist posture had improved from positions of 15- to 30-degree ranges of motion to 0- to 15-degree ranges of motion. She had less fatigue at the end of the day and indicated that her left scapular pain had decreased considerably. The body map revealed changes in the left scapular area from a 3/5 to 1/5. Deidre's dedication to prevention was worth her efforts.

Two and one-half years later Deidre was again contacted to determine her musculoskeletal status and the extent of her ergonomic changes. She had implemented a number of further ergonomic design changes. Her office had purchased two ergonomic dental chairs with arm supports, a trunk support bar, and an adjustable lumbar pad that supported her as she moved. Deidre felt this "made all the difference in the world" as she had no low back pain now and much less shoulder and neck pain.

Deidre was now the dental hygiene supervisor and had hired an assistant who assumed the client-education duties. This gave her time to regularly perform her stretches between clients. Further, the office implemented an informal peer posture checkout. When hygienists viewed each other working in awkward positions they brought it to each other's attention. Deidre had the tendency to elevate her shoulders during work and was reminded by her peers to "lower" her shoulders. Finally, she had begun walking at home, had continued with therapy and strengthening exercises and was delegating heavy gardening chores to others. The pain scale revealed that her pain was 0 most of the time, but sometimes went up to 2 when she was under stress. She stated that her pain was now related to stress at home rather than work-related tasks.

SUMMARY

Dental hygienists are increasingly aware of the biomechanical, psychosocial, and personal risk factors that contribute to the development of MSDs. Although the inherent risks may not be completely eradicated, they can be effectively controlled to minimize the risk for developing an MSD in the present and future. Health care professionals need to truly understand the specific risks in order to provide practical solutions for dental hygienists in this busy business environment.

REFERENCES

Akesson, I., Johnsson, B., Rylander, L., Moritz, U., & Skerfving, S. (1999). Musculoskeletal disorders among female dental personnel-clinical examination and a 5-year follow-up study of symptoms, *International Archives of Occupational and Environmental Health, 72*(6), 395-403.

Akesson, I., Hansson, G.A., Balough, I., Moritz, U., & Skerfving, S. (1997). Quantifying workload in neck, shoulder and wrists in female dentists. *International Archives of Occupational and Environmental Health, 69*(6), 461-474.

Atwood, M. J., & Michalak, C. (1992). The occurrence of cumulative trauma disorders in dental hygienists. *Work, 2*(4), 17-31.

Balogh, I., Hansson, G.A., Ohlsson, K., Stromberg, U., & Skerving, S. (1999). Interindividual variation of physical load in a work task, *Scandinavian Journal of Work, Environment, and Health, 25*(1), 57-66.

Beach, J. C., & DeBiase, C. B. (1998) Assessment of ergonomic education in dental hygiene curricula. *Journal of Dental Hygiene Education, 62*(6), 421-425.

Bernard, B. (Ed.). (1997). *Musculoskeletal disorders and workplace factors.* DHHS (NIOSH) Pub. No. 97-141. Cincinnati, OH: Department of Health and Human Services, National Institute for Occupational Safety and Health.

Bramson, J., Smith, S., & Romangnoli, G. (1998). Evaluating dental office ergonomic risk factors and hazards. *Journal of the American Dental Association, 129,* 174-183.

Branson, B. G., Williams, K. B., Bray, K. K., McIlnay, S. L. & Dickey, D. (2002). Validity and reliability of a dental operator posture assessment instrument (PAI). *Journal of Dental Hygiene, 76*(IV), 255-261.

Chaffin, D. B., & Andersson, G. B. J. (1984). *Occupational biomechanics.* New York: John Wiley & Sons.

Cherniak, M. (1998). Vibration and dental equipment. In D. Murphy (Ed.), *Ergonomics and the dental care worker.* Washington, DC: American Public Health Association.

Conrad, J. C., Conrad, K. J., & Osborn, J. S.(1991). Median nerve dysfunction evaluated during dental hygiene education and practice (1986-1989). *Journal of Dental Hygiene, 65*(6), 283-288.

Ekenvall, L., Nilsson, B. Y., & Falconer, C. (1990). Sensory perception in the hands of dentists. *Scandinavian Journal of Work, Environment, and Health, 16*(5), 334-339.

Feuerstein, M. (1996). Workstyle: Definition, empirical support, and implications for prevention, evaluation, and rehabilitation of occupational upper-extremity disorders. In S. D. Moon & S. L. Sauter (Ed.), *Beyond biomechanics: Psychosocial aspects of musculoskeletal disorders in office work.* Bristol, PA: Taylor & Francis.

Hardage, J. L., Gildersleeve, J. R., & Rugh, J. D. (1983). Clinical work posture for the dentist: An electromyographic study. *Journal of the American Dental Association, 107*(6), 937-939.

Johnson, S. (1990). Ergonomic design of handheld tools to prevent trauma to the hand and upper extremity. *Journal of Hand Therapy, 3*(2), 86-93.

Kroemer, K. H. E., & Grandjean, E. (2001). *Fitting the task to the human.* Philadelphia: Taylor & Francis.

Lalumandier, J., & McPhee, S. (2001). Prevalence and risk factors of hand problems and carpal tunnel syndrome among dental hygienists. *Journal of Dental Hygiene, 75*(2), 130-134.

Luopajärvi, T. (1990). Ergonomic analysis of workplace and postural load. In M. Bullock (Ed.), *Ergonomic: The physiotherapist in the workplace.* New York: Churchill Livingstone.

MacDonald, G., Robertson, M. M., & Erickson, S.A. (1988). Carpal tunnel syndrome among California dental hygienists. *Dental Hygiene, 62*(7), 322-328.

MacDonald, G. (1987). Hazards in the dental workplace. *Dental Hygiene, 61*(5), 212-218.

McLean, L., Tingley, M., Scott, R. N., & Rickards, J. (2001). Computer terminal work and the benefit of microbreaks. *Applied Ergonomics, 32*(3), 225-237.

Meador, H. L. (1993). The biocentric technique: a guide to avoiding occupational pain. *Journal of Dental Hygiene, 67*(1), 38-51.

Michalak-Turcotte, C. (2000). Controlling dental hygiene work-related musculoskeletal disorders. *Journal of Dental Hygiene*, *74*(1), 41-48.

Michalak-Turcotte, C., & Atwood-Sanders, M. (2000). Ergonomic strategies for the dental hygienist—Part II. *Journal of Practical Hygiene, 9*(3), 35-38.

Moore, J. S., & Garg, A. (1995). The strain index: A proposed method to analyze jobs for the risk of distal extremity disorders. *American Industrial Hygiene Association Journal, 56*(5), 443-458.

Murphy, D. C. (Ed.). (1998). *Ergonomics and the dental care worker.* Washington, DC: American Public Health Association.

Nunn, P. J. (1998) Posture for dental hygiene practice. In D. Murphy (Ed.), *Ergonomics and the Dental Care Worker.* Washington, DC: American Public Health.

Oberg, T. (1993). Ergonomic evaluations and construction of a reference workplace in dental hygiene: A case study. *Journal of Dental Hygiene, 67*, 262-267.

Oberg, T., Karzina, A., Sandsjo, L., & Kadefors, R. (1995) Work load, fatigue and pause patterns in clinical dental hygiene. *Journal of Dental Hygiene, 60*(5), 223-229.

Osborn, J. B., Newell, K. J., Rudney, J. D., & Stoltenberg, J. L. (1990). Musculoskeletal pain among Minnesota dental hygienists. *Journal of Dental Hygiene, 64*(3), 132-138.

Palermud, G., Forsman, M., Sporrong, H., Herberts, P., & Kadefors, R. (2000). Intramuscular pressure of the infra- and supraspinatus muscles in relation to hand load and arm posture. *European Journal of Applied Physiology, 83*(2-3), 223-230.

Pattison, G., & Pattison, A. M. (1992). *Periodontal Instrumentation* (2nd ed.). Norwalk, CT: Appleton & Lange.

Ratzon, N. Z., Yaros, T., Mizlik, A., & Kanner, T. (2000). Musculoskeletal symptoms among dentists in relation to work posture. *Work, 15*(3), 153-158.

Rolander, B., & Bellner, A-L. (2001). Experience of musculoskeletal disorders, intensity of pain, and general conditions in work—the case of employees in non-private dental clinics in a county in southern Sweden, *Work, 17*(1), 65-73.

Sanders, M. J., & Turcotte, C.A (2002). Strategies to reduce work-related musculoskeletal disorders in dental hygienists: Two case studies. *Journal of Hand Therapy, 15*(4), 363-374.

Shenkar, O., Mann, J., Shevach, A., Ever-Hadani, P., & Weiss, P. L. (1998). Prevalence and risk factors of upper extremity cumulative trauma disorders in dental hygienists. *Work, 11,* 263-275.

Silverstein, B.A., Fine, L. J., & Armstrong, T. J. (1987). Occupational factors and carpal tunnel syndrome. *American Journal of Industrial Medicine, 11*(3), 343-358.

Sjogaard, G., Savard, G., & Juel, C. (1988) Muscle blood flow during isometric activity and its relations to muscle fatigue, *European Journal of Applied Physiology, 57,* 327-335.

Stentz, T. L., Riley, M. W., Stanton, D. H., Sposato, R. C., Stockstill, J. W., & Harn, J. A. (1994). Upper extremity altered sensations in dental hygienists. *International Journal of Industrial Ergonomics, 13,* 107-112.

Strong, D. R., & Lennartz, F. H. (1992). Carpal tunnel syndrome. *Certified Dental Assistant Journal, 20*(4), 27-39.

Werner, R., Armstrong, T. J., Birkus, C., & Aylard, M. K. (1997). Intracarpal canal pressures: The role of finger, hand, wrist, and forearm position. *Clinical Biomechanics, 12*(1), 44-51.

Wilkins, E. M. (1994). *Clinical practice of the dental hygienist* (7th ed.). Malvern, PA: Williams and Wilkins.

Ylippa, V., Bengt, B.A., Preber, H., & Sandelin, S. (1996). Determinants of work satisfaction among Swedish dental hygienists. *Scandinavian Journal of Caring Sciences, 10*(4), 247-253.

Ylippa, V., Bengt, B.A., & Preber, H. (1999). Factors that affect health and well-being in dental hygienists: A comparison of Swedish dental practices. *Journal of Dental Hygiene, 73*(4), 191-199.

Yoshida, H., Nagata, C., Mirbod, S. M., Iwata, H., & Inaba, R. (1991). Analysis of subjective symptoms of upper extremities in dental technicians. *Sangyo Igaku Japanese Journal of Industrial Health, 33*(1), 17-22.

APPENDIX 22-1

Interview for Determining Dental Hygienists' Work Practices

Personal Data

Name: ______________________________ Date: __________

Address: ______________________________

Phone: ______________________________ Age: ______ Gender: ______

Diagnosis: ______________________________

History of current diagnosis: ______________________________

____

____

Chief complaint: ______________________________

____

Medical History (please check and comment)

- ❒ Diabetes ______________________________
- ❒ Hormone abnormality ______________________________
- ❒ Kidney disorder ______________________________
- ❒ Endocrine disorder ______________________________
- ❒ Rheumatoid arthritis ______________________________
- ❒ Previous surgeries ______________________________
- ❒ Wrist fracture ______________________________
- ❒ Acute trauma ______________________________
- ❒ Family history of carpal tunnel syndrome ______________________________
- ❒ Pregnancy ______________________________
- ❒ Motor vehicle accident ______________________________
- ❒ Other musculoskeletal diagnosis ______________________________

____

____

Previous treatment for the present condition: ____

____

____

Employment History

Number of years practicing dental hygiene: ____________

Types of dentistry practiced: ____

____

Types of dentistry at present job(s):

Primary ____________ Secondary ____________

Number of years at present job(s):

Primary ____________ Secondary ____________

Number of days worked per week:

Primary ____________ Secondary ____________

Number of hours worked per day:

Primary ____________ Secondary ____________

Tasks performed at present job(s): ____

____

____

Workplace Practices

Average number of clients per day: ____________

Amount of time allotted per client:

Adults ____________ Children ____________

Percentage of clients with the following degrees of calculus:

Light ____________

Moderate ____________

Heavy ____________

Do you alternate scheduling clients with light and heavy calculus? ____________

Percentage of clients on whom you use the ultrasonic scaler: ____________

Percentage of clients whose teeth you polish: ____________

Frequency of sharpening instruments: ____________

Handle shape used most frequently (check):

❒ Round ❒ Hexagonal

❒ Octagonal

Do you rotate instrument delivery systems?

❒ Yes

❒ No

Handle size used:
❒ $^3/_{16}$ in or smaller
❒ Larger than $^3/_{16}$ in

Primary mode of instrument delivery:
❒ Side ❒ Rear ❒ Front

Primary operator position:
❒ 9 o'clock
❒ 12 o'clock
❒ 3 o'clock

Do you rotate operator positions?
❒ Yes ❒ No

Handle serration used most frequently (check):
❒ Smooth
❒ Long, parallel
❒ Crosswise
❒ Intermittent bands
❒ Waffle-iron
❒ Rubber-coated
❒ Other: ____________________

Please draw a sketch of your office set-up on back.

Musculoskeletal Symptoms

Please check if you have had any of the following conditions:
❒ Pain or swelling in the hands or wrist
❒ Numbness or tingling in the hands or wrist
❒ Tendency for your fingers to "lock"
❒ Weakness in your grip
❒ Discomfort in the elbow or forearm
❒ Discomfort in the shoulder
❒ Discomfort in the neck area

Please indicate the location of your discomfort. Feel free to include locations other than your primary diagnosis.

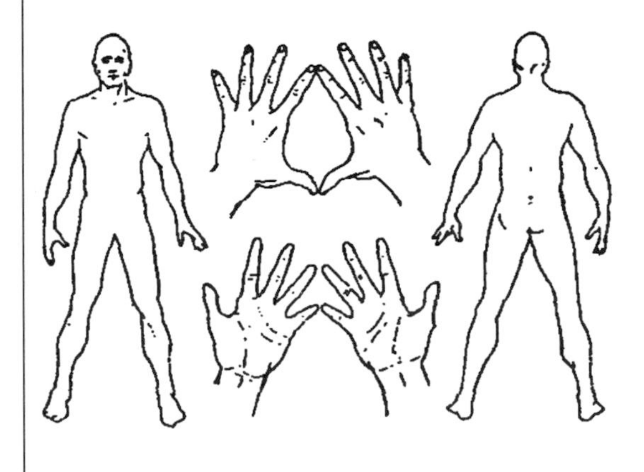

Which extremitites are involved?
❒ Dominant ❒ Nondominant
❒ Both

Have you ever noticed any of the following during work?
❒ Increased discomfort toward the end of the day
❒ Increased discomfort after clients with heavy calculus
❒ Difficulty in maintaining grasp of instruments
❒ Difficulty in detecting calculus
❒ Difficulty in judging the amount of pressure being used
❒ Dropping objects inadvertently
❒ Increased overall fatigue at the end of the day
❒ Shaking of the hands

Do any other activities induce similar discomfort?
❒ Typing ❒ Use of utensils
❒ Lifting or carrying ❒ Sports
❒ Brushing teeth ❒ Scrubbing
❒ Writing ❒ Opening jars

When do you experience your discomfort?
❒ Morning
❒ During work
❒ After work
❒ Evenings
❒ Interferes with sleep

What methods have you used to alleviate your discomfort?

- ❒ Shaking wrists
- ❒ Ice
- ❒ Heat
- ❒ Stretching
- ❒ Changing positions
- ❒ Taking more breaks
- ❒ Aspirin
- ❒ Splints
- ❒ Seeing fewer clients
- ❒ Vacation

Which of the above methods are effective? ______________________________

____

Briefly describe a typical day for you. ______________________________

____

____

What are your hobbies? ______________________________

____

How frequently do you perform your hobbies? ______________________________

If you have experienced musculoskeletal discomfort, do you feel that it has interfered with other aspects of your life? (Please check those that apply.)

- ❒ Household chores
- ❒ Dressing
- ❒ Grooming and bathing
- ❒ Cooking
- ❒ Child care
- ❒ Social recreation
- ❒ Job satisfaction
- ❒ Driving
- ❒ Writing
- ❒ Hobbies
- ❒ Energy level
- ❒ Positive attitude
- ❒ Relationships

Please describe aspects of your job that you enjoy and those that you do not enjoy.

____

____

____

Summary comments: ______________________________

____

____

____

Therapist's name: ______________________________ Date: ____________

CHAPTER 23

Managing MSDs in Performing Artists

Caryl D. Johnson

Life as a performing artist is intense, uncertain, demanding, and difficult. It stresses the body and mind and requires ability, training, talent, and commitment. This chapter refers to performing artists as those who present a work of art for the appreciation of an audience: dancers, singers, actors, mimes, clowns, and musicians. Their bodies or instruments are their tools; their workplaces are theaters, or concert halls, or any performing space. Although performing brings such benefits as personal satisfaction and professional feedback to these artists, the costs include musculoskeletal injuries that may threaten one's career (Brandfonbrener, 1999; Brodsky, 2001).

This chapter discusses the factors that contribute to the development of musculoskeletal disorders (MSDs) in both stage performers and instrumental musicians and provides an overview of the specific diagnoses common to groups of performers. A guide to musculoskeletal evaluation of the performing artist is presented, followed by two case studies that illustrate clinical intervention.

BACKGROUND ON PERFORMERS' CAREERS

When we speak of a performance, we think of the skill and technique involved in carrying out a dramatic or musical work. But to become a performer, the artist begins by conditioning, studying, and preparing to perform. Unlike a 9-to-5 job, the work of presenting a performance is a culmination of requisite years of training and preparation.

Performing artists' employment may also include teaching one's craft or working at nonartistic jobs such as waiting tables to meet financial needs, since job security is nearly unknown in this workplace. Life as a performer is one of predictable uncertainty, and survival requires self-assurance and coping skills. Success as a performer comes from opportunity, politics, financial backing, and luck, in addition to talent and skill. A majority of performers do not have health or disability insurance, since the availability or affordability of benefits is based on being employed.

TRAINING AND CONDITIONING PERFORMERS

Performing artists must spend many hours each day in training in order to prepare the body for the actions required to perform. Training parameters are the traditional technical approaches for each discipline that determine body positioning, motions used, and traditional patterns of movement. Practicing involves repetition, concentration, and consistency. The practicing of specific patterns results in conditioning the neuromuscular responses needed for speed, endurance, positioning, strength, and breathing. All performing artists must condition themselves to maintain the necessary stamina, muscle strength, coordination, and timing for their arts. Student performers practice to establish both traditional and physically practical techniques. Professional or amateur performers practice to maintain their technical skills. Serious performers will practice at least 3 hours each day and often much more. Wise teachers guide their students to make well-spaced incremental increases in practicing times.

Rehearsing for performance, another type of training, is specific to the work being performed. New instructions about performing a work must be learned, texts or music memorized, ensemble interactions made expert, and performance spaces made familiar. Preparing to perform requires hours of dedicated repetition and is usually carried out with other performers and coaches, directors, or conductors.

As performers undergo the rigors of training and performing, they inflict repeated microtrauma on their bodies, accumulating small injuries. These small injuries, when balanced with recovery time, lead to conditioning. If repeated microinsults are not followed by sufficient recovery time, overuse injuries result.

FACTORS THAT CONTRIBUTE TO MUSCULOSKELETAL INJURIES IN PERFORMING ARTISTS

Fatigue

Most MSDs in performing artists are manifestations of fatigue or inadequate recovery time after fatigue, whether physical or mental (Barr & Barbe, 2002; Horvath, 2001). Performers are prone to going beyond what is reasonable and healthful in their professional preparation, beyond performance conditioning, beyond whole-body conditioning, and beyond training (e.g., using poor or insufficient technical training to perform the chosen task). When the performer exceeds conditioning, he or she becomes fatigued. Emotional or physical fatigue may alter the neuromuscular control, the normal techniques of performing, and generate less efficient muscle synergies.

Repetition

Repeating a unit of music or a pattern of dance steps or a series of stage motions embeds the pattern in the mind and the "muscle memory." Although repetition is essential to learning or polishing performance skills, it can be carried to damaging extremes. Excessive repetitions can exceed conditioning and cause injury (Barron & Eaton, 1998; Harper, 2002; Hoppmann, 1998).

Awkward Posture

Certain instruments are played with the upper extremities in awkward and potentially damaging positions. For example, the flute and piccolo are played with the instrument supported at mouth level and to the right of the face. This requires the left arm to be horizontally adducted, the elbow flexed to approximately 100 degrees, and the wrist extended, while the right arm is abducted approximately 45 degrees, the elbow flexed to 100 degrees, and the wrist extended. Playing the guitar requires left wrist flexion (of varying degrees) while the forearm is supinated and right wrist flexion as it moves back and forth in radial and ulnar deviation (see the section on stringed instruments for details about the body demands of playing a stringed instrument). Positions such as those described cause biomechanical disadvantage and lead to chronic muscle imbalances (Berque & Gray, 2002).

Static Posture

Maintaining a body part, prop, or instrument in one place for long periods of time causes muscle fatigue, muscle recruitment, and increased tension in proximal stabilizing muscles (Barron & Eaton, 1998). Static posturing eventually decreases venous return (Hoppmann, 1998). Fatigue, muscle recruitment, and diminished venous return related to stasis can lead to injury.

Stress of Performing

Performing is stressful. Stage fright, or at least "stage nerves," is very real, as are the neurological responses to this psychological stress. Along with autonomic manifestations such as perspiration and dry mouth, involuntary muscle contractions (especially in the face, neck, and shoulders) make controlled performing more difficult (Ostwald, Avery, & Ostwald, 1998; Spahn, Ell, & Seidenglanz, 2001). If additional muscle groups are recruited, this increases the amount of work used for performing and at the same time decreases control of motor response. Stress can be a contributor to injury if it decreases endurance or control.

Lifting and Carrying to Transport Instruments and Equipment

Performers frequently carry instruments and performance equipment such as shoes, clothes, and scores. Although small equipment is manageable, transporting large instruments in heavy cases may contribute to injury from repeatedly lifting into and out of vehicles or over subway turnstiles. Jazz, rock, and club musicians who change venues may carry amplifiers, speakers, instruments, music stands, and even lights to a job. Many current styles of music further depend on electronic amplification equipment. This electronic equipment can be large, heavy, and awkward to lift, putting stress on the player's back and musculoskeletal system for which he is not conditioned.

Constrained Space

An important component of the work setting is space. All performers, both musicians and stage performers, require specific amounts of space to perform the motions of their art. Musicians are usually stationary in space while body parts and instrument parts are moving. If space limitations restrict playing motions, the player must modify his motions causing cocontractions and increased muscle tension. Stage artists perform with their whole bodies and require enough space for preparation, motion, and recovery from motion. Insufficient space for the required movement is a frequent cause of accidental injury. Unfortunately, most performers are unable to change their work setting and must learn to adapt to its constraints (Babin, 1999; Harper, 2002).

Changing Work Environments

Performers who are in traveling companies, or who tour alone, face uncertainties each time they change location (Ackermann, 2002). Each performing environment is different in terms of lighting, layout, sound and air conditioning systems, seating, stands, curtains, costumes, props, setup, temperature, and lighting. Unfamiliar stages, orchestra pits, backstage areas, and other work locations may be unsafe for the performer. Traveling performers also keep variable hours and face the stress of irregular schedules. The unknowns and unexpected circumstances facing a traveling performer often precipitate injury (Ackermann, 2002).

TYPES OF MUSCULOSKELETAL INJURIES IN PERFORMING ARTISTS

Musculoskeletal injuries are common events for performing artists. Injury may be related to training regimens, workplace hazards, or individual variables. If repeated motions are not balanced with recovery, or if good joint alignment, reasonable body placement, and sufficient strength are absent, injury may result. Continuing to practice or perform a task that is causing injury is the most common cause of extended disability in performers (Barron & Eaton, 1998).

Overuse or chronic injuries are seen more frequently than accidental injuries and affect both musicians and stage performers (Hoppmann, 1998; Sammarco & Tablante, 1998). The most common overuse injuries occur in muscle and tendon units and relate to overuse or lack of conditioning (Aronen, 1985; Barr & Barbe, 2002; Carvajal & Evans, 1998; Cayea & Manchester, 1998; Davies, 2002; Dawson, 2001; Horvath, 2001; Meinke, 1998). Acute and chronic inflammations seen in muscles, joints, or tendons often relate to repetitive actions. Bone injuries related to overuse are usually stress fractures related to jumping and are much more frequent in the lower extremity. Chronic ligamentous injuries in performing artists can result from repeated motion or weight bearing at a joint that is not well aligned. Ligament injuries may also result from lack of conditioning or technical skill.

INJURIES BY CLIENT GROUP

The treatment of performing artists is a specialized application of our skills as clinicians. To carry out effective treatment, the therapist must have a reasonable knowledge of instruments and instrument techniques, dance and dance techniques, gymnastics and acrobatics techniques, acting and mime performance techniques, and the physical demands of each type of performing. Exposure to methods of training and conditioning in these disciplines allows the therapist to be more specifically helpful to the artist. Familiarity with performance workplaces and their unique conditions can also increase the effectiveness of treatment.

Players of Woodwind Instruments

The flute, piccolo, clarinet, oboe, English horn, bassoon, and saxophone all consist of a column of air that vibrates and amplifies the sound initiated by the mouthpiece. The early forms of these instruments were wood tubes, and most are still made of wood—hence the term *woodwinds.* Pitch changes depend on the length and width of the column of air. Many of these instruments now have mechanical key systems that facilitate changing pitch (by assisting the change of tube length). Altering the speed of wind blown into the instrument changes volume and pitch. The most commonly used woodwinds are held to the mouth for playing. Woodwind instruments can be carried in hard or semirigid cases.

Injuries related to playing woodwinds often result from maintaining a static posture and holding or lifting the instrument for extended periods of time. Fatigue in the shoulder, elbows, and wrist may lead to shoulder bursitis, forearm tendinitis, and, in older players, degenerative joint problems and calcific tendinitis (Dawson, 1997; Spence, 2001; Thrasher & Chesky, 2001). Flutes, oboes, clarinets, and saxophones rest on the right thumb while they are being played, which stresses ligaments and sometimes leads to painful metacarpophalangeal (MCP) and carpometacarpal (CMC) joints in the thumb. This repeated joint stress might lead to stretching of ligaments, loss of joint alignment, and eventual CMC joint degeneration. Ligament attrition injuries can also result from the repeated finger and thumb abduction required to play larger woodwinds instruments (e.g., contrabassoon), since the keys are widely spaced on these instruments. The player with small hands is at a greater potential risk for ligament damage.

Players of Brass Instruments

The trumpet, trombone, French horn, and tuba represent the pitch range of the brass instrument family. Fewer players of brass instruments suffer from upper-extremity injuries brought about by playing their instruments (Dawson, 1997). All brass instruments are lifted to the mouth for blowing (playing). Many pitch changes are made by air pressure changes at the mouth. Forceful blowing has led to injuries related to intraoral and intraocular pressure. Compressive forces against the lips may alter tooth position.

Players of Percussion Instruments

Percussion instruments include many sizes and types of drums, timpani, the xylophone family of instruments, and cymbals. Percussion instruments have one or more parts, which resonate when struck. Sticks, mallets, brushes, and even hands are used for striking an instrument to make a sound. Tuning and pitch changes on percussion instruments are made deliberately by the player (as when the musician tunes the timpani) or by striking tuned parts of instruments (chimes, keys, metals bars, etc.).

Injuries to percussionists usually arise from repetitive playing, forceful playing, playing with wrists or thumbs in poor alignment, or playing for extended periods of time (Cayea & Manchester, 1998; Hoppmann, 1998; Zaza, Fleiszer, Maine, & Merchefske, 2000). De Quervain's disease may result from repeated use of drumsticks. Tendinitis of the forearm muscles may result from rapid alternation of radial and ulnar deviation at the wrist while using mallets or sticks. Shoulder bursitis or tendinitis may result from repeated cymbal clashing.

Playing drums with a rock band requires repeated forceful loud strokes of drumsticks (and foot) to provide forward motion and pulse in the music. Forceful strokes of the sticks bounce the wider end of the sticks repeatedly against the soft tissue in the palm. This can traumatize the soft tissues on palm and fingers and lead to chronic trigger fingers or trigger thumb.

Players of Keyboard Instruments

The structural element shared by the piano, organ, electronic keyboard, and the accordion (to name a few such instruments) is a keyboard that controls pitch changes of resonating strings, pipes, or speaker cones. The player usually sits in front of the keyboard(s) and reaches forward to touch the keys. Musculoskeletal problems in keyboard players are usually the result of a poor seated position relative to the keyboard (Pak & Chesky, 2001). Figure 23-1 demonstrates a typical seated posture while playing a piano.

Compression neuropathies can result from repeated excessive elbow or wrist flexion or wrist extension. These neuropathies include cubital, radial, and carpal tunnel syndromes (CTS). Lateral epicondylitis results from repetitive use of extensor tendons of both the fingers and the wrist. De Quervain's disease is another common finding in keyboard performers. It relates to forceful thumb use in abducted and extended positions. Repeated practicing of extended or awkward reaches on the keyboard, from thumb to fingers or finger to finger, can fatigue or even injure soft tissues in the hand.

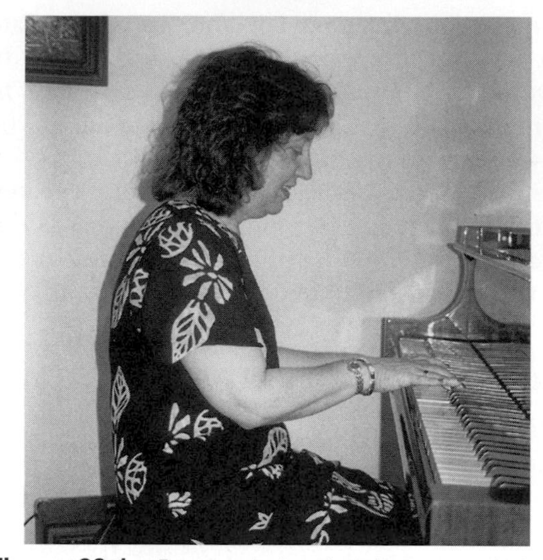

Figure 23-1 Person playing the piano; note lack of back support.

Figure 23-2, *A* and *B,* demonstrate the awkward finger reaches common in playing the accordion. These issues are exacerbated by the body's asymmetry while holding the instrument.

Players of Stringed Instruments

The violin, viola, cello, double bass, or guitar is basically a resonating box (body) with strings stretched tightly across it. The strings are set to vibrating by a bow, a pick, or a finger. Pressing down or "stopping" the string, which changes its length, changes the pitch of the string. The instrument body resonates and amplifies the sound of the string. Violins and violas are held under the chin near the left shoulder, guitars and lutes are held in front of the trunk, and cellos and double basses rest on the floor in front of the player. Bows are drawn across the strings when playing violins, violas, cellos, and double basses. Fingers are used to pluck on all stringed instruments.

The traditional position for playing violins and violas is probably the most frequent cause of upper-extremity injury in string players (Barron & Eaton, 1998; Berque & Gray, 2002; Hoppmann, 1998). These two types of instru-

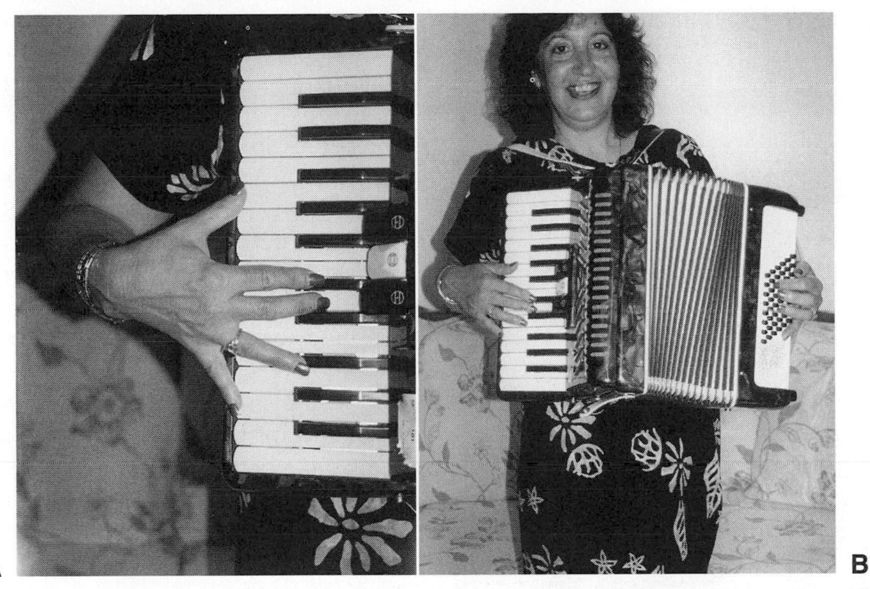

Figure 23-2 **A,** Extended finger reaches on the keyboard of an accordion. **B,** Postural asymmetry while holding the accordion.

ments are held in front of the left shoulder and under the chin by the left arm. The left arm supports the instrument while positioned in forward flexion and slight external rotation with supination. The right hand holds the bow. The right shoulder moves in adduction/abduction and forward elevation, while the elbow flexes and extends to move the bow across the strings. These arm positions are physically demanding and can cause inflammatory problems in either shoulder. Tendinitis of the wrist extensors or flexors results from playing beyond conditioned endurance levels and is seen in either hand (Hoppmann, 1998).

Guitars (and mandolins, ukuleles, harps, and other less common stringed instruments) are played with the fingers or picks. Traditionally, right-handed guitarists hold their instruments with the neck and fingerboard to their left while the instrument body rests across the right thigh (Figure 23-3, *A*). The left forearm supinates as the wrist flexes, and the fingers stop the strings (Figure 23-3, *B*). The right forearm is slightly pronated while the fingers or a pick initiate vibration of the strings. Some performers play with the right wrist flexed or move the hand back and forth into radial and ulnar deviation to strum. Sustained flexion in either wrist can make facile or continuous finger flexion both difficult and fatiguing. Tendinitis of the flexor tendons is a frequent problem in guitarists and harpists (Semmler, 1998).

Compression neuropathies of the upper extremity are seen in players of any type of stringed instrument. Cubital tunnel syndrome is caused by repetitive elbow flexion. CTS can result from repetitious finger flexion with the wrist flexed (Dawson, 1999).

Stage Performers: Dancers, Actors, Mimes, Acrobats

Stage performers present with both traumatic injuries and overuse injuries (Aronen, 1985; Brandfonbrener, 1999; Carvajal & Evans, 1998; Garrick & Lewis, 2001; Haight, 1998; Laws & Petrie, 1999; Sammarco, 1983). Accidental musculoskeletal injuries occur because stage performers are usually in motion in a limited space.

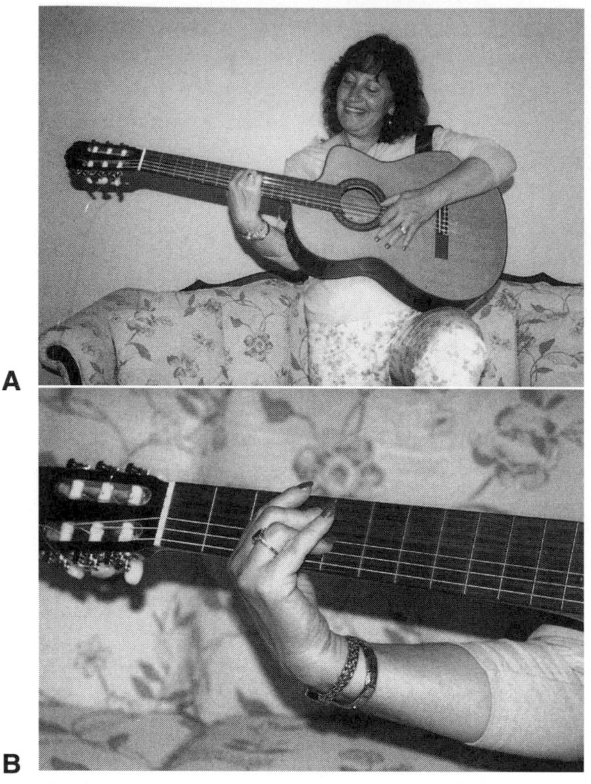

Figure 23-3 **A,** Guitar player (left-handed) protracts her shoulder while supporting the guitar and strumming with the left hand. **B,** Her wrist and fingers are flexed while stopping the strings.

Injuries can be related to the layout of stage space or insufficient space for the motion required. Stages are often "raked" or slanted to allow the audience to see to the back of the stage. This can affect motion, posture, and balance, and make performing more hazardous (Wenning & O'Connell, 1999). Lighting on and off stage can contribute to accidental injury to performers. Lighting that is too bright or directed across a path of movement (as may happen with spotlights) distracts and interrupts the split-second planning needed to move safely, and poor backstage lighting may impair space judgment. Too much or too little light can interfere with spatial awareness.

Stage performers also need a floor with some spring in it. Sometimes they must perform on an inelastic floor, which can cause shinsplints. To avoid this condition, many professional dance companies include in their contract that their dancers not be required to perform on cement (Sammarco & Tablante, 1998; Seals, 1983). Dancers, actors, and acrobats often suffer contact injuries with other performers or with portions of the stage sets. They may even be dropped or twisted by another performer (Solomon et al., 1999).

Overuse injuries such as tendinitis occur in stage performers, particularly dancers and acrobats, when they are not well conditioned. Inflammatory problems related to repetitive use include the following (Haight, 1998; Kirkendall, 1985; Krasnow & Kabboni, 1999; Sammarco & Tablante, 1998; Solomon, et al., 1999).

1. Bunions, a joint deformity related to weight bearing, foot shape, shoe fit, inadequate padding in shoe, or dance technique
2. Patellar tendinitis, or jumper's knee, a painful condition that results from repeated motion and impact during jumps
3. Ankle impingement syndrome
4. Achilles tendinitis and other inflammations around the ankle related to the muscles used in elevation or lifting the body into space
5. Plantar fasciitis, an inflammation caused by repetitive traction on a ligament or tendon in the sole of the foot

Dancers are subject to chronic inflammatory conditions of the hip related to the position of hip turnout traditional to classical ballet. Shoulder injury and impingements are seen in dancers or acrobats who bear body weight on the upper extremities or use motions exploiting shoulder flexibility. Elbows may dislocate, and wrists are subject to sprains and strains from flips, weight-bearing, and partnering (Harvey, 1983; Kahn, Brown, Way, Vass, Chrichton, Alexander et al., 1995; Solomon et al., 1999). For stage performers, the key risk factors to observe are posture, joint alignment, and conditioning.

EVALUATION OF PERFORMING ARTISTS

The following evaluation has been compiled from clinics that perform comprehensive evaluations of performing artists with musculoskeletal problems (Barron & Eaton, 1998; Hoppmann, 1998; Meinke, 1995; Newmark & Weinstein, 1995; Sammarco & Tablante, 1998).

History

Evaluation of the injured performing artist begins with obtaining a careful history including personal, medical, technical background, and training information. A complete report about this particular injury, type and location of injury or pain, how it may have happened, how long it has been going on (overuse), and any treatment that has already been provided is critical. Listening to the narrative as given by the client may also provide useful information about his or her emotional response to the injury.

Physical Examination for Overuse Injury

When performing an examination for overuse injury, it is important to note the following.

- Observe client's build and posture in relation to instrument or performing task.
- Note skeletal proportion, alignment, or development.
- Examine skin for callus or signs of inflammation.
- Note localized redness or swelling.
- If upper extremities are injured, measure grip and pinch strength.
- Perform manual muscle testing and provocative tests.
- Measure any limitations of active range of motion (AROM) or greater-than-normal AROM of joints.
- Observe joint stability, laxity, or abnormal normal alignments.
- Note performance equipment in use: assistive devices, glasses, straps, pads, taping, or other adaptive devices.

Client Performance Demonstration

The client must be evaluated while performing in order to address the various positions that the performer's body assumes during a typical session. (*Note:* This will be deferred for the client with accidental injury until he or she is sufficiently recovered to perform.) The therapist should observe the performer during live performance or at a location where he has acceptable performance conditions. The client must be observed from all angles: front, side, back, and oblique. The performer should be asked to demonstrate his or her customary warm-up and some of his current performing skills. Musicians may be asked to play something slow, something fast, and any piece or section of a piece that might have caused the presenting problem. Dancers and other stage performers may be asked to demonstrate parts of their routine including those that cause them discomfort. During the client's performance the therapist should make the following observations.

- Skill level
- Technique as it compares to standard technique
- Posture and motion during performance (Krasnow, Monasterio, & Charfield, 2001)
- Dynamic joint alignment
- Tension mannerisms
- Other causative factors

Workplace Environmental Evaluation

The workplace environment is equally important in understanding how the performer interacts with his instrument, the performing space, and equipment and props in his or her immediate environment (Babin, 1999; Harper, 2002). When evaluating a professional musician at his workplace, the treating professional should check the following environmental factors.

- The chair used: height, support for back, stability of chair
- Space between chairs
- Space for moving parts of instrument and body

- Viewing angle to music
- Viewing angle to conductor
- Adequacy of lighting

For example, with keyboard musicians, location of the player in relation to the keyboard, pedals, and music is frequently a factor in musculoskeletal problems. The therapist should check the height of the bench as related to the elbow and wrist angles. If the player sits too close to the keyboard, the elbows will be excessively flexed and the wrists may remain ulnarly deviated. If the musician sits too low, the wrists may be actively extended rather than in neutral. In both of these examples, additional muscle activity and tension cause inefficiency and fatigue. If the back is poorly supported or the shoulders are elevated, distal fine-motor actions can be less effective and more costly in terms of energy expenditure.

In the case of stage performers, including dancers, actors, or mimes, it is important to realize that all stage performers are in motion and must adapt to the stage constraints. Therapists should check the following factors related to their performance (Brandfonbrener, 1999; Brodsky, 2001; Bronner & Brownstein, 1997).

- Stage area in relation to body size
- Motion and speed of motion required
- Sets, curtains, and props in relation to motion and speed of motion
- Space backstage in relation to motion required
- Raking of stage
- Sufficiency of lighting
- Costumes: weight, limitations to body motion, and props being used

PRINCIPLES OF TREATMENT

Treatment is based on the type of injury, medical and surgical treatment, and necessary precautions. Performers are typically very anxious about their recovery, since injuries threaten them with the possibility of losing their performance abilities, job, and livelihood (Ackermann, Adams, & Marshall, 2002; Chamagne, 1998; Dommerholt, Norris, & Shaheen, 1998; Hoppmann, 1998; Krasnow & Kabboni, 1999; Medoff, 1999; Norris, 1993; Ramel & Moritz, 1998; Sugano & Laws, 2002).

Treatment of traumatic and overuse MSDs in performing artists follows the steps of recovery we already expect in other client populations (see Chapters 5 and 6 for further discussion).

Step I: Early Recovery

Goals of treatment include decreased pain, decreased swelling, protection of injured area, decreased inflammation (overuse injuries), and maintenance of health in uninjured body areas. Modalities include rest and immobilization of involved areas with or without splinting; heat or cold as indicated; passive and active assisted exercise to involved joints by protocol (traumatic) or active and assisted active exercise of involved joints (overuse); active whole body exercise for uninjured muscles and joints; nonsteroidal or steroidal antiinflammatory drug regimen; and client education about injury, wound care, dressings, and precautions (Leanderson, Eriksson, Nilsson, & Wykman, 1996; Lewis, 1998; Medoff, 1999).

Step II: Return to Protected Motion of Injured Areas

Goals of treatment include regaining active motion of injured area, avoiding increasing inflammation (flare reaction), protecting injured area as needed, and continuing to maintain strength and motion of uninvolved zones. Modalities include less-immobilizing splints; gentle active exercise of injured area; isometric exercises; upgraded resistance of uninjured muscles and joints; and client education about alignment, precautions, and body mechanics (Dommerholt et al., 1998).

Step III: Conditioning of Injured Area

Goals of treatment include a modified return to training or practicing, increased strength, endurance and speed, and preparation for a return to performance. Modalities include progressive resistive exercises for injured area graded to match level of recovery, upgrade of resistance and endurance training for uninjured body areas, and client education about a safe and productive return to work including precautions to avoid reinjury. At this level of recovery, the client with an overuse injury may also be encouraged to reexamine his or her technical skills and consider modifications in training or practice schedules, equipment, and technique. When treating the immature client, it is appropriate to include the teacher or coach in any such re-examination (Davies, 2002; Sugano & Laws, 2002; Stretanski, 2002).

Step IV: Back to Work

Goals of treatment include a safe return to the workplace; any necessary remedial work on range of motion, strength, speed, or endurance; and weaning of the client from the therapy environment. Modalities include (1) progression from low-intensity/high-repetition exercises to less repetition and high-intensity/faster-speed exercises, (2) resistance added as repetitions are reduced, (3) stress reduction training, and (4) a gentle stretch program combined with releasing exercises. Most performing artists need endurance, speed, and strength. Gymnasts and dancers also need flexibility. All performers need aerobic capacity (Ackermann, 2002; Frederickson, 2002).

WORKPLACE MODIFICATIONS

Stage performers may have little possibility for change at their workplace, since choreography usually includes other performers and is part of the larger work. Only temporary modifications can be expected, such as avoiding lifts or other minor changes. It is difficult to effect any change in stage configuration, backstage areas, or equipment. Occasionally, props or costumes can be improved, but this is completely dependent on cooperation with the director, producer, and other production personnel at the theater. Since modifications are for the most part minor, the performer should be instructed in ways to improve his or her safety and body use through body mechanics, body awareness, conditioning, and preparedness.

Musicians may or may not be able to change the configuration of seating, music stands, lighting, or space. Sometimes a small shift of seat location or angle, a cushion, a different music stand, or a new light can be used without disturbing other players or the conductor. With an improved awareness of biomechanics, an injured musician may have fewer overuse problems if he makes adjustments that improve his work habits. Rests, stretches, and good posture can also help avoid further injury.

ADAPTIVE EQUIPMENT

Certain types of musculoskeletal problems may be improved through the use of adaptive equipment (Horvath, 2001; Norris & Dommerholt, 1998; Okner, Kernozek, & Wade, 1997). Adaptive equipment refers to any device that increases the ease of performing a task. Start with a biomechanical analysis of the injurious work tasks, and then seek possible alterations in equipment or movement. Some instruments can be modified to facilitate playing, such as using plugs on flute keys. If the key is plugged, the finger does not have to be placed as precisely to fully close the hole. Violas can be built with a cutout of the left shoulder of the instrument in order to allow the left hand to reach over the strings. All adaptations should be done by well-qualified instrument makers who are experienced craftsmen. With rare exceptions, therapists are well advised to avoid attempting to change instruments. Splinting, which adapts the player to the instrument, may be an option.

Transporting Instruments and Equipment

Instrument cases are available to decrease the work of carrying. These cases are especially valuable for double bass, cello, percussion instruments, or bassoon. They are made of plastic or other light material and are designed to be light but sturdy. Other cases for heavier instruments can be carried on the back as well as beside the body. Assistive wheels can make it easier to move heavy or bulky instruments and equipment. They are either added to the instrument case or one can use a small dolly with wheels. Use of balanced backpacks is a better way to carry music, supplies, and equipment.

Lifting and Holding Instruments or Props while Performing

The work of instrument or prop weight-bearing is often the precipitating factor in overuse injury. There are assistive devices for lifting and holding instruments such as modified thumb rests and racks or supports, like the Fredke or English horn support. Instrumental weight bearing can be made less taxing with attachments or external supports. For example, several kinds of thumb supports are available for use on oboes, clarinets, and saxophones. Some thumb supports redistribute the instrument weight more evenly between thumb and wrist, whereas others spread the instrument weight to more forearm area than the thumb. Splinting can also be used for instrument weight-bearing assist (Johnson, 2003).

There are also external devices available to support part of the weight of an instrument. Saxophone players frequently make use of a neck support strap. Harnesses are available to help support the weight of bassoons and saxophones. Bassoonists use seat straps or endpins. Some woodwind players use an external stand to assist weight bearing. See the Resources at the end of this chapter for sources of woodwind weight-bearing assistive equipment.

Size of Instrument in Relation to Performer

If the therapist determines a mismatch between the size of the player and his instrument, he or she should investigate the availability of variable instrument sizes. Some stringed instruments are made in several sizes to match body size, such as violins that are sized as $\frac{1}{4}$, $\frac{1}{2}$, $\frac{3}{4}$, and full-sized violins. Some woodwind instrument keys can be modified or adapted to adjust to smaller hands or shorter fingers.

Tradition is an important factor with performers. Most instrumentalists will not wish to play an adapted instrument, even if it is ergonomically preferable. If a player presents with an instrument-related injury, it is easier to encourage him to consider an adaptation. (I try to encourage clients to try an adaptation until they are less symptomatic.)

The following two case studies illustrate the application of the treatment principles outlined previously. Both cases necessitated a temporary interruption of practicing and performance. Such interruptions are to be avoided or made as short as possible within the principles of safe treatment.

CASE STUDY 1

AE is a 31-year-old, right-handed piano student who suffered an acute injury to his left hand and forearm 1 week before his first visit to the doctor's office. He believed the injury was caused by extra practicing on one piece he was preparing to perform.

A hand surgeon referred him for evaluation, splinting, and treatment. The physician had placed him in a plaster volar mold wrapped in place with an elastic bandage, immobilizing his forearm, wrist, and hand. The thumb had not been immobilized. The physician's referral reported negative x-ray findings. History taking provided the following pertinent information.

The client is a pleasant but very worried young man of moderate height and weight. He is a full-time "preprofessional" student with minimal academic classes but many performing responsibilities at his conservatory. He has studied piano for 25 years, with a series of excellent teachers in both the United States and abroad, and is an experienced performer who is outgoing, assertive, and confident at the instrument.

He described his problem and its occurrence the following way: He was practicing a difficult contemporary piece for the piano in which there is a long section requiring the left hand to cross over the right and jab loudly accented notes above and between those notes being played by the right hand. He decided he would work out one part, repeating it until he could do it easily. As he usually does, he was practicing at full volume, late at night, after a full day of classes and practicing. He was tired but determined to learn this particular section. He stopped because his arms felt fatigued and a little painful on the ulnar border of his left wrist. Both hands felt a little more tired than usual.

The next morning, when he awoke, the client had extreme pain in his left wrist, in his hand, along the ulnar border of the forearm, and around the lateral epicondyle. He tried to rest his hand and did not practice that day, but the painful symptoms worsened. The next day he tried to practice and thought, at first, that the pain was better, but in the evening it became worse than ever. The following day he went to the nurse and was referred to a hand doctor.

The client reported no previous episodes of such pain, although he previously had felt aches in his forearms after long hours of practice. He plays a classical piano repertoire. He has made no recent changes in his musical life. AE's goal is to become a concert artist. He is currently preparing for a performance that will fulfill part of the requirements of his school. Customarily, he practices 5 to 7 hours daily. AE does some additional work to earn money, but none of it is demanding physically. He has made no recent changes in his lifestyle. AE reports that he never exercises. His family is musically inclined; a brother is a cellist. His father died just 2 months ago.

The physical examination showed no vascular or skin changes. His left wrist was painful to touch on the dorsum and when moved beyond midrange. Pain increased in resisted finger extension and wrist extension. He was more uncomfortable when he moved actively into ulnar deviation. There was minimal diffuse swelling around the wrist, the CMC joint of the thumb, and in the distal forearm, with tenderness to pressure over the dorsal wrist extensor compartments. Strength measurements were deferred. AROM measurements were normal except as limited by pain in full wrist flexion with no resistance and full pronation against minimal resistance.

Lateral epicondylitis and extensor tendon synovitis were diagnosed in AE. Treatment was begun with immobilization in a molded wrist cock-up splint, placing the wrist in 60 degrees of extension, neutral radial-ulnar deviation, and extending two-thirds of the length of the forearm. The splint was worn at all times except during meals and for three 15-minute periods each day when AE was to move through an active range of motion. He was begun on naproxen (Naprosyn) and told to discontinue practicing or playing the piano. His teacher was contacted, and the diagnosis and treatment plan were explained to her.

Two days later, he was seen again. His splint was checked, and he began regular treatments with heat and soft tissue mobilization to the forearm, wrist, and hand, and shoulder AROM exercises (no weight or resistance). He was also reinstructed to use the left arm as normally as possible even when wearing the splint. This first phase of treatment was continued for 3 weeks. By the end of the first week, AE's symptoms were beginning to resolve. He was seen three times a week for symptomatic treatment.

At the end of 3 weeks, AE was to wean himself from the splint under a protocol that began with removal of the splint for 1 hour at each mealtime and gradually increased this splintless time until, by the end of the fourth week, he donned the splint only when he felt pain. During the second 3 weeks, he began guarded isometric exercises to the involved muscle groups and increased the number of repetitions of his shoulder AROM exercises. His nonsteroidal antiinflammatory drug was continued through the second 3-week period.

The fourth week after beginning treatment, AE was allowed a guarded return to the keyboard. Limitations on practice included length of time at the keyboard (30 minutes) and which pieces were to be practiced. Piano practicing was preceded by shoulder AROM exercises used as a warm-up. He maintained this regimen daily, including Sundays. Visits to the therapist were reduced to once weekly until 6 weeks into treatment. At the end of 6 weeks, AE began phase three of treatment: graded resistive shoulder AROM exercises, with a resistance of 1 pound, and AROM of involved muscles against gentle manual resistance by the therapist.

From this point, the client progressed to upper-extremity exercises with increased resistance, increased lengths of time and a more difficult repertoire at the keyboard, and increased strengthening of the injured muscles. At approximately 3 months after injury, the client was cleared for a full 5-hour practice routine, was performing his exercises regularly with 3-pound weights, and was preparing a recital. Except for occasional twinges of discomfort, he was without problem and had learned a lesson: He was not able to practice in awkward or unconditioned hand positions for unlimited hours without injuring himself.

CASE STUDY 2

AG is a 20-year-old, left-handed young performer who works in a road company of a Broadway show. He presents for treatment after suffering an acute injury to his right knee that had been preceded by a 3-month history of increasing left shoulder pain. He works as an actor and dancer in a road company of a Broadway show. The client is a moderately built young man who expresses great concern about losing his job. At this time he has taken a leave of absence from his job while the company is on the East Coast and hopes to return to work in 6 weeks. He works in a show that performs a fairy tale, using imaginative staging, costuming, and choreography. His role requires him to perform acrobatics and dance while wearing a bulky costume. He has an important role and is on stage most of the show. It has been difficult to find and prepare an understudy, so he feels pressured to continue performing.

He describes the onset of his problem the following way: In his role he dances a long dance clad in a bulky, heavy costume with sleeves and padding that limit arm movement and make acrobatics more difficult to perform. He reports that it takes "so much more strength" to do flips and somersaults because of the costume. At the end of one scene, he moves along a platform atop a piece of scenery. Reaching with his left hand, he pulls each of three female dancers from another platform, located lower and to his right, and propels them into a turn as they move to his left. Then he jumps down from the platform, somersaults, and exits stage left. After a gradual onset and increase in left shoulder pain over the last few months, he began to try substitute motions to avoid stress to his shoulder. He found he could push off a little more with his right leg and use more trunk motion as he pulled the dancers into their turns. This seemed to help, and, although his shoulder did not get much better, it seemed to be no worse.

The evening he injured his knee he noticed as he moved onto the platform that the spotlights were in a slightly different place, making it difficult to see the dancers he was to spin. But they were all moved safely to his left. Yet, as he turned to jump down, the lights seemed to be in his eyes. As he landed he felt a sharp pain in his right knee. He found he could walk, albeit with pain, and partly bend his knees, and he managed to finish the performance. The next day his right knee was swollen and tender to the touch. Weight bearing required careful foot and ankle placement, and it was clearly impossible for him to go to work. Seen on an emergency basis, his x-rays demonstrated no bony injuries or abnormalities.

An orthopedic surgeon saw him, examined the knee injury as well as his painful left shoulder, and referred him to therapy for follow-up. His diagnoses were sprain of the medial collateral ligament of his right knee and impingement syndrome of the left shoulder.

Physical examination of the knee showed that the active range of motion without weight bearing was within normal limits except for slight limits in full knee flexion because of swelling and pain. The client was able to stand one-footed on his right leg, but weight-bearing knee flexion caused severe pain, as did lateral valgus stress. Palpable swelling was noted below medial patella, and his knee was tender to touch at the insertion site of the medial collateral ligament.

Physical examination of the shoulders showed an active range of motion within normal limits. This client was moderately hypermobile in his shoulders and elbows, as is often true of dancers and gymnasts. The left shoulder had a painful arc between 80 degrees and 110 degrees. Impingement testing as described by Neer and Welch was positive. Manual muscle testing demonstrated slight weakness in the scapular stabilizers and the supraspinatus. Palpable sites of increased muscle tone and tenderness were noted at the insertion of the levator scapula and at the superior scapular border. Overhead functional activities such as hanging clothes on a high rod and active motion of the left arm to the left in abduction and scaption were painful.

Treatment

Although his knee injury was acute and the shoulder injury related to overuse, the treatment plans for both involved joints had certain similarities. To decrease pain and inflammation, the shoulder was initially placed in a sling and the knee was taped. The physician started AG on antiinflammatory medication. Ice was applied to the knee for 15 minutes every 2 hours for 48 hours. He was to discontinue performing, participating in dance class, and rehearsing for 7 to 10 days. During this time, he was seen by the physical therapist that traveled with his company for modalities and soft-tissue mobilization.

After 7 days, the shoulder sling was discontinued, and a flexible knee support replaced immobilization taping, except when the client was dancing. Upper extremity and lower extremity active exercises were resumed for all uninvolved joints. Treatment included local heat and ultrasound followed by soft-tissue mobilization, joint releases, and gentle stretches. Range-of-motion exercises were carried out for the shoulder using a redaptor stick to provide assistance. Supine leg raises and seated knee extensions were used to begin strengthening the knee. Isometric strengthening was started for the scapula, rotator cuff muscles, and the quadriceps. Any exercise causing pain was discontinued for a few days, to be retried later.

At 2 weeks postinjury, the client was started on graded trunk strengthening exercises and was allowed to return to partial participation in dance classes. Restrictions included no elevation and no partnering. Before returning to class, he was observed while performing a full range of motion of the shoulder and knee to monitor joint alignment. The knee was checked in all positions of flexion while weight bearing, and he was to avoid jumping. He was instructed to avoid any painful motion of his injured shoulder or knee. Before each class, the client was to carry out a careful and extended warm-up period to increase his circulation and help avoid further injury. After class he was to stretch thoroughly and do slow AROM exercises before showering.

To regain his technical skills, the client was returned to full and regular dance classes. He also returned to practicing with a gymnastics coach to work on techniques for the acrobatic parts of his role. Strengthening exercises, both isotonic and isokinetic, were started for the scapular stabilizers of the rotator cuff and for the knee. After practice sessions to regain skills, any areas of discomfort or inflammation were treated with heat or ultrasound, soft-tissue mobilization, and stretching.

The client followed a graded plan to increase his endurance. Small increases in time for each portion of the workout were made every 5 days unless he complained of painful symptoms. Day six was a day for rest on which he cut back his time of practicing by one-third.

Technical and therapeutic workouts helped this client regain strength and endurance over a period of 6 weeks, but the necessary elements of speed, timing, and coordination with his fellow performers were still needed. To achieve this, he started to rehearse with the company again. His return to rehearsals was stressful, but he had an opportunity for part-time work when he was offered the chance to return as an understudy for his replacement. After 1 week of rehearsals he began to perform two or three of the eight weekly performances.

His return to pain-free dancing and acrobatics eventually allowed him to resume his job. To ensure his success, the following small changes were carried out in consultation with the company stage director: (1) The location of spotlights in the dance that caused his injury was changed to assure full vision, (2) the choreography was altered to reduce the need for use of his left arm as an assist to the other dancers as they turned, and (3) his costume was modified to remove some bulk and weight over his abdomen and arms.

SUMMARY OF IMPORTANT CONSIDERATIONS WHEN TREATING PERFORMING ARTISTS

These cases demonstrate that many factors contribute to the development of MSDs in performing artists. Common causes of musculoskeletal accidents and chronic injuries include physical factors such as body proportions, training and skill, strength and endurance, and kinesthetic awareness. However, the emotional factors, including fatigue, concentration, and performance stress, also make significant contributions to the degree of severity. Training or coaching influences the performing artist because some coaches encourage overly aggressive training or are poorly informed about the signs of MSDs in their students. Finally, workplace environment factors play an important role.

The guidelines for treatment include the following.

- Provide adequate conditioning for the performance task. Include proximal as well as distal conditioning.
- Focus treatment on establishing and maintaining requisite technical skills, physical preparedness, and emotional fitness.
- Be aware of the need for good alignment at all joints.
- Encourage the client to rest appropriately. Remember these clients tend to work even if injured. If an injury is not allowed to heal properly, it may become chronic and cause permanent disability.

CONCLUSION

Performing artists are a client population with unique talents, skills, and needs. Their dreams and enthusiasms make them dynamic clients. The therapist who provides care to them must be involved in their art, ready to understand their special life, and willing to devote time and study to serving them.

REFERENCES

Ackermann, B. (2002). Managing the musculoskeletal health of musicians on tour. *Medical Problems of Performing Artists, 17*(2), 63-67.

Ackermann, B., Adams, R., Marshall, E. (2002). Strength or endurance training for undergraduate music majors at a university? *Medical Problems of Performing Artists, 17*(1), 33-41.

Aronen, J. G. (1985). Problems of the upper extremity in gymnasts. *Clinics of Sports Medicine, 4*(1), 61-72.

Babin, A. (1999). Orchestra pit sound level measurements in Broadway shows. *Medical Problems of Performing Artists, 14*(4), 204-209.

Barr, A. E., & Barbe, M. F. (2002). Pathophysiological tissue changes associated with repetitive movement: A review of the evidence. *Physical Therapy, 82*(2), 173-187.

Barron, O., & Eaton, R. (1998). The upper limb of the performing artist. In R. Sataloff, A. Brandfonbrener, & R. Lederman (Eds.), *Performing Arts Medicine* (pp.231-260). San Diego, CA: Singular Publishing Group.

Berque, P., & Gray, H. (2002). The influence of neck-shoulder pain on trapezius muscle activity among professional violin and viola players. *Medical Problems of Performing Artists, 17*(2), 68-75.

Brandfonbrener, A. G. (1999). Theatrical patients in a performing arts practice. *Medical Problems of Performing Artists, 14*(1), 21-24.

Brodsky, M. (2001). Kabuki actors study. *Medical Problems of Performing Artists, 16*(3), 94–98.

Bronner, S., & Brownstein, B. (1997). Profile of dance injuries in a Broadway show: A discussion of issues in dance medicine epidemiology. *Journal of Orthopaedic and Sports Physical Therapy, 26*(2), 87–94.

Carvajal, S. C., & Evans, R. I. (1998). Risk factors for injury in the career female dancer: An epidemiologic study of a Broadway sample of performers. *Medical Problems of Performing Artists, 13*(3), 89–93.

Cayea, D., & Manchester, R. A. (1998). Instrument-specific rates of upper-extremity injuries in music students. *Medical Problems of Performing Artists, 13*(1), 19–25.

Chamagne, P. (1998). *Education physique preventive pour les musiciens*. Dijon-Quetigny, France: Darantiere.

Davies, C. (2002). Musculoskeletal pain from repetitive strain in musicians: Insights into an alternative approach. *Medical Problems of Performing Artists, 17*(1), 42–49.

Dawson, W. J. (1997). Common problems of wind instrumentalists. *Medical Problems of Performing Artists, 12*(4), 107–111.

Dawson, W. J. (1999). Carpal tunnel syndrome in instrumentalists: A review of 15 years' clinical experience. *Medical Problems of Performing Artists, 14*(1), 25–29.

Dawson, W. J. (2001). Upper extremity difficulties in the dedicated amateur instrumentalist. *Medical Problems of Performing Artists, 16*(4), 152–160.

Dommerholt, J., Norris, R. N., & Shaheen M. (1998). Therapeutic management of the instrumental musician. In R. Sataloff, A. Brandfonbrener, & R. Lederman (Eds.), *Performing Arts Medicine* (pp. 277–290). San Diego, CA: Singular Publishing Group.

Frederickson, K R. (2002). Fit to play: Musicians' health tips. *Music Educators Journal*, 38–44.

Garrick, J. G., & Lewis, S. (2001). Career hazards for the dancer (Review). *Occupational Medicine, 16*(4), 609–618.

Haight, H. (1998). Morphologic, physiologic, and functional interactions in elite female ballet dancers. *Medical Problems of Performing Artists, 13*(1), 4–13.

Harper, B. S. (2002). Workplace and health: A survey of classical orchestral musicians in the United Kingdom and Germany. *Medical Problems of Performing Artists, 17*(2), 83–92.

Harvey, J. S. (1983). Overuse syndromes in young athletes. *Clinics in Sports Medicine, 2*(3), 595–607.

Hoppmann, R. A. (1998). Musculoskeletal problems in instrumental musicians. In R. Sataloff, A. Brandfonbrener, & R. Lederman (Eds.), *Performing Arts Medicine* (pp. 205–229). San Diego, CA: Singular Publishing Group.

Horvath, J. (2001). An orchestra musician's perspective on 20 years of performing arts medicine. *Medical Problems of Performing Artists, 16*(3), 102–108.

Johnson, C. (2003). The musician. In M. Jacobs & N. Austin (Eds.), *Splinting the hand and upper extremity*. Philadelphia: Lippincott Williams & Wilkins.

Kahn, K., Brown, J., Way S., Vass N., Chrichton K., Alexander R., et al. (1995). Overuse injuries in classical ballet (Review). *Sports Medicine, 19*(5), 341–357.

Kirkendall, D. T. (1985). Physiologic aspects of gymnastics. *Clinics of Sports Medicine, 4*(1), 17–22.

Krasnow, D., & Kabboni, M. (1999). Dance science research and the modern dancer. *Medical Problems of Performing Artists, 14*(1), 16–20.

Krasnow, D., Monasterio, R., & Charfield, S. J. (2001). Emerging concepts of posture and alignment. *Medical Problems of Performing Artists, 16*(1), 8–16.

Laws, K., & Petrie, C. (1999). Momentum transfer in dance movement—vertical jumps: A research update. *Medical Problems of Performing Artists, 14*(3), 138–140.

Leanderson, J., Eriksson, E., Nilsson C., Wykman A. (1996). Proprioception in classical ballet dancers. *American Journal of Sports Medicine, 24*(3), 370–374.

Lewis, D. (1998). Health care for dance students at a performing arts academy: A dean's perspective. *Medical Problems of Performing Artists, 13*(3), 114–119.

Medoff, L. E. (1999). The importance of movement education in the training of young violinists. *Medical Problems of Performing Artists, 14*(4), 210–219.

Meinke, W. B. (1995). A proposed standardized medical history and physical form for musicians. *Medical Problems of Performing Artists, 10*(4), 137–139.

Meinke, W. B. (1998). Risks and realities of musical performance. *Medical Problems of Performing Artists, 13*(2), 56–60.

Newmark, J., & Weinstein, M. (1995). A proposed standard music medicine history and physical examination form. *Medical Problems of Performing Artists, 10*(4), 134–136.

Norris, R. (1993). *The musician's survival manual: A guide to preventing and treating injuries in instrumentalists.* S.l., International Conference of Symphony and Opera Musicians.

Norris, R. N., & Dommerholt, J. (1998). Applied ergonomics: Adaptive equipment and instrument modification for musicians. In R. Sataloff, A. Brandfonbrener, & R. Lederman (Eds.), *Performing Arts Medicine.* San Diego, CA: Singular Publishing Group.

Okner, M. A. O., Kernozek, T., & Wade, M. G. (1997). Chin rest pressure in violin players: Musical repertoire, chin rests, and shoulder pads as possible mediators. *Medical Problems of Performing Artists, 12*(4), 112–121.

Ostwald, P., Avery, M., & Ostwald L. D. (1998). Psychiatric problems of performing artists. In R. Sataloff, A. Brandfonbrener, & R. Lederman (Eds.), *Performing Arts Medicine* (pp. 337–348). San Diego, CA: Singular Publishing Group.

Pak, C., & Chesky, K. (2001). Prevalence of hand, finger, and wrist musculoskeletal problems in keyboard instrumentalists: The University of North Texas Musician Health Survey. *Medical Problems of Performing Artists, 16*(1), 17–23.

Ramel, E. M., & Moritz, U. (1998). Psychosocial factors at work and their association with professional ballet dancers' musculoskeletal disorders. *Medical Problems of Performing Artists, 13*(2), 66–74.

Sammarco, G. J. (1983). The dancer's hip. *Clinics in Sports Medicine, 2*(3), 485–505.

Sammarco, G. J., & Tablante, E. B. (1998). Foot and ankle in dance. In R. Sataloff, A. Brandfonbrener, & R. Lederman (Eds.), *Performing Arts Medicine* (pp. 301–319). San Diego, CA: Singular Publishing Group.

Seals, J. G. (1983). A study of dance surfaces. *Clinics in Sports Medicine, 2*(3) 557–561.

Semmler, C. J. (1998). Harp aches. *Medical Problems of Performing Artists, 13*(1), 35–39.

Solomon, R., Solomon, J., Micheli, L. J., & McGray, Jr. E. (1999). The "cost" of injuries in a professional ballet company: A five-year study. *Medical Problems of Performing Artists, 14*(4), 164–170.

Spahn, C., Ell, N., & Seidenglanz, K. (2001). Psychosomatic findings in musician patients at a department of hand surgery. *Medical Problems of Performing Artists, 16*(4), 144–151.

Spence, C. (2001). Prevalence rates for medical problems among flautists: A comparison of the UNT-Musician Health Survey and the Flute Health Survey. *Medical Problems of Performing Artists, 16*(3), 99–101.

Stretanski, M. (2002). Medical and rehabilitation issues in classical ballet. *American Journal of Physical Medicine and Rehabilitation, 81*(5), 383–391.

Sugano, A., & Laws, K. (2002). Physical analysis as a foundation for pirouette training. *Medical Problems of Performing Artists, 17*(1), 29–32.

Thrasher, M., & Chesky, K. (2001). Prevalence of medical problems among double reed performers. *Medical Problems of Performing Artists, 16*(4), 157–160.

Wenning, P. B., & O'Connell, D. O. (1999). Plantar stresses induced by inclined surfaces while standing. *Medical Problems of Performing Artists, 14*(4), 180–186.

Zaza, C., Fleiszer, M., Maine, F. W., & Merchefske, C. (2000). Beating injury with a different drumstick: A pilot study. *Medical Problems of Performing Artists, 15*(1), 39–43.

RESOURCES

Here are a few sources for instrument equipment.

David Gage String Instrument Repair
36 Walker Street
New York, NY 10013
212-274-1322

Mooradian Cover Company—Padded covers for instruments
65 Sprague Street
Boston, MA 02136
617-492-8930

Altus Handmade Professional Flutes
1-800-806-7965

Robertson and Sons Violin Shop, Inc.
3201 Carlisle NE
Albuquerque, NM 87110
505-889-2999 or 800 284-6546

The Abell Flute Company
111 Grovewood Road
Ashville, NC 28804
828-254-1004

Forrests Double Reed Specialists
1849 University Avenue
Berkeley, CA 94703
510-845-7178

APPENDIX 23-1

History Form for Use when Evaluating a Musician with a Musculoskeletal Disorder

Personal Data

Patient's name: ____________________ Date: __________

Date of birth: __________ Age: __________ Gender: __________

Instrument(s): ____________________

Referred by: ____________________

Referred for: ____________________

Medical Data

Patient description of problem (including duration and intensity of symptoms): __________

____

____

If patient has been referred, what was given as the diagnosis? __________

____

____

Was the patient ever evaluated or treated by other medical professionals? __________

When? In what sequence? Was any previous treatment successful? __________

____

____

____

Is patient being treated at the present time? __________

Body type: ____________________

Posture: ____________________

Does patient have a history of neck or back problems? __________

Does he/she exercise regularly? __________

Physical Examination Findings

____

____

____

____

Professional/Musical History

Type of performer (i.e., student, amateur, teacher, professional performer; full- or part-time):

____

____

Performing employment status (i.e., freelance, concertizing, theater pit, church, combination):

____

Years playing this instrument: ____________

Employed by: ____

Professional responsibilities and schedule or school where enrolled (include academic and music schools):

____

____

Schedule of academic and performance activities:

____

Teachers/training/technical background: ______________________________

Style of music played: ____

Professional/musical goals of patient: ______________________________

____

Any change of teacher, technique, work load, instrument setup, style that coincided with onset of symptoms:

____

Recent increases in practicing (may be related to competitions, performances, auditions, etc.):

____

Practicing habits (including comments on regularity, location, time of day, instrument, use of practice time):

____

____

Does patient believe the problem relates to a specific piece of music or a specific technical challenge?

____

Psychosocial/Lifestyle History

Does the patient have a family that includes other performers? ______________________

____

Does the patient have a nonmusic job? Could it relate to his/her problem? ______________

____

Has the patient suffered any recent trauma, emotional or physical? ________________

____

Evaluation with Instrument

Technical correctness and proficiency: ______________________________

____

Posture and body mechanics: ______________________________

____

Can patient demonstrate techniques that he/she feels cause his/her problem? ___________

____

CHAPTER 24

Addressing Musculoskeletal Disorders at Computer Workstations

Judy Sehnal

THE AUTOMATED OFFICE ENVIRONMENT

The use of computers in the workplace was once associated with clerical job functions. However, as technology has moved forward, computers have quickly become standard equipment in offices, schools, retail businesses, laboratories, design firms, and other environments. Computers now are used by more people in a larger variety of capacities than ever before. It has been estimated that more than 80 million computers were in use in 1991 and more than 100 million by year 2000 (Tittiranonda, Burastero, & Rempel, 1999). The proliferation of computers in the workplace is due at least in part to their versatility and capacity for detailed operations. Computers and software can handle many operations previously performed by manual procedures. Computers add value to business operations by increasing productivity, quality, and customer service.

With an increase in the frequency, intensity, and popularity of computer use inside and outside of work and at home, the incidence of work-related illnesses and injuries has increased. With more computer users seeking treatment, healthcare professionals are seeing more clients with computer-related musculoskeletal disorders (MSDs). Although therapists provide the necessary treatment, preventive services are ultimately more cost effective. This chapter provides background on MSDs in the automated office environment and elsewhere. Proactive and reactive approaches to addressing this issue are addressed.

The Changing Office Environment: Why MSDs Occur

A commonly asked question is why computer operators develop MSDs when, historically, those using typewriters did not experience these problems. The answer to this question is multifaceted.

Keyboard Design

The design of the keyboard is one factor in the incidence of MSDs among computer operators (Barry, 1993; Bureau of National Affairs, Inc., 1994). Standard typewriter keyboards and most contemporary keyboards conform to the QWERTY keyboard layout, referring to the letter-number-symbol sequence of the keys. The top row of alpha keys in this layout begins on the left with the letters QWERTY. This layout was designed to distribute keystrokes over the entire keyboard and thereby prevent jamming of keys as typists' keyboard skills and speed increased. Thus, manual and even electric typewriters provided a built-in system to pace workers. In addition, the typewriter requires inputting interruptions for paper replacement and correction of errors. Finally, many typists were trained on technique and appropriate use of the typewriter.

The standard computer keyboard still conforms to the QWERTY layout. However, the advanced technology of computers can handle unlimited inputting speed. From a biomechanical perspective, this presents a dilemma in that faster typing and inputting speeds are supported technologically by the system but not physically by key layout. This technology has also eliminated the opportunity for work interruptions and changes of posture related to paper changes and error corrections. In addition, the keys of the computer keyboard are closer to the work surface, making the work surface more accessible to the wrist and forearms for support. The result is a greater propensity for awkward and sustained postures during computer keyboard use.

Work Practices

The computer itself probably is no more demanding of workers than older equipment replaced or supplemented by computerization, such as manual typewriters, accounting machines, keypunch machines, and switchboards. However, the capacity of computer equipment allows people to work faster and, perhaps, more intensely.

Because task variety is reduced, yielding to increased repetitiveness of some job tasks and decreased postural changes, computer-related physical discomfort is likely to arise from long periods (more than several hours per day) of highly routine duties. Problems of visual or postural discomfort reported by computer users are probably not related to any intrinsic property of computers but rather to how the computer is used. Individual characteristics of stature, work habits, the nature of the job, and the design of the equipment and workplace each play a role in affecting worker comfort.

Job Design and Psychosocial Factors

In addition to the differences between typewriter and computer keyboard use, the advent and development of computer technology has changed significantly the way many jobs are done. Work practices, work methods, sequence of tasks, and intensity of visual attention are some factors that have changed. Today's computer-intensive jobs tend to require less physical body movement and more cognitive attention and concentration.

Psychosocial factors weigh heavily in the development and management of MSDs. Technological advances may be accompanied by a limited sense of competence and control that may manifest in physical symptoms (Carayon & Smith, 2000; Karasek & Theorell, 1990). These concerns affect motivation and job satisfaction.

The importance of psychosocial factors, workplace organization, and work systems design as a potential cause of employee injury was reinforced by the National Institute for Occupational Safety and Health (NIOSH) report (1992), which identified seven key psychosocial factors that indicate upper-extremity musculoskeletal injury and symptoms. Among these factors are fear of being replaced by a computer, jobs that have a variable workload, increasing work pressure, lack of production standard, lack of job diversity with little decision-making opportunity, high information processing demands, surges in workload, uncertainty about one's job future, lack of co-worker support, and lack of supervisor's support (see Chapters 8 and 12 for further discussion).

Faucett and Rempel (1994) investigated musculoskeletal symptoms among newspaper employees who use computers daily, examining the independent and combined effects of posture at the computer workstation and psychosocial work factors related to job characteristics and interpersonal relationships. Researchers found that more hours per day of computer use and less decision latitude on the job were significant risk factors for the development of MSDs. They postulated that greater psychologic workload may contribute to musculoskeletal symptoms by increasing background muscle activity, muscle strain and fatigue, intolerance of physical discomfort, and anxiety. Work stress, especially time pressure, may increase the speed and force of keying and may compound the effects of a workstation that is not ergonomically adjusted to fit the individual employee. In contrast, control over job decisions may act to buffer the effects of a maladjusted workstation. Greater work stress raises general symptom awareness and may make symptoms less tolerable.

There is also an association between musculoskeletal symptoms and the relationship with the supervisor. When the supervisory relationship is good, better workstation ergonomics is associated with less severe symptoms. When the supervisory relationship is not good, better workstation ergonomics is associated with more severe symptoms.

Most (1999) found that ergonomic interventions are more effective when psychosocial aspects of the jobs are evaluated. Biomechanical or physiologic approaches alone did not explain the cause of the increase in MSDs in a large call center operation. Other factors, including work organization and work systems design (including worker control), needed to be addressed in order to reduce psychologic strain. Further, a difference in supervisors' and employees' perceptions of job demand impacted the pain experienced by the employee.

Computer Operation Job Description

Many types of businesses are well suited to computer operations, and some have become extremely computer-dependent. Among the more common such industries are insurance, banking, mail-order sales, clerical work, and telephone operations.

New hardware and software products are expanding traditional computer applications. For example, police officers have access to criminal and other databases on the road via computers installed in their police vehicles. It is reasonable to expect that in this current climate of technologic development, the use of computers in traditional and other settings will continue to expand.

Job functions specific to computer operations can be identified through a functional job analysis. Individuals who use computers for any purpose are required to perform a combination of the following job tasks.

- Inputting information
- Operating input devices (keyboard, mouse, trackball, pen, tablet)
- Calling up information from the computer and reading it from the display
- Reviewing information on the screen
- Referencing source documents
- Entering or recalling text or graphic information, controlling text for errors, keying in corrections, and designing layout
- Paying attention visually
- Scanning visually (display, source documents)

The frequency, duration, and intensity of inputting and other job functions varies from job to job and from setting to setting. It has been estimated that a typist, typing 60 words per minute for 7 hours, may actually perform 126,000 repetitions with the hands (Ross, 1994). Data-entry work is characterized by continuous inputting, whereas customer service and sales work more commonly require intermittent inputting. Work speed in data entry is high; it is not uncommon for a worker to perform 8000 to 12,000 keystrokes per hour (Grandjean, 1987). Mital, Kilbom, and Kumar (2000) estimate data entry keystrokes at 35 per minute, or 2100 per hour, or 140,000 per day, or 2,940,000 per month, or 32,900,000 strokes per year. The repetitiveness of individual finger movements for a touch typist is controlled in part by distribution of the workload across all fingers. Even so, it is clear that repetition is a risk factor associated with computer-related tasks.

Employers and regulatory bodies that have attempted to develop guidelines for ergonomic programs have used definitions of *light, moderate,* and *heavy computer use* to identify, prioritize, and target high-exposure jobs. In many cases, these definitions are based on hours of use per day. In fact, the U.S. Occupational Safety and Health Administration (OSHA) has proposed the use of time intervals as a measure of risk (U.S. Department of Labor, OSHA, 1994). Some companies have determined that ergonomic exposure in jobs requiring 4 or more hours of input per day is sufficient to warrant attention. Nevertheless, ergonomic exposure or risk in jobs that do not meet this criterion must still be considered. For example, intense inputting for less than 4 hours can be injurious. On the other hand, intermittent inputting over long periods of time may not be a significant exposure.

In addition to actual computer use, there are other tasks common to computer-intensive jobs that may contribute to ergonomic risk. Some of these tasks are telephone use, writing, filing, and calculator use. Sorting, stapling, staple removal, and hole punching are other job functions that may pose ergonomic risk in the office environment.

COMPUTERS AND MSDS

Cost and Incidence of MSDs

Potential cost exposures for computer-related claims are significant. Most computer-oriented operations have experienced at least one computer-related injury. The average cost of claims generated by computer-related injuries or illnesses ranges from $6000 to $35,000. Although many claim cost estimates include medical expenses paid and anticipated, most do not include costs associated with time away from work or employee replacement or training.

There is little direct information available on the incidence and cost of upper-extremity and computer-related MSDs. Statistical data available from the U.S. Department of Labor, Bureau of Labor Statistics (BLS) report the incidence of MSDs and lost and restricted time related to MSDs as a whole. Categories of MSDs are not specified, although data by business type are available. According to BLS data, the number of reported MSDs rose from 23,000 in 1981 to 223,600 in 1991 (a ninefold increase over 10 years). These figures represent 18% of all occupational illnesses in 1981 and 61% of all occupational illnesses in 1991, respectively (Webster & Snook, 1994). The BLS *Survey of Occupational Injuries and Illnesses, 1992* (U.S. Department of Labor, BLS, 1994) indicated that most workplace illnesses were disorders associated with repeated trauma (approximately 282,000), such as carpal tunnel syndrome (CTS). Furthermore, trade, finance, and service industries together accounted for almost all of the 1991 to 1992 increase in injury and illness rates (Murray, 1994). These are the industry groups in which we see phenomenal growth in automation and computer ergonomic exposure. According to BLS data, as shown in Table 24-1, the number of repeated trauma cases increased to 332,000 in 1994 and has steadily decreased through 2001. However, the number of repeated trauma cases reported by the industry groups that would be considered office operations has remained relatively steady and, in fact, in some cases (e.g., business and health services), has actually shown a general increase. In contrast, the number of recordable repeated trauma cases reported in manufacturing has steadily decreased since 1993 (BLS, 1995, 2001).

Workplace Injuries and Illnesses Related to Computer Workstations

A variety of MSDs has been associated with working in an automated office, and particularly with computers. Common diagnoses that may be associated with work in the automated office environment include CTS, tendinitis, tenosynovitis, and de Quervain's disease (also see Chapters 5, 6, and 7). CTS has, unfortunately, become a catch-all category but clearly is not the only disorder that occurs in this environment. In fact, there are many cases in which the general aches, pains, and discomforts that are reported cannot be specifically diagnosed. Visual problems reported among these workers include eyestrain, burning or itching eyes, blurred or double vision, deteriorations of visual acuity, and headaches (Bergqvist & Knave, 1993).

The incidence of these disorders by occupation has not been definitively established. However, Leavitt and Taslitz (1993) refer to three studies that address incidence and risk. In one study of 2876 telephone operators, 86% reported neck or back pain, 78% indicated arm or shoulder pain, and 14% developed cysts on hands or wrists; in 9%, CTS was medically diagnosed. A

Table 24-1
Recordable Cases of Repeated Trauma (000s)

				Finance					**Service**			
	Total	Mfg	Trade	Fin	Srv	Ins Car	Ins Ag	Bus Srv	Eng	Lgl	Educ	Hlth
1992	281.8	219.9	20.2	11.4	17.3	0.5	0.8	2.9	1.9	1.0	0.5	6.5
1993	302.4	226.9	22.5	14.4	23.3	0.4	0.6	4.8	1.8	1.5	1.2	8.5
1994	332.1	248.9	26.0	13.1	27.2	0.5	1.1	5.7	2.4	1.5	1.7	9.6
1995	308.2	230.9	23.7	11.2	26.8	0.4	1.0	6.0	2.5	1.3	1.1	10.1
1996	281.1	203.9	22.8	12.4	28.2	0.3	1.2	6.2	2.7	1.7	0.8	11.4
1997	276.6	198.6	23.1	13.1	27.1	0.5	1.1	5.2	2.6	0.9	0.8	10.2
1998	253.3	180.9	20.9	12.0	27.0	0.4	1.4	5.8	2.4	1.1	0.8	11.9
1999	246.7	172.4	19.1	11.5	27.7	0.4	0.6	4.7	3.0	0.8	0.7	12.7
2000	241.8	163.9	20.4	14.9	29.1	0.6	0.9	4.7	3.2	1.0	0.7	13.5
2001	216.4	141.0	18.4	12.4	30.6	0.4	0.9	6.8	2.9	1.0	0.8	13.3

Bus Srv, Business services; *Eng,* engineering and management services; *Educ,* educational services; *Fin,* finance, insurance, and real estate; *Hlth,* health services, *Ins Ag,* insurance agents, brokers, and services; *Ins Car,* insurance carriers; *Lgl,* legal services; *Mfg,* manufacturing; *Srv,* services; *Trade,* wholesale and retail trade.
Source: U.S. Department of Labor Bureau of Labor Statistics (BLS)

study of 533 communications workers reported upper-extremity musculoskeletal disorders in 22% of all workers, with the hand-wrist area most frequently involved (12% of participants). A 5-year study of 15 occupational groups, including butchers and meat cutters, found data-entry operators to be at the second greatest level of risk for developing CTS, followed by dental hygienists.

A report on CTS by the Work Loss Data Institute (2001) indicates that the prevalence of CTS increases by 56.77% in data entry and typing positions. In contrast, a Mayo Clinic study identified no correlation between computer work and CTS, finding that CTS in computer users to be similar to that in the general population (Stevens, Witt, Smith, & Weaver, 2001). Possible reasons contributing to the discrepancy in findings include differences in sample size and diagnostic criteria.

MSDs associated with the automated office environment most commonly affect anatomic structures of the fingers, hand, forearm, and upper arm (Kroemer, 1992). Disorders of the neck and back, which have gone more or less unreported in the past, are surfacing now with greater frequency. The causal relationship between muscular activity and MSDs remains uncertain. If a causal relationship between work activities and MSDs is presumed, the exact job factors are not well defined (Kroemer, 1992).

Hales, Sauter, Peterson, Fine, Putz-Anderson, (1994) found that 22% of 573 directory assistance operators at U.S. West Communications met the case definition for potential work-related upper-extremity MSDs. The most common disorders were tendon-related (15%), probable muscle-related (8%), probable nerve entrapment (4%), ganglion cyst (3%), and joint-related (3%). The hand-wrist was the area most affected, followed by the neck, elbow, and shoulder.

NIOSH (1992) conducted a survey and found that 40% of 834 newspaper employees reported symptoms suggestive of MSDs. The hand-wrist was the most common area identified in complaints (23%), followed by the neck (17%), elbow and forearm (13%), and shoulder (11%).

Ergoweb (2001) recognizes the danger in generalizing and summarizes the data as follows.

- Approximately 22% to 40% of computer operators experience MSDs.
- The body areas primarily affected by computer activity are the neck, wrist, elbow, and shoulder.

- Eye and low-back complaints can be significant but were not included in studies that delineated categories of injuries.
- The most common injury or illness is tendonitis, followed by muscle strain or sprain.

From a risk-management perspective, it is advisable to focus on proactive early identification of those symptoms and related exposures. Without an active, effective program, the preventable and treatable aches and pains may go unrecognized and develop into more serious problems that may be more difficult or perhaps impossible to remedy.

Symptoms

The symptoms of MSDs in the office environment include discomfort, pain, tingling, numbness, swelling, weakness, and loss of dexterity (see Chapter 6). Symptoms occur at varying levels of intensity, from mild to severe. Any symptom at any level should be heeded as a possible warning sign, particularly if it occurs with any degree of severity, regularity, or consistency. In the office worker, the earliest indication of a potential developing MSD can be discomfort. The discomfort may begin or persist during periods of heavy workload. Discomfort and pain may be generalized or specific and may develop over varying periods of time. Additional symptoms usually occur in a specific identifiable body location.

Intervention

There are three approaches to intervention. The first is *prevention*. Issues of comfort in the workstation must be addressed before symptoms develop. This can be done through engineering design and training programs supported by routine follow-up.

A second approach is *symptomatic treatment*. Workstation modification or alternative work assignments may be necessary as physical corrections. Medical intervention may include modalities (e.g., application of ice), medication (antiinflammatory drugs), splints, work restrictions, or rest. Wrist splints may be effective for night use. However, when splints are used in the workplace, symptoms may be masked or diverted to other areas of the body. Close communication between the therapist and involved medical providers is necessary.

The third approach is *surgery*, a treatment method that, in many instances, can be avoided through effective training programs or effective intervention at the first report of symptoms. Early identification of symptoms and early intervention are necessary. Surgery is a last-resort treatment (see Chapter 3 for further discussion).

From an occupational health perspective, the most effective intervention for all work-related disorders is prevention. A proactive health and safety program with a strong emphasis on ergonomics is an effective tool. Early identification of worker discomfort and hazardous conditions is a key ergonomic program element and requires a clear understanding of the symptoms and risk factors associated with work-related disorders.

When reported early enough, most cases of work-related injury or illness involve short-term discomfort and not permanent injury. Scalet (1987) states, "Almost all of these complaints can be alleviated or avoided by proper attention to the workstation, the work environment, and the design of work."

Risk Factors

The adverse health effects of many workplace hazards do not become immediately apparent but may take years to develop. Although we cannot yet predict specific injuries, we are able to identify common risk factors associated with MSDs in the automated office environment. Tittiranonda et al. (1999) associate specific risk factors, including repetitive and sustained exertions, forceful exertions, awkward postures, and localized mechanical stresses, with computer work (for a complete discussion of risk factors, see Chapter 10).

Static Posture

Static positioning has become an issue of equal importance to repetitive motion in office work.

Numerous office workers spend many hours each day performing work at the computer, with little opportunity to move around or change position. During inputting, motion is greater in the distal joints of the upper extremity, although the proximal musculature statically supports the distal movements. When the hands and fingers are not actively keying, the entire upper extremity often is in a static "ready" position. Stiffness and fatigue occur in response to static postures, even when good principles of body mechanics are applied. Task variation and workstation exercises can be effective in reducing or eliminating static postures. It is important that employees vary tasks as much as their jobs will allow, in order to achieve changes of position. Employees should take scheduled breaks. It has been advised that employees who regularly work at computers for 4 or more hours daily be encouraged to perform stretches or some alternate tasks each hour.

Awkward Posture

The rules of good body mechanics suggest that neutral body postures are most efficient and effective. Awkward postures bring the body out of alignment and are less efficient and effective. All joints move through a specified range of motion. Postures in the middle of the range of motion are generally considered to be neutral postures. Postures at the end of the range can be considered awkward. Common awkward postures observed in the office environment involve the neck, back, shoulders, and wrists. For example, back flexion is observed as the computer operator leans forward away from the back of the chair. Neck extension occurs when the monitor is too high and the operator must look up to the screen. Wrist extension occurs when the keyboard is too low and the wrists rest on the work surface or the edge of the keyboard. Wrist flexion occurs when the keyboard is too high. When the keyboard is too far away, shoulder flexion allows the operator to reach the keys. Awkward postures include asymmetric postures. Asymmetric posture caused by neck or trunk rotation occurs when the computer monitor is located off-center relative to the keyboard. Awkward postures can occur as a result of poor work habits, poorly designed furniture and equipment configuration, and other factors.

Prolonged awkward postures of the head, neck, and upper extremities can contribute to complaints of pain, parathesias, and numbness, having the following three major consequences (Novak & MacKinnon, 1997).

1. Placing increased pressure on nerves by increasing pressure in entrapped nerve sites or by placing tension on nerves. For example, wrist flexion and extension has been shown to increase pressure within the carpal canal, thus increasing pressure on the median nerve. Elbow flexion increases pressure within the cubital tunnel, causing increased pressure on the ulnar nerve.
2. Placing muscles in shortened position. Over time, muscles will adaptively shorten. When the shortened muscle is stretched, local discomfort can occur. A shortened muscle can also compress a nerve (e.g., tightness of the pronator teres muscle can cause compression of the median nerve in the forearm).
3. Creating muscle imbalance that results in musculoskeletal misalignment. Anatomic, biomechanical, and physiologic changes in the muscles cause muscle weakness. For example, a head-forward and scapular-abducted position as might occur when the computer is located too far from the user can cause muscle imbalance in the cervicoscapular region. Tightness of the pectoralis minor and scalene muscles may compress the brachial plexus. Weakness of the middle and lower trapezius and serratus anterior may cause overuse of the upper trapezius and levator scapulae. There are several entrapment sites in the upper extremity commonly cited for their ability to compress the median nerve, ulnar nerve, radial nerve, and brachial plexus (see Chapters 5 and 6).

Repetition

The most common occurrences of repetitive movements involve the fingers, wrists, and neck. High-frequency keystroke is responsible for repetitive finger movements in many input-intensive jobs. Repetitive wrist movements can be observed as operators reach for some keys, particularly function keys. Repetitive neck movements occur as the visual reference point changes from monitor to document to keyboard.

Amounts of actual input vary from job to job, but in many cases inputting is intermittent (as described in the Computer Operation Job Description section of this chapter). Repetitive movements can be related to other than computer job functions. Stapling, staple removal, hole punching, filing, and sorting tasks all require significant repetitive movements of various joints.

Force

Force is another factor that creates muscle fatigue and stress. Applying too much force to the keyboard creates unnecessary pressure and shock to the complex hand, wrist, and arm structures, including tendons and nerves. Current standards recommend an upper limit "make" force (actuation force) of 1.5 N (ANSI, 1988). Feuerstein, Armstrong, Hickey, and Lincoln (1997) measured keyboard force to determine whether office workers who report more severe levels of musculoskeletal symptoms of the upper extremities demonstrate higher levels of keyforce in comparison to controls with less severe symptoms. Cases generated significantly higher keyboarding forces (3.5 N) than controls (2.8 N). Both groups exerted more force than actually required to operate the keyboard (0.72 N). These results suggest that generation of excessive force while working on a computer keyboard may contribute to the severity of upper-extremity symptoms.

Gerard, Armstrong, Franzblau, Martin, and Rempel (1999) reviewed typing force studies and report that these studies found that, on average, subjects exerted between 2.5 and 7.9 times as much force as required to activate the keys. The results of their study investigating the effects of keyswitch stiffness on typing force, finger electromyography, and subjective discomfort suggest that increasing actuation force causes typing and EMG to increase. Subjective discomfort was higher for the keyboard with height actuation force.

Force can also be a factor in noncomputer job tasks, including stapling, staple removal, hole punching, and filing. In addition, many workers use unnecessarily tight grips on pens and pencils. Light touch and skillful use of many fingers may reduce muscle fatigue and strain significantly.

Physical Contact or Mechanical Stress

Prolonged physical contact with the work surface or equipment can impair blood circulation and nerve function. Common examples of physical contact include wrists "planted" on the work surface or edge of the keyboard during inputting, forearms resting on the edge of the work surface, elbows resting on the armrests of the chair, and front edge of the chair seat pressing on backs of thighs or on the backs of legs at the knee.

Temperature Extremes

Temperature and humidity are also important environmental elements that clearly influence worker comfort and performance. Computers contribute additional heat and changes in air movement. Temperature variation in the office environment is generally not extreme. However, temperatures that are out of the range of normal comfort can affect posture. In cold environments, for example, circulation slows as blood vessels contract and posture becomes stiff. The strength of a muscle performing static work is reduced when muscle temperature is lowered below 30° C (86° F) (Phillips, 2000). Workers may feel restless and become easily distracted in an office that is too cold. Optimum summertime temperature ranges are 23° C to 26° C at 50% relative humidity. The range for wintertime is

20° C to 23.5° C at 50% relative humidity (Weir, 2000).

Workers may feel lethargic or tire quickly in an office that is too warm. An increase in ambient temperature may produce the following physiologic effects (Grandjean, 1988).

- Increased fatigue, with reduced efficiency in both physical and mental tasks
- Rise in heart rate
- Rise in blood pressure
- Reduced digestive organ activity
- Slight increase in core temperature and sharp rise in temperature of the skin
- Increase in blood flow through the skin (from a few ml/cm^3 of skin tissue per minute to 20 to 30 ml). The increased blood flow to the skin is a thermal regulatory adaptive response to transport heat to the skin, thereby cooling the body, and it occurs at the expense of blood supply to the musculature, compromising performance and efficiency of the motor system.
- Increased production of sweat

COMPONENTS OF AN OFFICE ERGONOMICS MANAGEMENT PROGRAM

In its *Ergonomics Program Management Guidelines for Meatpacking Plants*, OSHA (U.S. Department of Labor, OSHA, 1991) identified four major components of an effective ergonomics program that still form the rubric to many programs: (1) work site analysis, (2) hazard prevention and control, (3) medical management, and (4) training and education. These guidelines are comprehensive and applicable to office workers (see Chapter 14 for a complete discussion of the components). Components of these guidelines significantly applicable to the office environment address equipment, furniture, and job design. Recommendations are made for ongoing review and adjustment of equipment, furniture, and job specifications, as well as ergonomic review of proposed equipment and furniture purchases, new job functions, and changes in job functions. Employee involvement is also critical. Consideration of employee feedback regarding health, safety, and other job issues, and employee representation on the company's health and safety committee are key elements.

Educating office workers about health and wellness issues in the workplace and what they can do to achieve a comfortable environment is directed toward empowering workers to take responsibility for themselves and have some control over the work environment. Workers should be sensitive to their own limitations, whereas supervisors should be alert to differences among employees. Problems must be dealt with individually on a case-by-case basis. Complaints of discomfort must not be ignored.

There are various methods of providing training. A train-the-trainer approach is outlined in Table 24-2. Using this approach, individuals are selected to be trained as local resources who will be responsible for providing ergonomic awareness training to computer users and for performing routine workstation assessments. Trainee selection is critical to the effectiveness of such a program. It is important that the individuals selected have a genuine interest in the subject, have an ability to relate well to others, and have management support to carry out training and workstation assessment responsibilities.

WORKSTATION ASSESSMENT

Process

A workstation assessment is an evaluation of how a job is performed, taking into account the physical characteristics of the workstation as they relate to the performance of job functions. The purpose of a workstation assessment is to identify job performance factors or workstation features that may contribute to injury and to recommend corrective actions to eliminate or minimize these exposures and risk of injury. The first step in developing an effective workstation assessment program is to understand job tasks and workstation components. A typical workstation is composed of a variety of pieces of furniture and equipment. Some components of a typical workstation are listed in Box 24-1. Each of these components has its own characteristics, dimensions, and function. Information regarding where each piece is located and how it is used provides the basis of ergonomic workstation assessment.

It is important to observe the person performing job functions at the workstation for at least one full work cycle. The focus of a workstation assessment is primarily on the person's body posture and secondarily on the workstation configuration and the person and workstation interact. The following factors are considered during the workstation assessment process.

- Components of the physical workstation (including furniture, equipment, tools, and materials)
- Location, dimensions, and adjustability of the workstation components
- Job functions
- Work flow (including schedules, breaks, overtime, productivity standards)
- Body posture
- Lighting
- Noise

Key elements in the workstation assessment process are communication and timely response to requests for assistance. A recognized and

Table 24-2
Proposed Agenda for Train-the-Trainer Program

Time	Event
8:30-8:45	**Introduction** Facilitator(s), participants Participants' expectations of session Objectives, roles, and responsibilities
8:45-9:30	**Ergonomics training program** Program components
9:30-9:45	**Ergonomics** Definition Research facts Trends in the workplace Effects: productivity, quality, safety, profit
9:45-10:15	**Basic sciences and ergonomics** Anatomy and functional relationships Anthropometry and furniture and equipment design Body mechanics Ergonomic risk factors
10:15-10:30	**Break**
10:30-12:00	**Basics of workstation ergonomics** Workstation components and configuration Workstation assessment Checklists and other forms Workstation assessment demonstration (analysis of videotape/on-site assessment)
12:00-1:00	**Lunch**
1:00-2:30	**Basics of workstation ergonomics (continued)** Problem solving: simple practical changes Accessory use Follow-up and referral
2:30-2:45	**Break**
2:45-3:30	**Facilitation and training techniques** Presentation Typical questions and responses
3:30-4:00	**Discussion and questions**

Source: Developed by J. Sehnal for The Hartford, 1992.

BOX 24-1
Components of a Typical Workstation

Chair
Desk, work surface
Monitor
Central processing unit
Keyboard
Inputting devices
Document holder
Wrist rest
Footrest
Telephone
Calculator
Shelves
File cabinets
Waste can
Power cords
Lighting
Manuals
Paper
Writing utensils
Baskets (in-out)
Eyewear

organized method of recording and communicating workstation recommendations must be established. It is imperative that the employee understands the reasons for adjustments and is actively involved in making suggestions for the problem-solving process. Because the feasibility and practicality of alternative solutions varies, it is necessary to evaluate the advantages and disadvantages of each possibility before choosing and implementing one option. Optimally, the supervisor should also be actively involved in this process.

Protocol

A typical protocol for the workstation assessment process in a corporate computer ergonomics program is described in this section. Proactively, workstation assessments can be performed to identify exposures and implement corrective actions prior to the potential development of symptoms as part of the surveillance requirements of an effective program. Reactively, a timely workstation assessment must be performed in response to any report of symptoms or injury. The initial assessment should be performed within 2 to 3 days of the injury report.

Follow-up workstation assessments should be performed within 2 weeks of the initial assessment. Subsequent follow-ups can be scheduled at intervals determined individually by need. Follow-up can be discontinued after two symptom-free reviews or when maximum symptom improvement has been reached and no further workstation or job performance changes are required.

Follow-up is critical to the success of workstation assessment. The education and assessment involved in an ergonomic program must be ongoing. How this is achieved will probably differ somewhat at each location. In most cases, when an employee reports discomfort, the supervisor (if not already notified) and the local ergonomics resource person should be notified.

After the initial individual workstation assessment is completed, it is necessary to verify that the recommended changes were made. The changes must be reviewed within 1 to 2 weeks to determine their effectiveness. If the recommended changes were not made, it is necessary to determine why. The situation should be reassessed and action taken to ensure that the necessary changes are made. Follow-up assessments need not be as detailed or time-consuming as the initial assessment, but they must be thorough. Follow-up assessments can be documented on a workstation assessment form or in another format.

Feedback on the effectiveness of changes is a necessary component of the follow-up process. Both the employee and the supervisor are expected to provide this feedback. The medical department or personnel department may be included to complete the communication loop in the organization.

When symptoms are reported early, workstation or work-style changes are, in most cases, effective in eliminating the symptoms. However, some cases are not so easily resolved. These may require multiple workstation assessments and modifications.

In summary, critical components of an effective workstation-assessment protocol are as follows.

- Communication
- Timely response
- Thorough observation
- Ongoing education
- Feedback
- Follow-up

Documentation

Documentation of all workstation-assessment activity is necessary. Initial workstation assessment establishes the basis for subsequent follow-up assessments and helps determine the efficacy of intervention; an auditable paper trail demonstrates ergonomic program activity and implementation. A sample of a detailed workstation assessment form is provided in Appendix 24-1. This form provides a mechanism to document current job function, body positions, workstation features, comments relative to ergonomic concerns, possible causes and possible solutions, and recommended changes. Recommendations are recorded on the workstation assessment form. Changes that require assistance for implementation can be recorded on a work request form. Distribution of the workstation assessment form and the work request form can assist in the communication process.

Workstation checklists can also be used as self-assessment tools. A sample is provided in Appendix 24-2. This kind of checklist can be completed by every employee at the time of initial ergonomics awareness training and at least annually thereafter. The checklist should be reviewed by the supervisor with the employee to ensure that the review is accurate and complete and that necessary corrective actions have been taken.

Ergonomic Guidelines for Video Display Terminal Operators

Application of principles of good body mechanics eliminates or minimizes risk of injury in any workplace. Suggestions regarding posture and position of equipment in the office environment are based on principles of good body mechanics for seated work. The ergonomic guidelines for computer operators outlined in Box 24-2 are useful to computer operators as an educational tool and to those performing workstation assessments as an evaluation guide.

The optimal body position for computer operators is illustrated in Figure 24-1. Although the 90/100-90-90 posture (hips, knees, ankles, and elbows at 90 degrees) is recommended by many ergonomists, there is little evidence to indicate that one posture is optimal for all people or for all tasks. There is no one perfect posture for all office workers and no one posture can be maintained all day long. The most effective way to maintain comfort while working at a computer workstation is to use neutral postures and to change postures frequently throughout the day. Workers should be encouraged to move through a range of comfortable postures.

BOX 24-2
Ergonomic Guidelines for Video Display Terminal (VDT) Operators

Optimal Body Position for Seated VDT Work

1. Trunk upright with ears, shoulders, and hips in vertical alignment
2. Shoulders in symmetric, nonelevated position
3. Arch in back supported by back of chair or cushion insert
4. Feet flat on floor or on a footrest
5. Thighs supported evenly on chair and approximately parallel with floor
6. Upper arms close to the sides of the body
7. Forearms approximately parallel to floor
8. Wrists in neutral position

Optimal Equipment Position

1. Top line of monitor screen slightly below eye level or lower
2. Monitor screen at approximately 20 to 26 in from user's eyes
3. Keyboard and monitor positioned in alignment in front of user (when monitor is primary visual reference)
4. Keyboard (height) positioned such that home row (ASDF) is approximately at elbow level
5. Mouse (height) positioned at elbow level and as centrally as possible
6. Document holder located near monitor at same height and distance as is screen from user
7. Work surface at height to allow appropriate arm, wrist, and hand position while also allowing adequate leg space
8. Chair: seat and backrest height and angle adjusted to allow comfortable posture
9. Shelf height and location within comfortable reach
10. All frequently used equipment, manuals, and so on within comfortable reach

Note: The preceding criteria are provided as generic guidelines for comfortable and safe VDT operation. Variations in specifications may be acceptable and should be determined individually.
Source: Developed by J. Sehnal for The Hartford, 1993.

Common Observations during Workstation Assessment

The workstation assessment process calls for identification of deviations from neutral postures as well as identification of conditions that might be contributing to reported symptoms. Some typical postural observations and their

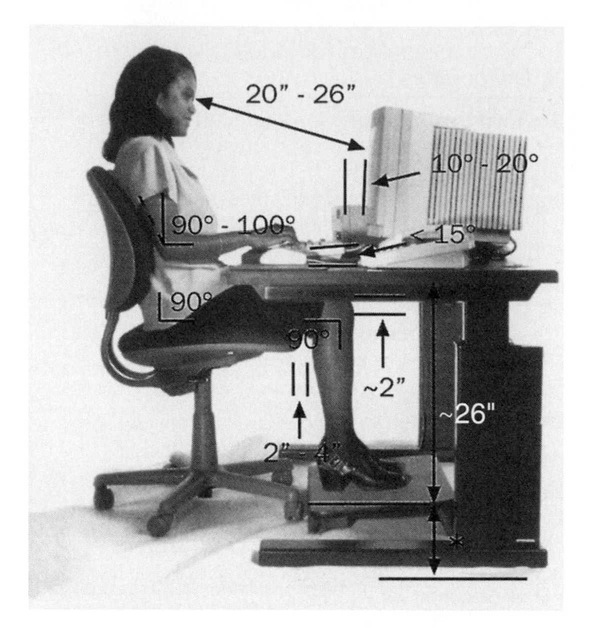

Figure 24-1 Optimal body position for computer operators. (Photo courtesy of The Hartford, ©2002.)

Table 24-3
Workstation Assessment: Possible Causes of Awkward Postures

Observation	Possible Causes
Elbows away from side of body	Work surface too high
	Keyboard too far away
Feet on base of chair	Chair too high
Sitting on leg crossed under other leg on chair	Chair too high
	Seat pan angle inappropriate (i.e., too far down)
Sitting forward on chair away from back	Seat pan angle inappropriate (i.e., too far down)
	Chair too high
	Keyboard too far away
	Screen too far away
Wrist resting on sharp edge or surface of desk	Keyboard too far away
	Work surface too high
Wrist in extension	Wrist resting on work surface
	Keyboard angle too steep
Head and neck extended	Screen too high
Excessive turning or twisting of head and neck or trunk	Asymmetric position of video display terminal or components
	Poor chair support
	Unsatisfactory position of hard copy
	Unsatisfactory position of equipment or files

possible causes are presented in Table 24-3. Typical discomforts or symptoms and contributing causes are presented in Table 24-4. Note that these lists are not exhaustive and are not intended to be used to determine "cookbook" solutions. The observations and possible causes are examples of those commonly determined through the workstation assessment process.

FURNITURE AND EQUIPMENT

Work Surfaces and Chairs

Work surfaces supporting computers vary greatly. In many situations, computers have been installed on existing work surfaces that may have been designed for clerical, noncomputer job functions. Typically, standard clerical desks are nonadjustable at $28\frac{1}{2}$ to 30 in high. Work surface heights within this range may be suitable for a large percentage of the population performing noncomputer tasks, but these heights are too high for many workers performing computer functions.

In other situations, computer furniture marketed for its purported ergonomic design may or may not be suitable for its users or for some job functions. In any case, a complete assessment requires a thorough examination of the work surface and other components of the workstation in order to identify dimensions, adjustability, and other features. The chair is perhaps the most critical element in the workstation as it provides the basis for proximal support and good posture

Computer Hardware

The computer workstation must be considered as a system. Many factors, including furniture, equipment (e.g., keyboards), workstation design,

Table 24-4
Workstation Assessment: Possible Causes of Symptoms

Observation	Possible Causes
Neck or shoulder discomfort or pain	Screen too high Hard copy too far from screen Screen off to side with keyboard central Work surface too high Mouse too far from keyboard Elbows bump armrests
Back discomfort	Chair too high or too low Backrest not used
Lower leg circulation cut off	Feet not supported Seat pan too deep Chair too high
General pain at back of wrist, top of forearm	Excessive wrist extension Keyboard too far away Keyboard too high Keyboard angle too steep
Wrist discomfort on little finger side	Overstretching to reach function, cursor, enter keys Striking keys with excessive force Elbows away from body
Numbness or tingling of little finger or on little finger side of hand	Pressure on elbow Pressure on underside of forearm Resting forearm, elbow, or little finger on work surface
Pain through thumb or thumb side of wrist	Repetitive spacebar strike Striking keys with excessive force Folding paper and using thumb to crease Writing with excessive grip force Writing with awkward thumb angle
Eyestrain	Screen too high Screen too far or too close Poor resolution or clarity Poor visual acuity Reflection caused by screen angle Reflection caused by screen position glare

the general work environment, work organization and practices, and performance pressures, must be considered in order to truly prevent or eliminate risks associated with MSDs. The design and specifications of the computer equipment itself must be considered in the workstation assessment process. Size or dimensions and location of computer components relative to the work surface and the computer user influence posture and comfort. The height, width, depth, and, in some cases, the weight of each of the components should be determined.

The current trend toward computer multitasking has led to an increase in the size of monitors. Cathode tube display (CRT) monitors are the traditional monitors that most people associate with computer use. They feature a curved glass display housed in a rather bulky and space-consuming box. Screen size usually is indicated as the diagonal measure in inches, similar to the system used for measuring televisions. The greater height and width of the monitor influences angle of vision (height of screen) and position of other equipment on the work surface (width of screen). Of perhaps more significance is the depth of the monitor. The average-size monitor (15-inch screen) measures approximately 16 to 18 inches deep. In some cases an additional 1 to 2 inches of work surface space is required for connecting cables from the back of the monitor. A comfortable eye-to-screen distance can be maintained when this size monitor is positioned on a 30-inch-deep work surface. However, 17-inch (and larger) monitors measure 20 to 22 inches deep. If positioned on a 30-inch-deep work surface, the eye-to-screen distance is reduced significantly, and, in some cases, the remaining work surface space is not adequate for the keyboard. Workers respond by using self-determined fixes, which commonly result in asymmetric positioning of the monitor or keyboard (or both). When this happens, body posture is seriously compromised.

Flat screen monitors are becoming more popular because they are far less space-consuming than CRT monitors, and some workers prefer the liquid crystal display (LCD). Screen size ranges from 12 to 21 inches, and these monitors usually measure only a few inches in depth. Plasma screens and plasma displays use different technology. Screen size ranges from 21 to 50 inches, and they are available in both normal (4:3 ratio) and wide-screen formats (19:9 ratio). They can be used for both computer and video input, and they allow switching between the two for presentations. As with all other accessories, there are pros and cons associated with their use. For example, flat-screen monitors use less work surface space, but they are more expensive, and the LCD screen is not comfortable to all users. A trial period is recommended prior to purchase.

Ergonomic Accessories

A variety of standard office accessories can be effective in improving comfort in the workplace. Some examples of these accessories include document holders, computer tables, keyboard trays, telephone headsets, electric staplers, glare screens, staple removers, task lights, a variety of writing utensils (pens), wrist rests, footrests, and pencil grips. Workstation factors and job functions must be considered in the determination of need for or potential effectiveness of ergonomic accessories. Requests for ergonomic accessories may be indicative of another ergonomic need for change, and therefore proactive workstation assessment is in order. If not used appropriately, an accessory can be ineffective or even injurious.

Products that meet a company's ergonomic and safety standards can be made available through company purchasing systems. Additionally, many office and ergonomic accessories are now available from vendors in the community. Some of these products are listed in Box 24-3. Many office and computer supply houses, as well as medical and rehabilitation suppliers, carry these products. A brief review of issues relative to common accessories is discussed.

Wrist Rests

A wrist rest is a common comfort aid designed to provide wrist support to computer operators

BOX 24-3
Common Office Products that Can Be Effective Ergonomic Accessories

Backrest
Cleaning pad (for glare filter)
Video display terminal foam cleaner
Document holder
Document holder accessories
Electric hole punch
Electric stapler
Monitor risers
Footrest
Glare screen
Headsets
Forearm cushion
Mouse pad
Pencil grip
Staple remover
Task light
Terminal stand or table
Wrist rest

and help users avoid direct body contact (arms, wrists) with the work surface. A wrist rest is intended to provide intermittent support—it is not intended to encourage users to position or "plant" their wrists on the wrist rest during all phases of inputting and typing. There should be some clearance between the wrists and the wrist rest during actual typing and inputting. Wrist rests are most beneficial when the keyboard and work surface are at an appropriate height.

Keyboard Trays

Installation of keyboard trays is a popular solution to work space and work surface height problems. Although keyboard trays, particularly adjustable models, offer flexibility in keyboard height and angle, they are not as stable as computer tables. The width of the keyboard tray selected must accommodate space for a mouse, trackball, or other input device, in addition to the keyboard. A keyboard tray extends the depth of the work surface that may accommodate larger monitors, but it also increases the distance to a writing surface, telephone, and other implements. A negative slope offered by some keyboard trays benefits some, but not all, users. After careful selection, a trial installation, offered by many suppliers, is recommended.

Ergonomic Guidelines for Workstation Design

The optimal workstation design applicable to *all* situations does not exist. Even taking into account the need for some standardization of furniture and equipment specifications in some organizations, particularly large ones, it is possible to make some general recommendations regarding work surfaces intended to support computers, as well as chairs and other equipment intended to support the individuals performing computer-intensive jobs. Some of these general recommendations also appear in Box 24-2.

The computer work surface height for adults should be adjustable in a range of 23 to 28 inches. The work surface should position the keyboard such that the home row (ASDF) is approximately level with the elbow. A non-adjustable computer work surface of 26 to 27 inches is acceptable if appropriate body position can be achieved through chair height adjustments or accessory use. Operator-adjustable work surfaces are recommended for shared or multiuser workstations and may also be an advantage in frequently changing environments.

The depth of the computer work surface must be adequate to allow aligned symmetric position of the keyboard and monitor. A minimum of 30 inches is required for computers with standard-size monitors that are up to 18 inches deep, and 36 inches for computers with larger monitors that exceed 18 inches deep. In some situations, a work surface less than 30 inches deep can be adapted to accommodate the computer.

The width of the computer work surface must be adequate to support the keyboard and other necessary equipment, including mouse, mouse pad, paperwork, document holder, telephone, and calculator. A minimum of 36 inches is required to support both the keyboard and the mouse.

Noninterfering and accessible storage space is required for the processing unit. In general, work surface space should be adequate to support all necessary equipment and supplies, placing frequently used items within comfortable reach.

The chair is perhaps the most critical component of the workstation because a stable, comfortable seated posture provides the basis of support for body movements, distal joint positions, and task performance. Critical chair features include the following.

- Easily height adjustable (range of 15 to 21 inches)
- Smooth-rolling casters
- Locking back
- Height-adjustable backrest
- Tension adjustment for chairs that recline

- Model available with and without arms
- Model available in smaller or larger size
- Independently adjustable seat and back angles
- Swivel
- Five-spoke base

Minimally, seat pan height and backrest adjustment features are required in office chairs. Availability of models with and without armrests and models in smaller or larger sizes is necessary. Even a well-designed chair can be too big or too small for the user or for the workstation. Other chair features to consider are seat pan tilt, height adjustable armrests, and width adjustable armrests. These features increase the individual adjustability of the chair, and the greater the chair's adjustment capabilities, the greater the number of people that will be able to sit on it comfortably. Adjustment features must be easily accomplished by the user. An adjustable chair is ineffective if the adjustments are too difficult for the user to make. User participation in chair selection and a trial period prior to purchase are recommended.

Lighting is a critical workstation feature that affects the computer user's ability to work comfortably. Inadequate lighting, excessive lighting, glare, and reflection in the monitor screen contribute to visual discomfort including eyestrain, burning or itching eyes, and blurred or double vision. The typical illumination level of office environments is 75 to 100 ft candles. The American National Standards Institute (ANSI) (1988) recommends only 18 to 46 ft candles in a computer workstation environment. Lower ambient lighting levels complemented by task lighting is an effective combination. The effects of overhead and outside light can be controlled by following these recommendations (see Chapter 11).

- Locate the monitor perpendicular to the window.
- Close drapes or blinds to reduce ambient lighting, glare, and reflection.
- Use low-watt lights (rather than high-watt).
- Reduce overhead lighting where possible; remove light bulbs if necessary.
- Consider the use of a glare screen on the monitor to reduce glare and reflection.
- Use indirect or shielded lighting where possible.
- Paint walls a medium or dark color with no reflective finish.
- Properly placed partitions can also help block excess light.
- Dimmer switches and diffusing cover panels can control man-made light.

Noise, like lighting, is an environmental factor that can affect the comfort and productivity of office workers. Typical sources of noise in an office environment are copiers, telephones, printers, people talking, and traffic. Sound levels in most offices are well below those permitted by law and are not high enough to cause permanent or temporary hearing loss (Weir, 2000). Although noise levels are not usually a health hazard in an office, they can interrupt, annoy, and distract, and higher noise levels can negatively affect performance and concentration. ANSI (1988) recommends maximum ambient sound pressure levels of 55 dBA. The Canadian Standards Association (Weir, 2000) recommends the following sound design goals: video conference facilities—30 dBA; executive offices and conference rooms—35 dBA; private offices—45 dBA; open-plan offices—45 to 48 dBA; and call centers—50 dBA.

To the extent possible, each person should be aware of how his or her own conversation and activities contribute to office noise. The following control measures can be effective.

- Schedule noisy activities when few people are around.
- Specify quiet products and equipment for office use.
- Maintain equipment and report problems quickly.
- Move loud equipment away from people.
- Shield, partition, sequester, or cover loud equipment.
- Recommend acoustical materials for walls, partitions, ceilings, and floors to absorb noise.

- Place equipment on rubber mats to absorb noise.

The criteria for workstation design can be met in a variety of ways and by various types of furniture. Adequate and accessible work-surface space for noncomputer job functions is also required for many jobs. The height of this work surface should be adjustable (range 24 to 30 inches). Adequate and accessible filing and storage space, as required by specific job functions, must be available. The caveat to any generic guideline is that the specific workstation design may need to be tailored to meet the needs of the specific job. The optimal goal is to build maximum adjustability and flexibility into a generic workstation design such that various job functions and individual staff variances can be accommodated.

CURRENT COMPUTER-RELATED ERGONOMIC ISSUES

As computer applications expand and hardware changes, we are faced with ever-changing challenges from an ergonomic perspective. The basic principles of workstation ergonomics, including application of good body mechanics and the assurance of comfort at the workstation, are universal to all applications. Four new and challenging applications in office ergonomics are addressed here.

Input Devices

The primary recognized input tool has been the keyboard because it is, perhaps, the most commonly used tool. As operating systems have become increasingly mouse driven, the mouse has also been recognized as a key input tool and as a potential contributor to work-related discomfort and ergonomic risk factors. Many of the newer computer applications are mouse driven, and this accounts for increased use of the mouse as a primary input device. Other input devices gaining rapid popularity are trackballs, joysticks, touch pads, and pens. Some laptop designs incorporate trackballs or mini-joysticks into their keyboards or inputting systems. Newer technology of pentops offers additional versatility in application. These pentops may engage a pen, keyboard, or mouse for inputting. Finally, improvements in technology have rendered voice-activated (or voice-recognition) systems productive methods.

From an ergonomics perspective, each of these tools offers its own set of advantages and disadvantages. No tool is universal for all applications, and, ergonomically, the perfect input device does not yet exist. Key factors in determining the appropriateness of a particular tool in a particular application are how it is used, along with frequency, duration, and intensity of use. It is important to know whether this tool is the primary or only input device used. Are neutral postures maintained during use, and is the individual comfortable during and after use? Each tool must be evaluated carefully, with consideration of how, where, and by whom it is to be used.

Keyboards

A variety of so-called ergonomic keyboards are currently on the market. According to the sales literature, these keyboards eliminate awkward postures demanded by standard keyboards and prevent the development of various MSDs. The true benefit of these keyboards, however, has yet to be scientifically determined.

The new alternative keyboards conform to a variety of designs that meet different combinations of ergonomic criteria. Some mimic the standard keyboard layout with variation in key placement. For example, the split keyboard, such as the Microsoft Natural Keyboard and the Kinesis keyboard, splits the standard keyboard layout, angling two groups of keys. Other models, including the Kinesis Maxim, the Goldtouch Split Keyboard, and the Comfort Keyboard System, actually split the keyboard into two adjustable pieces. Other features offered by various models include the following.

- A curved base with angled keys
- A detached numeric keypad

- A trackball located in the wrist rest
- Concave keypad sections
- A foot pedal for keystroke assignment
- A split keyboard with articulating sections
- Detachable palm rests

Other keyboard designs vary considerably from the standard keyboard. One model, called a chord keyboard, resembles a small musical instrument. It is cylindrical and hand-held. The fingers lie over buttons that activate the keyboard for inputting. Another model, Data Hand, consists of two boxlike units, one for each hand. A glove-shaped depression in each unit supports the hands. The fingertips lie in three-dimensional "wells," where they are surrounded by magnetic switches. These switches are activated by the fingertips in various combinations for inputting. The cost of these products varies as much as the design. A recent review identified prices in the range of $89 to $2095.

Some studies have been conducted to provide data on the efficacy of alternative keyboard design features. Tittiranonda, Rempel, Armstrong, and Burastero (1999) found that the use of split keyboards, such as the Apple Adjustable Keyboard used in the study, can reduce some posture-related risk factors associated with the development of MSDs (e.g., wrist extension and ulnar deviation) but did not eliminate all the risks. Computer operators may also be exposed to other risk factors, such as repetitive and forceful exertions during keying and awkward postures associated with mouse or telephone use, and mechanical stress related to resting the hand or wrist on the edge of the keyboard or work surface. Swanson, Galinsky, Cole, Pan, and Sauter (1997) identified an initial decline in productivity when subjects began typing on two of three alternative keyboards of the split keypad type, but the productivity losses were recovered within the 2-day evaluation period. Their results also indicated no significant differences between keyboard (alternative keyboards or traditional) conditions in discomfort and fatigue, and suggest a minimal impact of the keyboard design features on productivity, comfort, and fatigue, at least after 2 days of exposure. The authors suggest further study to determine potential performance and health benefits for keyboard users over a longer period of time.

Although little data exist to support the use of alternative keyboards as a means to correct physiologic problems, the presumption that keyboards cause MSDs is also unproven. Injured users maintain that keyboard manufacturers have known for many years that conventional keyboards are responsible for exposures that lead to such disorders and that the manufacturers deliberately withheld warnings of the dangers. Users also claim that alternative keyboard designs could have prevented users' injuries. Manufacturers demonstrate that combination of factors, including posture, workstation design, work practices, and the ways in which the workstation is used contribute to symptoms of MSDs related to keyboard use. Since data supporting these claims do not exist, the courts have ruled in favor of the manufacturers in the cases to date *(Gonzalez v. Digital Equipment Corp.,* No. 92-CV-5230 E.D.N.Y. June 16, 1998; *Geressy v. Digital Equipment Corp.,* No. 94-CV-1427 E.D.N.Y. Oral decision. April 29, 1997). Despite continued controversy on the subject, most manufacturers place warning labels on keyboards in an effort to reduce the probability of product liability lawsuits. An individual operator may find one keyboard more comfortable than another. However, until research determines the true effect of the new keyboard designs, alternative keyboards must not be considered a generic solution to a very complex problem.

Pointing Devices

The variety of inputting devices available includes mouse, trackball, stylus, touch pad, and joystick. There is no conclusive research indicating that any one device is better than another from an ergonomic perspective. Selection of input device is appropriately made with consideration of intended use, job functions, anthropometric characteristics of the user, and use preference. As with any tool it is important to select the appropriate tool for the task. For example, certain devices may be more sensitive for certain types of graphic work (e.g., stylus), others more effective for editing work (e.g., mouse, trackball, or touch pad), and still others for computer games (e.g., joystick).

Portable Computers and Laptops

With the growth of a mobile workforce and ongoing technological advances, the portable computer market is expanding rapidly. Certainly, the mobility of portable computers, laptops, and pentops is a significant advantage for many. However, by nature of their design, laptops are not ergonomically correct. Many laptops are one-piece units, which limits the adjustment potential. Independent angle adjustment of the monitor screen and keyboard can be achieved; however, independent height adjustment of screen and keyboard is not possible. When the screen is at a comfortable height, the keys are not, and vice versa. The keys on many laptops are located in the far portion of the computer itself, creating an unavoidable, hard wrist rest. The pointing device on a laptop may be located at the middle of the keyboard. As laptops become smaller and more portable, user postures may become more constrained. Ongoing ergonomic evaluation of portable computers and their use is necessary. The evaluation should include not only features of the computer hardware, but also how the equipment is used in and outside of the workplace, as well as carrying case design and function. This evaluation should address equipment design and function specific to portable computers. In addition to factors common to all computers (e.g., size, resolution, adjustment controls, keyboard sensibility and layout, compatibility for left- and right-handed users, alternate input device, overall comfort of use), specific factors to consider include the following.

- Weight
- Screen sensibility, pentops (feel, pen control)
- Pen size (diameter, length), accessibility, sensibility (touch), port (stability), and battery requirement
- Stand (for desktop use) availability, stability, height adjustability, and angle adjustability
- Battery size, weight, and accessibility
- Mouse, trackball compatibility
- Carrying case size and equipment accessibility
- Cable connections ease of use, accessibility, and noninterference with position of components
- Ease of desktop connection
- Usability: static holding

Although the success of portable equipment depends in part on design factors, user technique and training are also significant factors. Conventional desktop monitors and keyboards may be more appropriate for use in the office. Some circumstances may require availability of conventional equipment for use in the office. Comfort during use of a laptop can be enhanced through the following options.

- Place the laptop at a height and distance that allows comfortable keyboard access. Adjust font size and contrast to prevent eyestrain.
- Obtain an external keyboard and/or monitor, particularly if the laptop is used for more than 1 hour at a time.
- Use a mouse or other external pointing device.
- Use a wrist rest as necessary and if feasible given laptop design (and location of the keyboard).
- Avoid using the laptop on a high surface to avoid awkward shoulder, arm, and wrist postures and to avoid wrist and forearm resting on the edge of the laptop (Kay, 2001).

Kids and Computers

Children of all ages are spending more and more time on computers and computer-related equipment (i.e., desktop computers, laptop computers, video games, palm pilots, etc.) in school, at home, in libraries, in game centers, in department stores, and even in restaurants where electronic equipment is installed for entertainment.

Library catalogs are automated, middle school and high school teachers post assignments on web sites, school assignments require Internet searches, handwritten papers are no longer acceptable, and e-mail and instant messaging have become standard means of communication among children. Even though much of this exposure would be considered intermittent use, the potential for intense use and greater exposure is certainly there. For example, some school assignments require steady and extended computer use; children become absorbed in computer and video games and play for hours on end. Children who actively use computers, video games, and other tools of automation are susceptible to the same computer-related risks and MSDs as their adult counterparts.

Now is the time to address ergonomic issues associated with the use of computers and video games by children. Continuity of principles they learn now, as children, will be of great benefit to these children in their adult years.

Computer Use by Children

The National Center of Education Statistics (1994, 1995) indicates that that more than 56 million public and private school children will be enrolled in kindergarten through twelfth-grade schools by the year 2005, an increase of 14% from 1993. Their findings also suggest that over 60% of students have access to computers at school, and 30% have access to computers at home. These numbers, they report, are projected to increase in conjunction with the U.S. Department of Education's GOALS 2000 Program, which intends to ensure that every student has equal access to computers.

Estimates of computer use by children vary. A poll conducted by *USA Today*/CNN for the National Science Foundation (Henry, 1997) reported that students in grades 7 through 12 averaged 4 hours per week using a computer. Forty-four percent used a computer at least once a day. Computers were used for playing computer games (93%), writing school reports (89%), using the Internet (56%), or sending e-mail and communicating on the Internet (48%). Roper and Starch (1999) estimate the average American child is spending 1 to 3 hours daily in front of a computer. Jones and Orr (1998) found average daily use of computers to be 2.33 hours in their sample of high school students.

Incidence of MSDs among Children Using Computers

Evidence in the literature of MSDs in children is not abundant, but it does exist. Injuries associated with the use of computers or their accessories have been described, including joystick digit, mouse elbow, and a central palmar blister following rotation of the central console joystick of a video game in the palm of the hand (Mirman & Bonian, 1992; Osterman, Weinberg, & Miller, 1987; Wood, 2001). Cleary, McKendrick, and Sills (2002) report the development of hand-arm vibration syndrome in a 15-year-old boy who presented with a 2-year history of painful hands. His hands became white and swollen when exposed to the cold and subsequently red and painful on warming. There were no clinical or laboratory findings of an underlying connective tissue disorder. The onset of his symptoms was preceded by the prolonged use of a widely available computer game. He spent up to 7 hours a day playing this game, with a preference for driving games using the vibration mode on the hand-held control device. The authors provide no information regarding treatment and outcome but do suggest consideration of statutory health warnings to advise users and parents.

Jones and Orr (1998) surveyed high school students to determine the prevalence of computer-related musculoskeletal injuries, pain, and discomfort among students in high school computer-use classes. They found that 28%, 40%, and 41% of high school students, respectively, experience symptoms of hand discomfort, neck and back pain, and pain in other parts of the body related to computer use. The prevalence of self-reported symptoms of

CTS and medically diagnosed CTS among high school students was slightly greater than that reported among U.S. adults (4% versus 1.55%). In addition, hand discomfort and self-reported symptoms of CTS were reported more often by males than by females in their study. Reports of symptoms were also related to duration of computer use. An increase in hand discomfort occurred as use increased from 2 hours per day to 5 or more hours per day.

Jacobs and Baker (2002) studied the home computer use of American middle school children and found that more than half the sixth-grade children in their study reported musculoskeletal pain in at least one body part (neck, shoulder, elbow, wrist-hand, back) within the year prior to the study. The number of hours spent on the computer showed an association with overall musculoskeletal pain. Another interesting finding was that children who were able to touch type were 54% less likely to report musculoskeletal discomfort than those who were not able to touch type. Their data analysis suggests that computer use may be associated with musculoskeletal complaints in a population of middle school–aged children, and they suggest further study to understand similarities and differences between adult and children computer use and how computer use influences children's health.

The Problem

Risk factors associated with the use of computers and other automated equipment by children are the same as those associated with adult use of computers. Awkward postures, particularly static awkward postures, are perhaps magnified as children struggle to use computers positioned on standard adult furniture. Sensorimotor feedback is affected by postural instability and insecurity when children are seated on chairs with seat pans too high to allow the feet to reach the floor. Repetitive motion is increased as children look back and forth between keyboards and monitors that are positioned above eye level. Some children are pulled away from normal play and interpersonal interaction, threatening psychosocial skill development. As a sedentary activity, computer use reduces opportunity for physical activity, strengthening, and endurance development (Sellers, 1994).

Most computer equipment, computer accessories, and computer furniture are designed for adults according to adult anthropometric data. Although the availability of alternative equipment is increasing, most computer equipment available to children is standard, adult-size equipment. Laeser, Maxwell, and Hedge (1998) draw the following conclusions from a review of the literature.

- Existing educational furniture standards are no longer adequate for today's educational environments since they fit neither the size of the children nor the tasks being performed.
- The strong evidence pointing to the adverse affects of poor workstation design on the musculoskeletal system in adults is likely to apply to children, too.
- The literature provides a strong argument for reevaluating and improving the situations in which we ask children to work.

Based on research with adults, the authors hypothesized that a student's performance and overall seated posture will improve with a keyboard and mouse arrangement adjusted to fit the anthropometric needs of that student. Using an experimental design in which students worked on a computer on a standard desktop and then on a work surface that allowed the keyboard and mouse arrangement to be adjusted to fit the specific anthropometric needs of the user, they demonstrated that children do adopt at-risk postures when using computer equipment on adult-size furniture and that overall seated posture improved with a keyboard and mouse arrangement adjusted to fit the student. Their results also suggested a relationship between level of typing skill and posture. Better skilled, more experienced student typists demonstrated better neck posture. The results of their study provide evidence that children can distinguish between workstation arrangements that relate to their comfort, ease of use, and relationship to the computing task.

Failure to consider the special needs of children in designing computer workstations at schools occurs with surprising frequency. This author's experience illustrates this point. The original building project plans for new classroom computer workstations in a public elementary school (grades kindergarten through five) called for installation of fixed 30-inch-height, built-in casework (cubicles) with standard keyboard drawers mounted under the work surface. The keyboard tray would position the keyboard approximately 2 inches below the work surface, or at approximately 28 inches. The keyboard tray would not support the mouse, since the width was only sufficient to support the keyboard itself. The tables used as work surfaces for classroom work in the kindergarten class-rooms measured only 18 inches high, the standard height for kindergarten classroom furniture. According to the original design, the keyboard height for children in these classrooms would be 10 inches above the height of their standard work surfaces (tables)! The posture problem would be magnified by use of standard kindergarten chairs. This occupational therapist performed a simple walk-through with the principal of the school, and demonstrated the discrepancy between the existing furniture and the proposed furniture and to gather anthropometric information from the children (e.g., popliteal height, elbow height in seated position). The principal was quickly convinced of the need to change the plans. Convincing the Building Committee and the Board of Education was a greater challenge. After much debate, the decision was made to alter the plan, replacing fixed-height casework with height-adjustable mobile computer tables in each classroom. In addition to the ergonomic advantage to children using the equipment, the height-adjustable mobile computer tables offer more flexibility in educational programming. The equipment can be repositioned in a classroom or shared by classrooms as needed for special activities or projects. This scenario demonstrates a classic example of the application of adult standards, or possibly the only standards and guidelines available, to children. In this case, costly retrofitting was avoided by early occupational therapy intervention and incorporation of ergonomic recommendations in the design process.

Unique Needs of Children

Aside from obvious size differences between children and adults, other characteristics of children present unique challenges regarding computer workstation design. For example, children working on a computer, and especially playing video games, are likely to be more focused on the computer task and not likely to be aware of a need to take a break. They do not consider posture or how the computer is set up. For this reason, it is critical that the workstation be set up in such a way that ergonomically correct postures occur automatically. Adult supervision of computer use is a critical factor. Monitoring software for computers is available and might be considered. However, the effectiveness of these programs is not well established.

Children may be more responsive to visual cues, as opposed to written or verbal instruction, regarding proper position of the body and computer equipment. Therefore, pictures and posters illustrating proper technique and setup may be effective.

Younger children's hands are smaller than those of adults. Standard computer equipment designed for adults may simply be too big. Equipment and accessory alternatives should be considered, at least for special cases. For example, keyboards and other input devices are available in alternate sizes, shapes, and design, which may be more appropriate for smaller bodies.

Adjustability is very important in setting up a workstation that will be shared by students, family members, and others. User-adjustability (e.g., via cranks or electronic adjustment) is ideal but may not be practical in a school setting.

Manual adjustability assures the opportunity to make adjustments when necessary.

Typical Findings

Observation of children using computers in typical classrooms or computer laboratories yields common findings. Figure 24-2 illustrates a common situation. This eighth-grade student, who is of average build, is using a computer in the laboratory at his new middle school. The computer is located on a fixed-height, built-in work surface. The height of the work surface measures 30 inches. The chair offers only seat pan height adjustability. The backrest is not adjustable. The work surface, the keyboard, and the monitor are all too high.

In Figures 24-3 and 24-4, seated posture is slouched. The feet are dangling because the chair has been raised in an effort to reach the keyboard. The neck is extended, tipping the head back and the chin up toward the monitor. The wrists are flexed and rest on the sharp edge of the work surface.

Efforts to reduce the risk and improve this middle school student's comfort included the following changes. The chair was raised to its maximum setting and a footrest provided. The central processing unit was moved and the monitor placed directly on the work surface. Posture is improved, but the keyboard is still too high. Practical solutions to this problem are limited. Raising the chair, even it could be raised, becomes a safety hazard and would require a different footrest. Installation of a keyboard tray

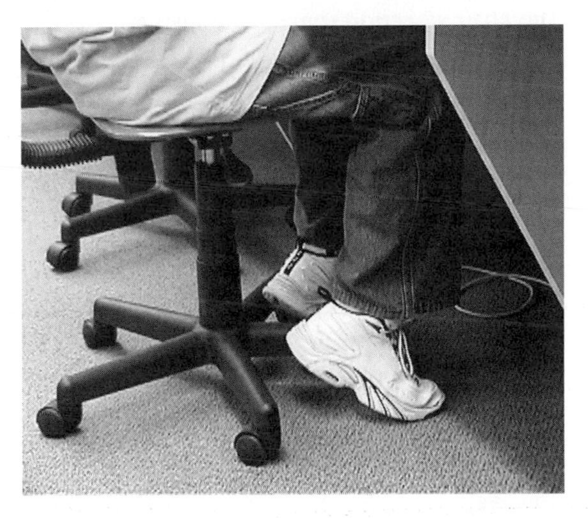

Figure 24-3 Detail of Figure 24-2 showing the student's feet dangling.

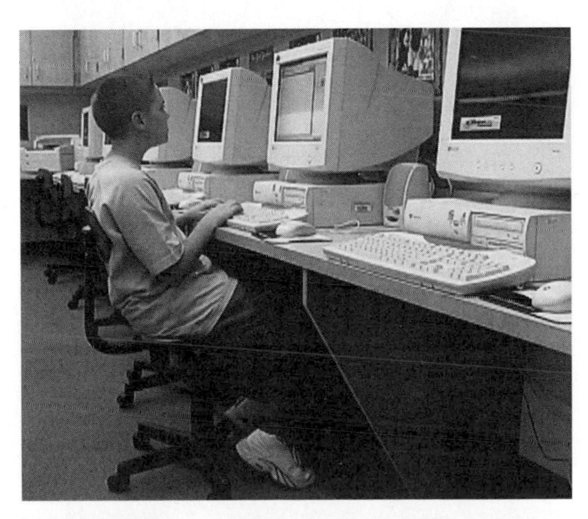

Figure 24-2 Student seated at a worksurface that is too high. Note the awkward posture.

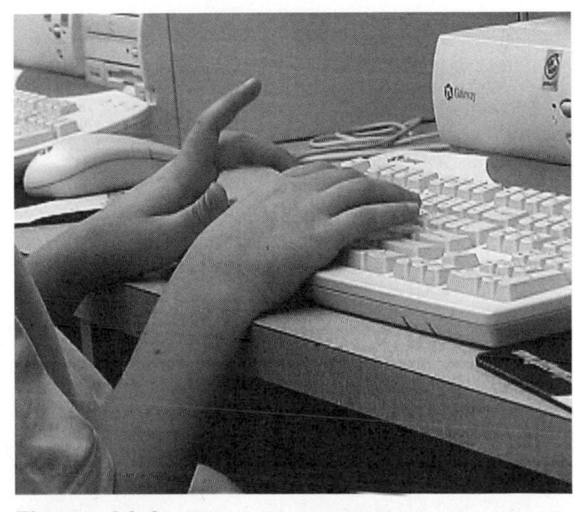

Figure 24-4 Detail of Figure 24-2 showing the student's wrists flexed and resting on the edge of the worksurface.

in the brand-new setting is impractical because of expense issues, durability concerns, and space (aisle width) factors.

The same school system selected height-adjustable computer tables for its elementary school computer laboratory (Figure 24-5). This furniture makes it possible to offer various work surface heights to accommodate the population of students in grades kindergarten through five. The chair selection remained consistent.

In another example, this first-grade student works at a computer positioned on a height-adjustable, mobile computer table in her classroom (Figure 24-6). Both the keyboard and mouse are positioned close to elbow level. The monitor is viewed with neutral neck posture. The chair provides adequate height adjustability, but the backrest provides no support. The observation of foot position, on the spokes of the chair, may be an indication that the chair (and possibly the work surface) is too high. If further investigation determined that to be true, table and chair height adjustments would be in order.

Games

If the use of standard computer equipment by children is considered a challenge, the use of electronic games by children can be considered an even greater challenge (Figure 24-7). To some extent, these games are used in less conventional settings. They are commonly added connections to televisions in living rooms, family

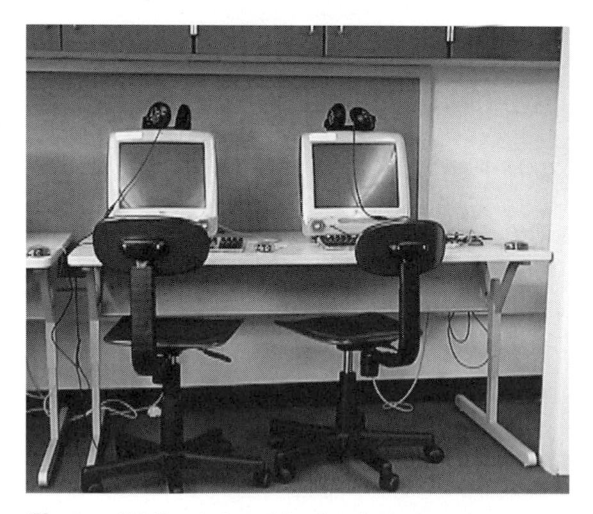

Figure 24-5 Adjustable furniture in a computer laboratory.

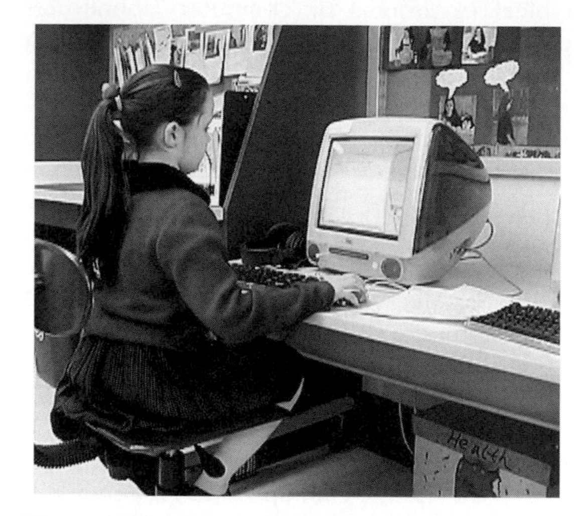

Figure 24-6 First grader at an adjusted workstation.

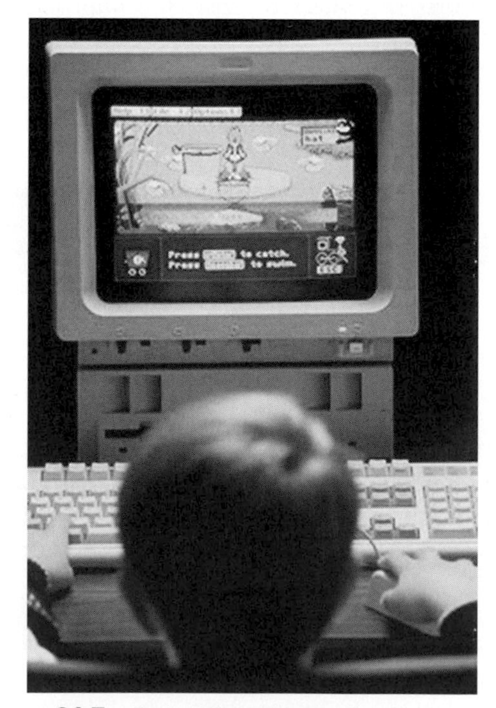

Figure 24-7 Typical electronic game setup.

rooms, bedrooms, and other locations. Children use these games while standing, sitting, or lying down. Picture the child sitting cross-legged on the floor, game pad in hand, looking up at the television screen located in the entertainment center. Or picture a teenager lying prone on the bed, propped up on elbows, game pad in hand, looking up at the television located on a tall dresser or on a wall-mounted TV stand. Even though the possible postural risks are endless, solutions are not impossible (see Chapter 18 for further discussion).

The Solution(s)

With careful planning and attention, risk factors associated with the use of computers and other automation by children can be avoided. Evidence of effective solutions is beginning to appear in the literature. Lucas (1997) presented an early education pilot project in hand health "as a proactive ergonomic solution to the present epidemic of cumulative trauma disorders." Nine hundred and fifty elementary students, ages 5 to 11, and their staff responded positively to a 20-minute program that introduced concepts of posture at the keyboard and basic upper-body stretches. It appears that wellness thinking and living can be learned at an early age to ensure that basic principles of work practice such as posture and upper-body stretches become a life skill. It is hoped this will minimize the occurrence of MSDs, especially in relation to the use of computers.

On an individual basis, the following recommendations (adapted from HealthyComputing.com) are made for children using computers and electronic games.

- Take stretch breaks every 15 minutes. Limit sustained computer use to 1 hour at a time.
- Hold the mouse, game pad, or joystick lightly.
- Keep the input or control device close and in front of you, not off to the side.
- Use programmable features (e.g., keyboard shortcuts or game pad programming to group common key sequences) to avoid repetitive key strike, like pushing the "fire" button.
- Change positions frequently.
- Watch your posture. Don't slouch or lean forward. Put the input or control device where you can use it with straight wrists.
- Make sure you are sitting comfortably.
- If you use a force-feedback game pad, take more frequent breaks.
- If you use voice-recognition software, rest your voice periodically.

The preceding examples address individual computer use issues. The following recommendations address ergonomic concerns relative to children and computer workstations on a larger scale.

- Evaluate current computer workstation setups to determine whether they are ergonomically correct. Look for height-adjustable work surfaces of sufficient width and depth dimensions. Look for supportive, adjustable chairs. Consider who the computer users are (e.g., high school students versus elementary school students; fifth-graders versus first-graders).
- To determine appropriate work surface height, measure from the floor to the elbow of the seated child.
- Educate children, parents, teachers, and school officials on ergonomics and how it applies to children. Include proper posture and movement, risk factors and how to avoid them.
- Advise parents, school officials, and other relevant parties regarding how to create a healthy workstation.
- Review plans for installation of computer workstations in existing classrooms and make recommendations.
- Review plans for new construction and make recommendations for computer workstation design.
- Use the many resources available, including the American Occupational Therapy Association web site for information on "Healthy Computing for Today's Kids" (2002).

Telecommuting

As many companies realize the benefits of portable computers, some are also realizing benefits from a relatively new and innovative work option called *telecommuting*. Telecommuting offers employees flexible work arrangements in which they work out of their homes or other remote locations. One author describes telecommuting as "moving the work to the workers, instead of the workers to work" (Smart Valley, 1994).

Telecommuting work arrangements lend themselves to many types of jobs. Telecommuting can work well in word processing, data entry, information management, writing, and research. Some companies have instituted telecommuting for customer-focused jobs such as technical support staff, customer service, catalogue sales, and travel agents. Less traditional approaches include human resource, finance, engineering, marketing, and manufacturing applications (Hamilton, 1987).

Although many telecommuting situations have evolved on an informal basis, some companies are developing and implementing formal telecommuting programs. In some cases, federal legislation such as the Clean Air Act Amendments of 1990, the Americans with Disabilities Act, and the Family Leave Act has sparked the initiative to develop these programs (Romano, 1994). As these programs are being developed, employers have recognized the need to address some issues that could become potential obstacles if not adequately handled. Among these issues are technical requirements, legal issues, security issues, tax issues, and ergonomic issues. For this reason, it is necessary to establish guidelines governing conditions of participation, equipment use, and liability issues (Beiswinger, 1994; Best, 1986).

- The application of principles of ergonomics in a telecommuting situation varies little from other applications. Development of specific ergonomic guidelines for personal computer use must be developed. These guidelines should provide recommendations for optimal body position and workstation configuration. The principles discussed elsewhere in this chapter apply.

Implementation of an ergonomics program in a telecommuting situation can be, in some ways, more challenging than in a traditional office environment. Unless the company selects and provides furniture for remote installation, there is likely to be more variety and less adjustability in what is being used. Further, home safety may be an issue related to overloaded circuits, power cords, lack of exits from one room, and organization of the office. It is more difficult to monitor job factors like schedules and breaks. In addition, monitoring and enforcement of the ergonomics program can be more difficult in a remote rather than an on-site location. Nevertheless, an active ergonomics program is necessary in the telecommuting environment to maintain a healthy workforce and to manage workers' compensation issues. Employers are responsible for home workstation safety under OSHA worker safety regulations. Home visits for workstation evaluation are not required but are advised to ensure the telecommuting worker's safety.

ERGONOMIC REGULATION

OSHA, under President Clinton's Democratic administration, promulgated an ergonomic standard for general industry, which was published in the Federal Register on November 14, 2000, with an effective date of January 16, 2001. This standard was promptly repealed by the Bush administration in January 2001. No other official, or enforceable, ergonomic regulation exists other than the general duty clause that generally provides for a healthy workplace (see Chapters 4 and 14). Voluntary standards have been adopted in California and Washington.

Although OSHA (1991) has not published a standard on office ergonomics or ergonomics of computer workstations, it has published an advisory document titled *Working Safely with Video Display Terminals.* This document offers some guidelines. This OSHA document covers health effects, interventions, and OSHA programs and services. Recommendations include the following.

- Work surface light about 28 to 50 ft candles

- Diffuse (indirect) lighting
- Height-adjustable work surface
- Chair height adjusted so feet rest firmly on the floor or on a footrest
- Top line of the display no higher than the user's eyes
- Keyboard positioned so forearms are parallel to the floor

ANSI/HFS 100-1988 American National Standard for Human Factors Engineering of Visual Display Terminal Workstation (ANSI, 1988) was written by the American National Standards Institute (ANSI) and The Human Factors Society (HFS). This voluntary standard specifies acceptable conditions for computer terminals, equipment and furniture, and environment in offices. Select standard office workstation dimensions are recommended, including height of work surface, width of work surface, viewing distance to the monitor, thickness of the work surface, knee room, seat height, seat pan depth, and so on.

The Ergonomics subcommittee of the Business and Institutional Manufacturers Association (BIFMA International, 1999) is developing a guideline for furniture intended for computer use in the United States and Canada. It applies the measurable principles and design requirements of ISO 9241 parts 3 ("Visual display requirements") and 5 ("Ergonomic requirements for office work with visual display units"). Topics addressed by this document include working postures, the work chair, and work surfaces. The BIFMA guidelines are available through BIFMA International at http://www.bifma.org.

The Canadian Standards Association (2000) released CSA-Z412 Guideline on Office Ergonomics in December 2000. CSA is a nonprofit organization that oversees the development of standards and guidelines and also application of standards through product certification, management systems registration, and information products. The Z412 Guideline is a comprehensive document that includes design of jobs, work organization, office layout, environmental conditions, and workstation design. Z412 presents a nine-step approach to a design process for achieving an optimal office environment. The nine steps address office design outcomes, consideration of the office as a system with organizational involvement, workers' characteristics and participation, job demands, job design, work organization, the office layout and design of work rooms, the office environment, individual workstation design, and education and training. The guideline is available from CSA.

As the term implies, voluntary standards are intended to provide guidance to those who choose to use them. They are not enforceable from a regulatory point of view.

Two of OSHA's 26-state occupational safety and health programs have adopted state ergonomics standards. California's ergonomics standard was adopted on November 14, 1996, and became effective in July 1997. The standard requires employers to establish an ergonomic program when at least two employees performing identical tasks have been diagnosed by a physician with repetitive motion injuries. Washington's ergonomics standard, adopted on May 26, 2000, requires a phased-in enforcement that begins on July 1, 2004. It is a proactive rule requiring employers with "caution zone jobs" to find and fix ergonomic hazards.

Other states have initiated prelegislative activities. Alaska held public meetings in January 2002 regarding a draft standard for general safety and health programs that included ergonomics. In response to the number of comments received from stakeholders concerning ergonomics, the Commissioner of Labor dropped the ergonomics provisions and is proceeding only with other aspects of the safety and health programs rule. Minnesota established an Ergonomics Task Force to recommend approaches to reduce work-related MSDs. In 1998, North Carolina's first safety and health standard aimed at reducing MSDs at work was proposed but has not been enacted.

Legislation addressing ergonomic standards was introduced in nine states during 2002.

California legislation calls for revision of the state's ergonomics standard. In Florida, legislation specifies levels of proof required in cases involving occupational disease or repetitive exposure for workers' compensation purposes. Legislation proposed in Kentucky would create a taskforce to study repetitive stress disorders. Massachusetts and Minnesota legislation would require adoption of an occupational safety and health standard. In Pennsylvania, legislation encourages Congress to revisit the issue of MSDs and to support meaningful legislation that addresses injuries caused by repetitive motion. Rhode Island legislation would establish a commission on ergonomics to develop ergonomic guidelines. A series of bills proposed calls for repeal or postponement of the ergonomic rules and tax credits for employers who comply with the rules (http://.nursingworld.org/gova/state/2002/ergo.htm). New Jersey legislation that would create an Ergonomics in Education Study Commission was approved in the Senate and is now awaiting consideration by the Assembly Education Committee (http://www.njsba.org/sb_notes/oct1702/NewSite/NewFiles/stateup.html).

SUMMARY

In summary, technology has created greatly enhanced possibilities for productivity and information processing. However, technology has also spurred a new era of work-related MSDs related to the automated office environment. The prevention of such MSDs through organizational and workstation design controls is critical to worker satisfaction and business success. This chapter has addressed ergonomic issues in the automated office including workstation assessment, intervention, training, and regulatory compliance issues.

REFERENCES

American National Standards Institute (ANSI) (1988). ANSI/HFS 100-1988. *American national standard for human factors engineering of visual display terminal workstations.* The Human Factors Society: Santa Monica, CA.

Barry, J. (1993). A review of ergonomic keyboards. *Work, 3*(4), 21–25.

Beiswinger, G. L. (1994). The home office: A practical guide. *D & B Reports, 43*(1), 38–40.

Bergqvist, U., & Knave, B. (1993). Eye discomfort and work with visual display terminals. *Scandinavian Journal of Work, Environment, and Health, 20*(1), 27–33.

Best, F. (1986). No place like home. *Management World, 15*(6), 9–12.

BIFMA International. (1999). BIFMA: Ergonomics guideline for VDT furniture used in office work spaces. 2680 Horizon Drive SE, Suite A-1, Grand Rapids, MI 49546-7500, http://www.bifma.org.

BLS. (1995). Workplace injuries and illnesses in 1994. Washington, DC: U.S. Department of Labor, Bureau of Labor Statistics, USLD 95-508.

BLS. (2001). Workplace injuries and illnesses in 1999. Washington, DC: U.S. Department of Labor, Bureau of Labor Statistics.

Bureau of National Affairs, Inc. (1994). Keyboard design examined. *Job Safe Health, 433,* 1–2.

Carayon, P. & Smith, M.J. (2000). Work organization and ergonomics. *Applied Ergonomics, 31,* 649–662.

Cleary, A. G., McKendrick, H., & Sills, J. A. (2002). Hand-arm vibration syndrome may be associated with prolonged use of vibrating computer games. *British Medical Journal, 324*(February), 302.

Canadian Standards Association. (2000). CSA-Z412 Guideline on Office Ergonomics. © by CSA, 178 Rexdale Blvd., Toronto, Ontario, M9W 1R3.

Ergoweb, Inc. (2001). Workplace ergonomics. 93 W. Main, P.O. Box 1089, Midway, UT 84049; 1-888-ERGOWEB; www.ergoweb.com.

Faucett, J., & Rempel, D. (1994). VDT-related musculoskeletal symptoms: Interactions between work posture and psychosocial factors. *American Journal of Industrial Medicine, 26,* 597-612.

Feuerstein, M., Armstrong, T., Hickey, P., & Lincoln, A. (1997). Computer keyboard force and upper extremity symptoms. *Journal of Occupational and Environmental Medicine, 39*(12), 1144–1152.

Gerard, M. J., Armstrong, T. J., Franzblau, A., Martin, B. J., & Rempel, D. M. (1999). The effects of keyswitch stiffness on typing force, finger electromyography, and subjective discomfort. *American Industrial Hygiene Association Journal, 60,* 762–769.

Grandjean, E. (1987). *Ergonomics in computerized offices.* New York: Taylor & Francis.

Grandjean, E. (1988). *Fitting the task to the man.* New York: Taylor & Francis.

Hales, T. R., Sauter, S. L., Peterson, M. R., Fine, L. J., Putz-Anderson, V., Schleifer, L. R., et al. (1994). Musculoskeletal disorders among visual display terminal users in a telecommunications company. *Ergonomics, 37*(10) 1603–1621.

Hamilton, C. (1987). Telecommuting. *Personnel Journal, 66*(4), 91-101.

Healthy Computing for Today's Kids. (2002). AOTA—The American Occupational Therapy Association, Inc. Publication available on AOTA web site at *www.AOTA.org*.

Henry, T. (1997). Today's teens embrace technology. *USA TODAY/CNN*, April 23, 4D.

Jacobs, K., & Baker, N. A. (2002). The association between children's computer use and musculoskeletal discomfort. *Work, 18,* 221-226.

Jones, C., & Orr, B. (1998). Computer-related musculoskeletal pain and discomfort among high school students. *American Journal of Health Studies, 14*(1), 26-30.

Karasek, R. & Theorell, T. (1990). *Healthy work.* Basic Books, Inc.: New York

Kay, E. (2001). Ergonomics for the laptop user. *ErgoSense*, 19.

Kroemer, K. H. E. (1992). Avoiding cumulative trauma disorders in shops and offices. *Journal of the American Industrial Hygiene Association, 53,* 596-604.

Laeser, K. L., Maxwell, L. E., & Hedge, A. (1998). The effect of computer workstation design on student posture. *Journal of Research on Computing in Education, 31*(2), 173.

Leavitt, S. B., & Taslitz, N. J. (1993). *Computer-related injuries: Legal and design issues.* Chicago: The BackCare Corporation.

Lucas, G. M. (1997). Hand care begins with prevention in elementary schools. *Work, 9,* 267-273.

Mital, A., Kilbom, A., & Kumar, S. (Eds.). (2000). *Ergonomics guidelines and problem solving.* New York: Elsevier.

Mirman, M. J., & Bonian, V. G. (1992) "Mouse elbow": A new repetitive stress injury. *Journal of the American Osteopathic Association, 92,* 701.

Most, I. G. (1999). Psychosocial elements in the work environment of a large call center operation. *Occupational Medicine: State of the Art Reviews, 14*(1), 135-147.

Murray, T. E. (1994). Survey of occupational injuries and illnesses for 1992. *Workers' Compensation Report 11.01.* New York: American Insurance Services Group, Inc.

National Institute for Occupational Safety and Health. (1992). Study of communication workers at U.S. West Communications. Cincinnati: NIOSH, HETA, 89-299-2230.

Novak, C. B. &, Mackinnon, C. B.(1997). Repetitive use and static postures: A source of nerve compression and pain. *Journal of Hand Therapy, 10,* 151-159.

Occupational Safety and Health Administration. (1991). Working safely with video display terminals (Revised). Retrieved at http://www.osha-slc.gov.

Osterman, A. L., Weinberg, P., & Miller, G. (1987). Joystick digit (to the editor). *Journal of the American Medical Association, 257*(6), 782.

Phillips, C. A. (2000). *Human factors engineering.* New York: John Wiley & Sons, Inc.

Romano, C. (1994). Business copes with the clean air conundrum. *Management Review, 83*(2), 34-37.

Roper Starch. (1999). *1999 America Online/Roper Starch Cyberstudy* (CNT-154). Nov. 11. New York: Roper Starch Worldwide Inc.

Ross, P. (1994). Ergonomic hazards in the workplace. *American Association of Occupational Health Nurses Journal, 42,* 171-176.

Scalet, E. A. (1987). *VDT health and safety issues and solutions.* Lawrence, KS: Ergocyst Associates, Inc.

Sellers, D. (1994). *ZAP! How your computer can hurt you and what you can do about it.* Berkeley: Peachpit Press.

Smart Valley, Inc. (1994). *Smart Valley telecommuting guide* (Ver. 1), 1.

Stevens, J. C., Witt, J. C., Smith, B. E., & Weaver, A. L. (2001). The frequency of carpal tunnel syndrome in computer users at a medical facility. *Neurology, 56*(11), 1431-1432.

Swanson, N. G., Galinsky, T. L., Cole, L. L., Pan, C. S., & Sauter, S. L. (1997). The impact of keyboard design on comfort and productivity in a text-entry task. *Applied Ergonomics, 28*(1), 9-16.

Tittiranonda, P., Burastero, S., & Rempel, D. (1999). Risk factors for musculoskeletal disorders among computer users. *Occupational Medicine: State of the Art Reviews, 14*(1), 17-38.

Tittiranonda, P., Rempel, D., Armstrong, T., & Burastero, S. (1999). Workplace use of an adjustable keyboard: Adjustment preferences and effect on wrist posture. *American Industrial Hygiene Association Journal, 60,* 340-348.

U.S. Department of Labor, Bureau of Labor Statistics. (1994). *Survey of occupational injuries and illnesses, 1992* (Summary 94-3). Washington, DC: Bureau of Labor Statistics.

U.S. Department of Labor, Occupational Safety and Health Administration. (1991). *Ergonomics Program Management Guidelines for Meatpacking Plants* (OSHA 3123). Washington, DC: US Government Printing Office.

U.S. Department of Labor, Occupational Safety and Health Administration. (1994). *Draft ergonomic protection standard summary of key provisions.* [Unpublished document]

Webster, B. S., & Snook, S. H. (1994). The cost of compensable upper extremity cumulative trauma disorders. *Journal of Occupational Medicine, 36,* 713-717.

Weir, B. (Ed.). (2000). *Canadian Standards Association CSA-Z412 guideline on office ergonomics.* © by CSA, 178 Rexdale Blvd., Toronto, Ontario, M9W 1R3.

Wood, J. (2001). The "how" sign—a central palmar blister induced by overplaying on a Nintendo console. *Archives of the Disabled Child, 84,* 288.

Work Loss Data Institute (2001). Determinants of return-to-work. www.worklossdata.com/PR_RepCTS.htm.

SUGGESTED READINGS

Carlson, C. R. (1990). An experiment in productivity: The use of home terminals. *Journal of Information Systems Management, 7*(4), 36–41.

Grant, C. (2000). Office ergonomic resources on the world wide web. *Applied Occupational and Environmental Hygiene, 15*(1), 5–7.

Jauchem, J. (1993). Alleged health effects of electric or magnetic fields: Additional misconceptions in the literature. *Journal of Microwave Power and Electromagnetic Energy, 28*(3), 140–155.

Lind, J. S. (2002). Musculoskeletal disorders among video display terminal operators. *Applied Occupational and Environmental Medicine, 17*(1), 18–21.

National Safety Council. (1993). *Ergonomics: A practical guide* (2nd ed.). Chicago: National Safety Council.

Sauter, S. L. (1990). *Improving VDT work: Causes and control of health concerns in VDT use.* Lawrence, KS: The Report Store.

Sehnal, J. P., & Christopher, R. C. (1993). Developing and marketing an ergonomics program in a corporate office environment. *Work, 3,* 22–30.

Tillman, P., & Tillman, B. (1991). *Human factors essentials: An ergonomics guide for designers, engineers, scientists, and managers*. New York: McGraw-Hill.

Venturino, M. (Ed.). (1990). *Selected readings in human factors.* Santa Monica, CA: Human Factors Society, Inc.

Woodson, W. E., Tillman, B., & Tillman, P. (1992). *Human factors design handbook* (2nd ed.). New York: McGraw-Hill.

Work Loss Data Institute. (2001). Carpal Tunnel Syndrome linked to computer work. http://www.worklossdata.com/PR_RepCTS.htm 9/21/01.

RESOURCES

http://www.tifaq.com
http://www.tifaq.org/kids/kids.html
http://engr-www.unl.edu/ee/eeshop/rsi.html
http://www.ur-net.com/office-ergo
http://ergo.human.cornell.edu/
http://data.bls.gov/cgi-bin/surveymost
http://data.bls.gov/labjava/outside.jps?survey=sh
http://www.cot.org
http://www.ctdnews.com
http://www.geocities.com/HotSprings/Villa/6113/index.html
http://ergo.human.cornell.edu/Mbergo/schoolguide.html
http://ergo.human.cornell.edu/Mbergo/intro.html
http://www.healthycomputing.com/kids/gaming.html
http://www.healthycomputing.com/kids/;Healthy Computing.com for Kids
http://www.orosha.org/cergos/; Computer Ergonomics for Elementary School
http://www.aota.org/featured/area6/links/link02af.asp; Healthy Computing for Today's Kids (AOTA Consumer Info—Consumer Fact Sheets)

APPENDIX 24-1

WORKSTATION ASSESSMENT FORM

WORKSTATION ASSESSMENT

NAME: ______ Position: ______ Tel. ______ Bldg/Flr ______

Date of Referral: ______ by ______ Dept. ______ Supv. ______ Tel. ______

Date of WSA: ______ by ______

Chief Complaint: ______

Right Handed: ______ Left Handed: ______ Ambidextrous: ______

CURRENT POSITION Start Date ______ FT PT Schedule: ______ Overtime: Yes No

DUTIES: input: ______ % writing: ______ % other ______ frequency: ______

touch typist: yes __ no __ prior typing training: yes __ no __ schedule: ______

special skills: ______

other: ______

scheduled breaks: yes __ no __ taken consistently ______ when ______

workstation shared: yes __ no __ with whom ______ supv. ______ when ______

OBSERVATION CHECKLIST*	Date	f/u Date	f/u Date
1. Posture			
Neck			
Shoulders			
Back			
Arms			
Wrist			
Legs			
Feet			
2. Chair			
Height			
Seat			
Back			

COMMENTS: (concerns, causes, possible solutions)

______
______
______
______
______
______
______
______
______
______
______
______

3. Desk				
Height				
Work space				
Leg room				
4. Equipment				
VDT location				
VDT height				
VDT angle				
Keyboard location				
Keyboard angle				
Document holder				
Telephone location				
Tel. receiver/headset				
Calculator location				
Calc. height/angle				
Mouse				

5. Other

____

____

____

		DATE		f/u 1 DATE		f/u 2 DATE	
		current	rec.	current	rec.	current	rec.
WORKSURFACE __________ (type)	Height						
CHAIR __________ (type)	Height						
	Seat pan						
	Back						
KEYBOARD	Location						
	Position						
DISPLAY	Height						
	Position						
EQUIPMENT	Footstool						
	Wrist rest						
	Doc holder						
	Glare screen						
	Headset						

RECOMMENDATIONS

Date	f/u Date	f/u Date	
			Work station adjustments as indicated
			Work practice change:
			Ergonomic accessories:
			Other:
			Follow-up:

cc: Employee _____ Supervisor _____ Personnel/EHC _____
*Use + for OK, - for problem
f/u = follow up.

APPENDIX 24-2

Workstation Checklist

Chair

Is individual sitting up straight?	❒ Yes	❒ No
When sitting, are thighs parallel to floor?	❒ Yes	❒ No
When sitting, are feet resting firmly on floor?	❒ Yes	❒ No
Is seat pan adjusted so that front of seat pan is up?	❒ Yes	❒ No

Actions taken: ______________________________

Computer Screen

Is top line of screen slightly below eye level?	❒ Yes	❒ No
Is computer screen glare-free?	❒ Yes	❒ No
Is computer screen clean?	❒ Yes	❒ No

Actions taken: ______________________________

Keyboard, Calculator, and Mouse

Is keyboard as close to edge of desk as practical?	❒ Yes	❒ No
Is keyboard angle adjusted to middle or lowest position?	❒ Yes	❒ No
Is keying done without pen, pencil, or other tool in hand?	❒ Yes	❒ No
Is mouse at keyboard height and close to keyboard?	❒ Yes	❒ No

Actions taken: ______________________________

Body Position

Are shoulders in a relaxed position?	❒ Yes	❒ No
While inputting information, are:		
Forearms parallel to floor or slightly angled?	❒ Yes	❒ No
Wrists in neutral (close to straight) position?	❒ Yes	❒ No
Upper arms close to side of body?	❒ Yes	❒ No

Is body position changed throughout the day? ❒ Yes ❒ No

Actions taken: ______________________

General

Are equipment, supplies, files, and manuals easily accessible? ❒ Yes ❒ No

Is the floor area free of clutter? ❒ Yes ❒ No

When talking on phone, is phone supported by hand instead of neck? ❒ Yes ❒ No

Actions taken: ______________________

Name of employee and extension: ______________________

Name of supervisor and extension: ______________________

Date: ______________________

Source: Developed by J. Sehnal for ITT Hartford, revised 2001.

Index

A
A beta fiber, 104
A delta fiber, 104
Abdominal depth, 233*f*, 288
Abductor digiti quinti, 83*f*
Abductor pollicis brevis, 81*f*
  intrinsic atrophy in carpal tunnel syndrome, 330-331
Abductor pollicis longus, 80*f*
Abnormal nerve conduction velocity, 335*f*, 335-336
Academic sensibility, 94
Accident investigation process, 304-306
Achilles tendinitis, 480
Acoustic streaming, 104
Acrobat, 479-481
Acromioclavicular joint
  biomechanical risk factors for, 139*t*
  injury to, 143
Activity descriptors, 285-289
Activity modification in inflammation phase, 102
Activity tolerance, 89-91, 90*t*
Actor, 479-481
Acupuncture, 112
Acute inflammation in performing artist, 477
Acute tendon injury, 68
Adaptation to shiftwork, 260
Adaptive equipment for performing artist, 483-484
Adaptive failure of muscle, 183-185*f*, 183-186
Adaptive strategies for older worker, 440-442
Adjustment factors, personality and, 274-276, 277*f*
Administrative controls in injury reduction, 303-307
  in dental hygiene profession, 461*t*, 461-462
  early return to work and modified duty in, 306-307
  injury reporting and accident investigation process in, 304-306
  new employee conditioning and training in, 304
  productivity standards and paced work in, 307
  sociopolitical atmosphere and employee morale in, 303-304
Administrator, 303
Adolescent, ergonomic considerations for, 399-402, 400*f*, 401*t*
Adson's maneuver, 107
Adverse neural tension assessment, 94, 95*f*
Age-related changes in health and disability, 437-440
Aging of tendon, 66
Aging population
  musculoskeletal disorders and, 12
  older worker and, 437-447
    adaptive strategies for, 440-442
    age-related changes in health and disability, 437-440
    assessment of, 443-444
    ergonomic issues and, 442-443
    psychologic issues of, 444-445
Aging workforce, 20
Alternative duty, 307, 383
American Conference of Government Industrial Hygienists, 56, 56*f*
American National Standards Institute, 56-57, 283
Americans with Disabilities Act, 21-22, 57, 283-284
  preemployment examinations and, 327-330
Amplitude, 161*t*
Anastomosis, potential compression and entrapment at, 82-83
Anger, chronic pain and, 276
Angiofibroblastic tendinosis, 68, 116
Ankle impingement syndrome, 480
Anterior interosseous nerve, 81*f*
Anterior interosseous syndrome, 119*b*, 120
Anterior shoulder instability, 143
Anthropometrics, 230-232, 232-234*f*
  to evaluate individual workers, 288
  of tool length, 248
  women's, 157
Antiinflammatory medication, 102-103
  for cubital tunnel syndrome, 114
  effect on tendons, 66
  for pronator syndrome, 119
  for supraspinous tendinitis, 111
Apfel 19-item pick-up test, 97
Applique needle, 425
Approach strategies, 274
Arcade of Frohse, 80*f*
Armrest, 236, 310
Arthritis, 132-148
  of acromioclavicular joint, 143
  anatomical design of joint and, 132-133
  biomechanical risk factors for, 138-139*t*
  carpal boss and, 141
  compressive loading injuries and, 133-134
  diagnosis of, 136-137
  of distal radioulnar joint, 142
  of elbow, 142-143
  of finger interphalangeal joints, 137-139
  of glenohumeral joint, 143-144
  of joint stabilizing structures, 134
  medical management of, 144
  of metacarpophalangeal joint, 139-140
  myofascial responses to, 134
  of radiocarpal joint, 140-141
  of thumb carpometacarpal joint, 140
  upper-extremity arthritis as, 134-135, 135*b*

References followed by *b* indicate a box; references followed by *f* indicate a figure; references followed by *t* indicate a table.

work-relatedness of, 144–145
of wrist pisiform-triquetral joint, 141–142
of wrist triangular fibrocartilaginous complex, 141
Arthrokinetic inhibition, 134
Artificial light sources, 255
Assessment
of contracture, 138–139*t*
outcome, 363–386
approach to program evaluation in, 363–364
case study in, 384–386, 385*t*
compilation of musculoskeletal disorder injury information system and, 364–366, 365*t*, 366–367*f*
cost accounting and return-on-investment analysis in, 381–384, 382*f*
determination of company losses and, 366–370, 368*t*
goal-setting process in, 370–373, 372–373*f*, 374*b*
issues in, 374–375
qualitative measures in, 375–377
quantitative measures in, 377–380, 379*f*, 380–381*t*
periarticular muscle-tendon unit, 137
of posture, 214–217
Activity, Tool and Hand assessment tool in, 213–214
computerized motion analysis systems for, 217
postural analysis tools in, 214–215, 215–216*t*
posture targeting in, 212–213, 213*f*
self-analysis checklist for, 214
range-of-motion, 92
of strength, 92–93, 94*t*
workplace, 283–298
activity descriptors in, 285–289
biomechanical aspects of, 290–294
computer workstation, 525–529
ergonomic assessment in, 289–290
essential job functions and, 284–285
historical background of, 283–284
marginal job functions and, 285
performing artist and, 481–482
psychosocial aspects of, 294
Attenuation, 219
Attitude rating scales, 377
Australia, musculoskeletal disorders in, 7–9
Avoidance strategies, 274
Awkward posture
biomechanical and physiologic perspectives on, 207–208*f*, 207–211
computer workstation and, 500–501
concepts related to neutral posture and, 205–207
in dental hygiene instrumentation, 452*t*, 453, 466*t*, 466
performing artist and, 475
Axial loading test
of distal radioulnar joint, 142
in upper-extremity joint injury, 136, 138–139*t*
Axillary interval, 78
Axillary nerve, 79*f*
Axon regeneration, 100
Axonotmesis, 76
Axoplasmic transport, 71–73, 72*f*, 75

B

Baby food, 414–415
Back, home activities and, 390*b*, 392
Back pain
backpack use in children and adolescents and, 399–400
in child care worker, 406, 409
in computer operator, 507*t*
in dental hygienist, 451, 457
laundering and, 397–398, 398*t*
in parent, 407
standing workstation and, 236
Back school, 344
Background noise
computer workstation and, 510–511
older worker and, 443
Backpack use in children and adolescents, 399–400, 401*t*
Backrest of chair, 236, 310
Balance, older worker and, 439
Balance theory of job design and stress, 269
Baltimore Therapeutic Equipment Work Simulator, 336, 337*t*
Bamboo knitting needles, 430
Base of chair, 236
Bathing of child, 415
Bicipital tendinitis, 109*b*, 111–112, 112*f*
in dental hygienist, 458, 458*t*
key restrictions in, 99*t*
Biomechanical risk factors, 191–229
cool temperatures in, 223–224
in dental hygiene instrumentation, 455
dynamic factors in, 217
force in, 199–204
external and internal force considerations in, 199–201, 200*t*
frictional, 201–202, 202*t*
gloves and, 202–203
measurement of, 203
psychophysical methods in estimation of, 203–204, 204*f*
research on, 201
in gardening, 420–421, 421*t*
in joint injury, 138–139*t*
measuring and reporting of exposures, 193–194
mechanical compression in, 218
posture in, 204–217, 205*t*
awkward postures and, 205–211, 207*f*, 208*f*
computerized motion analysis systems and, 217
film and video-based systems for assessment of, 214–217
postural analysis tools and, 214–215, 215–216*t*
posture targeting and, 212–213, 213*f*
self-analysis checklist and, 214
static postures in, 211–212
psychosocial risk factors and, 156–157
repetition in, 194*f*, 194–199
fatigue model of, 196*f*, 196–197
hand activity level and, 198–199
measurement of, 198
research on, 197–198
tissue strain and, 195*f*, 195–196
vibration in, 218–223
effects on body, 220
measurement of, 222–223
physical concepts of, 219–220
recommendations for decreasing, 223
research in, 221–222
segmental, 220–221
whole-body, 220

Biomechanics
in ergonomic job analysis, 290–294
of knitting, 429
of peripheral nerve, 73, 74*f*
of tendons, 65–66
in using tools, 242
Biopsychology, 273
Biothesiometer, 96
Blood flow, nerve compression and, 73–74, 75*f*
Blood-nerve barrier, 71
Blood supply
of nerve, 71
of tendon, 64–65
Body
effects of vibration on, 220
tissue strain in repetition and, 195*f*, 195–196
Body map, 464
Body mechanics
in child care, 410–411
home activities and, 390*b*, 392
backpack use in children and adolescents, 399–400
cleaning and, 395*t*, 396–397
cooking and, 393–394, 394*t*
laundering and, 397–399, 398*t*
Bone cyst, 134
Borg CR-10 scale, 204, 204*f*
Borg Rating of Perceived Exertion, 204, 204*f*
Bottle feeding, 414–415
Botulinum toxin, 126
Brachial plexus, 78, 79*f*
Brachioradialis, 80*f*
Brass instrument player, 477
Breast cancer, 257
Breastfeeding, 414–415
Bunion, 480
Bursitis, 69*f*, 69–70
olecranon, 115, 115*f*
subacromial, 69–70, 112
Buttocks-to-popliteal length, 232*f*, 288
Byl Cheney-Boczai sensory discriminator test, 97

C
C fiber, 104
Canadian Occupational Performance Measure, 89
Canadian Standards Association, 521
Car seat, 413–414, 414*f*
Carpal boss, 141
Carpal tunnel syndrome, 119*b*, 121–122
in computer operator, 497–498
in dental hygienist, 448, 457, 458*t*, 459
force and, 201
intrinsic atrophy and, 330–331, 331*f*
in keyboard player, 478
North American cases of, 9
repetition and, 197
segmental vibration and, 221–222
sensibility loss in, 331–333, 332*f*
in string player, 479
Carpometacarpal joint injury, 140
biomechanical risk factors for, 138*t*
in musician, 477
Carrying of child, 408, 413
Cartilaginous loose body, 134
Case study
of dental hygienist, 463–467, 466*t*
in muscle fatigue, 187–188
outcome evaluation and, 376, 384–386, 385*t*
of performing artist, 484–488
in reducing injuries, claims, and costs, 313–321
Cervical disc stenosis, 108–109
Cervical radiculopathy, 107*b*
Cervicobrachial region
cervical disc and foraminal stenosis and, 108–109
potential compression and entrapment in, 76–78, 79*f*
thoracic outlet syndrome and, 106–108, 106–108*f*, 107*b*
Chain piecing in quilting, 425
Chair
in computer workstation, 506–507
for seated workstation, 235–236, 236*t*
Changing table, 415
Checklist
for biomechanical risk factors, 193
for computer workstation assessment, 528–529
Chest depth, 288
Child
computer use and, 513–519, 517*f*, 518*f*
ergonomic considerations for, 399–402, 400*f*, 401*t*
Child care equipment, 411*t*
Child care ergonomics, 405–418
bathing child and, 415
bedtime and napping and, 415–416, 416*f*
body mechanics and, 410–411
carrying child and, 413
child care workers and preschool teachers, 405–406
dressing and changing child and, 415
feeding child and, 414–415
job analysis in, 407–409
lifting and lowering child and, 411–413, 412*f*
parents and family providers, 406–407
performing chores and, 416
play time and family recreation and, 416, 417*f*
risk factors in, 409*b*, 409–410, 410*b*
transporting child and, 413–414, 414*f*
Child care worker, 405–406, 408
Chin tuck, 309
Chronic bursitis, 112
Chronic disease, older worker and, 438
Chronic inflammation in performing artist, 477
Chronic pain
anger and, 276
older worker and, 439
Chronic tendinitis, 68
Circadian rhythms, shiftwork and, 256, 259
Circular knitting needles, 430
Cleaning of house, 395*t*, 396–397
Clearance, ergonomic design and, 231
Clothes dryer, 398, 398*t*
Codman shoulder pendulum exercise, 309
Coefficient of friction, 202, 249
Cognitive appraisal of stress, 273–274
Cold pack, 103
Cold temperatures, 223–224

Cold treatment, 103-104
Collagen
in tendons, 63-64, 64*f*
viscoelastic properties of peripheral nerve and, 73
Collateral ligaments, 133
injuries to, 134
metacarpophalangeal joint injury and, 139
translational stability testing of, 136
Communication, injury prevention program and, 345-346
Company losses, 366-370, 368*t*
Compression band, 321-322
Compression loading test, 136, 138-139*t*
Compression neuropathies, 71-83
anastomosis and, 82-83
biomechanics of peripheral nerves and, 73, 74*f*
cervicobrachial region and, 76-78, 79*f*
classification of nerve injuries in, 76, 77*f*, 78*t*
dorsal radial sensory nerve compression and entrapment in, 122-123
Guyon's tunnel syndrome in, 122
in keyboard players, 478
median nerve and, 80-81, 81-82*f*
nerve anatomy and physiology in, 71-73, 72*f*
neural reorganization secondary to compression in, 75-76
pathology of, 73-75, 75*f*
radial nerve and, 78, 80*f*
in string players, 479
ulnar nerve and, 81-82, 83-84*f*
Compression tests, 96
Compressive loading injury, 133-134
of radiocarpal joint, 140-141
Computer games, 518*f*, 518-519
Computer hardware, 507-508
Computer mouse, 170-171, 171*f*
Computer operation job description, 496-497
Computer workstation, 494-529
assessment of, 502-506, 503*b*, 505*b*, 506*f*
awkward posture and, 500-501
children and, 513-519, 517*f*, 518*f*
computer hardware and, 507-508
computer operation job description, 496-497
cost and incidents of musculoskeletal disorders and, 497, 498*t*
ergonomic accessories for, 508*b*, 508-509
ergonomic design of, 509-511
ergonomic regulation and, 520-522
ergonomics management program for, 502, 503*t*
force and, 501
input devices and, 511
job design and psychosocial factors, 495-496
keyboard and, 494-495, 511-512
physical contact and mechanical stress and, 501
pointing devices and, 512-513
portable computers and laptops, 513
repetition and, 501
static posture and, 499
telecommuting and, 519-520
temperature extremes and, 501-502
work practices and, 495
work surface and chair in, 506-507
workplace injuries and illnesses related to, 497-499
Computerized motion analysis systems, 217
Concise Exposure Index, 214
Conditioning
in cubital tunnel syndrome, 115
of performing artist, 474-475, 483
Conducting of outcome evaluations, 374-380
case studies in, 376
checklists and attitude rating scales in, 377
focus groups in, 376
interviews in, 376, 377
narrative records in, 375-376
surveys in, 377
Confidence interval, 194
Connective tissue of peripheral nerve, 71
Consensus diagnostic classifications for musculoskeletal disorders, 33
Constrained space, performing artist and, 476
Consultant in injury prevention program, 342
Contact stresses
computer workstations and, 501
in dental hygiene instrumentation, 452*t*, 453
Containers for gardening, 422, 423*f*
Contour of tool handle, 245, 246*f*
Contracture assessment, 138-139*t*
Contrast ratio, 253
Cooking, ergonomic principles in, 393-396, 396*f*, 397*f*
Cool temperatures, 223-224
Coping
with age-related vulnerabilities, 440
with stress, 273-274
Corticosteroids, 102-103
for bicipital tendinitis, 111
effect on tendon, 66
Cost accounting, 381-384, 382*f*
Cost-benefit analysis, 53-54, 54*t*
Cost-effectiveness of worksite programs, 380-384, 382*f*
Costoclavicular compression test, 107
Costoclavicular interval, 78
Costoclavicular space, 79*f*
Costs, injury severity and, 301
Counterforce bracing of elbow, 116, 117*f*
CR-10 scale, 204, 204*f*
Crawford small parts test, 97
Creep test, 66
Crib, 415-416, 416*f*
Cross-bridge, 207
Cross-friction massage, 116
Cross stretch, 105
Cryotherapy, 103
Cubital tunnel syndrome, 113*f*, 113-115, 114*b*, 115*f*
in dental hygienist, 458*t*, 459
in keyboard player, 478
in string player, 479
Culturally diverse workforce, 20-21, 21*b*
Cumulative trauma disorders, 9, 106-126
anterior interosseous syndrome in, 119*b*, 120
bicipital tendinitis in, 109*b*, 111-112, 112*f*
carpal tunnel syndrome in, 119*b*, 121-122
cervical disc and foraminal stenosis in, 108-109
cubital tunnel syndrome in, 113*f*, 113-115, 114*b*, 115*f*
de Quervain's disease in, 123*f*, 123-124, 124*b*
dorsal radial sensory nerve compression and entrapment in, 122-123

Cumulative trauma disorders—*cont'd*
  flexor tenosynovitis in, 120-121, 121*b*
  focal hand dystonia in, 125-126
  Guyon's tunnel syndrome in, 122
  by industry, 47*t*, 48*f*
  intersection syndrome in, 121*b*, 124
  lateral epicondylitis in, 115-117, 116*b*, 117*f*
  medial epicondylitis in, 116*b*, 118-119
  myofascial trigger points and, 112
  number of cases, 46*f*
  olecranon bursitis in, 115, 115*f*
  pronator syndrome in, 119*b*, 119-120
  radial tunnel syndrome in, 117-118, 118*b*
  rotator cuff tendinitis in, 109-111, 110*t*
  subacromial bursitis in, 112
  thoracic outlet syndrome in, 106-108, 106-108*f*, 107*b*
  trigger finger in, 124*b*, 124-125, 125*b*, 125-126*f*
Curved handle, 246-247
Cutaneous innervation
  by median nerve, 82*f*
  by ulnar nerve, 84*f*
Cutting
  cooking and, 394*t*
  quilting and, 425
Cycle time, 198
Cylindrical tools, 243, 243*f*
Cyst
  bone, 134
  ganglion cysts, 331, 331*f*

D
Damping, 219
Dancer, 479-481
Day care worker, 405-406
Daylight, 255
  shiftwork and, 259
de Quervain's disease, 123*f*, 123-124, 124*b*
  in dental hygienist, 458*t*, 459
  Finkelstein's test in, 334, 334*f*
  key restrictions in, 99*t*
  in keyboard player, 478
Decentralization of companies, 11-12
Decompression of nerve entrapment, 100
Deep-friction massage, 104-105
Deep heating, 104
Demand control models, 271-272
Dental hygienist, 448-473
  case study of, 463-467, 466*t*
  interview for determination of work practices, 470-473
  job analysis for, 448-451, 450*f*, 451*f*
  musculoskeletal disorders common to, 457-460, 458*t*
  neck and shoulder pain in, 209
  professional background and roles of, 449
  recommendations to reduce risks of, 460-462, 461*t*, 462-463*f*
  risk factors for musculoskeletal disorders in, 451-457, 452*t*
    work task factors in, 452-455, 453*f*
    worker risk factors in, 456-457
    workplace organization factors in, 455-456
Dental instruments, 449-450
Design limits, 231
Dexterity tests, 97
Diabetes mellitus, older worker and, 438
Digging, gardening and, 420, 421*t*
Digital force gauge, 203
Digital separators of tool, 245-246
Direct glare, 254-255
Direct injury costs, 369
Direct lighting, 255
Disability
  age-related changes in, 437-439
  discriminatory testing methods and, 329
Disc compressive force in laundering, 404
Discriminatory testing methods, 328-329
Distal interphalangeal joint
  anterior interosseous syndrome and, 120
  injury of, 137-139, 138*t*
Distal radioulnar joint injury, 138*t*, 142
Documentation of workstation assessment, 504-505
Dorsal cutaneous branch, 84*f*
Dorsal radial sensory nerve compression and entrapment, 122-123
Dorsal scapular nerve, 79*f*
Dorsal wrist syndrome, 141
Downsizing, 22
Dressing and changing of child, 415
Drop-arm test, 111
Dusting, 395*t*
Dynamic dimensions, 231
Dynamic factors, 217
Dynamic functional muscle testing, 168
Dynamic work, 211
Dynamometer, 93, 335, 335*f*

E
Early return to work, 306-307
Economic aspects
  cost-benefit analysis and, 53-54, 54*t*
  cost-effectiveness of worksite programs, 380-384, 382*f*
  in injury prevention program, 343, 348
  injury severity and, 301
  of musculoskeletal disorders, 50-53, 51*f*, 51*t*
Edema following stress test, 336, 337*f*
Elbow
  anterior interosseous syndrome and, 119*b*, 120
  awkward postures of, 205*t*, 209-210
  biomechanical risk factors for, 138*t*
  cubital tunnel syndrome and, 113*f*, 113-115, 114*b*, 115*f*
  flexion strength of, 207*f*, 207
  grip force and, 242
  injury of, 142-143
  lateral epicondylitis and, 115-117, 116*b*, 117*f*
  medial epicondylitis and, 116*b*, 118-119
  olecranon bursitis in, 115, 115*f*
  pain in dancer, 480
  pain in dental hygienist, 458*t*, 458-459, 459*f*
  pronator syndrome and, 119*b*, 119-120
  radial tunnel syndrome and, 117-118, 118*b*
  sites of nerve compression around, 113, 113*f*
Elbow height, 233*f*, 288
Elbow rest height, 232*f*, 288
Elbow span, 288
Elbow-to-fingertip length, 288
Elbow-to-fist length, 232*f*

Electrical filament lamp, 255
Electromyography, 91-92f
Electroneurometer, 335f, 335-336
Electronic database of musculoskeletal disorders, 364-366, 365t, 366-367f
Emotion-focused coping, 274
Emotion regulation, older worker and, 441
Emotional states, 276, 277f
Employee education and training, 322-323
  in injury prevention, 349-351, 350t
Employee interviews and surveys, 377
Employee morale, 303-304
Employee turnover, 383-384
Employment examinations, 324-341
  accuracy of, 326-327
  Americans with Disabilities Act and, 327-330
  ethical and legal rights in, 338-339
  support of medical exams in industry, 325-326
  typical components of, 327
  Upper Extremity Fitness for Duty Evaluation in, 330-338
    abnormal nerve conduction velocity in, 335f, 335-336
    accuracy of, 336-338, 338t
    epicondylar pain in, 333-334
    Finkelstein's test in, 334, 334t
    ganglion cysts in, 331, 331f
    intrinsic atrophy in, 330-331, 331f
    Phalen's test in, 334-335, 335f
    presence of edema following stress test in, 336, 337f
    Raynaud's phenomenon in, 333
    sensibility loss in, 331-333, 332f
    Tinel's sign in, 334, 334f
    triggering in, 333, 333f
    weakness of grip or pinch in, 335, 335f
Endoneurium, 71, 72f
Endorphins, 104
Endotenon, 64, 64f
Energy conservation, home activities and, 390b, 392-393
Engineering controls in reducing injury, 309-313
  in dental hygiene profession, 460, 461t
  in vibration exposure, 223
Entrapment syndromes, 71-83
  anastomosis and, 82-83
  biomechanics of peripheral nerves and, 73, 74f
  cervicobrachial region and, 76-78, 79f
  classification of nerve injuries in, 76, 77f, 78t
  in dental hygienist, 459
  dorsal radial sensory nerve, 122-123
  Guyon's tunnel syndrome in, 122
  in keyboard player, 478
  median nerve, 80-81, 81f, 82f
  nerve anatomy and physiology in, 71-73, 72f
  neural reorganization secondary to compression in, 75-76
  pathology of, 73-75, 75f
  radial nerve, 78, 80f
  in string players, 479
  treatment of, 99-102, 101f
  ulnar nerve, 81-82, 83f, 84f
Environmental factors
  in dental hygiene profession, 456
  ergonomic job analysis and, 154-155, 294
  in injury in performing artist, 476
  older worker and, 442
  quilting and, 424-427
  recommended levels of illumination and, 253-256, 254t
Epicondylar pain, 333-334
Epicondylitis
  lateral, 115-117, 116b, 117f
  medial, 116b, 118-119
Epidemiological model of musculoskeletal disorders, 268-269
Epineurium, 71, 72f
Epitenon, 64
Equal Employment Opportunity Commission, 57
Equipment
  child care, 411t
  in computer workstation, 506-511
    computer hardware and, 506-508
    ergonomic accessories in, 508b, 508-509
    ergonomic guidelines for workstation design and, 509-511
    work surfaces and chairs in, 506-507
  in dental hygiene instrumentation, 452t
  of performing artist, 476, 484
  workstation design and, 237-238, 238f
Ergonomic accessories for computer workstation, 508b, 508-509
Ergonomic assessment
  in dental hygiene profession, 463-464
  of older worker, 443-444
  of workplace, 289-290
Ergonomic disorders, 302
Ergonomic hazards, 302
Ergonomic risk factors, 151-280
  biomechanical, 191-229
    awkward postures and, 205-211, 207-208f
    computerized motion analysis systems and, 217
    cool temperatures in, 223-224
    dynamic factors in, 217
    film and video-based systems for assessment of, 214-217
    force in, 199-204, 200t, 202t, 204f
    measuring and reporting of exposures, 193-194
    mechanical compression in, 218
    postural analysis tools and, 214-215, 215-216t
    posture targeting and, 212-213, 213f
    repetition in, 194-196f, 194-199
    self-analysis checklist and, 214
    static postures and, 211-212
    vibration in, 218-223
  in child care, 409b, 409-410, 410b
  difficulties in identification of, 155-157
  expanded definition of ergonomics and, 152
  in home activities, 389-390
  job design and, 230-264
    anthropometrics in, 230-232, 232-234f
    hand and powered tools and, 238-251. *See also* Tools.
    lighting in workplace and, 251-256, 252t, 253t, 254t
    machine pacing and worker control in, 262
    shiftwork and, 256-260
    work breaks and, 261-262
    working hours and overtime in, 260-261
    workstation design and, 232-238, 236-238f
  musculoskeletal disorder etiology models and, 152-155, 153f
  origins of ergonomics, 151-152
  personal, 157-158
  physiologic, 160-190

Ergonomic risk factors—*cont'd*
physiologic—*cont'd*
case study in, 187-188
fatigue without recovery and, 170*t*
global muscle inhibition and, 169*t*
hyperresponsivity and, 167*t*, 170-172, 171*f*
muscle activation and, 163
muscle overload and, 167*t*, 176-177, 177*f*
neural distress and, 167*t*, 172-176, 173*f*, 177*f*
recovery model in, 186-187
surface electromyography and, 163-168, 164*f*, 165*f*
task-specific muscle inhibition with compensation and, 168*t*, 183-185*f*, 183-186
task-specific muscle inhibition without compensation and, 167-168*t*, 178-183, 179*f*, 181*f*, 182*f*
terminology in, 160-162, 161*t*
psychosocial, 265-280
concepts and definitions in, 265-266
coping and cognitive appraisal in, 273-274
demand control models and, 271-272
immune responses to workplace stress, 273
models of stress and health, 267-269, 268*f*
objective and subjective sources of stress, 269-270, 270*t*
personal and adjustment factors in, 274-276, 277*f*
quality of life and, 276-277
stress and work environments and, 266-267
workplace stress research and, 270-271
Ergonomic solution, 302
Ergonomics
of child care, 405-418
bathing, 415
bedtime and napping, 415-416, 416*f*
body mechanics and, 410-411
carrying child, 413
child care workers and preschool teachers, 405-406
dressing and changing child, 415
feeding child, 414-415
job analysis in, 407-409
lifting and lowering child, 411-413, 412*f*
parents and family providers, 406-407
performing chores and, 416
play time and family recreation, 416, 417*f*
risk factors in, 409*b*, 409-410, 410*b*
transporting child, 413-414, 414*f*
defined, 230
expanded definition of, 152
global trends in, 11-12
home activities and, 389-404
backpack use in children and adolescents and, 399-400, 401*t*
body mechanics in, 392
cleaning and, 395*t*, 396-397
cooking and, 393-396, 396*f*, 397*f*
development of musculoskeletal disorders in, 389-390
energy conservation in, 392-393
handwriting and, 401*t*, 401-402
joint protection principles in, 390-392
laundry and, 397-399, 398*t*, 404
video gaming and, 400-401, 401*t*
in industrial developing countries, 10-11
in injury prevention program, 352-353
of leisure activities, 419-433
gardening and, 420-425, 421*t*, 422-425*f*
general considerations in, 419-420
knitting and, 428-432, 430-433*f*
quilting and, 424-428, 426-428*f*
musculoskeletal disorder etiology models and, 152-155, 153*f*
national strategies for injury prevention and, 301-307
origins of, 151-152
Ergonomics equation, 310
Ergonomics Program Standard, 303
Ergonomics standards, 55
Ergonomics team, 313
Essential job functions, 284-285
Ethical issues in preemployment examinations, 338-339
Ethnographic interview, 19, 25-28
Europe, musculoskeletal disorders in, 8
Exercise
mechanical demands on tendons and, 66-67
stretching, 308-309
for dental hygienist, 462-463*f*
in injury prevention program, 354-358
for knitter, 431-432, 432*f*,
for quilter, 427-428, 428*f*
for tendinitis, 105
Exposure intensifier, 194
Exposure measures, 13
Extended workday, 260-261
Extensor carpi radialis brevis, 80*f*
Extensor carpi radialis longus, 80*f*
Extensor carpi ulnaris, 80*f*
Extensor digiti quinti, 80*f*
Extensor digitorum communis, 80*f*
Extensor indicis proprius, 80*f*
Extensor pollicis brevis, 80*f*
Extensor pollicis longus, 80*f*
External forces, 199-201, 200*t*
External stressors, 154
Extreme postures, 206
Extrinsic biomechanical risk factors, 191
Extrinsic vascularity of tendon, 64
Eye height, 232*f*, 233*f*
Eyestrain in computer operator, 507*t*

F

Faces pain rating scale, 90
Falls, older worker and, 443
Family child care provider, 408
Fasciculation, electromyography and, 91
Fatigue
in child care worker, 406
home activities and, 392-393
leisure activity ergonomics and, 419-433
gardening and, 420-425, 421*t*, 422-425*f*
general considerations in, 419-420
knitting and, 428-432, 430-432*f*
quilting and, 424-428, 426-428*f*
muscle fiber recruitment patterns in, 200
in performing artist, 475
physiologic risk factors for, 160-190
case study in, 187-188
fatigue without recovery and, 168*t*
global muscle inhibition and, 169*t*

hyperresponsivity and, 167*t*, 170-172, 171*f*
muscle activation and, 163
muscle overload and, 167*t*, 176-177, 177*f*
neural distress and, 167*t*, 172-176, 173*f*, 177*f*
recovery model in, 186-187
surface electromyography and, 163-168, 164*f*, 165*f*
task-specific muscle inhibition with compensation and, 168*t*, 183-185*f*, 183-186
task-specific muscle inhibition without compensation and, 167-168*t*, 178-183, 179*f*, 181-182*f*
terminology in, 160-162, 161*t*
Fatigue model of repetition, 196*f*, 196-197
Fatigue without recovery, term, 168*t*
Feeding of child, 414-415
Fibrillations, electromyography and, 91
Fibroplasia, 98
Film-based systems for posture assessment, 214-217
Finger
awkward postures of, 205*t*
dental hygienist and, 458*t*, 459, 459*f*
interphalangeal joint injury, 137-139
keyboard player and, 478, 479*f*
mechanical compression of, 218
pain in computer operator, 507*t*
string player and, 478-479, 480*f*
trigger, 124-125, 124-125*b*, 125-126*f*
triggering in tenosynovitis, 333
Finger loops, 218
Finger rings of tool, 246, 246*f*
Fingertip height, 288
Finkelstein's test, 123, 334, 334*t*
Flat screen monitor, 508
Flexibility
of injury prevention program, 346
in work structure, 11-12
Flexible support, 321-322
Flexor carpi radialis, 81*f*
Flexor carpi ulnaris, 83*f*, 84*f*
Flexor digiti quinti, 83*f*
Flexor digitorum profundus, 81*f*, 83*f*
Flexor digitorum superficialis, 81*f*, 82*f*
Flexor paratendinitis, 99*t*
Flexor pollicis brevis, 81*f*, 83*f*
Flexor pollicis longus, 81*f*
Flexor tenosynovitis, 120-121, 121*b*
Flicker in fluorescent lighting, 255
Floor surfaces, 237
performing artist and, 480
Fluorescent lighting, 255
Focal hand dystonia, 70, 125-126
Focus group, 376
Foot breadth, 232*f*
Foot length, 232*f*
Foot pain, standing workstation and, 236
Foot placement and lower limb positioning, 311
Football carry, 413
Footrest
of chair, 236
standing workstation and, 237
Foraminal stenosis, 108-109
Force, 199-204
computer workstations and, 501
in dental hygiene instrumentation, 452*t*, 452-453, 466*t*
in ergonomic job analysis, 292
external and internal, 199-201, 200*t*
frictional, 201-202, 202*t*
gloves and, 202-203
measurement of, 203
psychophysical methods in estimation of, 203-204, 204*f*
research on, 201
Force gauge, 203
Forced vibration, 219
Forearm
anterior interosseous syndrome and, 119*b*, 120
pain in dental hygienist, 458*t*, 458-459
pronator syndrome and, 119*b*, 119-120
radial tunnel syndrome and, 117-118, 118*b*
Forward functional reach, 233*f*
Free vibration, 219
Frequency and acceleration, 219
Frictional forces, 201-202, 202*t*
Front carry, 413
Front-loading washing machine, 398
Function tests in upper-quadrant screen, 94*b*
Functional Analysis of Movement with Electromyography, 168, 177
Functional dimensions, 231
Functional overhead reach, 232*f*, 233*f*
Functional pain, 276
Functional sensibility, 94, 97
Fundamental cycle, 198

G
Gamekeeper's thumb, 139
Gaming, ergonomic principles in, 400-401, 401*t*
Ganglion cyst, 331, 331*f*
Gardening ergonomics, 420-425, 421*t*, 422-425*f*
Gardening products, 424
Gardening tools, 423-424, 423-424*f*
Gender, personal risk factors and, 157
General adaptation syndrome, 266
Gerotechnology, 393
Glare, 254-255
Glenohumeral joint
biomechanical risk factors for, 139*t*
injury of, 143-144
Global appreciation for musculoskeletal disorders, 10
Global muscle inhibition, 169*t*
Globalization, 11
Gloves
ergonomic job analysis and, 293
grip force and, 202-203
in knitting, 431, 431*f*
Goal-setting process in outcome assessment, 370-373, 372-373*f*, 374*b*
Golgi tendon organs, 65
Grip, weakness of, 335, 335*f*
Grip force, 240-241
in ergonomic job analysis, 292-293
gloves and, 202-203
vibration and, 222
Grip strength, 93, 241, 242
Guyon's tunnel, 82, 84*f*
Guyon's tunnel syndrome, 114*b*, 122

H

Hand
  anthropometric data for, 234*f*
  carpal tunnel syndrome and, 119*b*, 121-122
  de Quervain's disease and, 123*f*, 123-124, 124*b*
  dental hygiene profession and, 450*f*, 450-451, 454, 459, 459*f*
  dorsal radial sensory nerve compression and entrapment, 122-123
  flexor tenosynovitis and, 120-121, 121*b*
  focal hand dystonia and, 125-126
  Guyon's tunnel syndrome and, 122
  intersection syndrome and, 121*b*, 124
  keyboard player and, 478, 479*f*
  knitting and, 432*f*
  string player and, 478-479, 480*f*
  trigger finger and, 124-125, 124-125*b*, 125-126*f*
Hand activity level
  osteoarthritis and, 135
  repetition and, 198-199
  voluntary standard for mono-task jobs, 56, 56*f*
Hand-Arm Vibration analysis tool, 216*t*
Hand-arm vibration syndrome, 218-219, 221
Hand breadth, 288
Hand piecing in quilting, 425
Hand-skin temperature, 224
Hand span, 288
Hand stitching in quilting, 425
Hand Tool Analysis Method, 251, 252*b*
Hand tools, 238-251
  cylindrical, 243, 243*f*
  dental, 449-450
  digital separators in, 245-246
  ergonomic selection of, 250-251, 252*b*
  finger rings in, 246, 246*f*
  handle diameter and span, 243
  handle length in, 247-248, 248*f*
  handle orientation in, 246-247, 247*f*
  handle surface, texture, and materials of, 248-249
  inappropriately sized, 244-245, 245*f*
  operation and activation of, 250
  optimal shape of, 245
  precision, 244, 244*f*
  prehension patterns and, 239-241, 239-242*f*
  principles for use of, 241-242
  slipperiness of, 249
  surface pattern of, 249
  tool position and, 250
  tool weight and balance in, 250
  two-handled, 243-244, 244*f*
  vibration absorption of, 249-250
Hand-wrist osteoarthritis, 135
Handheld digital force gauge, 203
Handle of tool
  contour of, 245, 246*f*
  design for home activities, 395-396, 396*f*
  diameter and span of, 243
  length of, 247-248, 248*f*
  orientation of, 246-247, 247*f*
  surface, texture, and materials of, 248-249
Handwriting, ergonomic principles in, 401*t*, 401-402
Hard floor surfaces, 237
Harmonic vibration, 219
Harvesting, gardening and, 420, 421*t*
Hatha yoga simple twist, 428, 428*f*
Healing, 98
Health
  age-related changes in, 437-439
  models of, 267-269, 268*f*
Health outcomes, 13
Health screening, 383
Healthcam, 214-217
Hearing, older worker and, 439
Heat treatment in cubital tunnel syndrome, 115
Heberden's nodule, 458*t*, 459
Height
  of chair, 235, 236*f*
  of workstation, 235, 237, 237*f*
High repetitive job, 198
High-vibration tools, 450, 454
Hip breadth, 232*f*, 288
Hip carry, 413
Hip height, 288
History
  musculotendinous *versus* neural disorders and, 89, 91
  of performing artist, 481, 491-493
Hoeing, gardening and, 420, 421*t*
Home activities ergonomics, 389-404
  backpack use in children and adolescents and, 399-400, 401*t*
  body mechanics in, 392
  child care and, 416
  cleaning and, 395*t*, 396-397
  cooking and, 393-396, 396*f*, 397*f*
  development of musculoskeletal disorders and, 389-390
  energy conservation in, 392-393
  handwriting and, 401*t*, 401-402
  joint protection principles in, 390-392
  laundry and, 397-399, 398*t*, 404
  video gaming and, 400-401, 401*t*
Hook grasp, 239
Hot pack, 104
Human relations approach to management, 17
Hyperresponsivity of muscle, 161*t*, 167*t*, 170-172, 171*f*
Hypovascular watershed area, 70

I

Ice massage, 103
Illumination, 252-253, 254*f*
  in computer workstation, 510
  dental hygienist and, 456
  in injury in performing artist, 480
  older worker and, 442
  quilting and, 426-427
  recommended levels of, 253-256, 254*t*
  terminology in, 252*t*, 252-253, 253*t*
Immune response to stress, 273
Impact vibration, 219
Impingement, 109-111, 110*t*
Impingement test, 111
Inappropriately sized tools, 244-245, 245*f*
Indemnity, 369
Indirect glare, 254-255

Indirect injury costs, 369-370
Indirect lighting, 255
Industrial epidemic, 3
Industrial Revolution, 16
Industrially advanced countries, 10-11
Industrially developing countries, 10-11
Inflammation
  in performing artist, 477
  treatment of, 102-104, 103*f*
  wound healing and, 98
Information and communication technology, 12
Infraspinous tendinitis, 111
Inhibition of muscle, 161*t*
Injury
  computer use-related, 497-499
  neural reorganization after, 76
  reducing injuries, claims, and costs, 299-323
    case studies in, 313-321
    in dental hygienist, 460-462, 461*t*, 462-463*f*
    early return to work and modified duty in, 306-307
    engineering controls in, 309-313
    injury reporting and investigation process in, 304-306
    issues in determination of injury, 299-300
    management-employee education and training in, 322-323
    national strategies for, 301-303
    new employee conditioning and training in, 304
    physical comfort aids and, 321-322
    productivity standards and paced work in, 307
    relationship of costs to injury severity, 301
    sociopolitical atmosphere and employee morale in, 303-304
    work practice controls in, 307-309
    worker *versus* supervisor perceptions in, 300-301
  in stage performers, 474-493
    adaptive equipment for, 483-484
    awkward posture and, 475
    background of performers' careers and, 474
    brass instrument players and, 477
    case studies in, 484-488
    changing work environments and, 476
    constrained space and, 476
    dancers, actors, mimes, and acrobats, 479-481
    fatigue and, 475
    history in, 481, 491-493
    keyboard players and, 478, 478*f*, 479*f*
    lifting and carrying instruments and equipment, 476, 484
    percussionists and, 477-478
    physical examination for overuse injury in, 481
    principles of treatment for, 482-483
    repetition and, 475
    static posture and, 475
    stress of performing and, 476
    string players and, 478-479, 480*f*
    training and conditioning and, 474-475
    types of injury in, 476-477
    woodwind players and, 477
    workplace environmental evaluation and, 481-482
    workplace modifications and, 483
  tendon response to, 67*t*, 67-69
Injury cost trend analysis, 382*f*, 382-383
Injury data, 44-46, 45-46*f*, 47-48*t*, 48*f*
  determining company losses and, 366-370, 368*t*
  tracking system for, 364-366, 365*t*, 366-367*f*
  use of, 49-50
Injury prevention
  in dental hygienist, 460-462, 461*t*, 462-463*f*
  early return to work and modified duty in, 306-307
  implementation of program for, 342-363
    communication and, 345-346
    employee training and education and, 349-351, 351*t*
    ergonomics and, 352-353
    money factor in, 343-344
    people involved in, 342-343
    presentation style in, 350-352
    providing services in, 345
    selling of, 347-349, 362-363
    stretching and warming up in, 354-358
    time factor in, 344
  injury reporting and accident investigation process in, 304-306
  job design and, 230-264
    anthropometrics in, 230-232, 232-234*f*
    hand and powered tools and, 238-251. *See also* Tools.
    lighting in workplace and, 251-256, 252*t*, 253*t*, 254*t*
    machine pacing and worker control in, 262
    shiftwork and, 256-260
    work breaks and, 261-262
    working hours and overtime in, 260-261
    workstation design and, 232-238, 236-238*f*
  national strategies for, 301-303
  new employee conditioning and training in, 304
  outcome assessment in, 363-386
    approach to program evaluation in, 363-364
    case study in, 384-386, 385*t*
    compilation of musculoskeletal disorder injury information system and, 364-366, 365*t*, 366*f*, 367*f*
    cost accounting and return-on-investment analysis in, 381-384, 382*f*
    determination of company losses and, 366-370, 368*t*
    goal-setting process in, 370-373, 372-373*f*, 374*b*
    issues in, 374-375
    qualitative measures in, 375-377
    quantitative measures in, 377-380, 379*f*, 380-381*t*
  productivity standards and paced work in, 307
  sociopolitical atmosphere and employee morale in, 303-304
  Upper Extremity Fitness for Duty Evaluation in, 330-338
    abnormal nerve conduction velocity in, 335*f*, 335-336
    accuracy of, 336-338, 338*t*
    epicondylar pain in, 333-334
    Finkelstein's test in, 334, 334*t*
    ganglion cysts in, 331, 331*f*
    intrinsic atrophy in, 330-331, 331*f*
    Phalen's test in, 334-335, 335*f*
    presence of edema following stress test in, 336, 337*f*
    Raynaud's phenomenon in, 333
    sensibility loss in, 331-333, 332*f*
    Tinel's sign in, 334, 334*f*
    triggering in, 333, 333*f*
    weakness of grip or pinch in, 335, 335*f*
Injury review process, 305-306
Innervation
  median nerve, 81*f*, 82*f*
  of tendons, 65
  ulnar nerve, 83*f*

Innervation density tests, 95–96
Input devices, 511
Instruments
dental, 449–450, 454, 456, 466*t*
of performing artist, 476, 484
Internal forces, 199–201, 200*t*
International Classification of Diseases, 9th Revision, 31–32, 32*t*
Interphalangeal joint
anterior interosseous syndrome and, 120
of dental hygienist, 459–460, 460*f*
injury of, 137–139
Intersection syndrome, 70, 99*t*, 121*b*, 124
Intervertebral disc pressure
calculation for laundering, 404
home activities and, 392
Interview
conducting of outcome evaluation and, 376, 377
of dental hygienist, 470–473
Intraarticular ligaments, 133
Intramuscular pressure
force and, 199
static posture and, 211
Intrinsic atrophy, 330–331, 331*f*
Intrinsic biomechanical risk factors, 191
Intrinsic vascularity of tendon, 64–65
Investigation process, 304–306
Iontophoresis, 103, 103*f*, 111
Isometric warm-up, 105

J

Jamar dynamometer, 335, 335*f*
Japan, occupational cervicobrachial disorder in, 6–7
Jar, opening of, 394–395
Jebsen-Taylor hand function test, 97
Job analysis, 283–298
activity descriptors in, 285–289
biomechanical aspects of, 192, 290–295
of child care work, 407–409
in dental hygiene profession, 449–451, 450–451*f*, 463–464
ergonomic assessment in, 289–290
essential job functions and, 284–285
historical background of, 283–284
of local external stressors, 154
marginal job functions and, 285
psychosocial aspects of, 294
Job content
in computer operation, 496–497
in dental hygiene profession, 455
Job design, 230–264
anthropometrics and, 230–232, 232–234*f*
balance theory of stress and, 269
computer workstation and, 495–496
hand and powered tools and, 238–251
cylindrical, 243, 243*f*
digital separators in, 245–246
ergonomic selection of, 250–251, 252*b*
finger rings in, 246, 246*f*
handle diameter and span, 243
handle length in, 247–248, 248*f*
handle orientation in, 246–247, 247*f*
handle surface, texture, and materials of, 248–249
inappropriately sized, 244–245, 245*f*
operation and activation of, 250
optimal shape of, 245
precision, 244, 244*f*
prehension patterns and, 239–241, 239–242*f*
principles for use of, 241–242
slipperiness of, 249
surface pattern of, 249
tool position and, 250
tool weight and balance in, 250
two-handled, 243–244, 244*f*
vibration absorption of, 249–250
lighting in workplace and, 251–256
computer workstation and, 510
dental hygienist and, 456
injury in performing artist and, 480
older worker and, 442
quilting and, 426–427
recommended levels of, 253–256, 254*t*
terminology in, 252*t*, 252–253, 253*t*
machine pacing and worker control in, 262
shiftwork and, 256–260
work breaks and, 261–262
working hours and overtime in, 260–261
workstation design and, 232–238
frequently used equipment and controls in, 237–238, 238*f*
seated workstations in, 235–236, 236*f*
standing workstations and, 236–237, 237*f*
workplace layout in, 234–235
workstation height in, 235
Job hazard analysis tools, 215–216*t*
Job security, 22
Job Strain Index, 215*t*
Job strain models, 271–272
Job stress
coping and cognitive appraisal in, 273–274
immune responses to, 273
methodologic issues in workplace stress research, 270–271
models of, 267–269, 268*f*
objective and subjective sources of, 269–270, 270*t*
personality and adjustment factors in, 274–276, 277*f*
work environment and, 266–267
Job tasks in dental hygiene profession, 449
Joint
anatomical design of, 132–133
protection principles for, 390*b*, 390–392
stabilizing structures of, 134
Joint injury, 132–148
of acromioclavicular joint, 143
anatomical design of joint, 132–133
biomechanical risk factors for, 138–139*t*
carpal boss in, 141
compressive loading injuries in, 133–134
diagnosis of, 136–137
of distal radioulnar joint, 142
of elbow, 142–143
of finger interphalangeal joints, 137–139
of glenohumeral joint, 143–144
home activities and, 390–392
of joint stabilizing structures, 134
medical management of, 144

of metacarpophalangeal joint, 139-140
in musician, 477
myofascial responses to, 134
of radiocarpal joint, 140-141
of thumb carpometacarpal joint, 140
upper-extremity arthritis as, 134-135, 135*b*
work-relatedness of, 144-145
of wrist pisiform-triquetral joint, 141-142
of wrist triangular fibrocartilaginous complex, 141
Jumper's knee, 480

K
Keyboard, 494-495, 511-512
Keyboard player, 478, 478*f*, 479*f*
Keyboard tray, 509
Kinematic posture measures, 217
Kitchen layout and storage, 393-394
Kitchen utensils, 394-396, 396*f*, 397*f*
Knee height, 232*f*, 233*f*
Knitting belt, 430, 430*f*
Knitting ergonomics, 428-432, 430-432*f*
Knitting needles, 429-430
Knuckle height, 233*f*, 288

L
Laboratory tests, 34
Lag time in reporting of injury, 306
Laptop computer, 513
Lateral epicondylitis, 115-117, 116*b*, 117*f*
in dental hygienist, 458*t*, 458-459
iontophoresis in, 103, 103*f*
key restrictions in, 99*t*
in keyboard player, 478
Lateral forearm pain, 90
Lateral grasp, 239, 240*f*
Lateral pectora nerve, 79*f*
Laundering, ergonomic principles in, 397-399, 398*t*, 404
Leg length, anthropometric, 232*f*
Leg pain
in computer operator, 507*t*
standing workstation and, 236
Legal issues in preemployment examinations, 338-339
Leisure activity ergonomics, 419-433
gardening and, 420-425, 421*t*, 422-425*f*
general considerations in, 419-420
knitting and, 428-432, 430-432*f*
quilting and, 425-428, 426-428*f*
Length-tension relationship, 207
Levels of cumulative trauma, 90*t*
Levi's model for psychosocial mediation of disease, 267, 268*f*
Lifting
of child, 408, 411-413, 412*f*
stage performer and, 476, 484
Lifting equation of NIOSH, 57, 215*t*
Ligament injury
collateral, 134
of metacarpophalangeal joint, 139
in performing artist, 477
Ligament of Struthers, 81
Light duty, 306-307
Light therapy for shiftworker, 259
Light touch in upper-quadrant screen, 93*b*
Lighting, 251-256
in computer workstation, 510
dental hygienist and, 456
in injury in performing artist, 480
older worker and, 442
quilting and, 426-427
recommended levels of, 253-256, 254*t*
terminology in, 252*t*, 252-253, 253*t*
Load sharing, 161*t*
Local external stressors, 154
Long-finger extension test, 116
Long thoracic nerve, 79*f*
Loss-control information systems, 367-369, 368*t*
Low-back pain
backpack use in children and adolescents and, 399-400
in child care worker, 406, 409
in dental hygienist, 457
laundering and, 397-398, 398*t*
in parent, 407
standing workstation and, 236
Low repetitive job, 198
Lumbricals, 81*f*, 83*f*
Luminance, 252-253

M
Machine pacing and worker control, 262
Machine piecing in quilting, 425
Macrophage, 98
Magnifying lens for knitting, 430, 431*f*
Management-employee education and training, 322-323
Manager of injury prevention program, 342-343
Marginal job functions, 285
Martin-Gruber anastomosis, 82
Massage, 104-105
in cubital tunnel syndrome, 115
for lateral epicondylitis, 116
for supraspinous tendinitis, 111
Maudsley's test, 116
Maximal holding time, 211-212
Maximum voluntary contraction, 452-453
McGill pain questionnaire, 90-91
Mechanical compression, 218
Mechanical stresses
computer workstations and, 501
in dental hygiene instrumentation, 454, 466*t*
Mechanism of injury, 305
Medial epicondylitis, 99*t*, 116*b*, 118-119
Medial-laxity, lateral-compression syndrome, 142
Median cutaneous nerve, 79*f*
Median nerve, 79*f*
adverse neural tension assessment of, 95*f*
anterior interosseous syndrome and, 120
carpal tunnel syndrome and, 121
potential compression and entrapment of, 80-81, 81-82*f*
pronator syndrome and, 119
Median nerve conduction study, 92*f*
Median nerve tension test, 108, 108*f*
Median pectora nerve, 79*f*
Medical examination before employment, 324-341
accuracy of, 326-327

Medical examination before employment—*cont'd*
Americans with Disabilities Act and, 327-330
ethical and legal rights in, 338-339
support in industry, 325-326
typical components of, 327
Upper Extremity Fitness for Duty Evaluation in, 330-338
abnormal nerve conduction velocity in, 335*f*, 335-336
accuracy of, 336-338, 338*t*
epicondylar pain in, 333-334
Finkelstein's test in, 334, 334*t*
ganglion cysts in, 331, 331*f*
intrinsic atrophy in, 330-331, 331*f*
Phalen's test in, 334-335, 335*f*
presence of edema following stress test in, 336, 337*f*
Raynaud's phenomenon in, 333
sensibility loss in, 331-333, 332*f*
Tinel's sign in, 334, 334*f*
triggering in, 333, 333*f*
weakness of grip or pinch in, 335, 335*f*
Mental health
demand control models and, 271-272
services for older worker, 445
Mesoneurium, 71, 72*f*
Metacarpophalangeal joint injury, 139-140
biomechanical risk factors for, 138*t*
in dental hygienist, 460
in musician, 477
Mid-shoulder height, 232*f*
Mill's stretch, 309
Milton Behavioral Health Inventory, 276
Mime, 479-481
Minigaps, 161*t*
Minnesota Multiphasic Personality Inventory, 276
Minnesota Rate of Manipulation Test, 97
Moberg pick-up test, 97
Mobility, seated position and, 310-311
Modified duty, 306-307
Modified Moberg pick-up test, 97
Modified pen grasp, 450, 450*f*
Modified Phalen's test, 335, 335*f*
Moment arm, 208, 208*f*
Monitor in computer workstation, 508
Mood, 266
Mopping, 395*t*
Morale, employee, 370
Motoneuron, 161*t*
Motor control strategy, 161*t*
muscle overload and, 176-177, 177*f*
neural distress and, 173-176
Movement adaptation syndrome, 168
Multiphasic health screening, 383
Multiple symptoms in musculoskeletal disorders, 36-38
Muscle
activation of, 163
adaptive changes in, 97
adaptive failure of, 183-185*f*, 183-186
hyperresponsivity of, 161*t*, 167*t*, 170-172, 171*f*
Muscle atrophy, 330-331, 331*f*
Muscle fatigue
leisure activity ergonomics and, 419-433
gardening and, 420-425, 421*t*, 422-425*f*
general considerations in, 419-420
knitting and, 428-432, 430-432*f*
quilting and, 425-428, 426-428*f*
physiologic risk factors for, 160-190
case study in, 187-188
fatigue without recovery and, 168*t*
global muscle inhibition and, 169*t*
hyperresponsivity and, 167*t*, 170-172, 171*f*
muscle activation and, 163
muscle overload and, 167*t*, 176-177, 177*f*
neural distress and, 167*t*, 172-176, 173*f*, 177*f*
recovery model in, 186-187
surface electromyography and, 163-168, 164*f*, 165*f*
task-specific muscle inhibition with compensation and, 168*t*, 183-185*f*, 183-186
task-specific muscle inhibition without compensation and, 167-168*t*, 178-183, 179*f*, 181*f*, 182*f*
terminology in, 160-162, 161*t*
Muscle overload, 167*t*, 176-177, 177*f*
Muscle spasm, 161*t*
Muscle spindle, 65
Musculocutaneous nerve, 79*f*
Musculoskeletal disorder injury information system, 364-366, 365*t*, 366*f*, 367*f*
Musculoskeletal disorders
aging population and, 12
in Australia, 7-9
biomechanical risk factors in, 191-229
awkward postures and, 205-211, 207-208*f*
computerized motion analysis systems and, 217
cool temperatures in, 223-224
dynamic factors in, 217
film and video-based systems for assessment of, 214-217
force in, 199-204, 200*t*, 202*t*, 204*f*
measuring and reporting of exposures, 193-194
mechanical compression in, 218
postural analysis tools and, 214-215, 215-216*t*
posture targeting and, 212-213, 213*f*
repetition in, 194-196*f*, 194-199
self-analysis checklist and, 214
static postures and, 211-212
vibration in, 218-223
common characteristics in, 30-31
computer workstations and, 494-529
assessment of, 502-506, 503*b*, 505*b*, 506*f*
awkward posture and, 500-501
children and, 513-519, 517*f*, 518*f*
computer hardware and, 507-508
computer operation job description, 496-497
cost and incidents of, 497, 498*t*
ergonomic accessories for, 508*b*, 508-509
ergonomic design of, 509-511
ergonomic regulation and, 520-522
ergonomics management program for, 502, 503*t*
force and, 501
input devices and, 511
job design and psychosocial factors, 495-496
keyboard and, 494-495, 511-512
physical contact and mechanical stress and, 501
pointing devices and, 512-513
portable computers and laptops, 513

repetition and, 501
static posture and, 499
telecommuting and, 519-520
temperature extremes and, 501-502
work practices and, 495
work surfaces and chairs in, 506-507
workplace injuries and illnesses related to, 497-499
in dental hygienists, 448-473
case study of, 463-467, 466*t*
interview for determination of work practices, 470-473
job analysis for, 449-451, 450*f*, 451*f*
musculoskeletal disorders common to, 457-460, 458*t*
professional background and roles of, 449
recommendations to reduce risks of, 460-462, 461*t*, 462-463*f*
work task factors in, 452-455, 453*f*
worker risk factors in, 456-457
workplace organization factors in, 455-456
diagnosis of, 31-39
consensus classifications for, 33
multiple symptoms and, 36-38
nonoccupational risks and, 39
protocols for, 34-36
regulatory definitions in, 33
research definitions in, 33
stages in, 38
symptom questionnaire survey in, 33-34
traditional system of, 31-33, 32*t*
electronic database of injury information, 364-366, 365*t*, 366*f*, 367*f*
etiology of
model of, 152-155, 153*f*
multifactorial, 155-157
in Europe, 8
flexibility in work structure and, 11-12
global appreciation for, 10
historical background of, 4-5
home activities and, 389-404
backpack use in children and adolescents and, 399-400, 401*t*
body mechanics in, 392
cleaning and, 395*t*, 396-397
cooking and, 393-396, 396*f*, 397*f*
development of, 389-390
energy conservation in, 392-393
handwriting and, 401*t*, 401-402
joint protection principles in, 390-392
laundry and, 397-399, 398*t*, 404
video gaming and, 400-401, 401*t*
individual worker perspective of, 15-28
beliefs and values about work and, 17
changing social context of work and, 19-22, 20*f*, 21*b*
definition of work and, 15-17
values of work culture and, 17-18
work culture assimilation and, 18-19
joint injury in, 132-148
of acromioclavicular joint, 143
anatomical design of joint, 132-133
biomechanical risk factors for, 138-139*t*
carpal boss in, 141
compressive loading injuries in, 133-134
diagnosis of, 136-137
of distal radioulnar joint, 142
of elbow, 142-143
of finger interphalangeal joints, 137-139
of glenohumeral joint, 143-144
of joint stabilizing structures, 134
medical management of, 144
of metacarpophalangeal joint, 139-140
myofascial responses to, 134
of radiocarpal joint, 140-141
of thumb carpometacarpal joint, 140
upper-extremity arthritis as, 134-135, 135*b*
work-relatedness of, 144-145
of wrist pisiform-triquetral joint, 141-142
of wrist triangular fibrocartilaginous complex, 141
new technology and, 12
in North America, 9
in older worker, 437-447
adaptive strategies for, 440-442
age-related changes in health and disability and, 437-440
assessment of, 443-444
ergonomic issues and, 442-443
psychologic issues of, 444-445
organizational issues in, 39-41
pathogenesis of, 30
in performing artists, 474-493
adaptive equipment and, 483-484
awkward posture and, 475
background of performers' careers and, 474
brass instrument players and, 477
case studies in, 484-488
changing work environments and, 476
constrained space and, 476
dancers, actors, mimes, and acrobats, 479-481
fatigue and, 475
history in, 481, 491-493
keyboard players and, 478, 478*f*, 479*f*
lifting and carrying instruments and equipment and, 476, 484
percussionists and, 477-478
physical examination for overuse injury, 481
principles of treatment for, 482-483
repetition and, 475
static posture and, 475
stress of performing and, 476
string players and, 478-479, 480*f*
training and conditioning and, 474-475
types of injury in, 476-477
woodwind players and, 477
workplace environmental evaluation and, 481-482
workplace modifications and, 483
peripheral neurovascular compressions and entrapment syndromes in, 71-83
anastomosis and, 82-83
biomechanics of peripheral nerves and, 73, 74*f*
cervicobrachial region and, 76-78, 79*f*
classification of nerve injuries in, 76, 77*f*, 78*t*
median nerve and, 80-81, 81*f*, 82*f*
nerve anatomy and physiology in, 71-73, 72*f*
neural reorganization secondary to compression in, 75-76
pathology of, 73-75, 75*f*
radial nerve and, 78, 80*f*
ulnar nerve and, 81-82, 83*f*, 84*f*

Musculoskeletal disorders—*cont'd*
personal risk factors in, 157-158
physiologic risk factors in, 160-190
case study in, 187-188
fatigue without recovery and, 168*t*
global muscle inhibition and, 169*t*
hyperresponsivity and, 167*t*, 170-172, 171*f*
muscle activation and, 163
muscle overload and, 167*t*, 176-177, 177*f*
neural distress and, 167*t*, 172-176, 173*f*, 177*f*
recovery model in, 186-187
surface electromyography and, 163-168, 164*f*, 165*f*
task-specific muscle inhibition with compensation and, 168*t*, 183-185*f*, 183-186
task-specific muscle inhibition without compensation and, 167-168*t*, 178-183, 179*f*, 181*f*, 182*f*
terminology in, 160-162, 161*t*
psychosocial factors in, 39-41, 265-280
concepts and definitions in, 265-266
coping and cognitive appraisal in, 273-274
demand control models and, 271-272
immune responses to workplace stress, 273
models of stress and health, 267-269, 268*f*
objective and subjective sources of stress, 269-270, 270*t*
personal and adjustment factors in, 274-276, 277*f*
quality of life and, 276-277
stress and work environments and, 266-267
workplace stress research and, 270-271
reducing injuries, claims, and costs in, 299-323
case studies in, 313-321
early return to work and modified duty in, 306-307
engineering controls in, 309-313
injury reporting and investigation process in, 304-306
issues in determination of injury, 299-300
management-employee education and training in, 322-323
national strategies for, 301-303
new employee conditioning and training in, 304
physical comfort aids and, 321-322
productivity standards and paced work in, 307
relationship of costs to injury severity, 301
sociopolitical atmosphere and employee morale in, 303-304
work practice controls in, 307-309
worker *versus* supervisor perceptions in, 300-301
regulatory perspective of, 44-59
cost-benefit analysis and, 53-54, 54*t*
economic and social aspects and, 50-53, 51*f*, 51*t*
injury/illness statistics and, 44-46, 45-46*f*, 47-48*t*, 48*f*
regulatory environment and, 54-57, 56*f*
underreporting and, 46-49
union contracts and, 58
use of injury data and, 49-50
workers' compensation and, 57-58
research in, 12-13
role of ergonomics in industrial developing countries, 10-11
tendonopathies in, 63-70
biomechanics of tendons and, 65-66
conditions related to, 69*f*, 69-70
factors affecting integrity of tendons in, 66-67
pathology of, 67
regional anatomy in, 63-65, 64*f*
tendon response to injury and, 67*t*, 67-69
terminology in, 29-30, 30*b*
treatment of, 89-131
activity tolerance and, 89-91, 90*t*
adaptive changes in nearby tissue and, 97
adverse neural tension assessment in, 94, 95*f*
in anterior interosseous syndrome, 119*b*, 120
in bicipital tendinitis, 109*b*, 111-112, 112*f*
in carpal tunnel syndrome, 119*b*, 121-122
in cervical disc and foraminal stenosis, 108-109
in cubital tunnel syndrome, 113*f*, 113-115, 114*b*, 115*f*
in de Quervain's disease, 123*f*, 123-124, 124*b*
in dorsal radial sensory nerve compression and entrapment, 122-123
electromyography in, 91, 91*f*
in flexor tenosynovitis, 120-121, 121*b*
in focal hand dystonia, 125-126
functional sensibility tests in, 97
in Guyon's tunnel syndrome, 122
history and subjective assessment in, 89
in inflammatory phase, 102-104, 103*f*
innervation density tests in, 95-96
in intersection syndrome, 121*b*, 124
in lateral epicondylitis, 115-117, 116*b*, 117*f*
in medial epicondylitis, 116*b*, 118-119
myofascial trigger points and, 112
in nerve compressions and entrapments, 99-102, 101*f*
nerve conduction studies in, 92, 92*f*
objective clinical assessments in, 92, 93*b*
in olecranon bursitis, 115, 115*f*
pain assessment and, 90-91
palpation in, 97
in proliferative phase, 104-105
in pronator syndrome, 119*b*, 119-120
provocative tests in, 96
in radial tunnel syndrome, 117-118, 118*b*
range of motion tests in, 92
in recovery stage, 105-106
related history and, 91
in rotator cuff tendinitis, 109-111, 110*t*
sensibility tests in, 94
stages of wound healing and, 98
strength assessment in, 92-93, 94*t*
in subacromial bursitis, 112
sympathetic signs of nerve injury and, 96-97
in tendonopathies, 98-99, 99*t*
in thoracic outlet syndrome, 106-108, 106-108*f*, 107*b*
threshold tests in, 94-95, 96*f*
in trigger finger, 124*b*, 124-125, 125*b*, 125-126*f*
visual inspection in, 92
in twentieth century, 5-7, 39-40
workplace setting and, 31
Musculoskeletal system
considerations in using tools, 242
effects of vibration on, 220
Musculotendinous disorders, 89*t*, 89-97
activity tolerance and, 89-91, 90*t*
adaptive changes in nearby tissue and, 97
adverse neural tension assessment in, 94, 95*f*
electromyography in, 91, 91*f*
functional sensibility tests in, 97
history and subjective assessment in, 89

innervation density tests in, 95-96
nerve conduction studies in, 92, 92*f*
objective clinical assessments in, 92, 93*b*
pain assessment and, 90-91
palpation in, 97
provocative tests in, 96
range of motion tests in, 92
related history and, 91
sensibility tests in, 94
strength assessment in, 92-93, 94*t*
sympathetic signs of nerve injury and, 96-97
threshold tests in, 94-95, 96*f*
visual inspection in, 92
Myers-Briggs Type Indicator, 275
Myofascial release, 105
in cervical disc and foraminal stenosis, 109
in cubital tunnel syndrome, 115
Myofascial response to joint injury, 134
Myofascial trigger points, 69, 112
hyperresponsivity of muscle and, 170-172, 171*f*
muscle overload and, 167*t*, 176-177, 177*f*
neural distress and, 167*t*, 172-176, 173*f*, 177*f*
palpation of, 97
physiologic risk factors and, 167-169*t*
Myotendinous junction, 64

N
Nanny, 408
Narrative records, 375-376
National Institute of Occupational Safety and Health
lifting equation of, 57, 215*t*
strategies for injury prevention, 301-303
National Safety Council, 56-57
Neck
awkward postures of, 205*t*, 208-209
pain in, 107*b*
in computer operator, 507*t*
in dental hygienist, 209, 458, 458*t*
Neck side-bending, 309
Needs-analysis survey, 371, 372*f*
Needs-discrepancy analysis, 370-371, 374*b*
Nerve
anatomy and physiology of, 71-73, 72*f*
considerations in using tools, 242
Nerve compression, 71-83
anastomosis and, 82-83
biomechanics of peripheral nerves and, 73, 74*f*
cervicobrachial region and, 76-78, 79*f*
classification of nerve injuries in, 76, 77*f*, 78*t*
in dental hygienist, 459
dorsal radial sensory nerve, 122-123
in Guyon's tunnel syndrome, 122
in keyboard player, 478
median nerve and, 80-81, 81*f*, 82*f*
nerve anatomy and physiology in, 71-73, 72*f*
nerve conduction studies in, 92, 92*f*
neural reorganization secondary to compression in, 75-76
pathology of, 73-75, 75*f*
radial nerve and, 78, 80*f*
in string players, 479
versus tendinitis, 89*t*
treatment of, 99-102, 101*f*
ulnar nerve and, 81-82, 83*f*, 84*f*
Nerve conduction studies, 92, 92*f*
Nerve gliding, 73, 74*f*
Nerve injury
neural reorganization after, 76
sympathetic signs of, 96-97
Nerve percussion, 96
Nerve regeneration, 100-102, 101*t*
Neural distress, 167*t*, 172-176, 173*f*, 177*f*
Neurologic effects of vibration, 220
Neuromuscular disorders, 89*t*, 89-97
activity tolerance and, 89-91, 90*t*
adaptive changes in nearby tissue and, 97
adverse neural tension assessment in, 94, 95*f*
electromyography in, 91, 91*f*
functional sensibility tests in, 97
history and subjective assessment in, 89
innervation density tests in, 95-96
nerve conduction studies in, 92, 92*f*
objective clinical assessments in, 92, 93*b*
pain assessment and, 90-91
palpation in, 97
peripheral neurovascular compressions and entrapment syndromes in, 71-83
anastomosis and, 82-83
biomechanics of peripheral nerves and, 73, 74*f*
cervicobrachial region and, 76-78, 79*f*
classification of nerve injuries in, 76, 77*f*, 78*t*
median nerve and, 80-81, 81*f*, 82*f*
nerve anatomy and physiology in, 71-73, 72*f*
neural reorganization secondary to compression in, 75-76
pathology of, 73-75, 75*f*
radial nerve and, 78, 80*f*
ulnar nerve and, 81-82, 83*f*, 84*f*
provocative tests in, 96
range of motion tests in, 92
related history and, 91
sensibility tests in, 94
strength assessment in, 92-93, 94*t*
sympathetic signs of nerve injury and, 96-97
tendonopathies in, 63-70
biomechanics of tendons and, 65-66
conditions related to, 69*f*, 69-70
factors affecting integrity of tendons in, 66-67
pathology of, 67
regional anatomy in, 63-65, 64*f*
tendon response to injury and, 67*t*, 67-69
threshold tests in, 94-95, 96*f*
visual inspection in, 92
Neuropraxia, 76
Neurotmesis, 76
Neurovascular entrapment syndromes of upper quadrant, 106
Neutral posture, 205-207
New employee conditioning and training, 304
Nine-hole peg test, 97
Ninhydrin sweat test, 97
Nintendo thumb, 400, 400*f*
NIOSH. *See* National Institute of Occupational Safety and Health.

Noise
  computer workstation and, 510-511
  older worker and, 443
Nonextreme postures, 206
Nonoccupational risks for musculoskeletal disorders, 39
Nonsteroidal antiinflammatory drugs
  for cubital tunnel syndrome, 114
  for pronator syndrome, 119
  for supraspinous tendinitis, 111
Nonwork risk factors in musculoskeletal disorders, 156
North America, musculoskeletal disorders in, 9

O

Objective stressors, 269-270, 270*t*
Occupation, defined, 276
Occupational cervicobrachial disorder, 6-7, 30
Occupational disorders, 8
Occupational health
  historical background of, 4
  regulatory perspective of, 44-59
    cost-benefit analysis and, 53-54, 54*t*
    economic and social aspects and, 50-53, 51*f*, 51*t*
    injury/illness statistics and, 44-46, 45-46*f*, 47-48*t*, 48*f*
    regulatory environment and, 54-57, 56*f*
    underreporting and, 46-49
    union contracts and, 58
    use of injury data and, 49-50
    workers' compensation and, 57-58
Occupational Safety and Health Act of 1960, 302
Occupational Safety and Health Administration, 56-57
  in control of ergonomic problems in workplace, 283, 520-522
  national strategies for injury prevention and, 301-303
  use of injury data from, 49-50
Occupational stress
  coping and cognitive appraisal in, 273-274
  immune responses to, 273
  methodologic issues in workplace stress research, 270-271
  models of, 267-269, 268*f*
  objective and subjective sources of, 269-270, 270*t*
  personality and adjustment factors in, 274-276, 277*f*
  work environment and, 266-267
Odds ratio, 193-194
Older worker, 437-447
  adaptive strategies for, 440-442
  age-related changes in health and disability, 437-440
  assessment of, 443-444
  ergonomic issues and, 442-443
  psychologic issues of, 444-445
Olecranon bursitis, 70, 112, 115, 115*f*
On-the-job stretching exercises, 308-309
Opening of jar, 394-395
Operator chair, 460
Opponens digiti quinti, 83*f*
Opponens pollicis, 81*f*
Organizational issues in musculoskeletal disorders, 39-41, 154-155
  dental hygiene profession and, 456
Organizational pause, 261
O'Riain wrinkle test, 97
Oscillatory vibration, 219
Osteoarthritis, 134-135, 135*b*
  of acromioclavicular joint, 143
  of carpometacarpal joint, 140
  of elbow, 143
  of finger interphalangeal joints, 137-139
  of glenohumeral joint, 144
  of metacarpophalangeal joint, 139-140
Outcome assessment of prevention programs, 363-386
  approach to program evaluation in, 363-364
  case study in, 384-386, 385*t*
  compilation of musculoskeletal disorder injury information system and, 364-366, 365*t*, 366*f*, 367*f*
  cost accounting and return-on-investment analysis in, 381-384, 382*f*
  determination of company losses and, 366-370, 368*t*
  goal-setting process in, 370-373, 372-373*f*, 374*b*
  issues in, 374-375
  qualitative measures in, 375-377
  quantitative measures in, 377-380, 379*f*, 380*t*, 381*t*
Output forces, 199-200
Ovaco Working Posture Analysis System, 213
Overflow, 161*t*
Overuse injury
  in performing artist, 476-477, 480
  physical examination for, 481
Overuse syndrome, 30
Overuse terminology, 67*t*, 67-68

P

Paced work, productivity standards and, 307
Pain
  assessment of, 90-91
  back
    backpack use in children and adolescents and, 399-400
    in child care worker, 406, 409
    in computer operator, 507*t*
    in dental hygienist, 451, 457
    laundering and, 397-398, 398*t*
    in parent, 407
    standing workstation and, 236
  chronic
    anger and, 276
    older worker and, 439
  elbow
    in dancer, 480
    in dental hygienist, 458*t*, 458-459, 459*f*
  epicondylar, 333-334
  finger
    in computer operator, 507*t*
    in dental hygienist, 458*t*, 459, 459*f*
  foot, 236
  forearm
    in dental hygienist, 458*t*, 458-459
    lateral, 90
  functional, 276
  leg
    in computer operator, 507*t*
    standing workstation and, 236
  in mild compressions, 76, 78*t*
  muscle activation and, 172

neck, 107*b*
in computer operator, 507*t*
in dental hygienist, 209, 458, 458*t*
in nerve entrapment, 106
older worker and, 444
posture-related, 170
referred, 69
shoulder
in computer operator, 507*t*
in dancer, 480
in dental hygienist, 209, 458, 458*t*
in string player, 479
thumb
in computer operator, 507*t*
in dental hygienist, 459-460, 460*f*
wrist, 333-334
in computer operator, 507*t*
in dental hygienist, 458*t*, 459
Palmar cutaneous branch, 82*f*
Palmar grasp, 239, 240*f*
Palmaris longus, 81*f*
Palpation of trigger points, 97
Paratendinitis, 67*t*, 67-68
Paratenon, 64
Pareto chart, 378, 379*f*
Patellar tendinitis, 480
Pathogenesis of musculoskeletal disorder, 30
Pectoralis minor space, 79*f*
Percussionist, 477-478
Percussive vibration, 219
Performing artists, 474-493
adaptive equipment for, 483-484
awkward posture and, 475
background of performers' careers and, 474
brass instrument players and, 477
case studies in, 484-488
changing work environments and, 476
constrained space and, 476
dancers, actors, mimes, and acrobats, 479-481
fatigue and, 475
history in, 481, 491-493
keyboard players and, 478, 478*f*, 479*f*
lifting and carrying instruments and equipment, 476, 484
percussionists and, 477-478
physical examination for overuse injury in, 481
principles of treatment for, 482-483
repetition and, 475
static posture and, 475
stress of performing and, 476
string players and, 478-479, 480*f*
training and conditioning and, 474-475
types of injury in, 476-477
woodwind players and, 477
workplace environmental evaluation and, 481-482
workplace modifications and, 483
Periarticular muscle-tendon unit assessment, 137
Perineurial diffusion barrier, 71
Perineurium, 71, 72*f*
Periodic stretching, 308
Peripheral compression neuropathies, 71-83
anastomosis and, 82-83
biomechanics of peripheral nerves and, 73, 74*f*
cervicobrachial region and, 76-78, 79*f*
classification of nerve injuries in, 76, 77*f*, 78*t*
in keyboard player, 478
median nerve and, 80-81, 81*f*, 82*f*
nerve anatomy and physiology in, 71-73, 72*f*
neural reorganization secondary to compression in, 75-76
pathology of, 73-75, 75*f*
radial nerve and, 78, 80*f*
in string players, 479
tendinitis *versus*, 89*t*
ulnar nerve and, 81-82, 83*f*, 84*f*
Peripheral muscle overloading, 172-176, 173*f*, 177*f*
Peripheral nerve, biomechanics of, 73, 74*f*
Personal protective equipment, 287
Personal risk factors, 157-158, 467
Personality, 266
adjustment factors and, 274-276, 277*f*
shiftwork and, 258
Phalen's test, 96, 334-335, 335*f*
Phonophoresis, 102-103, 111
Photometer, 252
Physical capacities testing, 383
Physical comfort aids, 321-322
Physical examination, 34
of performing artist, 481
of upper-extremity joint injury, 136
Physical performance, shiftwork and, 257-258
Physical size
as dental hygienist risk factor, 457
inappropriately sized tools, 244-245, 245*f*
Physiologic pain, 76, 78*t*
Physiologic risk factors, 160-190
case study in, 187-188
fatigue without recovery and, 168*t*
global muscle inhibition and, 169*t*
hyperresponsivity and, 167*t*, 170-172, 171*f*
muscle activation and, 163
muscle overload and, 167*t*, 176-177, 177*f*
neural distress and, 167*t*, 172-176, 173*f*, 177*f*
recovery model in, 186-187
surface electromyography and, 163-168, 164*f*, 165*f*
task-specific muscle inhibition with compensation and, 168*t*, 183-185*f*, 183-186
task-specific muscle inhibition without compensation and, 167-168*t*, 178-183, 179*f*, 181*f*, 182*f*
terminology in, 160-162, 161*t*
Physiologic Analysis Compilation, 168
Pianist, 478, 478*f*
Piecing of fabrics in quilting, 425
Piezoelectric accelerometer, 222
Pincer grasp, 239, 241*f*
Pinch gauge, 335, 335*f*
Pisiform-triquetral joint injury, 141-142
Pistol grip handle design, 247, 247*f*
for home activities, 395-396
Plantar fasciitis, 480
Plasma screen in computer workstation, 508
Pointing device for computer, 512-513
Polishing, 456
Polishing devices for dental hygienist, 450

Popliteal height, 232*f*, 288
Portable car seat, 413-414, 414*f*
Portable computer, 513
Positional posture, 291-292
Posterior impingement syndrome, 142
Posterior interosseous nerve, 80*f*
Postural analysis tools, 214-215, 215-216*t*
Postural stress syndromes, 170
Posture, 204-217, 205*t*
  Activity, Tool and Hand assessment tool and, 213-214
  awkward, 205-211, 207*f*, 208*f*
  backpack use in children and adolescents and, 399
  computer workstation and, 500-501
  computerized motion analysis systems for, 217
  in dental hygiene profession, 451, 452*t*, 453*f*, 453-454, 464
  ergonomic design and, 231
  film and video-based systems for assessment of, 214-217
  generation of muscle force and, 200
  handwriting and, 402
  performing artist and, 475
  postural analysis tools and, 214-215, 215-216*t*
  posture targeting and, 212-213, 213*f*
  self-analysis checklist and, 214
  static, 211-212
  in upper-quadrant screen, 93*b*
Posture targeting, 212-213, 213*f*
Potential lesion, 76, 78*t*
Power grasp, 239, 239*f*, 242
Power grip, 292
  carpometacarpal joint injury and, 140
  effects of wrist angle on, 200*t*
  osteoarthritis and, 135
Power lift, 413
Powered tools, 238-251
  cylindrical, 243, 243*f*
  digital separators in, 245-246
  ergonomic selection of, 250-251, 252*b*
  finger rings in, 246, 246*f*
  handle diameter and span, 243
  handle length in, 247-248, 248*f*
  handle orientation in, 246-247, 247*f*
  handle surface, texture, and materials of, 248-249
  inappropriately sized, 244-245, 245*f*
  operation and activation of, 250
  optimal shape of, 245
  precision, 244, 244*f*
  prehension patterns and, 239-241, 239-242*f*
  principles for use of, 241-242
  slipperiness of, 249
  surface pattern of, 249
  tool position and, 250
  tool weight and balance in, 250
  two-handled, 243-244, 244*f*
  vibration absorption of, 249-250
Precision grasp, 239, 240-241*f*, 242
Precision grip, 292-293
Precision tools, 244, 244*f*
Predictive value, 327
Preemployment examinations, 324-341
  accuracy of, 326-327
  Americans with Disabilities Act and, 327-330
  ethical and legal rights in, 338-339
  support of medical exams in industry, 325-326
  typical components of, 327
  Upper Extremity Fitness for Duty Evaluation in, 330-338
    abnormal nerve conduction velocity in, 335*f*, 335-336
    accuracy of, 336-338, 338*t*
    epicondylar pain in, 333-334
    Finkelstein's test in, 334, 334*t*
    ganglion cysts in, 331, 331*f*
    intrinsic atrophy in, 330-331, 331*f*
    Phalen's test in, 334-335, 335*f*
    presence of edema following stress test in, 336, 337*f*
    Raynaud's phenomenon in, 333
    sensibility loss in, 331-333, 332*f*
    Tinel's sign in, 334, 334*f*
    triggering in, 333, 333*f*
    weakness of grip or pinch in, 335, 335*f*
Prehension forces, 240-241, 453
Prehension patterns of tools, 239-241, 239-242*f*
Preschool teacher, 405-406, 408
Primary appraisal, 274
Private household worker, 408
Problem-focused coping, 274
Process safety management, 312
Productivity and labor costs analysis, 383-384
Productivity standards, 307
Proliferation phase of wound healing, 98
Pronator quadratus, 81*f*
Pronator syndrome, 119*b*, 119-120
Pronator teres, 81*f*, 82*f*
Pronator teres syndrome, 458*t*, 459
Proposal for injury prevention program, 348, 362-363
Proprioceptive wandering, 161*t*
Protective equipment for vibration exposure, 223
Protective sensory programs, 101
Protestant work ethic, 16
Provocative tests, 96
Proximal interphalangeal joint, biomechanical risk factors for, 138*t*
Psychiatric disorders, 40
Psychologic factors, 266
Psychoneuroimmunology, 273
Psychophysical methods in estimation of force, 203-204, 204*f*
Psychosocial factors, 39-41, 265-280
  biomechanical risk factors and, 156-157
  of child care, 405-407
    day care worker and, 405-406
    parent and, 406-407
  in computer operation, 495-496
  concepts and definitions in, 265-266
  coping and cognitive appraisal in, 273-274
  demand control models and, 271-272
  of ergonomic job analysis, 294
  immune responses to workplace stress, 273
  models of stress and health, 267-269, 268*f*
  objective and subjective sources of stress, 269-270, 270*t*
  older workers and, 444-445
  personal and adjustment factors in, 274-276, 277*f*
  quality of life and, 276-277
  stress and work environments and, 266-267
  workplace stress research and, 270-271
Psychosocial stressors, 266

Pulsed ultrasound, 104
 for supraspinous tendinitis, 111
Purdue pegboard test, 97
Pure risks, 367-368

Q

Qualitative measures in outcome assessment, 375-377
Quality of life, impact of musculoskeletal disorders on, 276-277
Quantitative measures in outcome assessment, 377-380, 379*f*, 380-381*t*
 cost accounting and return-on investment analysis in, 381-384, 382*f*
Quilting ergonomics, 425-428, 426-428*f*

R

Radial nerve, 78, 79*f*, 80*f*
Radial tunnel syndrome, 117-118, 118*b*
 in dental hygienist, 458*t*, 459
 in keyboard player, 478
Radiocarpal joint injury, 140-141
Raised bed gardening, 421-422
Raking, gardening and, 420, 421*t*
Range-of-motion, 92
 in cervical disc and foraminal stenosis, 109
 musculotendinous *versus* neural disorders and, 92
 in upper-extremity joint injury, 136-137, 138-139*t*
Rapid Entire Body Assessment, 214, 215*t*
Rapid Upper Limb Assessment, 193, 214, 216*t*
Rate coding, 161*t*
Rating of Perceived Exertion, 204, 204*f*
Raynaud's disease, 221
Raynaud's phenomenon, 221, 333
Reach, ergonomic design and, 231, 232, 232*f*
Recovery model in musculoskeletal disorders, 186-187
Recovery time
 dental hygiene instrumentation and, 454-455, 466*t*
 for static work, 196*f*, 196-197
Reduced employee turnover, 383-384
Referred pain, compression to trigger point and, 69
Reflective values, 253, 253*t*
Reflexes in upper-quadrant screen, 93*b*
Regeneration of nerve, 100-102, 101*t*
Regulatory definitions for musculoskeletal disorders, 33
Regulatory environment, 54-57, 56*f*
Regulatory perspective of musculoskeletal disorders, 44-59
 cost-benefit analysis and, 53-54, 54*t*
 economic and social aspects and, 50-53, 51*f*, 51*t*
 injury/illness statistics and, 44-46, 45-46*f*, 47-48*t*, 48*f*
 regulatory environment and, 54-57, 56*f*
 underreporting and, 46-49
 union contracts and, 58
 use of injury data and, 49-50
 workers' compensation and, 57-58
Rehearsing for performance, 475
Remodeling phase of wound healing, 98
Repetition, 194*f*, 194-199
 computer use and, 501
 in dental hygiene instrumentation, 452, 466*t*
 fatigue model of, 196*f*, 196-197
 hand activity level and, 198-199
 measurement of, 198
 performing artist and, 474-475, 478
 research on, 197-198
 tissue strain and, 195*f*, 195-196
Repetition rate, 198
Repetitive strain injury, 7-8, 30, 45*f*
Research
 in force, 201
 in mechanical compression, 218
 methodologic issues in, 270-271
 in musculoskeletal disorders, 12-13, 33
 in repetition, 197-198
 in static posture, 212
 in vibration, 221-222
Resistive tests, 94*t*
Rest and immobilization for performing artist, 482
Return-on-investment analysis, 381-384, 382*f*
Risk factors for musculoskeletal disorders, 249-280
 biomechanical, 191-229
  awkward postures and, 205-211, 207-208*f*
  computerized motion analysis systems and, 217
  cool temperatures in, 223-224
  dynamic factors in, 217
  film and video-based systems for assessment of, 214-217
  force in, 199-204, 200*t*, 202*t*, 204*f*
  measuring and reporting of exposures, 193-194
  mechanical compression in, 218
  postural analysis tools and, 214-215, 215-216*t*
  posture targeting and, 212-213, 213*f*
  repetition in, 194-196*f*, 194-199
  self-analysis checklist and, 214
  static postures and, 211-212
  vibration in, 218-223
 in child care, 409*b*, 409-410, 410*b*
 in computer use, 499-502
 in dental hygiene profession, 456-457, 464, 466*t*
 difficulties in identification of, 155-157
 in home activities, 389-390
 job design and, 230-264
  anthropometrics in, 230-232, 232-234*f*
  hand and powered tools and, 238-251. *See also* Tools.
  lighting in workplace and, 251-256, 252*t*, 253*t*, 254*t*
  machine pacing and worker control in, 262
  shiftwork and, 256-260
  work breaks and, 261-262
  working hours and overtime in, 260-261
  workstation design and, 232-238, 236-238*f*
 musculoskeletal disorder etiology models and, 152-155, 153*f*
 personal, 157-158
 physiologic, 160-190
  case study in, 187-188
  fatigue without recovery and, 168*t*
  global muscle inhibition and, 169*t*
  hyperresponsivity and, 167*t*, 170-172, 171*f*
  muscle activation and, 163
  muscle overload and, 167*t*, 176-177, 177*f*
  neural distress and, 167*t*, 172-176, 173*f*, 177*f*
  recovery model in, 186-187
  surface electromyography and, 163-168, 164-165*f*
  task-specific muscle inhibition with compensation and, 168*t*, 183-185*f*, 183-186

Risk factors for musculoskeletal disorders—*cont'd*
physiologic—*cont'd*
task-specific muscle inhibition without compensation and, 167-168*t*, 178-183, 179*f*, 181*f*, 182*f*
terminology in, 160-162, 161*t*
psychosocial, 265-280
concepts and definitions in, 265-266
coping and cognitive appraisal in, 273-274
demand control models and, 271-272
immune responses to workplace stress, 273
models of stress and health, 267-269, 268*f*
objective and subjective sources of stress, 269-270, 270*t*
personal and adjustment factors in, 274-276, 277*f*
quality of life and, 276-277
stress and work environments and, 266-267
workplace stress research and, 270-271
Risk-management systems, 367-369, 368*t*
Roos test, 107-108
Rotary cutter, 425, 427, 427*f*
Rotator cuff tendinitis, 99*t*, 109-111, 110*t*
Run chart, 365-366, 366-367*f*
Rupture of supraspinous tendon, 111

S
Safety committee, 312-313
Scalene triangle, 79*f*
Scapholunate interval
biomechanical risk factors for, 138*t*
injury of, 140-141
Scapular myalgia, 458*t*
Scar, 105
Screening examinations, 324-341
accuracy of, 326-327
Americans with Disabilities Act and, 327-330
ethical and legal rights in, 338-339
support of medical exams in industry, 325-326
typical components of, 327
Upper Extremity Fitness for Duty Evaluation in, 330-338
abnormal nerve conduction velocity in, 335*f*, 335-336
accuracy of, 336-338, 338*t*
epicondylar pain in, 333-334
Finkelstein's test in, 334, 334*t*
ganglion cysts in, 331, 331*f*
intrinsic atrophy in, 330-331, 331*f*
Phalen's test in, 334-335, 335*f*
presence of edema following stress test in, 336, 337*f*
Raynaud's phenomenon in, 333
sensibility loss in, 331-333, 332*f*
Tinel's sign in, 334, 334*f*
triggering in, 333, 333*f*
weakness of grip or pinch in, 335, 335*f*
Seat angle, 235
Seat pan, 235
Seated position
anthropometric data for, 232*f*
engineering controls for, 310-311
Seated workstation, 235-236, 236*f*
Secondary appraisal, 274
Seddon classification of nerve injuries, 76, 77*f*
Seeding, gardening and, 420, 421*t*
Segmental vibration, 219, 220-221
Selective fatigue, 161*t*
Selective optimization with compensation, 442
Selective polishing, 456, 462
Self-analysis checklist for posture assessment, 193, 214
Self-leading team, 21
Self-managed work team, 21
sEMG. *See* Surface electromyography.
Semmes-Weinstein monofilaments, 94, 96*f*, 331-333, 332*f*
Sensibility loss, 331-333, 332*f*
Sensibility tests, 94
Sensory reeducation program, 101
Sequential upper-limb tension test, 95*f*
Sewing machine, quilting and, 426
Sharpey's fibers, 64
Shiftwork, 256-260
Shiftwork tolerance, term, 256
Shoes, standing workstation and, 237
Shoulder
acromioclavicular joint injury and, 143
awkward postures of, 205*t*, 208-209
bicipital tendinitis and, 109*b*, 111-112, 112*f*
glenohumeral joint injury and, 143-144
laundering and, 398
myofascial trigger points and, 112
pain in
in computer operator, 507*t*
in dancer, 480
in dental hygienist, 209, 458, 458*t*
in string player, 479
rotator cuff tendinitis and, 109-111, 110*t*
subacromial bursitis in, 112
Shoulder breadth, 232*f*
Shoulder carry, 413
Shoulder height, 233*f*, 288
Shoulder-to-grip length, 288
Simulation of alternative duties, 383
Sit-stand options, 311
Sitting height, 232*f*, 288
Sitting position
dental hygienist and, 451
knitting and, 432
musician and, 482
quilting and, 426
video display terminal operator and, 505, 505*b*, 506*f*
Size
as dental hygienist risk factor, 457
inappropriately sized tools, 244-245, 245*f*
of instrument in relation to performer, 484
Sleep, shiftwork and, 256-257, 259
Sleep-wake disturbances, shiftwork and, 257
Slipperiness of tool, 249
Small force sensitive resistors, 203
Social aspects
of musculoskeletal disorders, 50-53, 51*f*, 51*t*
of shiftwork, 258, 259
Social context of work, 19-22, 20*f*, 21*b*
Sociopolitical atmosphere, 303-304
Soft-tissue massage, 104-105
Sollerman grip and function test, 97
Sound levels

computer workstation and, 510–511
older worker and, 443
Speculative risks, 367–368
Spherical grasp, 239, 241*f*
Splint, 321–322
in cubital tunnel syndrome, 115, 115*f*
to improve neural function, 101
in trigger thumb, 124–125, 125*f*, 126*f*
Spontaneous pause, 261
Spring scale, 203
Stage performers, 474–493
adaptive equipment for, 483–484
awkward posture and, 475
background of performers' careers and, 474
brass instrument players and, 477
case studies in, 484–488
changing work environments and, 476
constrained space and, 476
dancers, actors, mimes, and acrobats, 479–481
fatigue and, 475
history in, 481, 491–493
keyboard players and, 478, 478*f*, 479*f*
lifting and carrying instruments and equipment, 476, 484
percussionists and, 477–478
physical examination for overuse injury in, 481
principles of treatment for, 482–483
repetition and, 475
static posture and, 475
stress of performing and, 476
string players and, 478–479, 480*f*
training and conditioning and, 474–475
types of injury in, 476–477
woodwind players and, 477
workplace environmental evaluation and, 481–482
workplace modifications and, 483
Stain Index, 193
Stakeholders, needs-discrepancy analysis and, 370–371
Standing position
anthropometric data for, 233*f*
engineering controls for, 311
older worker and, 439
Standing workstation, 236–237, 237*f*
State ergonomic standards, 55
State-Trait Anxiety Inventory, 275–276
Static dimensions, 231
Static load, 161*t*, 182
Static posture, 211–212
computer use and, 500
in dental hygiene instrumentation, 452*t*, 453–454, 465, 466*t*
performing artist and, 475
in upper-quadrant screen, 93*b*
Static splinting, 102
Static work, 211
Statistical analysis, 378–380, 379*f*, 380*t*
Statue of Liberty stretch, 309
Stature, 233*f*, 288
Stereognosis tests, 97
Stirring, cooking and, 394*t*
Strain Index, 214, 215*t*
Strength
assessment of, 92–93, 94*t*
ergonomic design and, 231
Stress
child care worker and, 406
coping and cognitive appraisal in, 273–274
immune responses to, 273
methodologic issues in workplace stress research, 270–271
models of, 267–269, 268*f*
objective and subjective sources of, 269–270, 270*t*
older worker and, 441
performing artist and, 476
personality and adjustment factors in, 274–276, 277*f*
work environment and, 266–267
Stress-relaxation test, 66
Stress-strain curve, 65–66, 195, 195*f*
Stress test, edema following, 336, 337*f*
Stressors
external, 154
objective and subjective, 269–270, 270*t*
psychosocial, 266
Stretch-and-spray technique, 103–104
Stretching exercises, 308–309
for dental hygienist, 462–463*f*
in injury prevention program, 354–358
for knitter, 431–432, 432*f*,
for quilter, 427–428, 428*f*
String player, 478–479, 480*f*
Structural dimensions, 231
Subacromial bursa, 69, 69*f*
Subacromial bursitis, 69–70, 112
Subacromial impingement, 109–111, 110*t*
Subchondral bone cyst, 134
Subjective stressors, 269–270, 270*t*
Subscapular nerves, 79*f*
Sunderland classification of nerve injuries, 76, 77*f*
Superficial cutaneous branch, 80*f*
Superficial radial nerve compression, 118*b*
Supervisor of injury prevention program, 343
Supinator, 80*f*
Suprascapular nerve, 79*f*
Supraspinatus tendinitis in dental hygienist, 458, 458*t*
Supraspinous tendon impingement, 111
Surface electromyography, 160–190
case study in, 187–188
fatigue without recovery and, 168*t*
global muscle inhibition and, 169*t*
hyperresponsivity and, 167*t*, 170–172, 171*f*
internal forces and, 203
muscle activation and, 163
muscle overload and, 167*t*, 176–177, 177*f*
neural distress and, 167*t*, 172–176, 173*f*, 177*f*
recovery model in, 186–187
task-specific muscle inhibition with compensation and, 168*t*, 183–185*f*, 183–186
task-specific muscle inhibition without compensation and, 167–168*t*, 178–183, 179*f*, 181*f*, 182*f*
terminology in, 160–162, 161*t*
in understanding musculoskeletal disorders, 163–168, 164*f*, 165*f*
Surface of tool handle, 248–249
Surface pattern of tool, 249

Survey
in conducting of outcome evaluations, 377
needs-analysis, 371, 372*f*
symptom questionnaire, 33-34
Sweat test, 97
Symptom questionnaire survey, 33-34

T

Tactile gnosis, 97
Task-specific muscle inhibition with compensation, 168*t*, 183-185*f*, 183-186
Task-specific muscle inhibition without compensation, 167-168*t*, 178-183, 179*f*, 181-182*f*
Task stimulation, 93
Teknocyte, 98
Telecommuting, 519-520
Temperature
computer workstations and, 501-502
workplace evaluation and, 289
Tendinitis, 63, 67*t*, 67-68
bicipital, 109*b*, 111-112, 112*f*
eccentric exercise program for, 105
in lateral epicondylitis, 115-117, 116*b*, 117*f*
massage therapy for, 104-105
in medial epicondylitis, 116*b*, 118-119
nonsurgical treatment of, 98-99, 99*t*
patellar, 480
peripheral nerve compression *versus*, 89*t*
rotator cuff, 109-111, 110*t*
in stage performers, 480
in string players, 479
vibration and, 220-221
Tendon, 63-64, 64*f*
biomechanics of, 65-66
factors affecting integrity of, 66
response to injury, 67*t*, 67-69
vulnerable anatomic sites in, 67
Tendonopathies, 63-70
biomechanics of tendons and, 65-66
conditions related to, 69*f*, 69-70
factors affecting integrity of tendons in, 66-67
pathology of, 67
regional anatomy in, 63-65, 64*f*
tendon response to injury and, 67*t*, 67-69
treatment of, 98-99, 99*t*
Tenosynovitis, 67*t*, 67-68
in dental hygienist, 458*t*, 459
finger triggering and, 333
flexor, 120-121, 121*b*
key restrictions in, 99*t*
mechanical compression in, 218
tool handle orientation and, 246
Tenosynovium, 64
Tension neck syndrome, 458, 458*t*
Terminology
in lighting design, 252*t*, 252-253, 253*t*
in musculoskeletal disorders, 29-30, 30*b*
Texture of tool handle, 248-249
Thenar muscle atrophy, 331, 331*f*
Therapeutic interventions, 89-131
activity tolerance and, 89-91, 90*t*
adaptive changes in nearby tissue and, 97
adverse neural tension assessment in, 94, 95*f*
in anterior interosseous syndrome, 119*b*, 120
in bicipital tendinitis, 109*b*, 111-112, 112*f*
in carpal tunnel syndrome, 119*b*, 121-122
in cervical disc and foraminal stenosis, 108-109
in cubital tunnel syndrome, 113*f*, 113-115, 114*b*, 115*f*
in de Quervain's disease, 123*f*, 123-124, 124*b*
in dorsal radial sensory nerve compression and entrapment, 122-123
electromyography in, 91, 91*f*
in flexor tenosynovitis, 120-121, 121*b*
in focal hand dystonia, 125-126
functional sensibility tests in, 97
in Guyon's tunnel syndrome, 122
history and subjective assessment in, 89
in inflammatory phase, 102-104, 103*f*
innervation density tests in, 95-96
in intersection syndrome, 121*b*, 124
in lateral epicondylitis, 115-117, 116*b*, 117*f*
in medial epicondylitis, 116*b*, 118-119
myofascial trigger points and, 112
in nerve compressions and entrapments, 99-102, 101*f*
nerve conduction studies in, 92, 92*f*
objective clinical assessments in, 92, 93*b*
in olecranon bursitis, 115, 115*f*
pain assessment and, 90-91
palpation in, 97
in proliferative phase, 104-105
in pronator syndrome, 119*b*, 119-120
provocative tests in, 96
in radial tunnel syndrome, 117-118, 118*b*
range of motion tests in, 92
in recovery stage, 105-106
related history and, 91
in rotator cuff tendinitis, 109-111, 110*t*
sensibility tests in, 94
stages of wound healing and, 98
strength assessment in, 92-93, 94*t*
in subacromial bursitis, 112
sympathetic signs of nerve injury and, 96-97
in tendonopathies, 98-99, 99*t*
in thoracic outlet syndrome, 106-108, 106-108*f*, 107*b*
threshold tests in, 94-95, 96*f*
in trigger finger, 124*b*, 124-125, 125*b*, 125-126*f*
visual inspection in, 92
Thigh clearance, 232*f*, 288
Thoracic outlet, 76-78, 79*f*
Thoracic outlet syndrome, 106-108, 106-108*f*, 107*b*
in dental hygienist, 458, 458*t*
Thoracodorsal nerve, 79*f*
Three-jaw chuck grasp, 239
Threshold limit values, 56, 56*f*
Threshold tests, 94-95, 96*f*
Thumb
carpometacarpal joint injury and, 140
de Quervain's disease and, 123
keyboard player and, 478, 479*f*
pain in computer operator, 507*t*
pain in dental hygienist, 459-460, 460*f*
trigger, 124*b*, 124-125, 125*b*, 125-126*f*

trigger near, 70
video gaming and, 400*f*, 400-401
Thumb spica splint, 123, 123*f*
Time factor in injury prevention program, 344
Tinel's sign, 96, 334, 334*f*
Tissue strain, repetition and, 195*f*, 195-196
Tokyo Declaration, 10
Tonic vibration reflex, 220
Tool position, 250
Tools, 238-251
cylindrical, 243, 243*f*
dental, 449-450
digital separators in, 245-246
ergonomic selection of, 250-251, 252*b*
finger rings in, 246, 246*f*
gardening, 423-424, 423-424*f*
handle diameter and span, 243
handle length in, 247-248, 248*f*
handle orientation in, 246-247, 247*f*
handle surface, texture, and materials of, 248-249
inappropriately sized, 244-245, 245*f*
kitchen utensils, 394-396, 396-397*f*
knitting, 429-430, 430*f*, 431*f*
operation and activation of, 250
optimal shape of, 245
precision, 244, 244*f*
prehension patterns and, 239-241, 239-242*f*
principles for use of, 241-242
quilting, 427
redesign for older worker, 443
slipperiness of, 249
surface pattern of, 249
tool position and, 250
tool weight and balance in, 250
two-handled, 243-244, 244*f*
vibration absorption of, 249-250
Torque wrench, 203
Tracking database, 364-366, 365*t*, 366-367*f*
Training
of performing artist, 474-475
vibration exposure and, 223
Trait-treatment interaction, 378
Transactional model of job stress and health, 267-268
Transcutaneous electrical nerve stimulation, 104, 119
Translational stability testing, 136, 138-139*t*
Transporting of child, 413-414, 414*f*
Transverse carpal ligament, 82*f*, 84*f*
Trapezius myalgia, 458, 458*t*
Triangular fibrocartilaginous complex injury, 138*t*, 141
Triceps, 80*f*
Trigger design of tool, 250
Trigger finger, 70, 124*b*, 124-125, 125*b*, 125-126*f*, 333, 333*f*
key restrictions in, 99*t*
mechanical compression in, 218
Trigger points, 69
hyperresponsivity of muscle and, 170-172, 171*f*
muscle overload and, 167*t*, 176-177, 177*f*
neural distress and, 167*t*, 172-176, 173*f*, 177*f*
palpation of, 97
physiologic risk factors and, 167-169*t*
Trigger thumb, 99*t*, 333, 333*f*
Tripod grasp, 239
Tripod lift, 413
Tuning fork, 96
Two-handled tool, 243-244, 244*f*
Two-point discrimination, 95-96, 331
Type-A personality, 274-275

U
Ulnar nerve, 79*f*
compression of, 113*f*, 113-115, 115*b*, 115*f*
potential compression and entrapment of, 81-82, 83-84*f*
Ultrasonic scaler, 450
Ultrasound
for drug diffusion, 103
pulsed, 104, 111
Underreporting of musculoskeletal disorders, 46-49
Union
contracts with, 58
injury prevention program and, 343
United States Bureau of Labor Statistics website, 365
Unwinding, 105
Upholstery of chair, 236
Upper-arm length, 232*f*
Upper Extremity Fitness for Duty Evaluation in, 330-338
abnormal nerve conduction velocity in, 335*f*, 335-336
accuracy of, 336-338, 338*t*
epicondylar pain in, 333-334
Finkelstein's test in, 334, 334*t*
ganglion cysts in, 331, 331*f*
intrinsic atrophy in, 330-331, 331*f*
Phalen's test in, 334-335, 335*f*
presence of edema following stress test in, 336, 337*f*
Raynaud's phenomenon in, 333
sensibility loss in, 331-333, 332*f*
Tinel's sign in, 334, 334*f*
triggering in, 333, 333*f*
weakness of grip or pinch in, 335, 335*f*
Upper extremity joint disorders, 132-148
of acromioclavicular joint, 143
anatomical design of joint, 132-133
biomechanical risk factors for, 138-139*t*
carpal boss in, 141
compressive loading injuries in, 133-134
diagnosis of, 136-137
of distal radioulnar joint, 142
of elbow, 142-143
of finger interphalangeal joints, 137-139
of glenohumeral joint, 143-144
of joint stabilizing structures, 134
medical management of, 144
of metacarpophalangeal joint, 139-140
myofascial responses to, 134
of radiocarpal joint, 140-141
in string players, 479
of thumb carpometacarpal joint, 140
upper-extremity arthritis as, 134-135, 135*b*
work-relatedness of, 144-145
of wrist pisiform-triquetral joint, 141-142
of wrist triangular fibrocartilaginous complex, 141

Upper-leg length, 232*f*
Upper-limb cumulative trauma disorders, 106–126
  anterior interosseous syndrome in, 119*b*, 120
  bicipital tendinitis in, 109*b*, 111–112, 112*f*
  carpal tunnel syndrome in, 119*b*, 121–122
  cervical disc and foraminal stenosis in, 108–109
  cubital tunnel syndrome in, 113*f*, 113–115, 114*b*, 115*f*
  de Quervain's disease in, 123*f*, 123–124, 124*b*
  dorsal radial sensory nerve compression and entrapment in, 122–123
  flexor tenosynovitis in, 120–121, 121*b*
  focal hand dystonia in, 125–126
  Guyon's tunnel syndrome in, 122
  intersection syndrome in, 121*b*, 124
  lateral epicondylitis in, 115–117, 116*b*, 117*f*
  medial epicondylitis in, 116*b*, 118–119
  myofascial trigger points and, 112
  olecranon bursitis in, 115, 115*f*
  pronator syndrome in, 119*b*, 119–120
  radial tunnel syndrome in, 117–118, 118*b*
  rotator cuff tendinitis in, 109–111, 110*t*
  subacromial bursitis in, 112
  thoracic outlet syndrome in, 106–108, 106–108*f*, 107*b*
  trigger finger in, 124*b*, 124–125, 125*b*, 125–126*f*
Upper-limb test, 108, 108*f*
Upper-quadrant screen, 92, 93*b*

V
Vacuuming, 395*t*
Vapo coolant spray, 103
Vascular system
  effects of vibration on, 220
  of nerve, 71
  of tendon, 64–65
Ventilation factors, dental hygienist and, 456
Vertical growing in gardening, 423, 423*f*
Vibrating tool
  carpal tunnel syndrome and, 220–221
  dental hygienist and, 450, 452*t*, 454
  elbow osteoarthritis and, 143
Vibration, 218–223
  effects on body, 220
  measurement of, 222–223
  physical concepts of, 219–220
  recommendations for decreasing, 223
  research in, 221–222
  segmental, 220–221
  whole-body, 220
Vibration absorption of tool, 249–250, 293–294
Vibrometer, 332
Video-based systems for posture assessment, 193, 214–217
Video display terminal operator, 505, 505*b*, 506*f*
Video gaming, 400–401, 401*t*
Viscoelasticity of tendon, 66
Vision, older worker and, 439
Visual analog scale, 90
Visual inspection, 92
Volumeter, 336, 336*f*
Voluntary ergonomic standards, 55

W
Waist height, 233*f*
Warm-up program, 354–358
Wartenberg's syndrome, 122
Washington State Appendix B, 216*t*, 217
Watering, gardening and, 420, 421*t*
Weber's test, 95
Weeding, gardening and, 420, 421*t*
Weight of tool, 250
  in ergonomic job analysis, 292
  vibration and, 222
Weinstein enhanced sensory test, 94–95
Wheelchair, gardening and, 424–425, 425*f*
Whole-body vibration, 219, 220
Women's anthropometry, 157
Woodwind player, 477
Work
  beliefs and values about, 17
  changing social context of, 19–22, 20*f*, 21*b*
  definition of, 15–17
  impact of age-related changes in health and disability on, 439–440
Work activity analysis, 296–298
Work breaks, 261–262
Work culture
  assimilation of, 18–19
  values of, 17–18
Work environment
  performing artist and, 476
  stress and, 266–267
Work groups, 17–18
Work organization, 154, 266
  dental hygiene profession and, 465–467, 466*t*
Work practice controls, 307–309
  computer workstations and, 495
  in dental hygiene profession, 461*t*, 462–463*f*, 470–473
Work-recovery times for static work, 196*f*, 196–197
Work-related musculoskeletal disorders, 302
Work-related pause, 261
Work schedule, 256–262
  in dental hygiene profession, 449, 455–456
  shiftwork and, 256–260
  work breaks and, 261
  working hours and overtime, 260–261
Work structure flexibility, 11–12
Work surface of computer workstation, 506–507, 509
Work task risk factors
  in computer operation, 495
  in dental hygiene profession, 452*t*, 452–455, 453*f*, 464, 466*t*
Worker
  control of work pace, 262
  job analysis and, 287–288
  older, 437–447
    adaptive strategies for, 440–442
    age-related changes in health and disability, 437–440
    assessment of, 443–444
    ergonomic issues and, 442–443
    psychologic issues of, 444–445
  perception of work-related injury, 300–301
Worker demographics, 19–20, 20*f*

Workers' compensation, 39-40, 57-58
direct costs for, 52-53
use of injury data from, 50
Working hours and overtime, 260-261
Workplace
assessment of, 283-298
activity descriptors in, 285-289
biomechanical aspects of, 290-294
computer workstation and, 525-529
ergonomic assessment in, 289-290
essential job functions and, 284-285
historical background of, 283-284
marginal job functions and, 285
performing artist and, 481-482
psychosocial aspects of, 294
layout in workstation design, 234-235
lighting in, 251-256
in computer workstation, 510
dental hygienist and, 456
in injury in performing artist, 480
older worker and, 442
quilting and, 426-427
recommended levels of, 253-256, 254*t*
terminology in, 252*t*, 252-253, 253*t*
organizational factors in dental hygiene instrumentation, 455-456, 464, 466*t*
as setting of musculoskeletal disorders, 31
Worksite programs, 281-386
for computer operators, 502, 503*t*
employment examinations and, 324-341
accuracy of, 326-327
Americans with Disabilities Act and, 327-330
ethical and legal rights in, 338-339
support of medical exams in industry, 325-326
typical components of, 327
Upper Extremity Fitness for Duty Evaluation in, 330-338. *See also* Upper Extremity Fitness for Duty Evaluation.
implementation of, 342-363
communication and, 345-346
employee training and education and, 349-350, 351*t*
ergonomics and, 352-353
money factor in, 343-344
people involved in, 342-343
presentation style in, 350-352
providing services in, 345
selling of, 347-349, 361-362
stretching and warming up in, 354-358
time factor in, 344
job analysis and, 283-298
activity descriptors in, 285-289
biomechanical aspects of, 290-294
ergonomic assessment in, 289-290
essential job functions and, 284-285
historical background of, 283-284
marginal job functions and, 285
psychosocial aspects of, 294
outcome assessment in, 363-386
approach to program evaluation in, 363-364
case study in, 384-386, 385*t*
compilation of musculoskeletal disorder injury information system and, 364-366, 365*t*, 366*f*, 367*f*
cost accounting and return-on-investment analysis in, 381-384, 382*f*
determination of company losses and, 366-370, 368*t*
goal-setting process in, 370-373, 372-373*f*, 374*b*
issues in, 374-375
qualitative measures in, 375-377
quantitative measures in, 377-380, 379*f*, 380*t*, 381*t*
reducing injuries, claims, and costs, 299-323
case studies in, 313-321
early return to work and modified duty in, 306-307
engineering controls in, 309-313
injury reporting and investigation process in, 304-306
issues in determination of injury, 299-300
management-employee education and training in, 322-323
national strategies for, 301-303
new employee conditioning and training in, 304
physical comfort aids and, 321-322
productivity standards and paced work in, 307
relationship of costs to injury severity, 301
sociopolitical atmosphere and employee morale in, 303-304
work practice controls in, 307-309
worker *versus* supervisor perceptions in, 300-301
Workspace
kitchen layout and storage and, 393-394
in knitting, 429
performing artist and, 476
in quilting, 426, 426*f*
Workstation design, 232-238
anthropometrics and, 231
computer, 509-511
in dental hygiene profession, 456, 466*t*, 467
frequently used equipment and controls in, 237-238, 238*f*
for older worker, 443
seated workstations in, 235-236, 236*f*
standing workstations and, 236-237, 237*f*
workplace layout in, 234-235
workstation height in, 235
Worst-case analysis, 382
Wound healing, 98
Wright's maneuver, 107
Wrinkle test, 97
Wrist
awkward postures of, 205*t*, 210
carpal tunnel syndrome and, 119*b*, 121-122
computer operation and, 507*t*
de Quervain's disease and, 123*f*, 123-124, 124*b*
dorsal radial sensory nerve compression and entrapment, 122-123
effects of angle on power grip strength, 200*t*
epicondylar pain and, 333-334
flexor tenosynovitis and, 120-121, 121*b*
grip force and, 242
Guyon's tunnel syndrome and, 122
instrumentation techniques in dental hygiene profession and, 450-451, 451*f*
intersection syndrome and, 121*b*, 124
pain in dental hygienist, 458*t*, 459
pisiform-triquetral joint injury, 141-142

Wrist—*cont'd*
radiocarpal joint injury, 140-141
string player and, 479, 480*f*
triangular fibrocartilaginous complex injury, 141
Wrist extensor stretch, 309
Wrist flexor stretch, 309
Wrist rest, 509
Wrist splint, 117*f*
Writer's cramp, 70
Writing, ergonomic principles in, 401*t*, 401-402

Y
Yarn, 430

Z
Zeitbergers, 259